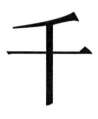

Sūn Sī-Miǎo 孫思邈

Bèi Jí Qiān Jīn Yào Fāng

Essential Prescriptions Worth a Thousand in Gold for Every Emergency

Volumes 2 - 4 on Gynecology

Sabine Wilms, Ph.D.

The Chinese Medicine Database
www.cm-db.com
Portland, Oregon

Bèi Jí Qiān Jīn Yào Fāng

Essential Prescriptions worth a Thousand in Gold for Every Emergency

備急千金要方

Sabine Wilms

Copyright © The Chinese Medicine Database
& Sabine Wilms

1923 NW Kearney
Portland, OR 97209 USA

COMP designation original Chinese work and English translation

Cover Design by Tiffany Howard
Artwork supplied by Makoto Mayanagi
Library of Congress Cataloging-in-Publication Data:

Sun, Si-Miao, fl.
    [Bei Ji Qian Jin Yao Fang. English]
    Bei Ji Qian Jin Yao Fang = Essential Prescriptions worth a
    thousand in gold for every emergency/ translation
    Sabine Wilms
            p. cm.
    Includes Index.
    ISBN 978-0-9799552-0-4 (alk. paper)
    Medicine, Chinese   I. Wilms, Sabine, 1968 II. Title: Essen
    tial Prescriptions worth a thousand in gold for every emergency.
    III. Title: Vol. 2-4 on Gynecology

International Standard Book Number (ISBN): 978-0-9799552-0-4
Printed in the United States of America

Contents

Appendixes

Indices

Preface by Nigel Wiseman

Sabine Wilms's translation of the gynecological sections of Sūn Sī-Miǎo's *Bèi Jí Qiān Jīn Yào Fāng* 備急千金要方 ("Essential Prescriptions worth a Thousand in Gold for Every Emergency") make a significant contribution to the Western understanding of East Asian medicine in many ways.

Sūn's gynecological materials are important historically for two reasons. First, they reflect the emergence of gynecology as a specialty in Medieval China. Never before had any medical scholar in China collected so much material dealing specifically with women's problems, in so much detail. Second, because of Sūn's open-mindedness to the whole gamut of healing practices in his time, he included in his texts many magical remedies and pragmatic herbal remedies alongside classical remedies of the theoretically based tradition of the *Nèi Jīng, Nán Jīng, Shāng Hán Lùn,* and *Jīn Guì Yào Lüè.* Important for Western readers is to bear in mind that in Sūn's time, magical remedies and pragmatic herbal remedies were still the basis of healing practices for the vast majority of people in China— theoretically based medicine was the medicine only of the educated elite. For these reasons, the material that Dr. Wilms presents provides English speakers in modern times with a magnificent window on the gynecological practices of 7th century China.

That window offers an especially clear view because of Dr. Wilms's training and experience. Her background in the history of medicine in China and anthropology enable her to give the most insightful explanations of the various practices on which Sūn reports, while her experience in the teaching of modern TCM enables her to highlight the relevance of Sūn's work for modern students and practitioners.

The inclusion of translations of relevant monographs of the *Shénnóng Běncǎo Jīng* 神農本草經 will be most appreciated by readers. This text is the earliest extant materia medica work of Chinese medicine. It is also the latest extant materia medica in Sūn Sī-Miǎo's time. Hence these monographs enlighten readers as to the contemporary usage of medicinal substances in Sūn's time. A unique feature of Dr. Wilms's translation lies in her choice of terminology of *A Practical Dictionary of Chinese Medicine* (PD). Chinese medical historians in the West generally translate terms so as to reflect their contemporary usage in the period on which they are writing, often to the neglect of reflecting the continuity of many terms and concepts over long periods, sometimes even to the present. Since PD terminology applies a source-oriented approach that reflects the original understanding of medical scholars who devised concepts, it can, by and large, be applied in the translation of works of any era. The use of PD terminology in the translation of Sūn's gynecological material enables modern Western readers to identify ideas and concepts still prevalent in the modern practice of Chinese medicine more readily than in historical works where terminology is not specifically chosen to reflect the continuity of medical thought.

Modern Chinese medicine represents an integration of what modern scholars consider to be the best elements of originally disparate traditions. Chinese students, being required to study the classics and understand the development of Chinese medical thought, naturally view their heritage in a complex historical perspective. Westerners, by contrast, receive little but the modern picture and are only starting to gain glimpses into medicine in China as it once was. Dr. Wilms's translation of Sūn's gynecological thought is a major breakthrough in presenting Chinese medical history in a way that is not only useful to historians, but also maximally enlightening for modern students and practitioners of traditional Chinese medicine. I hope she sets a new trend.

Nigel Wiseman,
Taiwan, September 2007

Preface by Arnaud Versluys Ph.D., L.Ac.

There are few masterworks in the history of Chinese medicine that enjoy such high regard as the *Qiān Jīn Fāng*. However, there are even fewer that despite such high esteem have previously received this little academic attention in the international Chinese medical community.

The *Qiān Jīn Fāng* is nowadays praised as the first clinical encyclopedia [1] and a milestone in the tradition of canonical formula literature. Historically, *Sòng* dynasty government editor Lín Yì has praised the comprehensiveness of the work, stating: "From the origins of script, to the times of *Suí*, regardless canon or prescription, all were collected invariably."[2]

Many a legend surrounds its author, Sūn Sī-Miǎo, as a spiritual persona, but only a limited number of attempts have been made to allow access to his factual life story. Sūn Sī-Miǎo lived in a time of great accomplishments and progress, and the Old Book on *Táng* mentions his wide range of interests: "… he is good at talking about Zhuāng, Lǎo and the hundred schools of doctrine, while on the side being fond of the Buddhist classics."[3] In folk and Daoist circles, he is revered as the King of Medicines, while his ethics display both Confucian and Buddhist influences. He practiced medicine with great compassion towards women, children and elderly.

The *Hàn* dynasty *Jīn Guì Yào Lüè* 金匱要略 (Essentials of the Golden Coffer) devotes three chapters on women's diseases at the end of the book, just before the addendum discussing various poisoning scenarios, vermin bites, and the waking of the dead. But one of the most remarkable aspects of Sūn Sī-Miǎo and his work is that he not only devotes three scrolls to the detailed description of women's diseases and their treatment, but that he placed these scrolls at the very opening of his book. This to comply with the laws of the *Dào* and show respect to the origin of life, or as he puts it: "… first women, children and then men and elderly, for this signifies homage to the root [of life]." [4] It is therefore befitting that when Dr. Wilms publishes the first translation and annotation of the *Qiān Jīn Fāng* in English, the first volume encompasses these very aforementioned chapters. She sets the tone for a series of encyclopedic volumes that will shed light on one of the more exciting chapters in the history of Chinese medicine.

Whenever I look at Dr. Wilms' accomplishments, I am humbled by her work ability and methodical mind. She is one of the hardest working scholars in the Chinese medicine sinologist community. Her contributions are hailed not only by linguists, anthropologists and historians but by Chinese medicine clinicians alike. This translation of the gynecology and obstetrics chapters of the *Qiān Jīn Fāng* along with a detailed introduction on Sūn Sī-Miǎo and the nature of his work have set a new benchmark in *Táng* dynasty medical literature research and as far as Western scholars and clinicians are concerned, is certainly worth its weight in gold.

Arnaud Versluys, PhD, MD (China), LAc
National College of Natural Medicine
Portland, OR, USA

[1] 任應秋 ed. 《中醫各家學說》, 上海：科學技術出版社. 1986: 190

[2] 李景榮 ed.《備急千金要方校釋》，北京：人民衛生出版社．1998: 10

[3] 劉昫，《舊唐書·孫思邈傳》，北京：中華書局．1975: 5094

[4] 李景榮 ed.《備急千金要方校釋》，北京：人民衛生出版社．1998: 85

Translator's Acknowledgements

This book would have been impossible without the help of countless individuals. I am deeply grateful to my patient doctoral dissertation supervisor of ten years, Donald J. Harper, for his meticulous sinological scholarship and uncompromising standards. Thanks also go to the other members of my doctoral committee: to Charlotte Furth, Mark Nichter, Anna Shields, and Elizabeth Harrison. Many Western scholars in the field of history of Chinese medicine provided inspirational and ground-breaking research, crucial advice, and interest in my project, including Christopher Cullen, Ute Engelhardt, Marta Hanson, T.J. Hinrichs, Elisabeth Hsu, Vivienne Lo, Makoto Mayanagi, Paul U. Unschuld, Lorraine Wilcox and Yi-li Wu.

During a much too brief research stay in 2001 at the, Academia Sinica in Taipei, many professors and colleagues, most notably Jender Lee (Lǐ Zhēn-Dé) 李貞德 and Lǐ Jiàn-Mín 李建民, gave so freely of their time that the foundations for this study were laid there in only six months.

The difficult process of transforming an academic dissertation into a readable book for a larger audience was made possible by the assistance of practitioners and authors in the practical field of Chinese medicine, especially Z'ev Rosenberg, Jason Robertson, Emmanuel Segmen, the contributors to several listserves on Chinese medicine, and to Arnauld Versluys who was so kind to write the preface. Thanks to my students at the Asian Institute of Medical Studies during Z'ev Rosenberg's herb walks here in Taos, and other alert listeners for their challenging questions. This study became a book under the faultless gaze of Nigel Wiseman, whose combined talents as mentor, author, translator, editor, and friend made the text terminologically consistent, clinically meaningful, and readable in English. I consider myself very lucky to have been able to work closely with him for a number of years, during which I have learned so much. His work has shown me that it might in fact be possible to translate a text from a vastly different time, culture, place, and language into modern English and still communicate something meaningful.

I also want to acknowledge my publisher, Jonathan Schell, for believing in this project and in the value of Chinese medical classics in general, for devoting weeks on end and sleepless nights to preparing files and finding typos, and for having such ambitious dreams of translating the mountains of classical texts into clinically useful books in modern English, bridging the gap between the academic and clinical worlds.

Special thanks to my family for sticking with me through a whole lot, to Linah Ababneh and Chieko Nakano for being the best friends anybody could ever wish for, to my goats, chickens, and apple trees for feeding me when I had no time to cook, to my neighbors for farming advice and help, to the universe for giving us galloping horses, fishing holes, raspberries, and squash blossoms, and to all the world's true teachers, healers, musicians, and sustainable farmers for nourishing our bodies, minds, and souls.

This book is dedicated to my favorite peach, my daughter Momo, whose birth provided the first spark for the topic, whose faith in me has been limitless, whose singing has kept me going, without whose help in milking goats, picking apples, and herding geese our farm would have fallen apart during the final stages of this book, and whose lack of patience and refusal to let me work too late has saved my sanity!

Publisher's Acknowledgements

For every path there is a door, which must be opened by choice, and at that door stands Coyote, guardian of the chosen path. Hok Pang Tang L.Ac., M.D. (China) was the guardian at my door -- I thank you for being the one. Scott Stuart L.Ac.: for burger and beer night; Chuck Bauman and Heather Agosta at the Jasmine Pearl: true friends and good tea; Brandon and Katye Landis: for the moral support; Norma Schell: mother and publisher before me; Steve & Georgia Schell: a home away from home; Sara Hazel N.D.: through tough life lessons comes growth; Sebastian Schell: the twinkle in my eye; Tom Schell: brotherly vigilance; Peter Falson: my clinch man; Arnaud Versluys PhD, L.Ac.: for putting up with me; Sue Westermin: my vision in the dark; all of my fabulous patients who, because of their belief in me, allowed this to happen; I thank you all and give thanks to the Universe for allowing me to help in this small way, bring the treasures from the past, to the here and now.

Publisher's Note

Terms:

We have used the terminolgy of the *Practical Ditionary of Chinese Medicine* (PD) by Nigel Wiseman and Féng Yè consistently throuohut the translation of the *Bèi Jí Qiān Jīn Yào Fāng*. For further understanding of the terms mentioned in this book please consult the PD.

Medicinals:

We thought hard about how, we would approach the dosages of medicinals, as represented in the *Bèi Jí Qiān Jīn Yào Fāng*. It is important to us that the dosages in the text reflect the literal translation. We have thus included as part of each formula the original measurement in Chinese, as recorded in the *Bèi Jí Qiān Jīn Yào Fāng*. But we also wanted to make the formulas from this book accessible to the modern clinician, after all this book is being translated for the modern clinical audience. In the formulas then, we give you the modern proportions for the herbs in grams. These modern proportions are not an attempt to translate the Chinese measurements, but will act as a guide for the modern clinician when thinking about using these formulas in their practice.

Weight

1 shǔ 黍 = 0.03g	1 shǔ 黍 = millet grain
1 zhū 銖 = 0.3g	1 zhū 銖 = 10 shǔ
1 fēn 分 = 1.8g	1 fēn 分 = 6 zhū
1 liǎng 兩 = 3g	1 liǎng 兩 = 24 zhū
1 jīn 斤 = 48g	1 jīn 斤 = 16 liǎng
1 shēng 升 = 24g	

Volume

1 dāo guī 刀圭 = 0.087 ml	1 dāo guī 刀圭 = 4 parasol tree seeds
1 cuō 撮 = 0.35 ml	1 cuō 撮 = 4 dāo guī
1 sháo 勺 = 3.5 ml	1 sháo 勺 = 10 cuō

1 gě 合	= 7 ml	1 gě 合 = 2 sháo
1 shēng 升	= 70 ml	1 shēng 升 = 10 gě
1 dǒu 斗	= 700 ml	1 dǒu 斗 = 10 shēng
1 hú 斛	= 7000 ml	1 hú 斛 = 10 dǒu

Length

1 fēn 分	= 0.3 cm	1 fēn 分	
1 cùn 寸	= 3 cm	1 cùn 寸	= 10 fēn
1 chǐ 尺	= 30 cm	1 chǐ 尺	= 10 cùn
1 bù 步	= 150 cm	1 bù 步	= 5 chǐ
1 lǐ 里	= 540 m	1 lǐ 里	= 1800 chǐ

We also thought our reader would like to look up the different reocurring ways that herbs are prepared throughout the text. We have included this information in the pinyin index.

Future Work:

The *Bèi Jí Qiān Jīn Yào Fāng* is a vast compendium of *Táng* dynasty Chinese medical knowledge that spans 30 volumes. This 3 volume translation on Gynecology is the first book of a 10 volume set on the *Bèi Jí Qiān Jīn Yào Fāng* that the Chinese Medicine Database and Dr. Sabine Wilms will be translating.

1

Bèi Jí Qiān Jīn Yào Fāng

備急千金要方

Prolegomena

3

Prolegomena

1. Introduction

This work investigates the medical treatment of the female body in medieval China. Its core consists of a translation of the three volumes on "prescriptions for women" (婦人方 *fù rén fāng*) from Sūn Sī-Miǎo's *Bèi Jí Qiān Jīn Yào Fāng* 備急千金要方 (Essential Prescriptions worth a Thousand in Gold for Every Emergency, in the following pages abbreviated as *Qiān Jīn Fāng* 千金方). Composed in the early seventh century, this text is in China regarded as its "first encyclopedic medical text, with continuing scientific significance and clinical value up to modern times, venerated by physicians in China and abroad." Its thirty volumes cover over two hundred topics, and contain over five thousand entries in the form of essays and prescriptions.

It begins with a preface in one volume, which discusses general guidelines regarding medical ethics, training, diagnosis, treatment, individual medicinals, compounding drugs, contraindicated foods etc. This is followed by three volumes on prescriptions for women, and one volume each on pediatrics, on the diseases of the seven orifices (that is, conditions of the eyes, nose, mouth, tongue, lips, teeth, throat and face), on wind poison and leg *qì*, and on the various winds. Next are two volumes on cold damage, which preserve the content of Zhāng Zhòng-Jǐng's 張仲景 *Shāng Hán Lùn* 傷寒論 (On Cold Damage). Since they constitute one of the earliest received versions of this text, they are of great value for research on Cold Damage theory. They are followed by one volume on each of the ten viscera and bowels, one volume on thirst and urinary problems, and one volume each on abscesses, on hemorrhoids and fistulas (concluding with a systematic discussion of the treatment and prevention of leprosy that reflects Sūn Sī-Miǎo's original ideas and personal experience), on resolving toxins and various other problems, and on emergency treatments. The following volume on dietary therapy contains information on the medicinal applications of household fruits, vegetables, grains, and meats, such as their natures and flavors, their therapeutic efficacies and usages, and dietary restrictions. Next is a volume on cultivating health and prolonging life that includes advice on an eremitic lifestyle, massage, regulating qì, dietary methods, "the various prohibitions of the Yellow Emperor," and "supplementing and boosting through sexual intercourse." The *Qiān Jīn Fāng* concludes with a volume on vessel theory and pulse diagnostics, and two volumes on acupuncture and moxibustion. Therein, we find a reference to three five-colored charts of the channels and acumoxa points on the human body, called *Míng Táng Sān Rén Tú* 明堂三人圖 (Three-Figure Chart of the Hall of Brightness) that presumably accompanied the original text, but have unfortunately been lost. The *Qiān Jīn Fāng* also contains the first reference to the "Ouch Point" (阿是穴 *ā shì xué*), which is still used today.

As a whole, the *Qiān Jīn Fāng* has proven to be a goldmine of information about what was apparently the most sophisticated level of medical theory and practice in the early *Táng* dynasty. The depth of Sūn Sī-Miǎo's medical knowledge is expressed in the theoretical essays, the conceptualization and organization of etiologies, and the complexities of the medicinal prescriptions. The most outstanding feature of the text, however, is its comprehensiveness, reflected particularly in the diversity of therapeutic techniques. These include such internal applications as medicinal decoctions, powders, pastes, jellies, or wines, external applications like ointments, hot compresses and suppositories, fumigations, baths, beauty treatments, physical manipulations, acupuncture and moxibustion, as well as religious methods like talismans, exorcistic rituals, and spells.

The medical contributions of the *Qiān Jīn Fāng* might not be quite as relevant and directly applicable in the modern clinical context as the *Shāng Hán Lùn*, which spawned an entire field of medical specialization in China, or as important theoretically as the classics *Huáng Dì Nèi Jīng* 黃帝內經 (Yellow Emperor's Inner Classic) and the *Nàn Jīng* 難經 (Classic of Difficult Issues). Sūn Sī-Miǎo's official recognition in the following centuries can be seen in the fact that the *Qiān Jīn Fāng* and its sequel, the *Qiān Jīn Yì Fāng* 千金翼方 (Supplemental Prescriptions Worth a Thousand in Gold), were two of only eleven medical texts to be meticulously revised and printed in the twelfth century by the imperially sponsored Office for the Correction of Medical Texts. The regular appearance of reprints until the present as well as the composition of a detailed explication in thirty volumes during the *Qīng* dynasty also testifies to Sūn Sī-Miǎo's continuing influence in Chinese medical circles. Today, annotated editions of this text are still found in the historical sections of well-stocked TCM bookstores in Asia, and lengthy excerpts are ubiquitous in Chinese TCM textbooks on a variety of medical fields.

It has been identified convincingly as the most influential text in the transmission of Chinese medicine to Japan and therefore the foundational text in the creation and development of Japanese Kampō 漢方 medicine. Miyashita Saburō points out that, contrary to numerous claims, the *Qiān Jīn Fāng* was not the earliest Chinese text to be transmitted to Japan. In the year 701, such texts as the *Sù Wèn* 素問 (Plain Questions), *Zhēn Jiǔ Jiǎ Yǐ Jīng* 針灸甲乙經 (Systematized Classic of Acupuncture and Moxibustion) and *Xiǎo Pǐn Fāng* 小品方 (Prescriptions of Minor Degree) are already recorded in Japan, whereas the *Qiān Jīn Fāng* is not recorded until 897. Nevertheless, its pivotal role in Japan is clearly reflected in the amount of quotations that are found in such Japanese collections of Chinese medical texts as the *Ishimpō* 醫心方 (Prescriptions at the Heart of Medicine), composed in 984 by Tanba no Yasuyori 丹波康賴. There, it is the second most extensively quoted text after Cháo Yuán-Fāng's *Zhū Bìng Yuán Hòu Lùn* 諸病源候論 (On the Origins and Symptoms of the Various Diseases, below abbreviated as *Bìng Yuán Lùn* 病源論), and provides the highest number of prescriptions. Its continuing influence throughout the Kamakura and Muromachi periods is obvious from the extensive usage of Sūn Sī-Miǎo's prescriptions in medical compendia from these periods. Moreover, Miyashita lists over twenty editions of Sūn Sī-Miǎo's writings to have been transmitted from China to Japan, and ten Japanese translations, published from the seventeenth to the mid-nineteenth century alone.

The monumental impact of Sūn Sī-Miǎo's work on the development of Chinese medicine has long been recognized in China in numerous and extremely varied publications. These reflect not only his enduring popularity, but also the diverse motivations that continue to stimulate his promotion for a wide range of audiences. To give only a few examples, at one end of the spectrum lies a short, but lavishly illustrated booklet entitled *Yào Wáng Sūn Sī-Miǎo* 藥王孫思邈 (Sūn Sī-Miǎo, King of Medicine) that was published in 1990 by the Shǎn-Xī Committee for the Compilation of Records on Public Health. Graced with prefaces by such honoraries as the director of the national Office of Public Health, the president of the Shǎn-Xī Province Office of Public Health, and the honorary president of the Shǎn-Xī Province Research Institute for Chinese Medicine and Pharmacology, it contains a brief twenty-page informational section and over fifty pages of illustrations. These display everything even remotely related to Sūn Sī-Miǎo, such as photographs of the well in which he reportedly cleaned his medicinal drugs, the gorgeous views and his favorite herb-gathering trails surrounding his purported hermitage on Mount Tài-Bó 太白山, artistic renderings of his legendary heroic acts, commemorative statues, temples, and rocks, the steaming food carts of vendors in the hustle and bustle of an anniversary celebration by his temple, two Americans admiring an exhibition in Beijing, commemorative stamps, scholarly conventions, and even the withered tree in whose shade Sūn Sī-Miǎo reportedly studied in his tender youth. While offering some historical background in the introductory essays, this booklet is obviously aimed at the promotion of tourism by reinforcing and encouraging the local concentration of a popular cult of Sūn Sī-Miǎo as the deified "King of Medicine" (藥王 yào wáng), whose origins Paul Unschuld has dated to the fourteenth or fifteenth centuries.

Addressing a more scholarly audience with historical interests is the biography by Gān Zǔ-Wàng 干祖望, entitled Sūn Sī Miǎo Píng Zhuàn 孫思邈評傳 (A Critical Biography of Sūn Sī-Miǎo). Authored by a practicing physician of great national fame, its stated goal is to establish Sūn Sī-Miǎo, on the basis of Marxist principles and a critical historical analysis, as one of China's eminent physicians and a key figure in the development of a modern scientific medicine in China. Nevertheless, it must be pointed out that this book is also to a large extent based on sources that are too far removed from Sūn Sī-Miǎo chronologically to be historically sound. Moreover, Gān's attempt to present Sūn Sī-Miǎo as an enlightened materialist with a modern scientific gaze forces him into questionable arguments. Thus, he explains for example Sūn Sī-Miǎo's encounter with a dragon who bestowed on him a "Classic for Ingesting Water" as a meeting with a person surnamed Lóng 龍 (Dragon). It is also clearly ahistorical for Gān to claim that Sūn Sī-Miǎo was merely citing an ancient legend—with the implication that such an enlightened scholar as Sūn Sī-Miǎo would not have believed that himself—when he advertises a pill prescription for the treatment of seasonal epidemics by stressing its origin from a demon king. Supernatural etiologies occur frequently not only in medieval medical texts by such "enlightened" medical authors as Sūn Sī-Miǎo and Cháo Yuán-Fāng, but as a widely accepted explanation throughout the entirety of Chinese history, especially in the treatment of epidemics. Thus, it is misleading to ignore an aspect of medieval medicine that was obviously considered an integral part by Sūn Sī-Miǎo himself and important enough for him to devote the majority of the final two volumes in the Qiān Jīn Yì Fāng, entitled "Classic of Prohibitions" (Jìn Jīng 禁經), to it. As such, certain parts of Gān's book might be of greater value to a researcher interested in the ideological creation of post-Maoist "traditional" Chinese medicine than to researcher of medieval medical literature or practice.

An equally celebratory but much less political picture is painted by the academic articles found in the January 1983 issue of Zhōng Huá Yī Shǐ Zá Zhì 中華醫史雜誌 (Chinese Journal of Medical History). Occasioned by the 1300-year anniversary of Sūn Sī-Miǎo's death, the entire volume is devoted to his medical achievements. Since the information in these articles is based largely on Sūn Sī-Miǎo's own writings, the journal does indeed present a clear and, for the most part, accurate overview of Sūn Sī-Miǎo's achievements and major innovations in a variety of medical fields. It includes brief but informative writings on such topics as Sūn Sī-Miǎo's social and intellectual background, his achievements in philosophy, medical theory, pharmacology, gynecology and pediatrics, geriatrics, bone setting, preventive medicine, ethics, foreign influences on his work, and his significance in Japan. Taken as a whole, the authors in this volume argue convincingly for the pivotal status accorded to Sūn Sī-Miǎo by contemporary Chinese medical historians and practitioners. It is only unfortunate that the brevity of the entries forces the authors to limit their presentations to basic summaries of the content and mere suggestions for future research, rather than engaging in in-depth analyses of the wealth of information found in the various volumes of the Qiān Jīn Fāng.

Lastly, Zhōu Yī-Móu's 周一謀 book-length study of Sūn Sī-Miǎo's techniques of health preservation, entitled Shòu Xīng Sūn Sī-Miǎo Shè Shēng Jīng Yào 壽星孫思邈攝生精要 (Essentials for Preserving Life by the Star of Longevity Sūn Sī-Miǎo) attempts to reconstruct the minutest details of Sūn Sī-Miǎo's life. Based primarily on evidence from Sūn Sī-Miǎo's own writing, which is taken at face value, it discusses the medicinal plants he grew, mountains he climbed, clothing he wore, sexual practices he engaged in, ethical values he followed, and texts he studied. This book appears to be aimed at providing readers with the concrete practical information to understand — and possibly emulate — the healthy lifestyle that Sūn Sī-Miǎo practiced, which purportedly enabled him to live to the great age of over one hundred years. It reads almost like an interesting variation on modern self-help literature based on medieval medical sources. A critical Western reader is unlikely to accept references in Sūn Sī-Miǎo's own writings, largely unsupported by the historical biographies, as sufficient proof that he actually engaged in these practices. This should not detract from the fact, however, that this book can still supply colorful details to allow us to envision certain aspects of medieval elite life that are neglected in other accounts like the biographies in the dynastic histories. More importantly, it also succeeds in illustrating the significance of life-prolonging practices and their wide-ranging applications in the gentry's life. It can therefore certainly be employed as a meaningful angle from which to investigate daily life in traditional China. Given the importance accorded to "nurturing life" (養生 *yáng shēng*) by Sūn Sī-Miǎo himself, it is only fitting that his contributions in this field should receive the praise and attention of an entire book. Indeed, it is not unlikely that this topic constitutes the apex of Sūn Sī-Miǎo's personal medical experience and erudition, a fact not gone unnoticed by Zhōu Yī-Móu, one of China's leading scholars of early medical history.

In conclusion, Sūn Sī-Miǎo is well-known and often cited by medical historians and physicians in China for his role in the development of medieval medicine. Nevertheless, this interest is often motivated by a practical concern for the applicability of his writings in a contemporary clinical context as well as nationalistic attempts to prove the great age of certain contemporary medical practices or the superiority of so-called "traditional Chinese medicine" in general. Consequently, such research agendas have sometimes led to the exclusion or denial of certain aspects of Sūn Sī-Miǎo's understanding of medieval medicine while overemphasizing others. To give just one example, many historical studies have confirmed the significance of religious healing modalities, whether in the context of Buddhism, Daoism, or folk religion. In contemporary Chinese scholarship that is aimed at stressing the scientific nature of TCM, these tend to be deemphasized, decried as "superstition" (迷信 *mí xìn*), ignored, or even denied.

In spite of this popularity in China and Japan, the *Qiān Jīn Fāng* and its illustrious author have remained shrouded in obscurity in the West. No translation has been published except for minor excerpts in English and the French translation of the two volumes on acupuncture by Catherine Despeux. In addition, the only major academic studies to focus on Sūn Sī-Miǎo and his work are a critical biography by Nathan Sivin and one article by Paul Unschuld. The field of medieval Chinese medicine is only beginning to receive Western scholars' attention. This is partly due to concerns that the received versions of medical literature predating the *Sòng* period frequently suffered from extensive revisions and were therefore of questionable historicity. Nevertheless, recent research on the Dūn-Huáng 敦煌 material has made available alternate versions of such classics as the *Sù Wèn* 素問, *Shāng Hán Lùn*, *Xīn Xiū Běn Cǎo Jīng* 新修本草經 (Newly Revised Classic of Materia Medica), and *Mài Jīng* 脈經 (Pulse Classic). In addition, the *Ishimpō*, a ninth-century Japanese compendium of early medieval Chinese medical literature, provides an alternative source for quotations from many major texts, allowing for republications of the received classics that approximate a form predating the *Sòng* revisions. As the following chapter will show, existing scholarship on medieval Chinese medicine is still at such an early stage that any general conclusions would be premature. Such text-oriented approaches as Catherine Despeux and Frédéric Obringer's study of the cough (La maladie dans la Chine mediéval: La toux), Catherine Despeux's translation of the acupuncture volumes in the *Qiān Jīn Fāng*, Ute Engelhardt's study of classical *qìgōng* (Die klassische Tradition der Qi-Übungen), or Stephan Stein's study of early literature on *yǎng shēng* (Zwischen Heil und Heilung) are extremely valuable. They indicate the need for more research of this sort in other fields of medical knowledge as well as for subsequent interpretation of the material introduced therein. The current study is intended as a step in a similar direction, translating the three volumes on prescriptions for women in the *Qiān Jīn Fāng*. Convincing arguments for the validity of studying the medical treatment of the female body can be found in much anthropological literature. Before addressing these issues, the next chapters will provide some background regarding the author and the text and a brief summary of the content of the volumes translated here.

2. Sūn Sī-Miǎo and the Qiān Jīn Fāng

To understand and evaluate the content of the three volumes translated here, we must first contextualize the text by assessing the background from which it originated. This chapter will therefore begin by analyzing the available and historically reliable information regarding the author's life and work. Clarifying the circumstances under which the *Qiān Jīn Fāng* was composed, it will situate it in the tradition of early medieval prescription literature and describe its editorial history and the differences between currently available editions.

2a. Summary of Sūn Sī-Miǎo's Life and Work

To this day, Sūn Sī-Miǎo is the object of a large popular cult as the deified "King of Medicine" (藥王 *yào wáng*), venerated particularly on his supposed birthday, the 28th day of the fourth lunar month. Locations associated with his life and work attract more than a hundred thousand pilgrims yearly. Given his fame and popularity throughout the centuries, historically verifiable facts are surprisingly hard to come by. As is not uncommon for a Chinese historical figure, we know close to nothing about those aspects of his personal life unrelated to public events or figures. In an attempt to separate the historical persona of Sūn Sī-Miǎo from the hagiographical embellishments in legends composed many centuries after his death, the information in this chapter is based primarily on two sources: I will reconstruct the basic facts of Sūn Sī-Miǎo's life as they are recounted in the official two histories, the Jiù Táng Shū 舊唐書 (Old Táng History), completed during the *Jìn* 晉 dynasty in 945 under the direction of Liú Xù 劉昫, and the Xīn Táng Shū 新唐書 (New Táng History), completed during the *Sòng* 宋 period in 1060 under the direction of Ōu-Yáng Xiū 歐陽 修. While their historical reliability is highly questionable from a modern academic standpoint, these two texts are still our most reliable and factual sources, since the authors of these imperially-sponsored biographies had access to the histories in the *Táng* archives and went to great lengths to ensure what they considered the historical accuracy of their accounts.

It does need to be noted, however, that both of these texts were not only composed several centuries after Sūn Sī-Miǎo's death, but are widely known to have used sources of questionable authenticity. The *Sòng* scholar Ōu-Yáng Xiū already claimed that the political unrest at the time of the composition of the *Jiù Táng Shū* had greatly hindered the compilers' access to many sources that had since become available in the *Sòng*. Thus, he was able to convince the *Sòng* emperor Rén Zōng 仁宗 to commission a revision, which took from 1045 to 1060 to complete and resulted in the *Xīn Táng Shū*. According to Nathan Sivin's meticulous and highly skeptical investigation of Sūn Sī-Miǎo's Táng Shū biographies, verifiable facts regarding Sūn Sī-Miǎo's life can be summed up in the following statement:

In the case of Sun, our warrantable knowledge, based on the incontrovertible testimony of a well-placed witness, at least allows us to set him in his time: Sun was in the Emperor's retinue in 673, and stated at the time that he was born in 581; despite the great age which these dates imply, he was in excellent condition, body and mind. Nothing else survives the process of elimination.

It is certainly commendable to take the information from the two *Táng* histories with a grain of salt, given both the internal contradictions and the distance between the dates of their composition and Sūn Sī-Miǎo's lifetime. Nathan Sivin considers the *Xīn Táng Shū* to be more reliable because it was written at a time of peace when the authors had access to additional sources of information. Nevertheless, a close comparison between the two biographies reveals that both texts are based on the same sources, namely the *Shí Lù* 實錄 (True Records) and *Guó Shǐ* 國史 (History of the States) from the *Táng* imperial archives. Thus, the *Xīn Táng Shū* fails to provide additional information, but, to the contrary, was abbreviated and condensed to conform to the stylistic requirements of the literary *gǔ wén* 古文 movement. In a similar vein, Sivin admits that "there is not a single discrepancy in the two biographies of such a nature as to suggest that the HTS [i.e., *Xīn Táng Shū*] editors had access to new archival material." While the standards for historiographical writing in medieval China obviously fall short of our modern demands, we can assume that the authors of both biographies based their accounts on what they considered reliable evidence, including personal interviews with locals from his home town, and eliminated material that they were unable to verify. Thus, I regard Sūn Sī-Miǎo's biographies as containing often exaggerated, but nevertheless highly relevant information that we can use to reconstruct a fairly realistic image of Sūn Sī-Miǎo's life, character, and cultural background. An inaccurate date or official rank, or a fabricated conversation, should not cause us to "throw the baby out with the bath water" and disregard the insights that can be gained into Sūn Sī-Miǎo's education, political engagement, social circle, or reputation.

These terse accounts are supplemented with three roughly contemporaneous biographies: in the *Tài Píng Guǎng Jì* 太平廣記 (Extensive Records of the Tài Píng period), which was completed in 977 by Lǐ Fǎng 李昉; in the *Xù Xiān Zhuàn* 續仙傳 (Further Biographies of Immortals), which was composed by Shěn Fén 沈汾 and cited in the 10th century Daoist encyclopedia *Yún Jí Qī Qiān* 雲笈七籤 (Seven Bamboo Slips from a Cloud Satchel); and, our earliest extant source, in the *Huá Yán Jīng Chuán Jì* 華嚴經傳記 (Records of the Transmission of the Avatamsaka Sutra), composed by Fǎ Zàng 法藏 (643-712), where Sūn Sī-Miǎo is recorded as a specialist on the Buddhist Avatamsaka Sutra.

Sūn Sī-Miǎo's biography in the *Jiù Táng Shū* is translated in full in the appendix at the end of this book, so the following paragraphs merely summarize the major events in his life: Sūn Sī-Miǎo was born in Huá-Yuán 華原 in Jīng-Zhào 京兆, located in modern Yào County 耀縣 in Shǎn-Xī Province 陝西, near the *Táng* capital Cháng-Ān 長安. He immersed himself so studiously in classical Confucian, Daoist, and Buddhist literature from the tender age of seven on that the governor Dú-Gū Xìn 獨孤信 recognized him as a child prodigy (聖童 *shèng tóng*). He commented, however, on his capabilities: "Regrettably, his talent is so great that his suitability is diminished and he will be difficult to employ." In addition to the information that Sūn Sī-Miǎo's talent was already recognized by the authorities in his youth, Dú-Gū Xìn's rank here suggests that this interview took place between 537 and 540, which would place Sūn Sī-Miǎo's birth year in the 520's or 530's. As Sivin points out, this story is a commonly found motif in *Táng* biographies and therefore highly suspect as historical evidence.

Due to the scandalous nature of the government during the reign of Emperor Xuān of the Zhōu 周宣帝 (578-579), Sūn Sī-Miǎo led the eremitic lifestyle of a true sage who would seclude himself during times of corrupt leadership, on Mount Tài-Bó 太白山 (modern Zhōng-Nán-Shān 終南山, part of the Wǔ-Gōng mountain range 武功山 in Shǎn-Xī Province). In this, he followed in the footsteps of individuals of moral integrity from ancient times who "advanced and retreated according to the ideals of propriety and deferential renunciation." He declined the honor of an appointment by Emperor Wén of the Suí 隋文帝 as an Erudite of the National University 國子博士 when Wén was still regent, that is, between 580 and 589. At this time, Sūn Sī-Miǎo predicted that a sage ruler would emerge after fifty years whom he would then be willing to assist with his prescriptions. When the *Táng* Emperor Tài-Zōng 太宗 assumed the throne in 627, he did indeed respond to an imperial summons to the capital. He astounded the emperor with his youthful appearance and remained in the government's service for a total of almost fifty years, but declined several honorary titles. He was finally allowed to retire in 674 on the pretext of ill health. If we consider the first story of his interview with Dú-Gū Xìn true, this is understandable since it would make him about 150 years old at this time.

Among his disciples were such eminent *Táng* figures as the physician and alchemist Mèng Shēn 孟詵 and the literary genius Lú Zhào-Lín 盧照鄰. In the preface to a poem, Lú characterizes Sūn Sī-Miǎo in the following way: "Miǎo's way harmonizes the past with the present. He has studied the arts of [calendrical and astrological] calculation to the utmost extreme. His eminent discussion of Orthodox Oneness is on a par with the ancient *Zhuāng-Zǐ* 莊子 [a reference to his familiarity with Daoist teachings]. His deep penetration of non-duality is on a par with the contemporary Vimalakirti [a reference to his familiarity with Buddhist teachings]. His astrological prognostications and measurements of the masculine and feminine are on a par with Luò-Xià Hóng 洛下宏 and Ān-Qí Shēng 安其生 [legendary masters of esoteric techniques, of astrology and materia medica respectively]." Sūn Sī-Miǎo is, moreover, credited with curing Lú Zhào-Lín from a "malign condition that physicians had been unable to treat," which is the only reference in the official biographies that Sūn Sī-Miǎo actually practiced medicine. The quotations that are attributed to Sūn Sī-Miǎo and cited in the biographies represent him as an enlightened scholar and eloquent intellectual, well-versed in an impressive range of classical texts, and shifting from moral exhortations based on *Shī Jīng* 詩經 (Classic of Poetry) quotations to cosmological and medical theory reminiscent of the *Huáng Dì Nèi Jīng*. In the only quotation with medical content, for example, Sūn Sī-Miǎo states that the physician's act of harmonizing the human body with the constancies of the universe by medicinal prescriptions, needles, and stones in the quest for health and longevity is equal to the sage-king's governing by patterning the affairs of human society after the heavenly cycles.

Besides information regarding his birth date, which will be discussed in the next paragraph, the remainder of the biography is devoted to substantiating the editors' claims of Sūn Sī-Miǎo's supernatural abilities: His great age of several hundred years is verified in interviews with residents from his home town and by the vivid nature of his recollections of events that occurred during the Northern Qí 北齊 and Northern Zhóu 北周 Dynasties, that is, in the second half of the sixth century. His extraordinary skills in physiognomy and prognostication go as far as predicting an event in the life of his not-yet-born grandson. Lastly, it is recorded that Sūn Sī-Miǎo died in 682. As customary for a true immortal, he requested and received a simple funeral, after which his physical appearance remained unchanged and stiff as wood a month later. The biography concludes with a short list of his writings and the fact that his son obtained the distinguished rank of Vice Director of the Imperial Secretariat.

While the year of Sūn Sī-Miǎo's death is generally agreed upon as 682, more controversy surrounds his date of birth. Most current scholars adopt as true what the biographies record as his own words: "Sun himself said that he was born in the *xīn yǒu* 辛酉 year of the Kāi Huáng 開皇 period (581-600), and that he was presently 93 years old." Since there was no *xīn yǒu* year during this period, the editors of the encyclopedia *Sì Kù Quán Shū* 四庫全書 (Complete Texts in the Four Treasuries) have proposed to read it as *xīn chǒu* 辛丑 instead. This would place his date of birth at 581 or 582, an argument now widely accepted in spite of the obvious contradictions with other statements in the biographies. An alternative is provided by Gān Zǔ-Wàng who devotes an entire chapter arguing for 541 as Sūn Sī-Miǎo's birth year instead since it fits more closely with the other events recounted in the biography. Whether he died at the age of 101 or 141, the *Táng* historians' belief in his supernatural longevity suggests that his contemporaries and successors gave credence to his deep insights into the workings of the human body and the universe, applied to his own body.

In conclusion, the official *Táng* histories identify Sūn Sī-Miǎo as a man of great intellectual talent with a profound and well-rounded education in the Confucian, Daoist and Buddhist literature. Simultaneously, he appears to have been a master of highly technical and esoteric matters like calendrical calculations, astrology, and physiognomy. To prove his moral integrity, they emphasize that he refused to serve in an immoral government and that he declined honorary titles when he did serve in the role of a court erudite. The quotations in the biographies function to illustrate his outstanding literary skills, his substantial political involvement and prestige at the *Táng* court, and his intimate connections with the eminent scholars of his time. Besides his worldly accomplishments, the biographers also stress that he possessed sagely illumination and supernatural powers, lived as a hermit in various stages of his life, and cured a prominent member of the elite of a "malign illness that physicians were unable to treat," the only reference in the biographies to any medical activities. His insights into the workings of the cosmos were regarded as so deep that he was not only able to predict the future and assist the emperor in guiding the country, but also to physically affect his own body in such a way that he preserved it from the decline of old age and from decay after his death.

This combination of attributes points directly at the milieu of the so-called "masters of prescriptions," 方士 *fāng shì*, namely specialists in natural philosophy and occult thought who distinguished themselves in early China through their possession of technical prescription literature, 方書 *fāng shū*. In particular, the constellation of technical skills related to divination and cosmology and the vagueness about concrete events in Sūn Sī-Miǎo's life suggests placing him in the subcategory of specialists in the art of immortality. Since "immortality is demonstrable only by something not happening,... the immortal is characteristically eremitic, and he emerges into public view only in the rarest of circumstances." Kenneth DeWoskin notes that the *fāng shì's* greatest influence fell between the second century BCE and the fourth century CE and that the term itself then came to be used with an increasingly deprecatory meaning. Nevertheless, the social group to which this term originally referred clearly continued to exert significant influence at court and in society at large. Ultimately, Sūn Sī-Miǎo's skills and reputation situate him among the respectable members of this group, while his classical education and ethical standards distance him from the lower stratum of its opportunistic members who were "taken to task for their ambitions, incompetence, excess, and dishonesty, all of which are forged in to the standard charge levied against the fang-shih."

As his categorization in the various biographies shows, the image of Sūn Sī-Miǎo as a Daoist immortal soon came to outweigh the more conventional aspects of his life: In the *Jiù Táng Shū*, he is still found in the category of "[masters of] prescriptions and technical skills" (方技 *fāng jì*), which was used in the *Táng* histories to refer to physicians, astrologers, physiognomers, and diviners. In the *Xīn Táng Shū*, he is moved to the section for "recluses" (隱逸 *yǐn yì*), a category for true hermits that, at least in pre-*Táng* times, specifically excluded individuals who found 'reclusion' within the court. The placement of Sūn Sī-Miǎo in this category could signify either a change in the meaning of this term, or, much more likely, the widespread perception of Sūn Sī-Miǎo as a true recluse, in spite of the fact that he apparently spent a large part of his active life in attendance of the *Táng* emperors at the capital. Finally, in the *Tài Píng Guǎng Jì* and *Xù Xiān Zhuàn*, he is listed among the "immortals" (神仙 *shén xiān*), which indicates that Sūn Sī-Miǎo's deification was already well under way in the late tenth century. By the fourteenth century at the latest, he had become the object of a popular cult to the "god of medicine." In that context, he is to this day perceived as an eccentric recluse who, accompanied by a tiger and a dragon, lived out his life in solitude in a mountain cave, devoted to the pursuit of immortality, alchemical experimentation, and the collection of medicinal substances.

For additional information regarding Sūn Sī-Miǎo's cultural background, motivation, and attitude towards medicine, we have his own writings, in particular the preface to the *Qiān Jīn Fāng*. As the following discussion will show, they suggest his membership in a social class that newly emerged in the early *Táng* period. According to David McMullen, it was "an aristocratic scholar community from which official scholars were drawn . . . distinct by virtue of their education in the Confucian canons and in historical and philosophical texts."

If we limit our account to the official biographies discussed above, the absence of specific information regarding Sūn Sī-Miǎo's medical practice, such as references to his training, sustained clinical practice, or official medical titles is conspicuous. This might prevent us from identifying him clearly as a practicing physician in the sense of Robert Hymes' definition:

> I identify someone as a doctor primarily by evidence that he practiced medicine regularly as an occupation (for example, mention of payment or description in terms associated with artisanry such as chi [*jì*] 技, i [*yì*] 藝, or kung [*gōng*] 工), and evidence that his contemporaries identified him to a significant extent by his involvement in medicine. These criteria apply to some who were active as conventional scholars or officials. I count them as physicians if the sources give medicine a weight equal, or nearly equal, to their other activities.

Sūn Sī-Miǎo's own writings show, however, that he certainly did play a central role in what Joseph Needham regards as the key to the professionalization of doctors in early China, namely "the passage from the wu [巫 *wū*], a sort of technological servitor, to the shi [士 *shì*], a particular kind of scholar, clad in the full dignity of the Confucian intellectual, and not readily converted into anyone's instrument." Nathan Sivin suggests a second angle from which to consider the status of physicians in Chinese history:

> The basic Chinese distinction was between the relatively few literate, well-born physicians who left the enormous written record, and the plebeian practitioners of every stripe, generally illiterate for most of Chinese history, who cared for the overwhelming majority of the population.

In the early centuries of the Common Era, the scholar-gentleman's traditional aversion to professional specialization, expressed most famously in Confucius' warning that "the gentleman not become a vessel" (君子不器 *jūn zǐ bú qì*), conflicted more and more with the demands for technical knowledge in increasingly complex fields of practical occupation such as medicine. Sūn Sī-Miǎo's preface to the *Qiān Jīn Fāng* eloquently expresses the way in which he attempted to solve this tension. As "the first Chinese author to have devoted a separate section of a paradigmatic nature to questions of medical ethics," Sūn Sī-Miǎo proposed that it is not only possible but mandatory for the ideal physician to combine medical practice with the Confucian education and moral values that had become the defining features of a medieval scholarly elite. In the following centuries, medically-inclined members of the elite argued for the respectability of professional medical practice by interpreting medicine as an extension of the Confucian virtues of humaneness and righteousness. Sūn Sī-Miǎo's list of intellectual and ethical requirements for a true "great physician" (大醫 *dà yī*) was frequently cited in these discussions. Found at the very beginning of the *Qiān Jīn Fāng*, it is significant enough to quote it here at length:

The Professional Practice of the Great Physician

Whenever someone intends to become a Great Physician, he must acquaint himself with the *Sù Wèn* 素問, the *Jiǎ Yǐ* 甲乙 [i.e., *Zhēn Jiǔ Jiǎ Yǐ Jīng* 針灸甲乙經 by Huáng-Fǔ Mì 皇甫謐], and the *Huáng Dì Zhēn Jīng* 黃帝針經 [Acupuncture Classic of the Yellow Emperor, a reference to the *Líng Shū* 靈樞 (Divine Pivot)]; with flow and drainage in the Hall of Brightness [a standard reference to the location of the acupuncture and moxibustion points], the Twelve Vessels, the Three Sections and Nine Symptoms [a reference to the techniques of pulse taking], the Five Viscera and Six Bowels, the openings and holes on the exterior and interior of the body; with the properties and clinical applications of the materia medica; and with every part of the theoretical and prescription literature by Zhāng Zhòng-Jǐng, Wáng Shū-Hé 王叔和, Ruǎn Hé-Nán 阮河南, Fàn Dōng-Yáng 范東陽, Zhāng Miáo 張苗, Jìn Shào 靳邵, and others.

Moreover, he must completely comprehend the techniques of prognosticating people's fortune and fate with *yīn* and *yáng*, the various schools of physiognomy, plastromancy, Five Portents, *Yì Jīng* 易經 [Classic of Changes], and Six Stem divination. He must familiarize himself thoroughly with all of these equally. Only then can he become a great physician. Otherwise, he will be like a traveler at night without eyesight, blindly stumbling to his death.

Next, he must thoroughly study these prescriptions, searching out and pondering their underlying patterns. Only when he fixes his mind on them, pinching them tightly as if with tweezers and grinding them like ink stones, will he be able to begin to speak of himself as [a practitioner of] the Way of Medicine.

Moreover, he must have waded and hunted through the general literature. Why is that? If he has not read the Five [Confucian] Classics, he does not know of the Way of Humaneness and Righteousness. If he has not read the Three Histories, he does not know the affairs of the past and present. If he has not read the various masters of philosophy, he is unable when observing things to discern them in silence. If he has not read the Buddhist sutras, he does not know of the virtues of compassion, sympathy, joy, and abandonment. If he has not read the *Zhuāng Zǐ* 莊子 and *Lǎo Zǐ* 老子, he is unable to shoulder perfection in his physical activities [that is, nurture the true body of perfection and prevent the loss of life force through everyday activities, a reference to Daoist longevity practices]. Consequently, he will hold on to superstitious fears, whether in good or bad fortune, and he will cause offenses and pollution everywhere. With regard to the Five Phases, astrological positions, and the celestial patterns of the Seven Luminaries [either the sun and moon and five planets, or the seven stars of the Big Dipper], he must investigate these in depth as well. If he can be well-versed in these, there will be no obstacles and hindrances in his Way of Medicine, and it will be characterized by perfection of skill as well as perfection of beauty.

Continuing in a similar vein, the second chapter on the "Absolute Sincerity of the Great Physician" outlines the ethical requirements for a "Great Physician." This includes such aspects as a self-possessed and concentrated attitude when seeing patients, a dignified appearance, equal treatment of all patients without attention to their wealth, gender, status, nature of ailment, or potential rewards, utmost devotion to easing the suffering of one's fellow humans regardless of one's own physical discomforts, abstention from the enjoyment of luxurious fabrics, music, and liquor when practicing, and not criticizing one's fellow physicians.

These paragraphs raise questions that cannot be fully answered, given the current state of research on medieval Chinese medicine and the limitations of this work: What was the basis of Sūn Sī-Miǎo's own understanding of medicine; practical experience, textual knowledge, or a combination of the two? Who exactly was Sūn Sī-Miǎo addressing in this preface and ultimately, who was the intended readership for his entire medical writings? Learned scholar-gentlemen who dabbled in medical literature out of philosophical interests and a pious concern to provide for the health of their families and friends, as Robert Hymes proposes as the most likely answer for the following Sòng period? Or should we read this as a carefully worded attempt by a member of the educated elite to appeal to a core group of literati physicians in professional practice who were trying to set themselves apart from ordinary practitioners engaging in medicine as a craft, as suggested by Paul Unschuld?

An increasing number of studies have broadened our knowledge regarding the social history of Chinese medicine from the Sòng dynasty on. However, in the case of medieval China the social status and background of practicing physicians on the one hand and the involvement of the literate elite in the actual practice of medicine on the other hand are still largely unknown. Sūn Sī-Miǎo clearly played a key role in the obscure transformation from the early Chinese "masters of pre-scriptions" (方士 fāng shì) to the virtuous "literati physicians" (儒醫 rú yī) whose rise Hymes situates between the Sòng and Yuán periods and Chén Yuán-Péng between the Northern and Southern Sòng.

The lack of any references in the official biographies as well as his own writings to an apprentice-ship or teacher to support Sūn Sī-Miǎo's claims to medical authority is certainly notable. On the other hand, Sūn Sī-Miǎo provides ample evidence for the importance of a textual transmission of knowledge in the passage translated above: His list of required knowledge begins with the most outstanding examples of the then current medical literature, ranging from medical theory and acupuncture and moxibustion manuals to prescription collections very much like his own. Next, he recommends, in an order that must have been significant, the mastery of the varieties of divina-tory practices, then a thorough study of his own prescriptions, and finally the traditional classical subjects of literature, history, philosophy, and cosmology. Moreover, the following description of medical etiquette obviously describes a man involved in the professional practice of medicine.

Regarding the status of physicians several centuries after Sūn Sī-Miǎo's lifetime, between the Sòng and Yuán periods, Robert Hymes has argued that "medicine as a field of knowledge, as intel-lectual endeavor [italics inserted], was widely valued and respected among the Sòng elite," but was not accepted as a proper occupational choice for an elite gentleman until the social changes of the Yuán dynasty. During that time, the scarcity of teaching and government positions, which had been the traditional occupations of the elite, forced some literati to look for an alternative profes-sion. Hymes' assertion that medical scholarship may not necessarily be equated with medical practice must certainly be borne in mind in a careful analysis of Sūn Sī-Miǎo's involvement in medicine. Nevertheless, his findings apply to elite attitudes from the Sòng dynasty on and there-fore cannot be accepted uncritically for Sūn Sī-Miǎo's lifetime. Thus, we cannot assume that the reservations of Sòng literati regarding medicine as a professional choice were necessarily shared by their Táng predecessors. Our current state of knowledge on medieval Chinese medicine does not allow for any concrete answers to the above questions about the extent of Sūn Sī-Miǎo's own or his readership's medical practice.

What emerges from an analysis of Sūn Sī-Miǎo's own writing — supported by the content of his *Táng Shū* biographies — is the image of a thoroughly respectable elite gentleman faithful to traditional morality who is arguing, on the basis and within the framework of these traditional values, for a "broaden[ing of] the criteria for what is and what is not suitable for a man of the ruling class." It is impossible at this point to reconstruct the extent to which Sūn Sī-Miǎo himself actually practiced the form of medicine he advocated in his writings as a professional. What is significant, however, is that Sūn Sī-Miǎo's vision laid the foundations from which scholars in the following centuries were able to construct the ideal "scholar-physician," able to engage in professional medical practice without a loss of prestige. It might be that it was precisely Sūn Sī-Miǎo's eminent social standing and reputation that allowed him to question the traditional Confucian disdain for technical knowledge in a medieval world that necessitated or at least encouraged increasing specialization and an expansion of intellectual horizons for China's governing elite. Most certainly, Sūn Sī-Miǎo's preface was influenced by the early *Táng* fascination with literary composition as a learned activity that "set value on an effortless command of the inherited tradition and on dexterity in composition."

2b. The Qiān Jīn Fāng in the Context of Prescription Literature

The preceding discussion has shown that both the external facts of Sūn Sī-Miǎo's life and his own writings place him firmly in the ranks of an early medieval scholarly elite with traditional Confucian values and aspirations. This is further supported by the facts that his calligraphy was among the finest pre-*Sòng* examples from the imperial collection to be carved into stone during the *Sòng* dynasty and that his poetry was included in the prestigious collection *Quán Táng Shī* 全唐詩 [Complete Táng Poetry]. While the *Qiān Jīn Fāng*, as one of his most important works, must be seen as a product of this environment, it is now necessary to also interpret it as a medical text in an established tradition of technical prescription literature. As will become obvious below in the context of the "prescriptions for women," even a cursory glance at the actual text proves that it was not an isolated product of Sūn Sī-Miǎo's personal creativity and medical expertise, but rather an encyclopedic collection of prescriptions that were also found in many other medical texts. Ute Engelhardt's study of the chapter on dietetics (食治 *shí zhì*) comes to a similar conclusion, pointing out the close textual parallels to materia medica literature as well as to interdictions concerning foodstuffs found in texts like the *Jīn Guì Yào Luè* 金匱要略 (Essential Prescriptions of the Golden Coffer) and *Ishimpō*. In the spirit of early *Táng* scholarship, it was intended to serve as a comprehensive reference work based on Sūn Sī-Miǎo's extensive bibliographic research. Thus, Sūn Sī-Miǎo probably saw himself as merely transmitting a large, but incoherent and disorganized body of often well-known prescriptions, which he compiled, reorganized, and explained in short essays based on the cosmological, etiological, and therapeutic ideas espoused in the contemporaneous theoretical medical literature.

Due to the vicissitudes of time, we have only fragmentary knowledge about this corpus of prescription literature regarding women's health before the *Sòng* period. It is therefore impossible to assess Sūn Sī-Miǎo's exact role in the process of creating a systematic and theoretically grounded gynecological literature, let alone practice. Nevertheless, it is clear that Sūn Sī-Miǎo was firmly rooted in and representative of a textual tradition of prescriptions related to women's health. The archaeological discovery and recent scholarship on the Mǎ-Wáng-Duī 馬王堆 medical manuscripts enables us to trace this tradition all the way back to the early *Hàn* dynasty. Donald Harper's thorough treatment of the medical manuscripts from Mǎ-Wáng-Duī has significantly sharpened our understanding of the significance and use of prescription literature, of the relationships between different realms of technical expertise such as astrology, medicine, and *yīn-yáng* cosmology, and of the people who propagated this knowledge, the so-called "masters of prescriptions" (*fāng shì*). As Harper points out, the possessors of a "Way of Medicine" (醫道 *yī dào*) were linked to other specialists of natural philosophy and occult learning such as divination, astrology, demonology, or *yīn-yáng* cosmology on the basis of their access to and familiarity with a written knowledge regarding the natural and supernatural world.

This continüm of knowledge is still reflected in Sūn Sī-Miǎo's collection of what he considered representative of medicine. Thus, his medical writings combine the theoretical concepts of correlative medicine with Daoist alchemical preparations and life-prolonging exercises (to which he devotes an entire volume in the *Qiān Jīn Fāng*, entitled 養生 *yǎng shēng*, "nurturing life"), complex medicinal prescriptions and materia medica knowledge, and astrological taboos and demonological spells. The oft cited biography of the famous early *Hàn* physician Chún-Yú Yì 淳于意 shows the essential role texts played in the transmission of knowledge and the status of a physician as part of an esoteric teacher-disciple lineage. According to Nathan Sivin, medicine was transformed from:

> … a hereditary family's transmission of a patrimony…into a new medicine, a free-for-all between every conceivable variety of practitioner, but with medical prestige newly concentrated at the top of the social scale, and the ranks of the doctors at the apex increasingly closed against incursions by the lower orders.

The corpus of technical literature found at Mǎ-Wáng-Duī, for which a terminus ante quem of 168 BCE has been determined, was presumably authored by medical specialists coming from this milieu. It includes the earliest example of prescriptions for women in a silk manuscript on the subject of childbirth, entitled *Tāi Chǎn Shū* 胎產書 (Book of the Generation of the Fetus). This short text consists of two charts for predicting the child's future and burying the placenta, as well as prescriptions for placenta burial, conception, manipulating the child's gender, easing birth, and promoting the child's health. Most notable, though, is a month-by-month description of gestation, which also includes instructions for the mother's diet and activities. This information is found in a much expanded but at times almost literal version in the *Qiān Jīn Fāng*, entitled 徐之才逐月養胎方 *Xú Zhī-Cái Zhú Yuè Yǎng Tāi Fāng* (Xú Zhī-Cái's month-by-month prescriptions for nurturing the fetus). It is quoted in the *Bìng Yuán Lùn* and *Ishimpō* as well and will be discussed in more detail below.

Apart from these instructions regarding pregnancy and childbirth, prescriptions specifically addressing women's health are not found elsewhere in the Mǎ-Wáng-Duī medical manuscripts, with the exception of a small section on prescriptions for women's hemorrhoids in the *Wǔ Shí Èr Bìng Fāng* 五十二病方 (Prescriptions for Fifty-Two Diseases). This is not surprising given the fact that the texts were selected as an elite gentleman's highly valued accoutrement for his journey to the netherworld. It is significant, however, that an entire text, devoted primarily to the ritual aspects of childbirth but also containing instructions for the mother's pregnancy, was included. Compared to later periods, this might indicate that at this early point in time, men tended to be less directly involved in women's healthcare, with the exception of the above-mentioned areas. This is also supported by Jender Lee's research on a female sphere of healing between the *Hàn* and *Táng* periods.

For the following centuries until the composition of the *Qiān Jīn Fāng*, our knowledge of a literature devoted to women's health is severely limited by a lack of primary sources. Most texts from this period are known to us only from references in the bibliographic catalogues or isolated quotations in preserved texts. The most important source of fragments is the Japanese compendium

Ishimpō, a compilation of medieval Chinese medical texts completed in 982 by Tanba no Yasuyori. In the context of prescriptions for women, found in volumes 21-24, this text is of the greatest significance: Besides quotations from the *Qiān Jīn Fāng* and *Bìng Yuán Lùn*, the section related to women's health consists most notably of quotations from two texts that have not been preserved elsewhere, the *Chǎn Jīng* 產經 (Classic of Childbirth) and the *Xiǎo Pǐn Fāng*.

The *Chǎn Jīng* is recorded in the bibliographic catalogue of the *Suí* dynasty, the *Suí Zhì* 隋志 (Annals of the Suí Period), as a work of one volume by Dé Zhēn-Cháng 德貞常. According to Mǎ Dà-Zhèng 馬大正, it provides proof for the high standards and sophisticated knowledge in the medical management of childbirth during the *Suí* dynasty. The various citations of this text in the *Ishimpō* present a wide range of childbirth-related prescriptions similar to those found in the *Qiān Jīn Fāng*. In addition, they include a lengthy quotation at the beginning of the twenty-second volume (on pregnancy-related conditions) that offers detailed instructions for the correct behavior of a woman in pregnancy, exact descriptions and illustrations of the channels prohibited for acupuncture in each month, and, most importantly, a month-by-month description of gestation. This particular citation is striking for its similarity to the description of gestation found both in the Mǎ-Wáng-Duī manuscript as well as in the later *Qiān Jīn Fāng*.

The following volume, concerning the actual management of childbirth and related ritual actions, again contains extensive quotations from the *Chǎn Jīng*, this time of a predominantly ritualistic nature. They describe the correct way for a woman in labor to face and position herself, depending on the astrological constellation at the time of delivery, to avoid offending baleful stars or spirits and to align herself with the auspicious flow of heavenly *qì*. They also offer information about particularly inauspicious times for delivery, depending on the branch designation of the year, the mother's age, the mother's birth year, or the daily branch designation. When delivering in any of these inauspicious times, the text warns, special precautions have to be taken to avoid disaster, in particular to prevent the mother's blood or any other childbirth-related substances from touching the ground.

Lastly, the *Chǎn Jīng* citations prescribe the proper position of the birth hut in relation to the month of childbirth, and contain an invocation to congregate a variety of guardian spirits and to propitiate dangerous goblins, talismans to swallow in case of stalled labor or retained placenta, and instructions for washing, preparing, and burying the placenta to ensure the health and good fortune of the newborn child.

As this brief summary shows, the *Chǎn Jīng* citations have proven to be invaluable evidence for any attempt at reconstructing the actual management of childbirth during the medieval period in China. This material can, moreover, be substantiated by later evidence from the Southern *Sòng* text *Wèi Shēng Jiā Bǎo Chǎn Yù Bèi Yào* 衛生家寶產育備要 (Essentials of Child Rearing for Protecting the Life of Treasures at Home) by Zhū Duān-Zhāng 朱端章.

In spite of the lack of primary sources, the continuity of content between the *Tāi Chǎn Shū* and the *Chǎn Jīng* suggests a continuous literary tradition related to the ritual management of childbirth. With regard to the *Qiān Jīn Fāng*, Sūn Sī-Miǎo most likely assumed that his readers would have separate instructions of this nature at hand and therefore limited his information predominantly to medical treatments. While his prescriptions do include references to other modalities of healing such as physical manipulation or exorcistic rituals, his main focus and area of expertise were clearly the medicinal prescriptions. It is therefore likely that Sūn chose to exclude the details of the ritual aspects of childbirth from his prescription collection because he considered them to belong to the terrain of another type of healer, the 巫 *wū* (shaman) who might have been called upon by a

family in addition to, or as an alternative to, the physician or midwife. The significance of sha-
mans in medieval Chinese medicine in general, and the religious activities of female providers of
women's healthcare specifically, have been discussed in some detail by Chinese scholars. The importance of ritual healing, especially in such life-threatening situations as childbirth, must not be
underestimated. In addition, Sūn Sī-Miǎo's relative brevity with regard to the physical manipulations of hands-on intervention during delivery also suggests that childbirth, in both its physical and
religious aspects, was performed in a female sphere of healing from which male literati physicians
were largely excluded.

Another lost text extensively quoted in the *Ishimpō*, the *Xiǎo Pǐn Fāng* has elicited considerable
debate among scholars with regard to its date of composition. Most of them do agree, however,
that it predates the *Suí* dynasty by at least a century. It is recorded in the *Suí Zhì* as twelve volumes authored by the physician Chén Yán-Zhī 陳延之. Reconstructed by the modern scholar Zhù
Xīn-Nián 祝新年 from quotations in the received literature and the *Ishimpō*, it appears to have
been a brief reference guide, consisting mainly of medicinal prescriptions and short introductory
essays. Chén's own statements mark him as a well-known physician who might or might not have
held an official office but was a frequent visitor at court and gentry households. He composed the
Xiǎo Pǐn Fāng with the following intention:

> Those who do not wish to make the art of prescriptions their occupation but only want
> to prevent illness and save emergency [situations] should first study these Prescriptions
> of Minor Degree and in occasions of extreme urgencies and disaster, they can then apply
> them… Those who begin the study of treating illness in their youth should also first prac-
> tice this text and use it as their entry [into medicine].

The sections related to women's health are frequently quoted in and very similar in style to the
Qiān Jīn Fāng, but quite brief and not very comprehensive.

Another source for medieval prescriptions that realistically reflects the medical practices of the
time and is quite similar to the *Ishimpō* in the combination of medical and religious material are
the medical manuscripts discovered at Dūn-Huáng. It is impossible to date each manuscript individually and establish a precise chronology. Nevertheless, these short texts have proven invaluable
for providing unmediated access to medicine as it was practiced during the *Táng* dynasty since
they never suffered the revisions by the *Sòng* editors that have shaped our reading of the transmitted medical literature. Besides fragments of such transmitted classics as the *Sù Wén*, the *Mài Jīng*,
the *Shāng Hán Lùn*, and the *Běn Cǎo Jīng Jí Zhù* 本草經集注 (Collected Commentaries on the
Classic of Materia Medica), this material also contains several short manuscripts with gynecological prescriptions:

The *Fù Kē Dān Yào Fāng Shū* 婦科單藥方書 (Book of Gynecological Prescriptions of Simple
Medicinals) from the *Táng* period contains prescriptions for being "stung by evil" (人被惡刺 *rén
bèi è cì*), infertility, incessant menstruation, stalled labor, postpartum pain, death of the fetus in the
abdomen, heart pain, and red and white diarrhea. As the title implies, the prescriptions all use a
single medicinal ingredient.
Another text, the *Qiú Zǐ Fāng Shū* 求子方書 (Book of Prescriptions for Seeking a Child), offers
interesting insights into what the medical category of fertility treatments covered in household
use: Treatments for the husband's wind vacuity and physical exhaustion are found next to treatments for the [wife's] genital cold, widened vagina, and [vaginal] bleeding during intercourse, as
well as prescriptions for enlarging the male [genitals], for "making women happy and men strong"
(a medicinal powder to be applied to the tip of the penis, which is then inserted into the vagina),

for lack of offspring, for strengthening *yáng* and supporting *yīn*, for giving birth to a male [child], and lastly pregnancy taboos. Most of the prescriptions share the fact that they are applied to the genitals or contain instructions for successful intercourse. They are therefore more reminiscent of sexual cultivation literature than the chapter on "seeking children" in the *Qiān Jīn Fāng*, which interprets lack of offspring as a medical condition caused by the "Five Taxations and Seven Damages and the hundred illnesses of vacuity and emaciation," and is limited to medicinal decoctions and a vaginal suppository.

A third Dūn-Huáng text, entitled *Tóu Mù Chǎn Bìng Fāng Shū* 頭目產病方書 (Book of Prescriptions for Head, Eye, and Childbirth Diseases) contains a number of fairly simple prescriptions for a variety of obstetrical emergencies and postpartum conditions. These are in no apparent order, but interestingly include a Sanskrit spell for the treatment of difficult childbirth, to be copied [by the woman in labor?] onto birch bark in one breath while burning incense in front of an image of the Buddha and holding pure water in one's mouth.

The *Qiān Jīn Fāng* certainly includes individual sections with a constellation of prescriptions similar to the Dūn-Huáng material, that is, containing only a few, commonly-available household ingredients, listed in no specific order, and without specific etiologies or clearly differentiated symptoms. Nevertheless, this only serves to illustrate the progress that has been made in other sections towards a true medical specialization in "prescriptions for women," containing elaborate prescriptions with literally dozens of medicinal ingredients, highly specific lists of symptoms, and a theoretically-based classification scheme. Unfortunately, research on medieval Chinese medicine is insufficient at this point to determine to what extent these differences reflect an individual author's creative innovations and medical sophistication, access to economic resources, developments over centuries that merely surface at an arbitrary point in time from a fortuitous archaeological discovery, or even regional specializations. And, of course, the situation is further obscured by the fact that certain aspects of women's healthcare remained in the hands of female practitioners who might have transmitted their knowledge only orally or to personal apprentices.

A last example of prescription literature predating the *Qiān Jīn Fāng* is found in Zhāng Zhòng-Jǐng's *Jīn Guì Yào Luè*. This text from the Eastern *Hàn* period contains three short chapters on "Pulses, Symptoms, and Treatments of Women's Diseases in Pregnancy" (婦人妊娠病脈証治 *fù rén rèn shēn bìng mài zhèng zhì*), "Pulses, Symptoms, and Treatments of Women's Postpartum Diseases" (婦人產後病脈証治 *fù rén chǎn hòu bìng mài zhèng zhì*), and on "Pulses, Symptoms, and Treatments of Women's Miscellaneous Diseases" (婦人雜病脈証治 *fù rén zá bìng mài zhèng zhì*). Mǎ Dà-Zhèng's evaluation of this text as the earliest gynecological text in China is debatable since it contains no more than a selection of superficial pulse descriptions, simple prescriptions, and a few acupuncture methods. Very frequently, Zhāng Zhòng-Jǐng fails to offer a specific prescription for a condition. Instead, he merely refers the reader to the relevant prescription found in the general, that is, nongendered, sections of the text that do not address specifically female conditions. In volume 21, for example, he states: "[In cases of] hard stool, vomiting, and inability to eat, Minor Bupleurum Decoction is indicated. For the prescription, see the section on vomiting." This practice illustrates the author's attitude that, with minor exceptions, women's conditions could be treated with the same prescriptions that applied to men. This notion was soon proven to be outdated by the creation of 婦科 *fù kē* as a "specialization for women" a few centuries later. Sūn Sī-Miǎo confronts exactly this attitude in the very first sentence of the section on gynecology:

> The reason why women have special prescriptions is that they are different because of pregnancy, childbirth, and flooding damage. Therefore, women's diseases are ten times more difficult to treat than men's.

Moreover, although the structure and likely intention of this text superficially resembles the *Qiān Jīn Fāng*, the two texts are worlds apart in terms of the complexity and sophistication of their contents. It is tempting to interpret this as a reflection of the primitive state of medical knowledge regarding women's health during the Eastern *Hàn* dynasty, but it is entirely possible that it also reflected each author's personal interest. Thus, Zhāng Zhòng-Jǐng is much more well-known as the author of the *Shāng Hán Lùn*, one of the fundamental classics of Chinese medicine, whose account of cold damage diseases far surpasses Sūn Sī-Miǎo's own account of cold damage diseases in the *Qiān Jīn Fāng* (volumes 9 and 10).

To complete this discussion of prescription literature related to women's health, mention should be made of Wáng Xī's 王燾 *Wài Tái Mì Yào* 外台秘要 (Essential Secrets from a Border Official/ the Palace Library). This prescription collection is very similar in content and structure to the *Qiān Jīn Fāng* and was composed roughly a hundred years later in 752 CE. The prescriptions related to women's health are found in volumes 33 and 34, a large proportion of which consist of literal quotations from the *Qiān Jīn Fāng*. The only major difference between the two collections occurs in the section on childbirth where the *Wài Tái Mì Yào* quotes many of the same ritual taboos, prognostications, and instructions that we find recorded in the *Ishimpō*. In addition, it includes the twelve childbirth charts that are also reproduced in the *Sòng* period text *Wèi Shēng Jiā Bǎo Chǎn Yù Bèi Yào*, and several talismans to swallow for the treatment of retained placenta and stalled labor. An extensive section on "seeking a child," including such detailed information as inauspicious times for sexual intercourse, turns out to be a quotation from the *Qiān Jīn Fāng*, found there in volume 27 on "nurturing one's nature" in section 8 on "supplementing and boosting through sexual intercourse." A detailed comparative analysis of the gynecological prescriptions in these two texts lies outside the scope of the current book. However, the *Wài Tái Mì Yào* does not appear to express any new developments in terms of therapeutic or etiological refinement, but merely a reworking of earlier material, based primarily on the *Qiān Jīn Fāng*. This suggests that the volumes on "prescriptions for women" in the *Qiān Jīn Fāng* did indeed constitute the most advanced gynecological text in medieval China, even a hundred years later.

Forming an integral part of the textual tradition outlined above, Sūn Sī-Miǎo's three volumes on women's health represent yet another compilation of prescriptions that were circulating in the hands of medically inclined literati. Unfortunately, Sūn Sī-Miǎo fails to provide us with information regarding his sources, with few exceptions like the quotation from "Xū Zhī-Cái's month-by-month prescriptions for nurturing the fetus." This contrasts with texts such as the *Ishimpō* where the origin of almost every single phrase is explicitly stated. Most modern editions of the *Qiān Jīn Fāng*, however, include the *Sòng* commentary that was produced by an editorial team under the direction of Lín Yì 林億. In this, we find frequent comparisons to similar or identical prescriptions from the work of other authors, such as Master Cuī 崔氏 (author of the *Yīng Yàn Fāng* 應驗方 [Prescriptions of Proven Efficacy] and the *Xiǎo Ér Lùn* 小兒論 [Discussion of Infants], both of which are lost), Hú Qià 胡洽 (author of the *Bǎi Bìng Fāng* 百病方 [Prescriptions for a Hundred Diseases], a lost text of three volumes), and Ruǎn from Hé-Nán 阮河南 (a reference to *Ruǎn Wén-Shū* 阮文叔, the author of the *Hé Nán Yào Fāng* 河南藥方 [Medicinal Prescriptions from Hé-Nán], a lost text of 16 volumes). The *Sòng* commentary also references such texts as the above-mentioned *Xiǎo Pǐn Fāng* and *Wài Tái Mì Yào*, as well as the *Zhǒu Hòu Fāng* 肘后方 (Prescriptions [to carry] Behind the Elbow, a lost text by Gé Hóng 葛洪) and the *Bì Xiào Fāng* 必效方 (Prescriptions of Absolute Efficacy, recorded in the *Jiù Táng Zhì* 舊唐志 [Annals of the Old Táng Period] as a text in ten volumes by Mèng Shēn 孟詵, and in the *Sòng Zhì* [Annals of the Sòng Period] as a text in three volumes by Shì Wén-Yòu 釋文宥). In many other instances, the *Sòng* commentary merely states that "another [version of this] prescription adds..." or that "another copy [of this prescription] replaces ... with...." These comments usually note either a divergence in the choice of ingredients, such as between similar drugs or between dried and fresh preparations, or in the amount of an ingredient. The *Sòng* commentary is noteworthy because it shows Sūn Sī-Miǎo to be representative of a shared tradition of medieval prescription literature with a surprising amount of overlap rather than an idiosyncratic practitioner who recorded his personal experience. In this light, we have to interpret occasional comments in Sūn Sī-Miǎo's text as to a prescription's "divine efficacy" (神效 *shén xiào*) or "divine results" (神驗 *shén yàn*) not as referring to Sūn Sī-Miǎo's own practice, but to the popularity and reputation of a prescription within this literary tradition. At one point, Sūn Sī-Miǎo even admits recording prescriptions for purely historical reasons:

> The ancients used mostly *Blessing Clouds Powder* and *Luster-Granting Pills* for seeking children, but modern people don't use them anymore. Although I have not tried them, their methods are worthy of our attention. Thus I have recorded them.

In contrast to the prescriptions, which Sūn Sī-Miǎo might have merely compiled and reorganized, it is feasible, if not likely, that substantial parts of the essays were composed by Sūn Sī-Miǎo himself. Often located at the beginning of a section, they introduce and summarize the following prescriptions, discuss general etiologies and treatment principles, or warn against heterodox and dangerous practices. As such, these essays might well be Sūn Sī-Miǎo's greatest contribution to the formation of a Chinese gynecology. They clearly serve as the foundation for all future gynecological writings by providing the prescription tradition with a theoretical structure and basis that it had lacked before. It therefore seems likely that Sūn Sī-Miǎo played a role in the formation of gynecological literature that is similar to what Ute Engelhardt suggests in the context of materia dietetica literature:

> In combining the basic pattern of the bencao [*běn cǎo* 本草] monographs with interdictions concerning foodstuffs, Sun Simiao appears to have written the first extant materia dietetica and with this, he has contributed to the establishment of an ensuing genre of materia dietetica.

What were the theoretical sources for Sūn Sī-Miǎo's knowledge of the medical treatment of women? To be sure, such classics as the *Huáng Dì Nèi Jīng* or the *Nàn Jīng* do contain occasional references to gender differences, but these are barely enough to fill a most extensively annotated and interpreted booklet on "Gynecology in the *Nèi Jīng*."

The only theoretical text before the *Qiān Jīn Fāng* that systematically refers to women's differences is Cháo Yuán-Fāng's *Zhū Bìng Yuán Hòu Lùn* from the early seventh century. Preceding the composition of the *Qiān Jīn Fāng* by only a few decades, it is China's first systematic collection of diseases and their origins, and contains a substantial section on women's conditions in volumes thirty-seven to fourty-four. A brief summary will give the reader an impression of the comprehensiveness of this text:

Volumes thirty-seven to thirty-nine cover "women's miscellaneous diseases" (婦人雜病 *fù rén zá bìng*), which discusses conditions related to wind strike and vacuity, convulsions, heart and abdominal pain, menstrual problems, vaginal discharge and spotting, abdominal accumulations, infertility and miscarriage, topical aches especially in throat, mouth, eyes and ears, cholera, swellings, seasonal diseases, sexual intercourse with ghosts, dreaming of intercourse with ghosts, the effects of traveling without male supervision, urinary problems, diseases of the reproductive organs and channels, and mammary and breast-feeding problems. Volumes fourty-one and fourty-two cover "women's diseases in pregnancy" (婦人妊娠病 *fù rén rèn shēn bìng*): After a long introductory essay on pregnancy, they discuss such topics as morning sickness, converting a female fetus into a male, pregnancy taboos, miscarriage, stirring fetus, abdominal, lumbar, and heart pain, malaria, diarrhea, vaginal discharge, *gǔ* 蠱 poisoning and flying corpse entering the abdomen, wind strike, spasms, fetal fright, ghost fetus, and intentional abortion. Volume forty-three on "women's diseases of childbirth" (婦人將產病 *fù rén jiāng chǎn bìng*) covers delivery techniques and medicinal prescriptions for such obstetrical conditions as retained placenta, stalled labor, breech presentation, the effects of different birthing positions (lying or squatting), death of child or mother during birth, and the first part of "women's postpartum diseases" (婦人產後病 *fù rén chǎn hòu bìng*). This discusses blood dizziness, heart pain due to postpartum blood ascending and knocking against the heart, retained lochia, premature birth, abdominal, lumbar, or heart pain, vacuity vexation and shortness of breath, general weakness, excessive sweating, wind strike, and wind vacuity convulsions and mania. Lastly, volume forty-four contains the second half of "women's postpartum diseases" (婦人產後病 *fù rén chǎn hòu bìng*), discussing menstrual problems, vaginal discharge, disinhibition (of blood, cold, or heat), vacuity cold and other forms of diarrhea, uterine prolapse, genital problems, digestive and urinary problems, fevers and chills, accumulations, dizziness, deafness, mouth and body sores, and lactation problems.

Even if not quoted literally by Sūn Sī-Miǎo, the information on women's diseases in the *Bìng Yuán Lùn* was of central importance for Sūn Sī-Miǎo's efforts to create a systematic and theoretically based organizational scheme for categorizing his gynecological prescription material. The *Bìng Yuán Lùn* appears to have been the only text that was able to provide Sūn Sī-Miǎo with a theoretical basis from which to approach the prescription literature and create a definition of female difference that was based on more than their reproductive functions.

2c. Editorial History of the Qiān Jīn Fāng

Before we can delve into the actual content of the *Qiān Jīn Fāng*, it is lastly necessary to review its editorial history to determine how accurately the available versions reflect Sūn Sī-Miǎo's original writing. The Japanese scholar Miyashita Saburō 宮下三郎 has traced the development and mutual influence of fifteen editions, including, however, only the major publications and, moreover, ending in the year 1915. For the contemporary period, even a cursory bibliographical search reveals almost yearly republications in China, Taiwan, and Japan, albeit of varying historical reliability and editorial quality. According to a critical edition from 1996, these amount to more than thirty major editions, which are all based on one or several of the following three source editions: First, a woodblock print edition sponsored by the *Sòng* government, second, the edition found in the Daoist Canon (道藏 *Dào Zàng*), and, lastly, various manuscripts and quotations from sources predating the *Sòng* revisions.

The most commonly used source text for contemporary editions of the *Qiān Jīn Fāng* is a *Sòng* copy that the medical historian Mǎ Jì-Xìng has determined to belong to the government-sponsored woodblock print edition from the Northern *Sòng Yě-Píng* 冶平 reign period (1064-68). It was published in thirty volumes, as part of a ten-year campaign by the Northern *Sòng* government to standardize, correct, and print medical classics in the context of "institutional and doctrinal reform of medicine [that] was part of an imperial agenda to spread good government with the intent of providing for the people's welfare and reforming unorthodox customs." For this purpose, an Office for the Correction of Medical Texts (校正醫書局 *jiào zhèng yī shū jú*) was established in 1057, which employed an editorial team under the direction of Lín Yì. Coming from this edition, the earliest still existing copy of the *Qiān Jīn Fāng* probably entered Japan during the Southern *Sòng* or *Yuán* period and was subsequently lost until its discovery in the early nineteenth century. It was then republished by the Edo Medical Bureau in 1849 in a photolithographed edition; the missing parts in the fourth volume were substituted from the *Yuán* edition. This text has been the source for such standard editions as the 1955 and 1982 editions by the People's Medical Publishing House 人民衛生出版社 in Beijing, the 1965 and 1974 editions by the National Medical Research Institute 國立醫藥研究所 in Taipei, the 1974 edition by the Japanese Daily News Agency 每日新聞開發公司, and the 1989 edition by the Oriekoto Publishing Company in Osaka. A reprint of the *Sòng* woodblock edition was also published during the *Yuán* dynasty, copies of which have been found in both China and Japan.

The second most commonly-available version of the *Qiān Jīn Fāng* is entitled 孫真人備急千金要方 *Sūn Zhēn Rén Bèi Jí Qiān Jīn Yào Fāng* (Essential Prescriptions worth a Thousand in Gold for Every Emergency by the Perfected Sūn). It is based on a text that was entered into the Daoist canon and apparently predates Lín Yì's revisions. However, the *Míng* period editor Qiáo Shì-Dìng 喬世定 cautions that "it was edited as a Daoist classic and therefore contains numerous inaccuracies and omissions." This is most noticeable with regard to the proportions of medicinal ingredients. In the Zhèng-Tǒng 正統 edition of the Daoist canon from 1445, it was placed into the *Tài Píng* 太平 section and the thirty volumes were divided into ninety-three. This version was the basis for several republications during the *Míng* period, such as the 1543 edition by Qiáo Shì-Dìng and the 1588 edition by a Mr. Zhu 祝, as well as many later republications, including the version found in the *Sì Kù Quán Shū* 四庫全書 collection. It is referred to in Chinese editions and in the translation below as the *Dào Zàng* 道藏 edition.

Adding substantially to these two sets of complete versions of the text, recent textual scholarship has made great progress towards approximating the original *Táng* version prior to Lín Yì's revisions. In several newer editions, Chinese scholars have managed to collate the *Sòng* photolithographic edition with fragmentary evidence from a variety of sources to more accurately reflect Sūn Sī-Miǎo's original text. They mainly utilize two types of textual sources predating the *Sòng* revisions: First, several manuscripts have surfaced that scholars have been able to access. They include a copy of Sūn Sī-Miǎo's preface and the first volume that were found in Japan and are apparently based on a version dating from the late *Táng* to early *Sòng* period. Entitled 真本千金方 *Zhēn Běn Qiān Jīn Fāng* (True Version of the Prescriptions worth a Thousand in Gold), this text is quite different from the *Sòng* version, but much closer to quotations found in the *Ishimpō*. It has therefore been determined to preserve a relatively early version of the *Qiān Jīn Fāng*. This text has recently been reprinted as an appendix to the 1995 edition of the *Sūn Zhēn Rén Qiān Jīn Fāng* 孫真人千金方 by People's Medical Publishing House.

More directly concerning the volumes that are the topic of this book, another manuscript dating from the *Sòng* period was discovered by a Chinese book collector in 1799. Entitled 新雕孫真人千金方 *Xīn Diāo Sūn Zhēn Rén Qiān Jīn Fāng* (Newly Carved Prescriptions worth a Thousand in Gold by the Perfected Sūn), it consists of twenty carefully-preserved volumes, including the gynecological sections in the second through fourth volumes. This version is referred to in Chinese editions and in the translation below as the *Sūn Zhēn Rén* 孫真人 edition. It was reprinted in 1995 as *Sūn Zhēn Rén Qiān Jīn Fāng* 孫真人千金方 by People's Medical Publishing House and is therefore widely available now. Given the considerable discrepancies with the *Sòng* version edited by Lín Yì, it is likely that this text constitutes an older *Sòng* version that predates — or is based on another text that predates — Lín Yì's revisions. It therefore provides an important corrective source that allows us to approximate the *Táng* original from another angle.

In addition, valuable evidence has been collected from quotations of the *Qiān Jīn Fāng* that are found in other medical texts predating the *Sòng* revisions, most importantly the *Wài Tái Mì Yào* from 752, which contains a total of 446 quotations, and the *Ishimpō* from 984, which contains a total of 480 quotations.

All of these sources have been taken into account in excellent contemporary critical editions, two of which are referenced extensively throughout the translation below: First, the 1996 edition by People's Medical Publishing House, produced under the direction of Mǎ Jì-Xìng and edited by Lǐ Jǐng-Róng 李景榮 et al., is referred to below as the *Rén Mín* 人民 edition. Secondly, the 1993 edition by Huá Xià Publishing Company 華夏出版社, edited by Liú Gēng-Shēng 劉更生 and Zhāng Duān-Xián 張端賢 et al., is referred to below as the *Huá Xià* 華夏 edition.

For the translation below of the three volumes on "prescriptions for women," I follow the methodologies employed by the editors of these last two editions. I have taken the *Huá Xià* edition as my main source text, comparing it carefully with the *Rén Mín* edition, with which it is for the most part identical. Wherever necessary, I have noted significant differences in the footnotes. As the editorial history of the *Huá Xià* edition states, this text has taken the *Sòng* photolithographic version as its primary source and collated it with those of the above-mentioned manuscripts that have been shown to predate Lín Yì's revisions, as well as quotations found in the *Wài Tái Mì Yào* and *Ishimpō*. In addition, it has used a Japanese text entitled *Chóng Kān Sūn Zhēn Rén Bèi Jí Qiān Jīn Yào Fāng* 重刊孫真人備急千金要方 (Republished Essential Prescriptions for Every Emergency worth a Thousand in Gold by the Perfected Sūn), published by the Kyoto physician Gotō Satoshi 後藤敏 in 1785. This version is based on a Japanese reprint of the Lín Yì edition, but has been consulted by the *Huá Xià* editors due to the high quality of its print, lack of mistakes, and meticulous annotation. In addition, I have noted any discrepancies to the *Sūn Zhēn Rén* edition in the footnotes. While the differences in the order and categorization of prescriptions are quite noticeable at times, this does not significantly alter the content, flow, or general character of the text. Moreover, the wording of the individual prescriptions is for the most part almost identical.

In conclusion, the original text of the *Qiān Jīn Fāng* remains impossible to reconstruct with absolute certainty. In many cases, however, recent research has managed to identify alterations of Sūn Sī-Miǎo's writings by the hand of Lín Yì's editorial team, as well as the omissions and inaccuracies found in the *Dào Zàng* edition, thus resulting in editions far more accessible and historically accurate than the formerly standard photolithographic *Sòng* edition, or the versions found in the *Dào Zàng* or *Sì Kù Quán Shū* collections. Therefore, we can be satisfied that, at least for the purposes of the current translation, we present an accurate impression of the medical treatment of women during the early *Táng* period based on the content of Sūn Sī-Miǎo's writing.

3. The Content of Sūn Sī-Miǎo's "Prescriptions for women"

The introductory essay of the section on "prescriptions for women" (*fù rén fāng*) in the *Qiān Jīn Fāng* begins with this oft cited statement: "The reason why women have special prescriptions is that they are different because of pregnancy, childbirth, and flooding damage [i.e., heavy vaginal bleeding]. Therefore, women's diseases are ten times more difficult to treat than men's." Placed at the very beginning of the main body of the *Qiān Jīn Fāng*, the significance of this statement cannot be overrated. The following information attempts to shed light on it from various angles:

A summary and brief interpretation of volumes two to four, which includes a case study that analyzes the prescriptions for "seeking a child" in more detail, is intended to give the reader an impression of the general nature, major themes, and issues of the text. Comparing the content and structure of Sūn Sī-Miǎo's "prescriptions for women" with earlier and later texts allows us to situate this text in the history of the development of gynecology in medieval China. In addition, it sheds light on Sūn Sī-Miǎo's various roles as an innovative author, as a preserver and transmitter of literary medical traditions, as a medical practitioner with a personal stance in advocating women's health, as a cosmologically-inclined practitioner of the arts of preserving and continuing life, and even as a advocate for oral traditions that transcended class or gender boundaries.

Although the categorical confusions, overlap between prescriptions, and contradictory statements found in these prescriptions indicate the preliminary state of knowledge about women's health in early medieval China, the material introduced in the following pages also points toward the sophisticated understanding of a gendered body with gender-specific etiologies and treatment needs that would emerge full-blown in the following *Sòng* dynasty. Sūn Sī-Miǎo's understanding of women's weaknesses and vulnerabilities was already far more comprehensive than what is included in a standard modern dictionary definition of obstetrics and gynecology as the "medical care of pregnant women (obstetrics) and of female genital diseases (gynecology)." As Sūn wrote in the sentence that follows the introductory statement quoted above, which also reflects the organization of prescriptions in the *Qiān Jīn Fāng*, Sūn Sī-Miǎo interpreted female difference under the categories of reproduction (consisting of fertility, pregnancy, childbirth, postpartum conditions, and lactation), miscellaneous treatments (including treatments for female genital diseases), supplementing and boosting, and a large section on menstruation and vaginal discharge.

It is impossible to discern at this point the extent to which Sūn Sī-Miǎo's placement of the "prescriptions for women" at the very beginning of the *Qiān Jīn Fāng* was motivated by a humanitarian concern for what he clearly perceived as the greater vulnerability and weakness of the female body, in both its physical and psychological aspects. It also appears that he consciously composed and organized the *Qiān Jīn Fāng* with the ultimate intention of preserving and prolonging life in the elite tradition of "nurturing life" (養生 *yǎng shēng*). Therefore, he placed women's health, interpreted as the foundation for the creation of life, at the beginning of the text, followed by pediatrics, and only then general medicine. This leads up to instructions for the preservation and prolongation of life based on diet, lifestyle, *qì* cultivation, and sexual cultivation, appended with technical instructions for pulse diagnostics and acumoxa therapy. Supporting this argument, he states in his introduction to volume five on pediatrics: ". . . For this reason [I have arranged] these prescriptions [by placing] those on women first, then those on children, and afterwards those on men and the elderly. This is the meaning of venerating the roots." Whatever Sūn Sī-Miǎo's motivations were, his treatment of women went far beyond ensuring their reproductive capabilities and reflects a genuine concern with what he saw as the special burdens suffered by the female body for the sake of continuing the family lineage.

3a. Reproduction

Tellingly enough, Sūn Sī-Miǎo's prescription collection starts with the treatment of reproductive problems. As the introductory statement quoted above shows, Sūn Sī-Miǎo considered the effects of childbearing to be the single most important factor in the etiology of women's diseases. The remainder of this first essay in the "prescriptions for women" refines this statement considerably. As additional causes for women's weak health, it mentions the onset of menstruation at the age of fourteen and external causes like immoderate food and drink, inappropriate sexual intercourse, and most notably, wind entering from below, that is, through the vagina. To complicate matters further, he states that "women's cravings and desires exceed their husbands' and they contract illness at twice the rate of men." Next, Sūn Sī-Miǎo lays out the significance of childbearing as "the adult role in women's destiny and fate," an elegant expression of the well-known Confucian attitude that defined women by their function of providing male descendants for the husband's family line or, in Margery Wolf's words, as a "rented womb." Because childbearing was "the basis of human affairs and the foundation of enlightened rule," the volumes on prescriptions for women should be "inspected by gentlemen of like intention" and "routinely copied and carried by servants engaged in childrearing."

Sūn Sī-Miǎo has now laid the foundations from which to launch the first aspect of his prescriptions for women, a treatment program for "seeking a child" (求子 qiú zǐ, i.e., enhancing fertility). Containing six essays, fourteen medicinal prescriptions, six moxibustion methods, and three "methods for converting a female [fetus] into a male," it comprises about six percent of the "prescriptions for women." Before offering treatments, though, Sūn Sī-Miǎo warns that even the best medicine is useless if the couple's basic destinies are mismatched (meaning that their birth signs do not follow the order of generation in the progression of the five phases) and the astrological constellations at the time of conceiving the fetus are inauspicious. If their birth signs are in harmony, however, they will still need to pay heed to Sūn Sī-Miǎo's medical advice and also guard against breaking taboos against sexual intercourse at inauspicious times to ensure their own and their offspring's future health and good fortune.

The Sòng editors insert a reference here to methods for determining the right time and day for "receiving a fetus" (受胎 shòu tāi), found later in the Qiān Jīn Fāng in volume 27 on "nurturing life" (yǎng shēng). It is interesting to note that these "methods for taboos and restrictions [on sexual intercourse]" are, in the Sūn Zhēn Rén edition, cited in the category for "seeking a child" and therefore considered part of the "prescriptions for women." Similarly, the Wài Tái Mì Yào and Ishimpō both devote considerable space to these taboos and prognostications about the child's and parents' future in the section on "seeking a child."

In a slight shift of emphasis, Sūn Sī-Miǎo lastly offers a purely medical etiology in the next essay, stating that "whenever people are childless, it is caused by the fact that both husband and wife suffer from the five taxations and seven damages and the hundred illnesses of vacuity and emaciation, with the disastrous result that the line of descendants is cut off." This seems to contrast the popular notions of his time, most notably the Bìng Yuán Lùn, which states: "When women are without child, there are three reasons: First, that the tombs have not been worshipped; second, that the husband's and wife's yearly fate [a reference to their astrological constellations] are in a relationship of mutual conquest; and third, the husband or wife's illness. All these cause childlessness. If it is a case of tombs not having been worshipped or the yearly fates conquering each other, there are no medicines that can benefit." Similar sentiments are expressed in the calendrical and astrological sections on childlessness in the Wài Tái Mì Yào, Ishimpō, and Qiān Jīn Fāng cited above.

Following this reference to nonmedical causes of childlessness, Sūn Sī-Miǎo then proceeds to discuss options for medical treatments. These are summarized here in a detailed case study to illustrate the treatment style and underlying etiological reasoning found in Sūn Sī-Miǎo's "prescriptions for women:"

Case Study: an Interpretation of Section 1, "Seeking a Child"

In order to prevent or treat the medical cause of infertility, which he has previously identified as the "five taxations, seven damages, and hundred diseases of vacuity emaciation," Sūn Sī-Miǎo proposes a complex treatment plan: First, the husband is treated for lack of offspring in conjunction with wind vacuity, clouded vision, and weakness and shortage of essential *qì* by supplementing his insufficiencies with "Seven Seeds Powder" (七子散 *qī zǐ sǎn*). The famous *Yuán* dynasty physician Zhū Zhèn-Hēng 朱震亨 (alt. Dān-Xī 丹溪) later developed this prescription into the "Five Seeds Pills for Abundant Descendants" (五子衍宗丸 *wǔ zǐ yǎn zōng wán*) that are still used today as a treatment for infertility. To return to the *Qiān Jīn Fāng*, the wife is treated for lifelong inability to give birth with a "uterus-rinsing decoction," to be ingested by the patient while she is wrapped in blankets. This preparation is supposed to induce sweating and cause the discharge of the illness in the form of accumulated blood, which will appear as cold red pus. Referred to as "this malign substance" in the uterus, the root of the illness is identified as an accumulation of cold blood, which causes pain below the navel, irregular menstruation, and inability to receive the fetus. Sūn Sī-Miǎo stresses the importance of consuming an entire preparation of this medicine, if possible, because the illness might otherwise not be completely eliminated. On the next day, the woman should be treated with a suppository consisting of pulverized drugs filled into a finger-sized silk bag and inserted into the vagina. This was to be applied repeatedly throughout the day while the patient was to remain in her chamber and rest until she discharged a "cold malign substance" in the form of green-yellow cold liquid, which again represented the illness being expelled below. The treatment should be concluded with "Fluorite and Asparagus Pills" (紫石門冬丸 *zǐ shí mén dōng wán*), to be taken until the sensation of heat in the abdomen indicated a successful completion of the treatment.

Next, Sūn Sī-Miǎo lists a number of fairly complex medicinal prescriptions for the treatment of infertility in conjunction with symptoms such as heat above and cold below, inhibited menstruation, the thirty-six illnesses of the lower burner, the myriad illnesses of vaginal discharge, and the twelve abdominal conglomerations. While the prescriptions differ based on the reason for infertility, such as the above-mentioned indications or a "blockage of the uterus that is preventing it from receiving the essence," they all share the goal of inducing a certain type of discharge below that indicates the expulsion of the illness, whether in the form of "long worms and green-yellow liquid," or "bean juice or snivel." Thus, it appears that in Sūn Sī-Miǎo's eyes, infertility was caused by an accumulation of cold blood in the uterus that was treated by expelling it below, sometimes in combination with a "scrubbing" of the uterus or internal organs. In the midst of these prescriptions, we find two prescriptions with significantly less ingredients, said to be "used by the ancients," but fallen out of use in Sūn Sī-Miǎo's times. The first one treats the husband for insufficiency of *yáng qì* and inability to cause transformation (i.e., in the woman's womb) or, if transformation did occur, failure to complete it. The second one seems like a rather standard treatment for women's infertility. Sūn Sī-Miǎo precedes these with the caveat that he has no personal experience using them, but has included them because of their popularity in ancient times.

Throughout this section, Sūn Sī-Miǎo's choice of drug ingredients reveals his underlying etiological ideas as well as treatment strategies. The following discussion of medicinal actions is based on the understanding of a substance's efficacy during the early *Táng* period. Thus, I follow the descriptions in materia medica literature roughly contemporaneous to the date of composition of the *Qiān Jīn Fāng*. For this purpose, I have relied on a critical edition of the *Shén Nóng Běn Cǎo*

Jīng 神農本草經 (Divine Farmer's Classic of Materia Medica), a *Hàn* period classic that was edited and annotated by Táo Hóng-Jīng 陶弘景 in the early sixth century. The edition used here includes this commentary, while attempting to reconstruct the original appearance of the text and can therefore serve as an accurate reflection of materia medica knowledge slightly prior to the time when the *Qiān Jīn Fāng* was composed.

According to the descriptions of the medicinal actions of drugs in this text, the prescriptions for treating infertility in the *Qiān Jīn Fāng* contain drugs like *pò xiāo* (朴消 Impure mirabilite), *mǔ dān* (牡丹 Bark of the root of Paeonia suffruticosa), and *táo rén* (桃仁 Seed of Prunus persica) that eliminate evil *qì*, break up accumulations, and treat blood stagnation. These are combined with drugs like *xì xīn* (細辛 Complete plant including root of Asarum heteropoides), *gān jiāng* (乾薑 Dried root of Zingiber officinale), *jié gěng* (桔梗 Root of Platycodon grandiflorum), and *shǔ jiāo* (蜀椒 Seed capsules of Zanthoxylum bungeanum) that are warming, treat wind, dampness, cough, and counterflow *qì* ascent, and precipitate *qì*, as well as drugs like *tiān mén dōng* (天門冬 Tuber of Asparagus cochinchinensis), *niú xī* (牛膝 Root of Achyranthes bidentata), *wǔ wèi zǐ* (五味子 Fruit of Schisandra chinensis), and *shān zhū yú* (山茱萸 Fruit of Cornus officinalis) that extend life and supplement insufficiencies, treat taxation damage and emaciation, nourish *yīn*, and boost essence and *qì*, in addition to the above characteristics of warming, moving blood, or eliminating wind and dampness. This choice of ingredients suggests an understanding of infertility as caused by the inhibited movement of *qì* and blood due to vacuity, leading to cold stagnation and accumulations in the abdomen of a substance that Sūn Sī-Miǎo refers to as "this malign substance." The frequent use of drugs like *xì xīn* 細辛 and *fáng fēng* (防風 Root of Ledebouriella divaricata) also indicates the notion that infertility might be caused by externally contracted wind-cold, which had to be dispersed and expelled by increasing the flow of blood and *qì* with supplementing, warming, and down-draining preparations.

In addition to medicinal prescriptions, the text lists several moxibustion techniques for treating women's infertility. The choice of moxibustion points is quite carefully differentiated by the particulars of the condition, such as general infertility, inability to have children because the mouth of the uterus is blocked, inability to complete a pregnancy due to miscarriage with abdominal pain and leaking of red discharge, blockage of the uterus so that she is unable to receive the [male] essence, or red and white leakage. Except for one use of Rán Gǔ, which is located on the ankle, the other points are all located in the area between the navel and the pubic bone (Guān Yuán, Bāo Mén, Qí Mén, and Quan Mén) and are for the most part still used today for the treatment of infertility.

Appended to the chapter on fertility is a short but significant section on manipulating the fetus' gender. As a brief introductory essay explains, the fetus is created by the interaction and mutual stimulation of *yīn* and *yáng*. According to the standard medical notions of the time, the shape of the fetus was not settled until the end of the third month of pregnancy, and the mother's behavior and environment could therefore affect the fetus' physical and psychological characteristics. This was the basis for the popular practice of "fetal education" (胎教 *tāi jiào*), discussed by Sūn Sī-Miǎo in the following chapter on pregnancy-related prescriptions. Regarding the fetus' gender, early medieval theories of conception and pregnancy were sometimes contradictory, suggesting either that the gender of the fetus was not yet fixed or that it could be transformed until the third month of pregnancy. By the *Sòng* period, sexual differentiation had become identified with conception in medical literature, and instructions for changing the fetus' gender were therefore eliminated from elite doctors' gynecological texts. On the other hand, instructions for influencing the gender of the fetus during the act of intercourse, as for example by timing it in relationship to the woman's menstrual cycle, become more important.

Being a prescription text with only short essays, the *Qiān Jīn Fāng* fails to provide a conclusive statement on this issue. Nevertheless, the prescriptions obviously reflect the belief that gender could be manipulated up to the third month of pregnancy, which, in most cases, meant converting a female fetus into a male. Besides a complex prescription of medicinals that mostly boost *yáng*, *qì*, blood, and essence, Sūn Sī-Miǎo also lists several instructions of a decidedly magical flavor, such as the advice to "take a crossbow string, place it in a crimson bag and have the pregnant woman carry it on her left arm" or to tie it around her waist below the belt. Another prescription calls for an ax to be hidden under the woman's bed. All of these actions needed to be performed secretly, a common feature in magical prescriptions. Interesting in this section is the curious combination of medical and magical thinking, but even the medicinal prescriptions include such ingredients as dog testicles and the head of a rooster from the top of the eastern gate.

In conclusion, the following points should be noted:

(1) This section includes prescriptions for treating male insufficiency of *yáng qì*, as well as a reference to prescriptions in the section on "nurturing life" that is aimed at men. This shows that responsibility for the inability to procreate was not placed exclusively with the woman, but was shared between husband and wife. The creation of the fetus was seen as an act performed by two equal partners, with *yīn* and *yáng* intermingling and stimulating each other. As the essay states, "*Yīn* and *yáng* blend in harmony, the two *qì* respond to each other, and *yáng* bestows and *yīn* transforms." Jender Lee has shown that in early medieval Chinese medicine, the treatment of infertility was shifted from sexual cultivation texts directed at men, called "texts of the bedchamber" (房中書 *fáng zhōng shū*), to medical prescription literature on women's health. In this context, increasing attention was focused on ensuring the woman's reproductive health before and during pregnancy with medicinal prescriptions, rather than on the avoidance of calendrical taboos at the time of conception.

(2) While the male cause for infertility is here simply diagnosed as insufficient *qì* (and treated in more detail in the section on "supplementing and boosting by sexual intercourse"), the woman's condition was carefully distinguished depending on a sophisticated diagnosis that took into consideration the appearance of abdominal masses, sensation of cold, menstrual irregularities, white or red vaginal discharge, and the anatomical shape of her reproductive organs.

(3) In all cases, treatment was directed at causing the discharge of cold blood, sometimes in connection with heat therapy, and the cleansing of the uterus with cold-expelling and precipitating medicinals. The stagnation and accumulation of pathogenic cold in the body's center was seen as caused by either the invasion of external wind-cold or a deep-lying insufficiency of *yīn*, blood, and *qì*, which in any case predisposed the patient to the former.

(4) The complexity of the medicinal prescriptions, requiring numerous non-household medicinal ingredients, suggests that this sphere of women's healthcare was not limited to the treatment by other female household members or local drug peddlers and midwives, but had also received the attention of concerned male literati like Sūn Sī-Miǎo.

(5) In addition to medicinal prescriptions, Sūn Sī-Miǎo also included magical treatments as well as references, in the very first paragraph, to the superior power of astrology and fate, against which even the finest physician was helpless. Thus, Sūn Sī-Miǎo recognized that, in this significant area of women's health, medicinal prescriptions did not exhaust his readers' need for different treatment modalities.

The second major category of the "prescriptions for women" in the *Qiān Jīn Fāng* covers pregnancy and comprises almost a quarter of the gynecological section. It is divided into three sections: "malign obstruction in pregnancy," "nurturing the fetus," and "the various diseases of pregnancy."

The comparatively short section on "malign obstruction in pregnancy" (妊娠惡阻 *rèn shēn è zǔ*) contains two long essays and four prescriptions. The first essay describes a method for determining whether a woman is pregnant and for predicting the gender of the fetus and the time of birth, by diagnosing the pulse. Several important ideas about conception, pregnancy, and fetal development can be deduced from this advice: The fetus is created through the harmonious intermingling of blood and *qì*, *yīn* and *yáng*. Pregnancy is diagnosed by detecting increased movement and blood flow in the pulse of either the heart vessel, which governs the flow of blood, or of the kidney vessel, which governs reproduction. By the fourth month, the fetus' gender is fixed and can be diagnosed by the characteristics of the pulse (deep and replete for a boy, big and floating for a girl). Sūn Sī-Miǎo also mentions several simpler methods for diagnosing the gender such as by inducing the woman to spontaneously turn to the left (for a boy) or right (for a girl) or finding lumps in the right or left side of the husband's chest. This section is reminiscent of folk advice given all over the world. It is significant that Sūn Sī-Miǎo chose to transmit this advice along with and as equal to what we would consider more properly medical and sophisticated methods of pulse diagnosis, which were by necessity the domain of an educated male physician with sufficient training and experience to distinguish such subtle differences. The remainder of this chapter concerns the etiology and treatment of "malign obstruction" in pregnancy in strictly medical terms. It defines the condition as a combination of physical and psychological symptoms caused by the presence of wind-cold, a pathological accumulation of fluids below the heart, as well as a general stagnation of *qì* and blood. These are in turn ultimately due to the quintessentially feminine problems of vacuity and emaciation from taxation damage, insufficiency of *qì* and blood, and additional weakness of kidney *qì*, potentially aggravated by exposure to wind.

The next section on "nurturing the fetus" (養胎 *yǎng tāi*) begins with an essay on "fetal education" (*tāi jiào*). This practice is aimed at creating a model Confucian descendant who is "long-lived, loyal and filial, humane, righteous, intelligent, wise, and free of disease." It prescribes the pregnant woman's ideal surroundings, activities (such as observing ritual performances, playing the zither, and reciting poetry), and composed mindset during the first three months of pregnancy, when the fetus "transforms in response to things, and its disposition and character are not yet fixed." This information is standard and similar to advice cited in many texts, from the *Tāi Chǎn Shū* from Mǎ-Wáng-Duī to the *Liè Nǚ Zhuàn* 列女傳 (Biographies of Exemplary Women) by Liú Xiàng 劉向. Following these instructions on fetal education, the *Qiān Jīn Fāng* contains a varied list of prohibited foods, with the more mundane goal of preventing miscarriage, childbirth complications, or physical deformities. Then, Sūn Sī-Miǎo quotes "Xū Zhī-Cái's month-by-month prescriptions for nurturing the fetus," the text we have already encountered in the *Tāi Chǎn Shū*, the *Bìng Yuán Lùn*, and the *Ishimpō*, where it is identified as a quote from the *Chǎn Jīng*. At times almost literally identical to the *Ishimpō* version, the quotation in the *Qiān Jīn Fāng* describes the monthly progress in the fetus' gestation and notes the foods and acupuncture channels prohibited in each month. It also includes two decoction prescriptions for each month, one for the treatment of pathologies likely to occur during that month and the other for the treatment of damage to the fetus. The last subsection of pregnancy treatments consists of "medicines for lubricating the fetus" (滑胎藥 *huá tāi yào*). This is an important category of prescriptions, taken during the final stage of pregnancy to prepare the mother and fetus for childbirth and to ease labor, which is still used today. As a whole, this section stands out for the nuanced descriptions of symptoms and the specificity and complexity of the prescriptions. This suggests that prescribing medicinal decoctions for nurturing the fetus and in preparation for delivery were two areas of women's medical care that educated medical practitioners, whether professional or amateur, were actively engaged in during Sūn Sī-Miǎo's lifetime.

The next chapter on the "various diseases of pregnancy" (妊娠諸病 *rèn shēn zhū bìng*) presents a more diverse treatment style: It contains ten sections on stirring fetus and repeated miscarriage; leaking uterus; child vexation; heart, abdominal, and lumbar pain and intestinal fullness; cold damage; malaria; [vaginal] bleeding; urinary diseases; diarrhea; and water swelling, containing a total of eighty-nine prescriptions and three moxibustion methods. The treatments in this section run seamlessly from complex medicinal prescriptions, often with more than half a dozen ingredients, to simple home remedies such as drinking infant's urine or water in which the husband's leather boots have been washed. Ingesting pulverized cow manure, grease from a cart's linchpin, or charred fingernails and matted hair are recommended side-by-side with physical manipulations such as applying abdominal compresses of roasted buffalo manure mixed with vinegar, or burning moxa on Qì Hǎi, a point still used today for the treatment of abdominal pain, painful or irregular menstruation, and vaginal discharge. Much to our regret, it is impossible to determine yet whether these different treatment modes — as well as the etiologies they were based on — reflected the practices of different types of practitioners, differentiated by gender, economic or social status, education, professionalization, family ties, or other factors.

Sūn Sī-Miǎo's treatment of childbirth, consisting of sections on childbirth complications, death of the child in the abdomen, breech birth, and failure to expel the placenta, might not be as comprehensive as a modern reader would expect, constituting only about six percent of the "prescriptions for women." But it still offers many insights into this sphere of women's healthcare, most notably by the virtual absence of multi-ingredient medicinal prescriptions. Instead, Sūn Sī-Miǎo offers standard advice such as prohibitions during labor against "having people visit from homes polluted by the filth of death or mourning," or against (presumably female) attendants that were either too numerous or overanxious, thereby upsetting the mother's state of mind.

He also includes a warning to "avoid the opposite branch month" and states that, "whenever childbirth is not done according to the birth charts, offenses and violations might occur that afterwards cause the death of both mother and child." This is a rather offhanded reference to an aspect of childbirth that has been shown to play a significant role in popular practices of the times in both elite and lower-class households. According to Jender Lee's research, these charts contained instructions for setting up the delivery hut, the direction to face and squatting position during delivery, and the placenta burial after delivery, in order to avoid offending the spirits. Already in use in the early *Hàn* period, as evidenced by the inclusion of a chart for the burial of the placenta and accompanying instructions among the Mǎ-Wáng-Duī manuscripts, these different charts were synthesized into single comprehensive twelve-month charts during the *Táng* period. Sun's attitude towards astrological taboos is highly telling and, according to Donald Harper, "exemplifies the attitude of certain physicians who balanced acceptance of iatromancy [i.e., medical divination] with pragmatic skepticism." In contrast, Charlotte Furth has emphasized the catholic nature of these rituals, stating that they were "the cultural property of elites as well as masses." It is also possible, though, that Sūn Sī-Miǎo saw his prescription collection in a more narrowly defined medical role and therefore perhaps assumed that households would find this information in other sources, such as the specifically obstetrical text *Chǎn Jīng* quoted in the *Ishimpō*.

Following this essay, Sūn Sī-Miǎo offers a number of short instructions for treating a stalled labor, including squirting vinegar in the woman's face, having the husband blow into her mouth, inserting balls made from pulverized *bàn xià* (半夏 Rhizome of Pinellia ternata) into her nostrils, or forcefully yanking her hair. These prescriptions are unnamed and neither differentiated by symptoms nor based on any apparent etiological theory or treatment principle besides arousing the woman or replenishing her exhaustion. References in later *Sòng* literature to women involved in the ritual roles of purifying the birth room as well as to the professionalization and high status of midwives strongly suggest what Charlotte Furth has called a "female sphere of healing."

This impression is supported by the following three sections, containing treatments for death of the child in the abdomen, breech birth, and failure to expel the placenta. Again, it appears that the messy and often physical management of childbirth complications was not an area that distinguished literati like Sūn Sī-Miǎo were too keen on attending. Instructions to swallow a magical number of *huái shí* (槐實 Fruit of Sophora japonica) seeds, to drink the husband's boiled urine, or to ingest an egg mixed with a pinch of salt to expel a dead fetus were hardly sufficient for a woman in a situation regarded as "resembling death." It is most likely that literati physicians, recognizing the limitations of medicinal prescriptions and acupuncture, left this area in the hands of women with extensive personal experience and no restraints of modesty. Their techniques are only alluded to briefly by Sūn Sī-Miǎo, as in instructions to prick the child's hand or foot with a needle or awl or to rub salt on the fetus' feet in the case of breech presentation. A number of prescriptions for retained placenta, finally, advise to ingest such substances as stove top soot, pulverized ink, or different types of dirt, such as that from under the center post of a house, mud from the bottom of a well, or ant hill dirt. Stating that "covering the top of the well with the husband's underclothes will expel [the placenta]" only leaves us hoping that other attendants of the childbearing woman had better advice up their sleeves.

With the last section of the first volume, entitled "precipitating the breast milk" (下乳 *xià rǔ*, i.e., promoting lactation), Sūn Sī-Miǎo is safely back in his territory of medicinal prescriptions: Already in early Chinese medical theory, breast milk was interpreted as a transformation of menstrual blood, which, during pregnancy, descended to nourish the fetus and, after birth, ascended to emerge as breast milk. Consequently, the obvious cause for an absence of fluid in the breast was an underlying etiology of "violent exhaustion of fluids and insufficiency of blood, due to the discharge of fluids and blood in childbirth," as Cháo Yuán-Fāng stated in the *Bìng Yuán Lùn* shortly prior to the *Qiān Jīn Fāng*. He already distinguished between the symptoms of "postpartum lack of milk in the breasts" (產後乳無汁 *chǎn hòu rǔ wú zhī*) and "postpartum spillage of breast milk" (產後乳汁溢 *chǎn hòu rǔ zhī yì*), albeit with an etiology considerably less sophisticated than, for example, his explanation of menstrual conditions. In contrast, Sūn Sī-Miǎo merely addressed the condition "lack of milk in the breasts" (乳無汁 *rǔ wú zhī*) in this brief section.

This absence of a differentiated diagnosis might indicate that issues related to breast-feeding were more commonly treated by midwives or other female caregivers and had only recently come to the attention of male medical authors. In any case, Zǎn Yīn's 昝殷 *Jīng Xiào Chǎn Bǎo* 經效產寶 (Birth Treasury of Proven Efficacy) from 853 shows that physicians' knowledge in this area increased considerably during the following few centuries. Thus, this text contains separate discussions of and prescriptions for the three categories of "postpartum lack of fluid in the breasts," "postpartum binding into abscesses in the breasts," and "postpartum spontaneous discharge of breast milk." By 1237, Chén Zì-míng's 陳自明 *Fù Rén Dà Quán Liáng Fāng* 婦人大全良方 (All-Inclusive Good Prescriptions for Women) differentiates between three types of "breast milk failing to flow" (乳汁不行 *rǔ zhī bù xíng*): In young women who experience distended breasts after their first birth, it is due to wind or heat and must be treated with clearing and disinhibiting medicines to make the milk flow. Women with an absence of milk after several births, by contrast, suffer from a lack of fluids and therefore need to be treated with moistening and enriching medicines to activate the flow. And lastly, women with milk in their breasts, but in scanty amounts, should take medicines that free the channels. Sūn Sī-Miǎo's choice of medicinals mostly suggests the first category, since the two most frequently occurring drugs in the prescriptions of this category, *shí zhōng rǔ* (石鐘乳 Stalactite) and *tōng cǎo* (通草 Pith in the stalk of Tetrapanax papyriferus), were both used medicinally in his time to "disinhibit the nine orifices" (利九竅 *lì jiǔ qiào*).

The second volume of Sūn Sī-Miǎo's prescriptions for women is almost exclusively devoted to women's postpartum care, comprising more than a quarter of the gynecological content in the *Qiān Jīn Fāng*. It is divided into seven sections on the postpartum conditions of vacuity detriment, vacuity vexation, wind strike, heart and abdominal pain, malign dew (that is, lochia), diarrhea, and strangury and thirst. It begins with an essay that explains the need for special postpartum care, and warns that therapy should consist only of supporting and supplementing, rather than moving and draining, treatments because of women's severe vacuity due to childbirth.

During the first hundred days postpartum, the new mother is considered to be in an extreme state of vulnerability, requiring constant vigilance, caution, and proscribed behavior (most notably social isolation) so as not to break any of the many postpartum taboos. In explaining these restrictions, Sūn Sī-Miǎo relates them not to women's ritual pollution from postpartum blood, but to women's susceptibility to "childbed wind," a condition similar to the Western condition of childbed fever, but as the name implies, directly related to an etiology of wind. The *Bìng Yuán Lùn* offers a strictly medical explanation for this condition: Childbirth stirs the blood and *qì*, taxes and injures the viscera and bowels, and, if women rise from bed before recovering, causes *qì* vacuity, which allows the cold *qì* of wind evil to invade.

Differing significantly from this medical interpretation, Sūn Sī-Miǎo states that this condition "is exactly the symptom related to a violation of the prohibitions," beyond the control of even the best physicians. He therefore advises to "not leave [women] without company at the time of delivery, [for] otherwise they might act without restraint and follow their whims, and then they are bound to violate the prohibitions." For the first hundred days postpartum, one must employ extreme diligence and "not [allow them to] indulge in their whims and thereby violate [the prohibitions] and offending [the spirits]." While any postpartum violation itself might have appeared "tiny like autumn down" at the time, it will cause a "disease larger than the Sōng-Shān 嵩山 or Tài-Shān 岱山 mountains" down the road, and make her fate "like a flickering candle."

Jender Lee has shown that this practice of postpartum social isolation is clearly linked to ideas about the polluting — and therefore ritually offensive — nature of birth and female blood, a common Daoist and Buddhist notion of the time. Yet, it can also be interpreted as a response to the dramatic changes in the new mother's social role, necessitating a liminal period of transition. As a third perspective on this practice, Lee notes that the custom could function, at least for elite women, as a period of rest and recuperation when they were relieved from the pressures of everyday life. Still practiced in contemporary Chinese communities today as "sitting out the month" (坐月子 *zuò yuè zǐ*), it includes such varied aspects as dietary prohibitions and restrictions on washing, leaving the house, sexual intercourse, and other activities. It is perpetuated by strict traditionally-minded mothers-in-law, but also by numerous modern self-help books with pictures of mouth-watering culinary delights and other ways of positively reinforcing the need for special attention and reward after the accomplishment of childbirth. In contemporary Taiwan, it has led to the establishment of private postpartum care centers, called "Centers for Sitting out the Month" (坐月子中心 *zuò yuè zǐ zhōng xīn*), where the burden of pampering new mothers has been turned over to paid personnel. The postpartum treatment of women in China is a fascinating and evocative topic that deserves a much more thorough investigation, whether from a medical, social, or religious angle, than it has received so far in either Chinese or Western scholarship.

A similar complexity in interpreting a new mother's postpartum status is reflected already in the *Qiān Jīn Fāng*. Postpartum practices appear, on the one hand, as restricting and isolating a ritually polluting member of the household, as is expressed by the need for caution, restraint, and control stressed in the introductory essay. The following prescriptions, on the other hand, focus on the special nurturance and protection required because of the physical depletion and vulnerability after childbirth. The special care for newly delivered women came to be actively promoted in medieval China by concerned male physicians and authors like Sūn Sī-Miǎo or Cháo Yuán-Fāng who emphasized that such infractions as premature sexual intercourse or the general taxation from childbirth were the primary reason for women's chronic illnesses for the rest of their lives. Consequently, Sūn Sī-Miǎo states in almost every single prescription in the following sections of this volume that the primary etiology is "postpartum vacuity emaciation" (產後虛瘦 *chǎn hòu xū shòu*). In this, he is following Cháo Yuán-Fāng's model of relating practically every symptom in his gynecological section to generalized vacuity, which is linked, implicitly or explicitly, to "taxation damage to *qì* and blood," the primary cause of which was childbirth.

To aggravate matters further, in Sūn Sī-Miǎo's eyes, this constellation of internal factors predisposed women to an invasion of wind-cold, the primary external agent cited for the majority of the conditions in this volume, because it caused women's blood to bind and congeal. This lead to their suffering from "accumulations and gatherings in the abdomen and from the myriad illnesses, arising unexpectedly, all the way until their old age, unable to recover even if treated with a myriad prescriptions." This theme is reiterated in volume four, in both the chapter on "supplementing and boosting" and the chapters on menstrual problems and vaginal discharge. The prescription for *Major Lycopus Pills* (大澤蘭丸 *dà zé lán wán*) for example, offers a page-long list of possible symptoms ranging from hernia, vaginal pain, numbness, and muscle spasms to mental confusion, digestive problems, skin eruptions, arthritis, dimmed eyesight, nasal congestion, convulsions, amenorrhea, infertility, and "instability of the ethereal and corporeal souls."

To return to the content of volume three, Sūn Sī-Miǎo's essays and treatment strategies provide evidence for the existence of conflicting medical ideologies with regard to women's postpartum treatment: On the one hand, he repeatedly warns that right after delivery "you may only use supporting and supplementing [treatments] and may not use moving or draining [treatments]," because they only aggravated women's postpartum weakness and depletion. Consequently, this type of prescription is exactly what is found in the first two sections in this volume on vacuity detriment and vacuity vexation, albeit with the note that one may only start taking them after the "malign substance" (i.e., lochia, the stale blood remaining in the uterus after childbirth) has been eliminated completely. This prohibition against employing strong drugs in a woman's weakened postpartum state is reiterated in the introduction to section three on wind strike: "In all cases of postpartum arched-back rigidity as well as the various wind diseases, you must not employ toxic medicines. It is only appropriate to act specifically with one or two ingredients. You may also not induce great sweating and must particularly avoid moving and draining [therapies that will induce] vomiting and diarrhea. They will invariably lead to her death."

Given the fact that the contraction of wind made a woman's fate fickle "as a flickering candle," however, the clinical need to actively treat a life-threatening condition with such intimidating symptoms as unconsciousness, seizures, hallucinations and insanity, heart palpitations, and panting — or, a cynical observer might add, the professional need to prescribe medicines with drastic and visible effects to awe his paying customers — promptly causes him to contradict his own advice. A mild prescription for toasted soybeans in liquor is followed by increasingly stronger preparations aimed at dispelling the external evils of wind and cold by inducing sweating, similar to the standard treatment for wind strike.

Most likely, this contradictory advice expresses a growing awareness of the need for women's spe-cial, gender-specific treatment, as opposed to the more traditional view that women's conditions could be treated with the same prescriptions as men, as seen in the maxim stated in the first essay on the "prescriptions for women": "In cases where the nodal *qì* over the four seasons has caused illness and where vacuity or repletion of cold or heat has caused worry, then [women are treated] the same as men."

But it is also a reflection of the difference between a treatment style that focused on expelling external pathogens with strong-acting medicinals and one that promoted a preventative medicine aimed at internally nourishing and balancing the body before any symptoms appeared. As an elite scholar deeply — and successfully, as evidenced by his advanced age — devoted to physical cultivation and life-prolonging techniques, Sūn Sī-Miǎo's loyalties in this dispute are obvious. He confirms this attitude when he quotes the *Shén Nóng Běn Cǎo Jīng* categorization of drugs in his chapter on "employing drugs:"

The highest [category of] medicinals... constitute the chiefs. Indicated for nurturing life, they cor-respond to heaven. They are nontoxic, can be taken constantly, and do not harm people when taken over a long time. When wanting to lighten the body, benefit *qì*, avoid aging, and extend one's years, base it on the highest category. The medium [category of] drugs...constitute the supports. Indicated for nourishing the body, they correspond to humanity. Some are toxic, some are not, and their appropriateness should be considered [on an individual basis]. When wanting to prevent illness and replenish vacuity and emaciation, base it on the medium category. The lowest [category of] drugs...constitute the assistants and conductors. Indicated for treating disease, they correspond to earth. They are mostly toxic and may not be taken for a long period of time. When wanting to expel cold or hot evil *qì*, break up accumulations and gatherings, and treat urgent conditions, base it on the lowest category.

Here, he clearly values life-prolonging drugs the highest, followed by drugs for supplementing vacuity, and lastly drugs for expelling external evils, breaking accumulations, and treating emer-gencies. Contrary to these ideals, and doubtlessly necessitated by the realities of medical practice, the prescriptions in the section on women do, however, contain mostly drugs and treatments that fit into the second or even third category.

A further complication related to this dilemma between the need to gently supplement women's postpartum vacuity and actively eliminate threatening pathogens appears in the next section on "malign dew" (惡露 *è lù*, translated in modern TCM as lochia), a technical term for the pathogenic blood remaining in a woman's uterus after childbirth. The symptoms addressed in this section show that an "incomplete elimination of malign dew" was associated with symptoms like severe abdominal and lumbar pain, [aversion to] cold and heat [effusion], and counterflow blood and *qì*, which might surge up into the lung and heart and cause shortness of breath, vexation, confusion, aching limbs, accumulating and binding *qì* and blood, and incessant vaginal bleeding. The choice of medicinals such as *dà huáng* (大黃 Root of Rheum palmatum), *táo rén* (桃仁 Seed of Prunus persica), *dà zǎo* (大棗 Mature fruit of Ziziphus jujuba), *wú zhū yú* (吳茱萸 Unripe fruit of Evodia rutaecarpa), *shēng jiāng* (生薑 Fresh root of Zingiber officinale), *dì huáng* (地黃 Root of Rehman-nia glutinosa), and *dāng guī* (當歸 Root of Angelica polimorpha) shows that this category of pre-scriptions was aimed at discharging pathogenic matter, directing *qì* downward, freeing blood, and promoting the free and correct flow of blood and *qì* in the body, as well as stabilizing the woman's overall condition.

The remaining two sections on postpartum diarrhea and postpartum strangury and thirst continue in a similar vein with medicinal prescriptions of varying length and complexity, including a prescription for *Lycopus Decoction* (澤蘭湯 *zé lán tāng*) with a total of twenty-one ingredients. In general, digestive problems are associated with a presence of cold in the uterus, and urinary problems with a presence of heat; the symptoms are treated accordingly.

In conclusion, the number of entries, differentiation of symptoms, and specificity of the prescriptions for treating postpartum conditions, sometimes with over a dozen ingredients, shows that the treatment of postpartum vacuity with medicinal decoctions, pills, and powders was an area in which medieval literati physicians had apparently gathered considerable expertise and were frequently consulted, able as they were to respond to a wide range of symptoms from general malaise and fatigue to raging insanity and convulsions. And in the unfortunate cases when their prescriptions proved unsuccessful, they were always able to cite Sūn Sī-Miǎo's caveat that even the most skillful physician was powerless if any of the numerous postpartum taboos had been broken and the illness was therefore due to supernatural causes. The extent of care and attention recommended for women to recover from the exertions of pregnancy and childbirth constitutes the single largest category in Sūn Sī-Miǎo's prescriptions for women. It is particularly noteworthy when compared with the relative neglect accorded to women during postpartum recovery in contemporary biomedical hospitals and the current practice in the USA for new mothers to return to work almost immediately after childbirth. The deep cultural differences in this attitude towards women's vulnerability after childbirth continue to be significant today. According to a sentiment still common in modern Taiwan, negligence after childbirth, crystallized in the prohibitions around "sitting out the month," could explain chronic health problems later that might be reversible only by another birth followed by a careful convalescence in accordance with the rules. Sūn Sī-Miǎo's abundance of prescriptions for postpartum recovery are merely an early expression of this same attention to the vulnerability and weakness of the female body after the taxations of pregnancy, labor, and delivery.

3b. Miscellaneous Treatments and Supplementing

The last chapter of the third volume, entitled "miscellaneous treatments" (雜病 *zá bìng*) covers conditions that lack a clear unifying etiology other than that they address specifically female health problems. It contains prescriptions for a variety of *qì* and blood diseases; one prescription for the iatrogenic effects of taking *liú huáng pills*; one prescription for intercourse with ghosts; two prescriptions and one moxibustion method for preventing pregnancy; more than thirty prescriptions and seven moxibustion methods for genital diseases such as coldness or openness of the vagina, prolapsed uterus, swelling, pain, or sores; and lastly fifteen prescriptions for conditions associated with or caused by sexual intercourse, including physical abuse during pregnancy to the point of near-death and several prescriptions for "wedding pain" (i.e., vaginal soreness from the first acts of intercourse).

The first section of the fourth and last volume on prescriptions for women contains prescriptions with the intended effect of "supplementing and boosting" (補益 *bǔ yì*). As some prescriptions state explicitly, this topic is related to the postpartum section discussed above, since vacuity and emaciation, the most common symptoms in this section, are generally seen as caused by childbirth. In addition to these, the prescriptions here treat such symptoms as general fatigue and lack of appetite, as well as conditions associated with the presence of cold, blood stagnation, and pain in the abdomen. The significance and wide-ranging effect of this etiology can be illustrated by the prescription for *Major Lycopus Pills* (大澤蘭丸 *dà zé lán wán*): It lists a whole page of symptoms that would exceed the imagination of most hypochondriacs and concludes that "there is no condition that cannot be treated with this [prescription]." Assuming that the number of ingredients is any indication for the medical sophistication of a prescription, this section represents one of the pinnacles of medieval physicians' treatment of women since several prescriptions contain over two dozen ingredients. This was probably related to the fact that such complex prescriptions were ideally suited to the style of medicine envisioned and practiced by educated literati like Sūn Sī-Miǎo. Moreover, postpartum supplementation was probably an area of women's healthcare where competition from other practitioners like midwives or (male and female) practitioners of manual or religious therapies was weaker than on such inherently female territory as the management of childbirth complications.

3c. Menstrual Irregularities and Vaginal Discharge

The remainder of the fourth volume is devoted to the treatment of menstrual stoppage (月水不通 *yuè shuǐ bù tōng*), vaginal discharge (帶下 *dài xià*) — ranging from life-threatening flooding (崩 *bēng*) to chronic spotting (漏 *lòu*), — and menstrual irregularities (月經不調 *yuè jīng bù tiáo*), which altogether constitute roughly one quarter of the "prescriptions for women." For the modern Western reader, the close connection between these pathological categories might not be obvious. Yet, as many prescriptions in this section show, the etiology, accompanying symptoms, and treatment of menstrual conditions and vaginal discharge overlap to a considerable degree and the placement of prescriptions in one or the other of these categories often seems arbitrary. An analysis of the historical development and etiological significance of this group of gynecological problems, often summarily referred to in Chinese as *dài xià*, will explain the difficulties Sūn Sī-Miǎo faced when compiling this section of his gynecological prescriptions. Since the category of *dài xià* — in the literal sense of "[diseases located] below the girdle" — was a key element in the formation of gynecology as a recognized and respected medical specialization in the following centuries, it is significant enough to be discussed in some detail here:

The most obvious link between the conditions of menstrual irregularity and vaginal discharge is the fact that both conditions often surface in the symptom of vaginal bleeding. Differentiated only by the timing of the bleeding in relation to the woman's menstrual cycle, it could be interpreted either as "red vaginal discharge" (赤帶 *chì dài*) or as menstrual fluid (月水 *yuè shuǐ*). A much stronger argument, however, crystallizes when we analyze the etiologies on which these categories are based. To complicate matters even further, it will be necessary to include in our discussion a third category of pathologies, namely abdominal masses or the "eight conglomerations" (八瘕 *bā jiǎ*), as they are referred to in the text. While not accorded a separate prescription section in the *Qiān Jīn Fāng*, this pathology does frequently appear as a key symptom in the section on vaginal discharge. It was clearly an important concern of literati physicians during this period, as is attested by the contents of contemporaneous medical texts: The *Wài Tái Mì Yào*, for example, lists twelve prescriptions for treating the eight conglomerations, as opposed to only ten for treating vaginal discharge and none at all for treating menstrual disorders; the *Ishimpō* contains four sections on menstrual disorders, two on vaginal discharge, and one on the eight conglomerations; the *Bìng Yuán Lùn*, lastly, devotes several sections to the varieties of abdominal masses, discussing the eight conglomerations in detail in a lengthy essay.

To understand the considerable confusion and overlap between the categories of vaginal discharge, menstrual irregularities, and abdominal masses in the *Qiān Jīn Fāng*, we need to take a closer look at the historical development of this etiological complex that is epitomized by the various uses of the term *dài xià*: As perhaps the earliest evidence for this term, the biography of the *Qín* period healer Biǎn Què 扁鵲 in the *Shǐ Jì* 史記 (Records of the Historian, most likely edited before 90 BCE) stresses his skills at treating women by referring to him as a 帶下醫 *dài xià yī* (physician of the region below the girdle). In a contemporary Chinese edition, a footnote glosses this term as "physician of gynecology" (婦科醫生 *fù kē yī shēng*) since "the conditions that trouble women (menstruation, vaginal discharge, pregnancy, and childbirth) are mostly related to the region below the girdling vessel [帶脈 *dài mài*]." It must be noted, however, that early medieval texts like the *Qiān Jīn Fāng* and *Bìng Yuán Lùn* do not yet emphasize the role of this vessel in their etiologies. Thus, the term must have originally referred not to the vessel in this location, but to the location of "below the girdle" itself. In the *Hàn* period text *Jīn Guì Yào Luè*, women's conditions are referred to as the "thirty-six diseases of women" (婦人三十六病 *fù rén sān shí liù bìng*) in the introduction. In the specific chapter on women, these are explained as "all being below the girdle" and summarized as "due to depletion, accumulated cold, and bound *qì*, causing the various [conditions of] interrupted menstruation . . ." In its most comprehensive meaning at this early period, Charlotte Furth has suggested, the term *dài xià* referred to "women's reproductive malfunctions in terms of an energy field holding the womb in place and regulating the flow of fluid discharges from the vagina." It might be significant, however, that the primary symptom of female pathology was, already at this early stage in the development of gynecology, identified as interrupted menstruation, a condition with potentially much broader consequences and connotations than a mere inability to reproduce.

The next text to attempt a categorization of women's symptoms by applying the structure of what it calls the "thirty-six diseases of *dài xià*" is the *Bìng Yuán Lùn*. Here, the entries on menstrual disorders immediately precede the entries on vaginal discharge, which are followed by sections on vaginal leaking, flooding (that is, profuse vaginal discharge or hemorrhaging), and various types of abdominal masses, concluding with an essay on the "thirty-six diseases of *dài xià*." The pathologies of menstrual inhibition and vaginal discharge are explained with almost identical etiologies: In both cases, the condition is ultimately caused by taxation damage to *qì* and blood, leading to physical vacuity and an invasion by wind and cold. This wind-cold lodges in the uterus and damages the channels, in particular the hand lesser *yīn* heart channel and the hand greater *yáng* small intestine channel, which are responsible for the descent of blood as menstrual fluid. Excessive cold causes the blood to congeal instead of flowing freely and being discharged as menstrual fluid (or turning into breast milk after childbirth or providing nurturance for the fetus during pregnancy). When *qì* is depleted and therefore unable to constrain and control blood, this pathology can easily turn into vaginal discharge in the various colors when "the blood in the channels is injured and therefore mixed with filthy fluids, forming vaginal discharge." The color of the discharge gives important etiological clues about which of the five viscera is primarily affected according to the five-phase association of viscera and colors, green pointing to the liver, yellow to the spleen, red to the heart, white to the lungs, and black to the kidneys. In the entry following the five entries on discharge in each of the five colors, an alternative etiological explanation links white discharge to the presence of excessive cold and red discharge to the presence of excessive heat.

The next entry, which introduces the pathological category of abdominal lumps, states that they are caused by an accumulation of cold *qì* and by a failure to disperse food and drink, causing them to lodge below the rib-sides instead. Several entries on specific types of accumulations repeatedly relate all of them to reproduction and menstruation, either because they are caused by childbirth-related depletion and weakness, or because they cause menstrual stoppage and interrupt women's ability to bear children. The *Bìng Yuán Lùn* then cites a list of "thirty-six diseases of *dài xià*," which is almost identical to Sūn Sī-Miǎo's list in the *Qiān Jīn Fāng*. The entry concludes with a reference to Zhāng Zhòng-Jǐng: "The thirty-six types of diseases mentioned by Zhāng Zhòng-Jǐng are all due to cold and heat and taxation damage in the uterus, causing [a woman] to suffer from vaginal discharge, arising inside the genitals...." Finally, supporting Furth's link of vaginal discharge, menstrual irregularities, and reproductive malfunctions, Cháo Yuán-Fāng concludes this volume with an essay on infertility. This is again related to taxation damage to *qì* and blood and an imbalance of heat and cold, causing wind-cold lodging in the uterus, blocked menstruation, flooding, or vaginal discharge. Faced with this confusion of categories based on symptoms related to menstruation, vaginal discharge, abdominal masses, and infertility, we might agree with Alfred North Whitehead that "classification is a halfway house between the immediate concreteness of the individual thing and the complete abstraction of mathematical notions... Classification is necessary. But unless you can progress from classification to mathematics, your reasoning will not take you very far."

Let us now turn to the *Qiān Jīn Fāng* and its medicinal prescriptions for the treatment of menstrual disorders and vaginal discharge. When interpreting the material from this clinical perspective, both categories are apparently interpreted as due to taxation damage. The resulting physical depletion then allows wind and cold to enter and impede the healthy flow of blood. Depending on the severity, this can surface merely as delayed or deficient menstrual flow, or it can lead to a total absence of menstruation. In that case, the menstrual fluid accumulates inside the abdomen and potentially forms painful masses or turns into vaginal discharge. While no clear-cut differentiation is possible, the prescriptions suggest a tendency by Sūn Sī-Miǎo to view menstrual problems mostly as a pathological inhibition or lack of the healthy and natural blood flow, that is, a problem of moving fluids around the body. By contrast, vaginal discharge is interpreted as a chronic problem of pathological leakage due to a general weakness of the body, requiring subtle differences in terms of treatment. These are, however, merely proportional differences since most prescriptions address both treatment aims and are intended to move blood as well as to supplement weakness.

In the first case of menstrual disorders, Sūn Sī-Miǎo predominantly employs strong blood-moving drugs like *táo rén* (桃仁 Seed of Prunus persica), *dà huáng* (大黃 Root of Rheum palmatum), and *shuǐ zhì* (水蛭 Dried body of Whitmania pigra), in conjunction with drugs for expelling pathogens like *xì xīn* (細辛 Complete plant including root of Asarum heteropoides) or *chái hú* (柴胡 Root of Bupleurum chinense). The potential use of such drugs, in TCM terminology summarized as "drugs that free the menses" (通經藥 *tōng jīng yào*), as abortifacients is well-recognized already in the early literature, but often not clearly distinguished. Sometimes, the list of symptoms associated with a blocked menstrual flow is, in fact, reminiscent of the Western category of morning sickness. The prescription for *Rehmannia and Chinese Angelica Pills* (乾地黃當歸丸 *gān dì huáng dāng guī wán*), for example, includes symptoms like "huffing and gasping and failure to eat and drink, ..., lack of interest in movement and activity; heaviness when lifting the limbs; only thinking of sleep and rest; desire to eat sour foods; and vacuity, jaundice, and emaciation." This category easily allowed a woman to present the symptoms of an unwanted pregnancy in such a way as to manipulate a physician to induce an abortion, without ever having to address the issue openly. On the other hand, amenorrhea was also recognized as a primary symptom of infertility. Other prescriptions therefore have the intended effect of inducing a pregnancy. In general, though, the prescriptions in this category are, at least on the surface, more concerned with the concrete and visible effect of freeing a blocked menstrual flow and therefore aim to stimulate the free movement of blood, *qì*, and fluids throughout the body.

While not clearly distinguished from the treatment of menstrual disorders except for the placement of prescriptions in one or the other category, the treatment of vaginal discharge points more towards a strategy of supplementing an underlying deficiency and strengthening the body as a whole. The prescriptions chosen by Sūn Sī-Miǎo therefore mostly contain strengthening, stabilizing, supplementing and *qì*-boosting drugs like *yǔ yú liáng* (禹餘糧 Limonite), *lóng gǔ* (龍骨 Os draconis), *rén shēn* (人參 Root of Panax ginseng), *lù róng* (鹿茸 Pilose antler of Cervus nippon), *dāng guī* (當歸 Root of Angelica polimorpha), and *sháo yào* (芍藥 Root of Paeonia albiflora). This category is clearly linked to fertility and the similarity to prescriptions for the treatment of seminal emission in men is noteworthy. Consequently, we find the warning in one prescription that "widows and virgins may not recklessly take this," and that "if she takes an excessive amount of this prescription, she will give birth to twins." In another prescription, absence of menstruation is mentioned merely as a secondary symptom and the root of the condition is a much deeper-lying disease: "After taking this medicine for fourteen days, she will discharge blood; after twenty days, long worms, and a clear or yellow liquid will come out; after thirty days, the illness will be expelled; and after fifty days, she will be fat and white." In cases of light but continuous vaginal discharge, it is referred to as "spotting discharge" (漏下 *lòu xià*); in its most serious form, it is called "center flooding" (崩中 *bēng zhōng*), indicating a heavy and unstoppable discharge of blood or other substances. The complexity of this situation is discussed in one of the rare explanatory essays: The health of a woman suffering from flooding is weakened severely, as if after childbirth. Therefore, strong medicinals for expelling pathogenic agents are contraindicated because they would tax her already endangered health even further. On the other hand, however, Sūn Sī-Miǎo offers the stern warning that "in the treatment of incessant leaking of blood, maybe caused by recent damage to the fetus or the fact that the residual blood after childbirth has not been dispersed but has solidified, which is preventing the entrance to the uterus from closing and is causing dribbling and dripping blood loss for several days and months without stopping, you may not yet use the various decoctions for interrupting the blood flow." In the ideal medical scenario, he suggests, "when the solidified blood has been dispersed, then the dribbling bleeding will stop on its own [since it is] also gradually being transformed, dispersed, and reduced." And yet again, Sūn Sī-Miǎo recognized the fact that life-threatening cases of excessive blood loss, such as from obstetrical complications, external injuries, or dental extractions, necessitated immediate action to stabilize the patient, which potentially ran counter to the advice above.

As this discussion shows, treatment strategies for vaginal discharge and bleeding had, by Sūn Sī-Miǎo's times, become quite numerous, diverse, and often conflicting. It is impossible to determine at this point to what extent the various strategies reflect developments over time or differences due to regional, class, or simply personal treatment styles. Nevertheless, it is not unreasonable to see in the contrasting statements above the seeds of a transformation of gynecology from "heroic" medical interventions aimed at immediate and visible results to a more refined awareness of the underlying causes of women's diseases, calling for long-term treatment aimed at restoring the body's strength and balance. In the framework of a specifically female-oriented medicine, this was based on the assumption that a woman's body, when restored to health with supplementing and stabilizing treatments, would naturally discharge pathological substances and resolve impediments in the free flow of blood and *qì*.

3d. Conclusion

The preceding pages have made it obvious that Sūn Sī-Miǎo's work is situated at a key point in the development of gynecology, when a clear awareness of the need for a separate treatment of female disorders had emerged. Nevertheless, a consensus, whether in theory or in practice, had yet to be formed on how this need was to be translated into etiological and therapeutic categories.

This is expressed not only in the contradictory treatment strategies discussed above, but also in the considerable confusion and overlap between etiological categories. Several centuries later, the physician and author Qí Zhòng-Fǔ 齊仲甫 criticized the treatment of vaginal discharge in the *Jīn Guì Yào Luè* in terms that could just as easily apply to the *Qiān Jīn Fāng*:

> The thirty-six types of diseases mentioned by Zhāng Zhòng-Jǐng are all due to cold and
> heat in the uterus and taxation vacuity, and are from there carried over to the genitals.
> The categorization of items is jumbled and confused and the prescriptions are all differ-
> ent. Nevertheless, [Zhāng] Zhòng-Jǐng's meaning is profound and not to be understood
> by foolish and shallow people. I fear that the writings are different, but the meaning is the
> same.

To illustrate this with the perhaps most obvious example, the lack of etiological distinctions between conditions associated with vaginal bleeding (referred to ambiguously as "flooding," *bēng*,
or "spotting," *lòu*) and vaginal discharge (*dài xià*) can be related to several factors: The term *bēng*
had two distinct meanings that were not clearly differentiated in early medical literature: Most
commonly called "center flooding" (崩中 *bēng zhōng*), it referred to a type of severe hemorrhaging that was related to "excessive taxation and activity damaging the viscera and bowels, leading
to vacuity of *qì* in the thoroughfare and controlling vessels and inability to control and restrain the
blood in the channels so that it is suddenly and violently discharged." Alternately, *bēng* was used
to refer to profuse vaginal discharge of different-colored fluids, as in the condition "five-colored
flooding" (五崩 *wǔ bēng*). It could therefore also surface as "profuse discharge like red juice" in
the case of "red flooding," a subcategory of "five-colored flooding" associated with the heart viscus by five-phase color correlation, or with the contraction of heat, in which case it was also called
"*yáng* flooding" (陽崩 *yáng bēng*). This was most commonly contrasted with "white flooding,"
a discharge of snivel-like fluids linked either to the contraction of cold or to disorders of the lung
viscus.

Similarly, the term *dài xià*, which usually referred to vaginal discharge, could also, in the form of
"red vaginal discharge," appear as bleeding when it was mixed with blood. Like in the etiology for
red flooding above, this was linked either to the presence of excessive heat or to depletion damage
in the heart viscus. A *Sòng* text shows the way this problem was finally resolved, clearly differen-
tiating between these symptoms:

> Incessant bleeding from the lower body is called 'center flooding.' A constant flow of foul
> fluids is what is referred to as 'vaginal discharge.' The loss of blood [associated with]
> center flooding is mostly caused by vacuity damage to the thoroughfare and controlling
> [vessels — and therefore related to the discharge of menstrual blood] or to damage to the
> constructive pathways. Cold in the girdling [vessel] and mixed discharge is mostly caused
> by instability below, complicated by an internal affliction with wind and cold.

During the *Sòng* period, the multiple and often overlapping or contradictory disease categories of
vaginal discharge were synthesized and reduced considerably. By contrast, menstrual disorders
came to be classified with an ever-increasing sophistication and attention to detail: Of the seven
new gynecological disease types proposed for the *Sòng* period by the contemporary medical historian Zhāng Zhì-Bīn 張志斌, three are concerned with varieties of menstrual problems. Moreover,
in addition to obstetrical complications, the categories of menstrual irregularities, painful menstruation, and menstrual stoppage are the three areas in gynecology that show the greatest innovation
in content from the *Táng* to the *Sòng* periods. The clarification and differentiation of menstrual
disorders began to take into account not only the timing and volume of the menstrual blood, but

also accompanying symptoms, their timing, and from the *Yuán* dynasty on, even the consistency and color of the blood. This can be related to a general development in gynecological literature where menstruation replaced vaginal discharge as the key symptom in gynecological diagnosis, "shifting the pathological sign from the foul to the unpredictable, from the physically repugnant to the measurably unreliable."

From the *Sòng* period on, the significance of menstruation and female bleeding for the diagnosis and treatment of the female body in Chinese medicine can hardly be overstated. It is perhaps best expressed in the well-known aphorism cited by practically every gynecological author from the *Sòng* period on that "blood is the root of women." As Chén Zì-Míng states in one of the greatest classics of Chinese gynecology, the *Fù Rén Dà Quán Liáng Fāng* 婦人大全良方, "Whenever treating disease, one first needs to discuss what [a particular case] is ruled by. In men, regulate their *qì*; in women, regulate their blood… Thus, in women, blood is the foundation. When *qì* and blood flow freely, their spirit is naturally clear."

To return to the beginning of this chapter and to Sūn Sī-Miǎo's statement regarding the need for "special prescriptions," *Sòng* gynecologists finally managed to integrate the diversity and complexity of treatments that had emerged in medieval China into a concise and yet comprehensive theoretical foundation. They succeeded in this by defining blood as the single underlying factor from which to approach the question of female difference.

4. Topics For Future Research

4a. General Issues

At least since the publication of *"The Mindful Body"* by Nancy Scheper-Hughes and Margaret M. Lock in 1989, it has been impossible for scholars to ignore the fact that medicine does not deal with an individual, physical, and objectively quantifiable human body as postulated by modern science, but with a complex and ever-changing combination of ideas, subjective experiences, and realities. This chapter will show that, in the case of female bodies in early China, the three bodies suggested instead by Scheper-Hughes and Lock — namely the phenomenological body, the social body, and the body politic — scratch merely the surface for understanding the many ways in which women and their healthcare providers interpreted and treated female bodies.

It is common knowledge by now that, in contrast to modern biomedical medicine, traditional Chinese medicine does not deal with a single and internally coherent explanatory model for interpreting the human body, but has always employed a number of often mutually contradictory concepts, depending on a variety of factors determined by the patient, her family, and the consulted healers. As Judith Farquhar points out:

> Not only the power to heal but also the complex power of knowledge in medical social life are derived from a collaboration between doctors and patients. This is not a submission of a sick body, a little piece of extradiscursive nature, to the power/knowledge of a medical master of nature; rather, it is an interlacing of two profoundly social specificities, in which the doctor's medical powers to embody and make history are brought to bear on the sufferer's contingent and active embodiment.

On the other hand, Francesca Bray reminds us in her study of reproductive technologies in late imperial China that any medical theories must always be rooted in the physical reality of the female body:

> When texts about bodies are what we have to work with, discourse and its political roots will loom larger in shaping our understanding of those bodies than it ever did in reality. It is important to remember, as Barbara Duden does, that the woman in the world cannot be detached from the woman beneath the skin.

While the nature of my primary sources, written texts by male, literate, elite physicians, admittedly limits the scope of the current exploration of early Chinese gynecology, it should at least suggest the possibility of posing interpretive questions that go far beyond what the author ever intended to communicate regarding the "woman beneath the skin."

Numerous studies have greatly enhanced our understanding of gynecology and the experience of women's bodies, in health and illness for the late imperial and early modern periods, based on such material as novels, case histories, or modern anthropological fieldwork. It is left to the reader's discretion to decide whether translating a medieval medical text on "prescriptions for women" might be a contribution to what Mark Nichter has described as the foundation of ethnomedicine, that is,

> ... the study of everyday life, perceptions of the normal and natural, the desirable and feared, and that form of embodied knowledge known as common sense as it emerges in efforts to establish or reestablish health as one aspect of well-being.

In the context of medieval China in general and Sūn Sī-Miǎo's prescriptions in particular, it is certainly beyond debate that "the afflicted body [is seen] as a space where competing ideologies are contested and emergent ideologies are developed through medico-religious practices and institutions, which guide the production of knowledge."

This rings particularly true in the context of the female body and the gendered medicine found in Sūn Sī-Miǎo's "prescriptions for women," since it is a case of a male literatus interpreting and giving advice, presumably to his male contemporaries, on how to respond to women's disorders and the particularities of the gendered body. Reinforced by culture-specific diagnostic techniques, most notably by limiting physical contact across gender boundaries, a male physician's diagnosis had by necessity to have been mediated through his female patient's personal testimony, rooted in her personal experience and reflecting her specific sense of embodiment. Nowhere in the *Qiān Jīn Fāng* — or, for that matter, elsewhere in medieval Chinese medical literature — can we find evidence of male doctors physically examining the intimate parts of women's bodies as part of a medical diagnosis. In stark contrast to the biomedical focus on anatomical structures and the concomitant objectification of women's bodies under the "medical gaze," Sūn Sī-Miǎo states in his summary on diagnosing symptoms: "The superior physician listens to sound; the mediocre physician examines the color [that is, the complexion]; the inferior physician diagnoses the pulse." Even in the contemporary Chinese context, Judith Farquhar has described the typical gynecological encounter in this way: "In contrast to the centrality of the pelvic examination in the Western practice of gynecology, with its fetishized arrangement of drapes over a disrobed body and asymmetrical placement of doctor and patient, the prototypical spatial arrangement of Chinese medical actors (their disposition in Bourdieu's sense of the word) is seated face to face at a corner of the table, talking."

Admittedly, it is impossible to reconstruct the exact nature of the patient-doctor encounter in medieval China. Nevertheless, Sūn Sī-Miǎo's detailed lists of highly personal symptoms such as the woman's emotional state including fears or dreams, subjective feelings in the limbs, or the color, consistency, and volume of menstrual blood, show once again that an accurate medical diagnosis and effective therapy had to be the result of the successful cooperation between patient and physician in a rather equal exchange of information. Again, it might help to cite what is perhaps the contemporary counterpart to medieval women's attention to their bodies. As Farquhar describes it:

> I have seen healthy and previously carefree young women who, having failed to conceive during the first year of marriage, became highly trained experts on their own bodily states when prompted by their doctors' questions. Slight feelings of chill or fever, headaches, periods of fatigue or irritability, the timing and colors of vaginal discharges, frequency and qualities of urination, and defecation are all monitored jointly by doctor and patient as they evaluate the effects of drugs and work towards increasing reproductive capacity.

This contrasts sharply with the Greek tradition where a male physician routinely examined female patients physically since he distrusted their words, and at the same time was forced to rely on female physicians for their intuitive knowledge regarding the female body. Thus, Lesley Dean-Jones has pointed out that, in the context of Hippocratic gynecology, "there is a paradox between on the one hand the Hippocratics' access to autopsia [that is, personal inspection] of women's bodies and their negative opinion of historia [that is, illness narratives] from women patients and, on the other hand, their comparatively frequent deference to the authority of women [medical authors]." She suggests that this constant "need [of male Greek authors] to cite female sources to validate their claims to knowledge" was due to their awareness that they lacked suneidesis, the "innate awareness of one's own body," when it came to understanding women's bodies, since they did not possess a uterus, the distinct anatomical organ that gynecology was intimately linked to.

As first described by Charlotte Furth and elaborated by Francesca Bray, "In dealing with women's bodies, Chinese physicians were not faced with this issue of understanding the other, because sex differences were conceived of as a question of degree rather than one of essential nature." It is important, however, not to be misled by what Charlotte Furth has so appropriately called the "androgynous body" and to draw the general conclusion made by Lisa Raphals, based mostly on nonmedical literature, that "men and women are medically identical, with few and specified exceptions involving sexuality and childbirth."

The perception and interpretation of identities, similarities, and differences between male and female bodies is a complex issue that has not been resolved in the early European context either. Contrast, for example, Dean-Jones' assertions above with a fourth century quotation by Nemesius, bishop of Emesa in Syria: "Women have the same genitals as men, except that theirs are inside the body and not outside it." This has led Emily Martin to the conclusion that in the European context, "from the ancient Greeks until the late eighteenth century...male and female bodies were structurally similar." In the Chinese case, Raphals' conclusion of the basic identity of male and female bodies is directly contradicted by the very first sentence in Sūn Sī-Miǎo's prescriptions, which explains the need for women's "separate prescriptions." Raphals' entire chapter on "yin-yang in medical texts" is based on only three sources, the *Wǔ Shí Ér Bìng Fāng* from Mǎ-Wáng-Duī, Chún-Yú Yì's biography in the *Shǐ Jì*, and references to *yīn-yáng* and gender in the *Huáng Dì Nèi Jīng*. In spite of this, it purports to represent the general attitude of Chinese physicians in later times, only slightly modified after the *Sòng* and *Míng* periods. She sums up her discussion, unfortunately without citing her sources, saying that "later texts pointedly state that the viscera of women and men are identical and stress the tacit equivalence of men and women from a medical viewpoint."

To be sure, Sūn Sī-Miǎo also states that, for illnesses other than those covered in his "prescriptions for women," women should be treated identically to men. However, a theoretical insistence on the basic identity of male and female bodies must always be balanced with an investigation of its application in clinical practice. And this is precisely where the significance of prescription literature lies: The conception of female difference by male literati in medieval China is, unfortunately, never addressed explicitly in the *Qiān Jīn Fāng* or other contemporaneous prescription texts. It is immediately apparent, though, that Sūn Sī-Miǎo deliberately placed the "prescriptions for women" at the very beginning of the text to stress the need for "separate prescriptions" for women. Thus, he obviously recognized the basic fact that women's bodies — and therefore ideas about their health, etiologies, vulnerabilities, and therapies, — differed substantially from men's, necessitating a separate category of medical knowledge.

In order to clarify this issue further, it may be helpful for future interpretive research to approach the text translated below from three angles, namely in terms of women's functional, physiological, and gendered difference, related to the etiological categories of reproduction, menstruation and vaginal discharge, and miscellaneous gendered diseases: The organization of the Chinese material into these three separate categories of female difference might appear artificial or farfetched at first sight, and there is indeed a fair amount of overlap between the sections. Nevertheless, the outline of the actual text indicates that Sūn Sī-Miǎo himself organized his information along very similar lines of thinking and seems therefore to have perceived female difference in related terms. Furthermore, the first paragraph in his introduction appears to adopt these three etiological categories as the justification for women's "separate prescriptions" by mentioning in the order of significance childbearing, menstruation, and other factors such as susceptibility to wind and emotional instability. In the following paragraphs, I indicate some directions for future research, suggested by other scholars' work in each of these categories:

4b. Reproduction

The first category, women's diseases related to reproduction, or in medical terms the categories of fertility, pregnancy, obstetrical complications, postpartum recovery, and lactation, represent by far the largest and at the same time the most obvious aspect of what any culture would recognize as "women's medicine," namely the difference in function between male and female bodies. On a most obvious level, the processes of conception, pregnancy, childbirth, and lactation are used as evocative metaphors for describing cosmic creation through the complementary interplay of *yīn* and *yáng*. In addition, the medical conceptualization of the male and female contributions to the creation of the fetus can inform our image of male and female roles in society at large. In this context, it is perhaps significant that the focus of fertility prescriptions changed from ritual, astrological, and other instructions regarding sexual intercourse, found in the medical category of "arts of the bedchamber" (房術 *fáng shù*) and directed at men, to medicinal prescriptions aimed at replenishing women's deficiencies and imbalances. In the contemporary context, Judith Farquhar has described the popularity and evocativeness of fertility prescriptions and fertility-boosting meals for middle-aged men in post-socialist China.

As is still the case in late imperial Chinese medicine, Sūn Sī-Miǎo's prescriptions see the father's reproductive role as limited to supplying essence during conception. The mother's role, on the other hand, includes not only the physical contribution of essence during conception, but also of blood, by nourishing the fetus during pregnancy in the uterus and when it turns to breast milk after childbirth. Furthermore, it also includes the moral responsibility of "fetal education," (*tāi jiào*) that is, molding the personality of the fetus by proper behavior and lifestyle during the course of pregnancy. This can be contrasted with the Western theory of a single seed supplied by the father, which was promoted by Aristotle, but debated by Galen who suggested that women also supplied a seed, albeit of a lesser kind.

Although not yet explicitly noted as such in the *Qiān Jīn Fāng*, from the *Sòng* period on, the notion of "fetal poison" (胎毒 *tāi dǔ*) directly linked maternal behavior during pregnancy to infant health, in particular to the high smallpox-induced infant mortality rate, through the potential pollution of the fetus from the heat of the mother's affects. Chinese reproductive theories have always emphasized the connections between body, psyche, and morality, since "a biological mother's fertility depended on her natural endowments but also on her behavior; the vigor, fortitude, and equanimity required of a good social mother were achieved in part through her conscious control of natural emotions whose roots lay in the equilibrium of the internal organs." In addition, Sūn Sī-Miǎo's prescriptions also reflect a clear precedence of the mother's health over the life of the fetus, and suggest a considerable freedom of choice accorded to women in the context of "regulating menstruation" for aborting unwanted pregnancies. While Charlotte Furth stresses that "the desire for an abortion could remain inarticulate and so relatively blameless," Francesca Bray's discussion of "Reproductive Hierarchies" modifies this somewhat by elaborating on a woman's power limitations due to hierarchies of age, status, and gender. Instead, she suggests that "flexibility of reproductive maneuver was restricted to high-ranking women and depended on exploiting the inequalities within female hierarchies." Challenging any orientalizing stereotypes of Chinese women as oppressed and powerless in the patriarchal Confucian family of traditional China, one only needs to contrast the above with modern Western discussions of abortion and pregnancy that stress, for example, "the legal double standard concerning the bodily integrity of pregnant and nonpregnant bodies, the construction of women as fetal incubators, the bestowal of 'super-subject' status to the fetus, and the emergence of a father's-rights ideology."

Finally, the topic of midwifery and the medical management of childbirth is a subject that has been explored successfully by innumerable scholars in an ever-growing range of cultures and time periods. Jender Lee has contributed invaluably to our understanding of actual practices in early and medieval China and to issues of women's involvement as providers of medical care, although her publications are unfortunately mostly in Chinese and have therefore been inaccessible to most Western scholars. Chinese scholars have also compiled early Chinese childbirth-related taboos, rituals, and popular customs from religious, medical, literary and other sources, and compared them to marriage and burial taboos. How these topics are reflected specifically in the *Qiān Jīn Fāng* is a question that certainly deserves future attention. The information contained there and translated below could doubtlessly add valuable insights, in particular to the topics of pollution and postpartum seclusion and taboos, which Jender Lee relates to the significance of childbirth as a social rite of passage for the new mother. Emily M. Ahern has written an entire article on "*The Power and Pollution of Chinese Women*" in the context of twentieth-century rural Taiwan, but Charlotte Furth stresses with regard to medical views on female pollution that "threatening symbols of female sexual power were replaced by benign symbols of female generativity and weakness that moderated pollution taboos and permitted an interpretation of gender based on paternalism, pity and protection." Jender Lee's research and the content of the *Qiān Jīn Fāng* appear to concur with this assessment.

This is an area that is obviously difficult to approach exclusively through the lens of male-authored elite medical texts from the medieval period. In light of the absence of women's voices or other perspectives on medieval childbirth, a critical application of modern ethnographical research, from Chinese as well as other Asian cultures, can at times sharpen our sensitivities to issues that would perhaps not be apparent otherwise and prevent us from unconsciously imposing our modern, ethnocentric views in instances where an author's underlying assumptions are not stated explicitly. Dorothea Sich, for example, contrasts the Western stereotype of pregnant women being "of good hope" and having to be protected diligently throughout pregnancy with the traditional Korean insistence on hard work right up to delivery. One can also cite here the common Southeast Asian practice of "mother roasting" (the practice of exposing the new mother to strong heat immediately after delivery), as described by Lenore Manderson in the Malaysian context, and other childbirth practices and beliefs, which have been studied, for example, among Thai and Hmong women. Moreover, research that stresses the social construction of the medical authority of childbirth can alert a discerning reader to power struggles between different categories of healers and actors that might have influenced the composition of prescriptions chosen by Sūn Sī-Miǎo in his obstetrical section.

4c. Physiology

To our modern eyes, reproduction is closely related to the second category of female difference discussed here, namely the features that set the female body apart physiologically. In the *Qiān Jīn Fāng*, they appear in the medical categories of menstruation and vaginal discharge. As the prescription translation below will show, fertility and the possibility of pregnancy was only a minor aspect in the treatment of menstrual irregularities, a highly evocative symptom of the female body's health understood in terms of the circulation of its vital fluids. Current anthropological publications on menstruation are as numerous and varied as those on childbirth and have undergone many refinements over the past two decades.

This development was perhaps at least partly stimulated by Emily Martin's publication of *The Woman in the Body*, an eye-opening feminist critique of the supposed objectivity of scientific writing about women's bodies. In this ground-breaking work, she compared, for example, the two analogous processes of menstruation, that is, the monthly shedding of the uterus, and the regular shedding of the stomach lining:

> One can choose to look at what happens to the lining of the stomachs and uteruses negatively as breakdown and decay needing repair or positively as continual production and replenishment. Of these two sides of the same coin, stomachs, which women and men have, fall on the positive side; uteruses, which only women have, fall on the negative."
> As if elaborating on the medieval Chinese view of the menstrual cycle, she suggests that "it might capture the sense of events better to say the purpose of the cycle is the production of menstrual flow.

And indeed, approaching the menstrual cycle from a positive angle, traditional Chinese medical literature can be said to express the view that "female health evoked metaphors of easy circulation, reliable periodicity and free flow of blood. These images resonated with an organismic cosmology of harmonious parts, orderly in their movements and interpenetrating without hindrance." Similarly, in the case histories of an eighteenth century German physician, "what distinguished women from men in the view of Storch and the authors he cites was not their monthly bleeding as such but solely the periodic nature of the bleeding or discharge of fluids from the body. Therefore, women, with their disposition to spontaneous discharges, were less threatened by plethora (overfullness), that is, illness, than men." The logical conclusion of this image is, of course, the common European therapy of bloodletting, an artificial discharge of blood performed to treat a large range of disorders, especially in men. Shigehisa Kuriyama has elaborated on this theme in his comparison of European bloodletting and Chinese acupuncture.

In spite of the fact that *Qiān Jīn Fāng* is primarily concerned with the clinical treatment of pathology, a careful reading of the prescriptions for women, as well as a detailed comparison with male-specific illness categories, could provide additional perspectives on questions about the significance of female blood and its loss, and on the extent to which menstruation was interpreted as a healthy discharge of excess rather than a pathogenic loss of vital fluid, as in contemporary biomedicine. In this context, Sūn Sī-Miǎo's elaborate and highly detailed section on the various types of vaginal discharge is certainly suggestive of medical ideas regarding women's health that centered to a large extent on the circulation of bodily fluids. This topic could benefit particularly from a detailed study of male-centered prescriptions, which would presumably express a perceived shortcoming in male physiology related to a male failure to discharge excess fluids regularly. Past studies on menstrual taboos have generally focused on the negative symbolism inherent in the "pollution" of female blood, such as in the evocative book title "*The Curse: A Cultural History of Menstruation,*" a collection of essays on the subject edited by Janice Delaney. Although coming from a context that couldn't be further removed in time or place, Elisa Sobo's interpretation of Jamaican menstrual taboos can alert us to the multiplicity of meanings and uses that a specific taboo can carry for the individual participant, depending on gender, age, social status, and a complex web of interpersonal relationships. This type of research should serve as a cautionary reminder for historians who might be tempted to read certain taboos, described only from a male perspective in early texts, as statements about women's oppression or liberation, as has often been done even by anthropologists working in the context of contemporary cultures.

4d. The Truly Gendered Body

Although they only constitute a small percentage of the gynecological prescriptions in the *Qiān Jīn Fāng*, the sections on "miscellaneous disease" and "supplementing and boosting" lastly offer yet another range of interpretative possibilities and insights. More directly than in the preceding two categories, some prescriptions in these sections point to a truly gendered body. Ideas about women's health and illness reflected here are rooted not in any functional or physiological differences, but in culturally constructed notions of gender-specific vulnerabilities and weaknesses that reflect the realities of gendered existence in medieval Chinese society. An assessment of what these prescriptions might imply for women's social status would certainly constitute a significant and needed contribution to our fragmentary knowledge about women in medieval China.

To cite just one example, the placement and treatment of a condition known as "intercourse with ghosts" (與鬼交通 *yǔ guǐ jiāo tōng*), a female pathological category found also in other medieval literature, raises a host of fascinating questions: In the *Bìng Yuán Lùn* it is explained in terms very similar to the pathology of wind evil as caused by depletion in the viscera that weakens the hold of the spirit and thereby allows ghosts to invade, manifesting as "inability to recognize people, speaking and laughing as if interacting with an invisible presence, and occasional crying and grief." Apparently, "intercourse" refers here not necessarily to sexual intercourse, but to any sort of interaction with supernatural entities. Contrary to cases of spirit possession, the ghost does not possess the host, but remains an external presence engaging the mind of the afflicted. In the *Ishimpō*, however, this interaction clearly has sexual overtones, evident from the etiology of the illness being "lack of intercourse between *yīn* and *yáng* [a common euphemism for sexual intercourse] causing deep and intense desires and wants." This is further supported also by the treatment, which here consists of advice to "make the woman have intercourse with a man, do not allow them to spill essence, day and night without stopping. If she tires, do not exceed seven days…"

Why does the pathological category of "intercourse with ghosts" strike our modern sensibilities as strange? What does it say about cultural values regarding sexual intercourse, lack thereof, women's vulnerabilities, and issues of control? Who was held responsible? Who determined the pathology and the appropriate treatment? Does the text reflect different layers of knowledge, potentially the elite male educated physician and his complex medicinal therapies versus illiterate (?) female healers, itinerant — male and/or female — drug peddlers, the patient, her parents, husband, mother-in-law or other social actors? How could different interpretations affect therapy, place blame, and empower or control the suffering woman? How is this related to notions of demonic possession or shamanism and ideas of women as vessels for male spirits? A comprehensive investigation of this topic will also have to address the role of dreams in Chinese culture, equivalents in male prescriptions for intercourse with (female) spirits, the physiological effects of lack of intercourse, the relationship between *yīn*, the supernatural, and femininity, etc.

Ultimately, the pathology of intercourse with ghosts and its links to sexuality could be usefully explored by comparison to medieval European concepts, such as the theory about suffocatio matricum by the German physician Alexander Seitz: Manifesting in the symptoms of loss of consciousness, failure to discern between good and bad, and the possibility of being buried alive, this condition was explained as due to the fact that women also produced semen that, if not emptied from the uterus during intercourse, could accumulate there and transform pathologically into noxious vapors that could cause the woman's hysterical suffocation from intoxication.

A careful analysis of the prescriptions and symptoms treated under the category of "supplementing and boosting" can also offer insights into the cultural construction of illness by suggesting recurring themes, specifically women's vulnerability to wind and the destabilizing effect of uncontrolled emotions. For examples from other cultures on approaching these concepts, we might look at the extensive anthropological literature on "culture-bound syndromes," in particular studies on hysteria in Victorian England, modern research on dieting and anorexia, and other specifically or predominantly female disorders such as latah in the Malay-Indonesian culture, susto in Hispanic-American cultures, or nerves in a variety of cultural contexts. Lastly, the possibility not only of women's resistance to the dominant medical ideology, but more poignantly of their conscious manipulation thereof for their own agendas, such as in self-initiated medicalization, also needs to be taken into consideration in any discussion of women's status as seen through male medical literature.

Given the complexity of these issues, the following translation is intended merely as a first step by providing a textual foundation. At times, I might indicate certain directions from which the data could be interpreted in the translation footnotes, but the reader should always bear in mind that these are never meant as conclusive statements. Until just recently, scholars have had to assert even the simple fact that "the history of women in imperial China, however invisible, was knowable." Dorothy Ko's study of the restrictions and freedoms experienced by elite women reading and writing in the seventeenth century, for example, shows that "the invention of an ahistorical 'Chinese tradition' that is feudal, patriarchal, and oppressive was the result of a rare confluence of three divergent ideological and political traditions — the May Fourth-New Culture Movement, the Communist revolution, and Western feminist scholarship." Since scholarship on the early history of Chinese gynecology, or the early medieval period in general, is still in the data-collecting stage, this book therefore refrains purposely from interpretations as to what a certain practice, condition, constellation of symptoms, or choice of treatment might have indicated in terms of women's status in society.

5. Conclusion

To conclude this introduction, when I set out on my initial dissertation research as an eager graduate student, I intended to compose a detailed history of the origins of Chinese gynecology, as a continuation into the deeper past of Charlotte Furth's exploration of gender and medicine from the *Sòng* period on. Given the lack of secondary research in this field, however, this soon proved to be impossible. It is my hope that this translation of one of the key texts in the formation of Chinese gynecology might draw the reader's attention to the potential and need for further research on some of the issued raised by this material, whether from a historical, medical, feminist, anthropological, or other perspective. As this book demonstrates, it has become impossible to cite a lack of primary data as an excuse for neglecting women's medical treatment in medieval China. During the past few decades, the meticulous work of Chinese historians and editors has provided the interested Chinese-literate reader with philologically sound critical editions of the major medical texts in the long history of medicine in China. Sinologists have finally accepted medicine, and science in general, as a legitimate field of academic inquiry, on a par with such traditionally valued disciplines as religion or philosophy. The achievements of medical anthropology, although primarily based on research in contemporary contexts, have indicated the potential of the human, and particularly the female, body, in medical and other treatments, as an evocative site for the negotiation of cultural values. This awareness of the significance of medicine as a source for historical information regarding a culture's notions about self, other, nature, society, gender, the universe, and many other significant topics, has sparked exciting research into the history of medicine both in China and the West. Nevertheless, much work remains to be done and this book most definitely raises more questions than it answers. Rather than devoting a separate lifetime of study to each of such topics as medieval medicine, gender, the clinical interpretation and significance of the "prescriptions for women," or the intellectual background and specific literary influences on Sūn Sī-Miǎo's writings, I hope that other scholars with training in these fields will respond to the information provided here with further publications.

Bèi Jí Qiān Jīn Yào Fāng

備急千金要方

Volume 2

卷第二

1. Seeking a Child 求子

LINE 1.1

(一) 論曰：夫婦人之別有方者，以其[1] 胎妊生產崩傷之異故也。是以婦人之病，比之男子十倍難療。(二) 經言：婦人者，眾陰所集，常與濕居。十四己上，陰氣浮溢，百想經心，內傷五藏，外損姿顏。月水去留，前後交互，瘀血停凝，中道斷絕。(三) 其中傷墮，不可具論。生熟二藏，虛實交錯，惡血內漏，氣脈損竭。或飲食無度，損傷非一，或瘡痍未愈，便合陰陽，或便利於懸廁之上，風從下入，便成十二痼疾，所以婦人別立方也。

(1) Essay: The reason why women have special prescriptions is that they are different because of pregnancy, childbirth, and flooding damage.[2] Therefore, women's diseases are ten times more difficult to treat than men's.

(2) It is a classic saying that "women are copious accumulations of *yīn* and are constantly inhabited by dampness."[3] From the age of fourteen on, [a woman's] *yīn qì* floats up and spills over, [causing] a hundred thoughts to pass through her heart. Internally, it damages the five viscera; externally, it injures the outward appearance. The discharge and retention of menstrual fluid is alternatingly early or delayed, stagnant blood lodges and congeals, and the central pathways[4] are interrupted and cut off.

(3) It is impossible to discuss the entirety of damages and losses[5] among these [conditions]. The raw and the cooked are deposited together,[6] vacuity and repletion intermingle with each other in confusion, malign blood[7] leaks internally, and the *qì* and vessels are injured and exhausted. Her intake of food and drink might have been intemperate, causing not just a single injury. Or she may have had sexual intercourse before [vaginal] sores have healed. Or she may have squatted over the privy without proper care, [allowing] wind to enter from below and thereby giving rise to the twelve intractable diseases. For these reasons, special prescriptions have been established for women.

---

1. The *Sūn Zhēn Rén* edition and a quotation in *Wài Tái Mì Yào* contain the additional phrase 血氣不調 "...the fact that their blood and *qì* are not balanced, and..." (《外台秘要》33).

2. 崩傷 *bēng shāng*: Literally referring to the collapse of earth, as in a landslide, the term *bēng* had by early *Táng* times become a technical medical term indicating a flood-like loss of blood and other varieties of vaginal discharge, caused by the collapse of the internal organs. As such, it was the most serious type of vaginal discharge, more severe than 賁 *bēn* (gushing) and 漏 *lòu* (spotting). In its modern TCM usage, the condition is explained as "heavy menstrual flow or abnormal bleeding via the vagina" (Wiseman and Féng, *Practical Dictionary*, p. 212; see also 謝觀《中華醫學大辭典》 p. 1288).

By contrast, medieval medical writers associated the term also with a collapse of the internal organs. According to the *Bìng Yuán Lùn* 病源論 for example, the etiology of 崩 involved the collapse of any or all of the five internal organs, thereby causing discharge in the corresponding colors (《病源論》 38:40-44). This usage is also employed by Sūn Sī-Miǎo in such expressions as 五崩 *wǔ bēng* (five-colored flooding), which refers to vaginal discharge in the five colors, or 崩中 *bēng zhōng* (center flooding). In the introductory statement above, the term is used in its broadest sense to refer to the variety of conditions related to vaginal discharge, which are also often summarized as 婦人三十六病 *fù rén sān shí liù bìng* (women's thirty-six diseases), as in (《千金方》 4:3), (《病源論》 38:50) and (《金匱要略》 1).

3.   The origin of this statement is unclear, but could quite possibly stem from an originally Sanskrit source because of its closeness to humoral theory. Sūn Sī-Miǎo's familiarity with Indian medicine is obvious from numerous references throughout the *Qiān Jīn Fāng* 千金方.

4.   中道 *zhōng dào*: While this is not a standard medical term, it most likely refers to the pathways in the central region of the body, related to the spleen and stomach and more commonly known as 水穀之道 *shuǐ gǔ zhī dào* (pathways of water and grains), which together comprise the center burner and govern the decomposition of water and grains. See for example 《難經》 31, translated in Paul U. Unschuld, *Nanching*, p. 347.

5.   In a gynecological context, the character 墮 *duò* has the strong connotation of "miscarriage," as in the compound 墮胎 *duò tāi*. In the phrase above, however, it can be understood in the more general sense of "losing" or "falling," or even in the sense of "breakdown," in which case it is pronounced *huì*.

6.   生熟二藏 *shēng shú èr cáng*: Based on the parallel construction of the next phrase, 虛實交錯, I read 藏 as a verb. Alternatively, 二藏 could denote the two organs of spleen and stomach since this section is concerned with the digestion of food in the central region of the body. In an interpretation less likely but more elegant perhaps for the modern reader, the *Rén Mín* edition has altered the entire sentence, based on the quotation of this sentence in *Wài Tái Mì Yào*: 生 *shēng* is read as 矣 *yǐ*, a sentence end particle of the preceding phrase (《外台秘要》 33). The following phrase then reads: 然五臟虛實交錯 Then vacuity and repletion in the five viscera alternate with each other in confusion. But since most other editions, such as the *Sūn Zhēn Rén* edition, the *Huá Xià* edition, as well as the *Dào Zāng* and *Sì Kù Quán Shū* editions, contain the first version, I see no reason to simplify the text in such a manner.

7.   惡血 *è xuè*: This is a common technical term referring to the blood that remains in a woman's body after childbirth. Also called 惡露 *è lù* (malign dew), it is considered a highly pathogenic substance, which must be discharged completely or it will cause permanent and serious health problems for the rest of the woman's life. See the Translator's note at the beginning of the chapter on "malign dew," chapter five of volume three on p. 318.

LINE 1.2

(一) 若是四時節氣為病，虛實冷熱為患者，故與丈夫同也，惟懷胎妊娠而挾病者，避其毒藥耳。其雜病與丈夫同，則散在諸卷中，可得而知也。 (二) 然而，女人嗜欲多於丈夫，感病倍於男子。加以慈戀愛憎嫉妒憂恚，染著堅牢，情不自抑，所以為病根深，療之難瘥。

(1) In cases where the nodal *qì* over the four seasons[1] has caused illness and where vacuity or repletion of cold or heat have caused worry, then [women are treated] the same as men, the only exception being that if they fall ill while carrying a fetus in pregnancy, you must avoid toxic medicines! In cases where their miscellaneous diseases are identical to men's, [the treatments] are dispersed throughout the various volumes and can be known from there.

(2) Nevertheless, women's predilections and desires exceed mens' and they contract diseases at twice the rate of men. In addition, when they are affected by compassion and attachment, love and hatred, envy and jealousy, and worry and rancor, these become firmly lodged and deep-seated. Since they are unable to control their affects by themselves, the roots of their diseases are deep and it is difficult to obtain a cure in their treatment.

1.   四時節氣 *sì shí jié qi*: According to the solar calendar, the Chinese year is divided into four seasons (四時 *sì shí*) and twenty-four nodes (二十四節 *èr shí sì jié*). "Nodal *qì*" refers here to a certain type of *qì* that causes illness because it appears out of its proper season.

LINE 1.3

(一) 故養生之家，特須教子女學習此三卷婦人方，令其精曉，即於倉卒之秋，何憂畏也。(二) 夫四德者，女子立身之樞機。產育者，婦人性命之長務。若不通明於此，則何以免於夭枉者哉。故傳母之徒亦不可不學。常宜繕寫一本，懷挾隨身，以防不虞也。

(1) Therefore, a specialist in nurturing life[1] should particularly instruct his[2] sons and daughters[3] to study these three volumes of prescriptions for women until they comprehend them thoroughly. Then what would there be to worry or fear even in the face of a harvest of unexpected surprises?[4]

(2) Now, the Four Virtues[5] are the pivot around which daughters set up their life. Bearing children is the adult role in women's destiny and fate. If you do not understand this clearly, how could you prevent premature and wrongful death? Neither, for this reason, can servants engaged in childrearing[6] afford not to study it.[7] Thus, they should routinely write out a copy and carry it on their person, clutched to their bosom, in order to guard against the unexpected.

1.   養生之家 *yǎng shēng zhī jiā*: A person engaged in longevity and good health practices, including breathing exercises, sexual cultivation, gymnastics, and diet. For a detailed discussion of the origin and extent of these practices in the early *Hàn* period, see Harper, *Early Chinese Medical Literature*, pp. 110-147.

2.   Throughout this translation, the male pronoun is used deliberately. Based on comments interspersed in this text and in consideration of the general cultural context, I have come to the conclusion that Sūn Sī-Miǎo was addressing his text to an elite male audience from a social background similar to his. As this paragraph shows, he intended these volumes to be used by literate male heads of household to interact in an informed manner with the

women under his roof and their predominantly female healthcare providers. To what extent this took the form of control or support, hierarchical instruction, mutually beneficial cooperation, or open or hidden rivalry must have depended on the individual context and a variety of factors such as the composition and social status of the household, the status of the patient within the family, and the education and skills of each male and female actor.

3. 　子女 *zǐ nǚ*: This expression is ambiguous and could be interpret either as "sons and daughters" or as "female offspring" (see 諸橋轍次，主編《大漢和辭典》 #6930-637, which gives both definitions).

4. 　倉卒之秋 *cāng zú zhī qiū*: The *Sūn Zhēn Rén* edition has 際 *jì* "occasion" instead of 秋.

5. 　四德 *sì dé*: A reference to the four womanly virtues, i.e., proper behavior (德 *dé*), words (言 *yán*), demeanor (容 *róng*), and work (功 *gōng*).

6. 　傅母之徒 *fù mǔ zhī tú*: The *Rén Mín* edition (p. 36, n. 2) explains this expression as 古代保育，輔導子女的老年男女 "elderly men and women charged with rearing and guiding the sons and daughters in elite households in ancient times." It paraphrases the compound as 傅，傅父；母，保姆 "tutors and nannies." See also (《辭源》 p. 247) for a similar reading.

7. 　While the connection between maternal health and the survival and welfare of children is fairly obvious (especially in the context of infertility), the importance of this text for child-rearing personnel is less clear. In my opinion, this does not only imply that the servants were supposed to educate children in the content of these prescriptions. More significantly, this points at the close links and overlapping responsibilities in elite households between mothers, their own healthcare providers, and their children's wet-nurses, nannies, and tutors. See 李貞德《漢唐之間的女性醫療照顧者》.

LINE 1.4

(一) 論曰：人之情性皆願賢己，而疾不及人。至於學問，則隨情逐物，墮於事業，詎肯專一推求至理。莫不虛棄光陰，沒歲無益。 (二) 夫婚姻養育者，人倫之本，王化之基。聖人設教，備論厥旨。後生莫能精曉，臨事之日，昏爾若愚。是則徒願賢己而疾不及人之謬也。 (三) 斯實不達賢己之趣，而妄徇虛聲以終無用。 (四) 今具述求子之法，以貽後嗣。同志之士，或可覽焉。

(1) Essay: It is the nature of people that they wish to consider themselves worthy and dislike not attaining the level of others.[1] In scholarship, if people follow their affects to pursue [material] things and slack off in their responsibilities and duties, how could they be capable of concentrating on the pursuit of the ultimate principle? Without exception, they will have wasted their precious time in vain and end their days without any gains.

(2) Now marriage and childrearing are the basis of human affairs and the foundation of enlightened rule.[2] The sages set out the teachings and completely discussed their purport. Among later generations, none are able to fully comprehend their meaning any more, and, on the day when they undertake a job, they are muddle-headed like simpletons. This is to commit the error of vanity, wishing to consider yourself worthy and disliking not attaining the level of others.

(3) In fact, it does not bring you closer to the goal of considering yourself worthy but is a reckless pursuit of hollow sounds, useless in the end.

(4) At present, I offer a description of the methods for seeking a child[3] in order to bestow descendants. Gentlemen of like intention might want to inspect them.

1.   This is an allusion to the Analects by Confucius (《論語》 4:17: 見賢思齊焉 "to see worthiness and to desire to equal it.")

2.   王化 *wáng huà*: Literally "a king's transformation," i.e., a true king's rule by the power of his virtuous example.

3.   求子 *qiú zǐ*: The medical category of fertility prescriptions.

LINE 1.5

(一) 論曰：夫欲求子者，當先知夫妻本命五行相生，及與德合，並本命不在子休廢死墓中者，則求子必得。若其本命五行相剋，及與刑殺衝破，並在子休廢死墓中者，則求子了不可得，慎無措意。縱或得者，於後終亦累人。(二) 若其相生並遇福德者，仍須依法如方，避諸禁忌，則所誕生兒子盡善盡美，難以具陳矣。

(1) Essay: Now, when wanting to seek a child, you must first ascertain that the husband and wife's basic destinies follow the mutual generation of the five phases[1] and match with [the astrological position of] virtue.[2] And if, in addition, their basic destinies are not situated at *zǐ xiū*, *fèi sǐ*, or *mù zhōng*[3], then their seeking a child is bound to be successful. If [however] their basic destinies are in a relation of mutual conquest among the five phases, if they run into [the astrological positions of] punishment and death,[4] or if they are located in *zǐ xiū*, *fèi sǐ*, or *mù zhōng*, then their seeking a child will be utterly impossible.[5] Take great care to make no mistakes when considering this! Even if [a child] is obtained, it will later also ultimately implicate other persons.

(2) If [their basic destinies] are mutually engendering and in addition meet with [the position of] auspicious virtue, you must still follow the methods in these recipes and avoid the various prohibitions and taboos.[6] Then, the child born will be of such utter goodness and beauty that it is difficult to describe exhaustively!

*   For the remainder of this translation, we have placed translation of the *Sòng* commentary in the footnotes, marked as "*Sòng* editors' notes," in spite of the fact that some modern Chinese editions treat these notes as an integral part of the *Qiān Jīn Fāng* text. It is, however, unlikely that they came from Sūn Sī-Miǎo's hand because they are generally not found in the *Sūn Zhēn Rén* edition, which predates the *Sòng* editions. These comments, which mostly compare the prescriptions in the *Qiān Jīn Fāng* with similar prescriptions in other texts, are significant for locating Sūn Sī-Miǎo's prescriptions in the textual tradition of prescription literature, most which has been lost since. Commentary from modern editions, when found helpful to the modern Western reader, is translated and identified as such in the footnotes.

1.   本命五行相生 *běn mìng wǔ xíng xiāng shēng*: This means that the husband's and wife's birth phases must be in a relationship where one engenders the other according to the order of generation in the cycle of the five phases. This is determined by astrological calculations based on the celestial stems and earthly branches of the day and year of their birth.

2.   與德合 *yǔ dé hé*: 德 *dé* "virtue/potency" refers here to an auspicious astrological position, signifying the potency of Heaven. The astrological position 天德 *tiān dé* (heavenly virtue) is, for example, mentioned as significant in instructions for the direction that a woman in labor should face for a safe childbirth. See *Ishimpô* 《醫心方》 23:1: "In the first month, the heavenly qì is moving south. The woman in childbirth should face south and sit by touching 丙 *bǐng* ground with her left knee. Greatly auspicious. Again, the heavenly dào is in 辛 *xīn* and the heavenly virtue in 丁 *dīng*..."

3.   子休廢死墓中: These are three astrological positions with the self-explanatory names of "ceasing children," "abolished to death," and "in the tomb's midst."

4.   刑殺 *xíng shā*: Parallel to "virtue" (德 *dé*) above, these terms are the most inauspicious positions in a person's astrological chart. The quotation of this passage in the *Ishimpô* has 煞 *shà* instead of 殺 *shā* (《醫心方》 28:21).

5.   The *Ishimpô* (《醫心方》 24:1), quoting the *Bìng Yuán Lùn*, lists three reasons for infertility: first, geomancy and problems with tombs; second, husband and wife's year destinies being in a relationship of mutual conquest; and third, physical disease of husband or wife. In the case of the first two reasons, it emphasizes, no medicines can help. See also (《病源論》 38:51).

6.   *Sòng* editors' note: "The methods for prohibitions and taboos, the time and day for conceiving the fetus, and the daily methods for calculating *wáng xiāng* and *guì sù* are found in volume 27." This volume contains prescriptions for physical cultivation and extending life. The various prohibitions regarding sexual intercourse are found in the last section, entitled "Boosting and Supplementing through Sexual Intercourse" (房中補益 *fáng zhōng bǔ yì*). The "methods for prohibitions and taboos" are also found in the *Sūn Zhēn Rén* edition where they are placed in the "prescriptions for women" directly following the essay above, as well as in *Wài Tái Mì Yào* (《外台秘要》 33) and *Yī Xīn Fāng* (《醫心方》 28:21), in both cases in the section on "seeking a child."

LINE 1.6

(一) 論曰：凡人無子，當為夫妻俱有五勞七傷，虛贏百病所致，故有絕嗣之殃。(二) 夫治之法，男服七子散，女服紫石門冬丸，及坐藥，盪胞湯，無不有子也。

(1) Essay: Whenever people are childless, it is caused by the fact that both husband and wife suffer from the five taxations and seven damages[1] and the hundred diseases of vacuity emaciation, with the disastrous result that the line of descendants is cut off.

(2) As for treatment methods, the male [partner] should take *Seven Seeds[2] Powder*, and the female [partner] should take *Fluorite and Asparagus Pills* and [be treated with] a suppository[3] and a uterus-rinsing decoction. Then they will most certainly have children.

1. 五勞七傷 *wǔ láo qī shāng*: This is a standard expression for debilitating conditions of vacuity taxation. See, for example, the list of "five taxations, six extremes, and seven damages" in the introductory essay on "the various symptoms of vacuity taxation diseases, A" (虛勞病諸候上 *xū láo bìng zhū hòu shàng*) in *Bìng Yuán Lùn* (《病源論》 3). The term "five taxations" is variably explained as taxation damage from prolonged staring, lying, sitting, standing, and walking in *Sù Wén* (《素文》 23), taxation of the five viscera 《病源論》 or as "mind taxation, thought taxation, heart taxation, spleen taxation, and kidney taxation" (*Bìng Yuán Lùn*, citing the *Qiān Jīn Fāng*). The "seven damages" are explained in the *Bìng Yuán Lùn* as food damage, anxiety damage, drinking damage, bedchamber damage, hunger damage, taxation damage, and damage from taxation of the channels and network vessels and construction and defense *qì* taxation *Bìng Yuán Lùn* (《病源論》 3:1). In the prescriptions for women in the *Qiān Jīn Fāng*, Sūn Sī-Miǎo uses the expression to refer to diseases of vacuity taxation and emaciation, as for example in *Qiān Jīn Fāng* (《千金方》 4:1).

2. 子 *zǐ*: While this character can also be read as "sons," I render it as "seeds" because the ingredients include seven types of seeds. However, the double meaning of the name and the medicinal use of numerous seeds 子 for the procreation of sons *zǐ* was no doubt intentional.

3. 坐藥 *zuò yào*: Literally "sitting medicine," it is an abbreviation for 坐導藥 *zuò dǎo yào*. While the term 導藥 *dǎo yào* (literally "abducting medicine"] is usually translated as enema (as in Wiseman and Féng, *English-Chinese Chinese-English Dictionary*, p. 442, entries on 導便 *dǎo biàn* or 導法 *dǎo fǎ*), a more accurate translation here is "suppository" since the medicine is not a fluid to be injected into the intestines via the anus, but a substance to be inserted into the vagina and held in for a longer period of time.

LINE 1.7a

七子散治丈夫風虛目暗，精氣衰少無子，補不足方

Seven Seeds Powder treats the husband's wind vacuity, with clouded vision, debilitation and scantness of essence and *qì*, and infertility; by supplementing insufficiency.

Seven Seeds Powder
七子散 *qī zǐ sǎn*

五味子 牡荊子 菟絲子 車前子 菥蓂子 石斛 薯蕷 乾地黃 杜仲 鹿茸 遠志（各八銖）附子 蛇床子 芎藭（各六銖）山茱萸 天雄 人參 茯苓 黃芪 牛膝（各三銖[1]）桂心（十銖）巴戟天（十二銖）蓯蓉（十銖）鍾乳（粉，八銖）。

五味子	*wǔ wèi zǐ*	Fruit of Schisandra chinensis	八銖 8 zhū	1g
牡荊子	*mǔ jīng zǐ*	Fruit of Vitex negundo L. var. cannabifolia	八銖 8 zhū	1g

菟絲子	tù sī zǐ	Seed of Cuscuta chinensis	八銖 8 zhū	1g
車前子	chē qián zǐ	Seed of Plantago asiatica	八銖 8 zhū	1g
菥蓂子	xī míng zǐ	Seed of Thlaspi arvense	八銖 8 zhū	1g
石斛	shí hú	Whole plant of Dendrobium nobile	八銖 8 zhū	1g
薯蕷	shǔ yù	Root of Dioscorea opposita	八銖 8 zhū	1g
乾地黃	gān dì huáng	Dried root of Rehmannia glutinosa	八銖 8 zhū	1g
杜仲	dù zhòng	Bark of Eucommia ulmoidis	八銖 8 zhū	1g
鹿茸	lù róng	Pilose antler of Cervus nippon	八銖 8 zhū	1g
遠志	yuǎn zhì	Root of Polygala tenuifolia	八銖 8 zhū	1g
附子	fù zǐ	Lateral root of Aconitum carmichaeli	六銖 6 zhū	.75g
蛇床子	shé chuáng zǐ	Fruit of Cnidium monnieri	六銖 6 zhū	.75g
川芎	chuān xiōng	Root of Ligusticum wallichii	六銖 6 zhū	.75g
山茱萸	shān zhū yú	Fruit of Cornus officinalis	三銖 3 zhū	.375g
烏頭	wū tóu	Main tuber of Aconitum carmichaeli	三銖 3 zhū	.375g
人參	rén shēn	Root of Panax ginseng	三銖 3 zhū	.375g
茯苓	fú líng	Dried fungus of Poria cocos	三銖 3 zhū	.375g
黃芪	huáng qí	Root of Astragalus membranaceus	三銖 3 zhū	.375g
牛膝	niú xī	Root of Achyranthes bidentata	三銖 3 zhū	.375g
桂心	guì xīn	Shaved inner bark of Cinnamomum cassia	十銖 10 zhū	1.25g
巴戟天	bā jǐ tiān	Root of Morinda officinalis	十二銖 12 zhū	1.5g
蓯蓉	cōng róng	Stalk of Cistanche salsa	十銖 10 zhū	1.25g
鍾乳粉	zhōng rǔ fěn	Stalactite, powdered	八銖 8 zhū	1g

上二十四味，治下篩。酒服方寸匕，日二，不知增至二匕，以知為度。禁如藥法。不能酒者，蜜和丸服亦得。

Finely pestle[2] and sift the above twenty-four ingredients. Take a square-inch spoon[3] in liquor twice a day. If no effect is noticed, increase to a maximum of two spoons, until an effect is noticed. Restrictions apply as in the general rules for taking drugs. If [the patient] cannot tolerate liquor, he may also take it in the form of pills mixed with honey.[4]

1.   The *Dào Zāng* and *Sūn Zhēn Rén* editions recommend five *zhū* instead. For the following translation, slight editorial variations in medicinal proportions and doses are overlooked. In general, I use the text of the *Huá Xià* edition, which is mostly identical with the *Rén Mín* edition. Major differences to other editions are noted.
2.   治 *zhì*: According to Donald Harper, this should be interpreted as 冶 *yě*, a metallurgical term that can mean "to hammer metal." Harper therefore renders it as "to smith" in the sense of finely pounding drugs, a labor-intensive technique for processing drugs. "…Sifting techniques were not common in medicine until after the *Hàn* period. Before that time,

long pestling was necessary to reduce the drug to a fine powder; and 冶 'smith' was borrowed from metallurgy to denote the pounding process. 冶 appears frequently in *Wǔ wēi* 武威 prescriptions, but it is rare in later medical literature (and when it does appear in the received literature it is regularly miswritten as 治. Evidently the word 冶 became obsolete once sifting simplified the process of pulverizing drugs (*Early Chinese Medical Literature*, p.223)." In the *Qiān Jīn Fāng*, the character is used consistently for the preparation of powders in the phrase "finely pestle and sift" (治篩下 *zhì shāi xià*). *Qiān Jīn Fāng* (《千金方》 1:7) on "compounding medicines" (合和 *hé hé*) states: "When sifting [drugs to prepare] medicinal pills, use heavy and tightly-woven thin silk cloth to make it fine, so that they are easily cooked with honey into pills. When sifting [drugs to prepare] medicinal powders, with herbal drugs use light, coarse silk, so they will not clump when taken in liquor. With mineral drugs, also use a fine silk sieve to [prepare them] like pill drugs. Whenever you have sifted [the drugs into a] medicinal powder or pill, always mix them again in a mortar, pounding them with a pestle several hundred times. It is best when you can see that the patterns of the colors are all mixed uniformly."

3. 方寸匕 *fāng cùn bǐ*. *Qiān Jīn Fāng* (《千金方》 1:7) on "Compounding medicines" explains: "As for a full square-inch spoon, make a spoon of a perfect one-inch square, scatter and disperse [the powder on it] and measure it by the amount that doesn't fall down."

4. *Sòng* editors' note: "Another version of this prescription adds eight *zhū* of *fù pén zǐ* (覆盆子 Fruit of Rubus chingii). Regarding methods for seeking children, other prescriptions are found in the chapter below on sexual cultivation." This is a reference to the various restrictions regarding the intake of drugs in general (e.g. diet, time, amount, and dosage), found in the preceding volume, particularly in section 8 on "Taking Drugs" (服餌 *fú ěr*). The sentence above is explained as "avoid raw and cold, vinegary and slippery foods, pork, chicken, fish and garlic, and oily noodles" in (張奇文《婦科雜病》 p. 49). The reference to the "chapter below on sexual cultivation" refers to *Qiān Jīn Fāng* (《千金方》 27:8) on "Supplementing and Boosting through Sexual Intercourse" (房中補益 *fáng zhōng bǔ yì*). The *Sūn Zhēn Rén* edition comments: "When practicing the methods of sexual intercourse, rely on the *Sù Nǚ Jīng* 素女經 [*Classic of the Plain Maiden*]: '[Conception] one day after the end of the menstrual flow will make a male [fetus], two days afterward a female, three days a male, four days a female. Outside of these, there will be no children. Performing it every day before noon and every night after midnight at *yáng* times will make a male. When making the semen descend, you want to obtain a distance of 0.5 *cùn* inside the jade gate [that is, insert the penis 0.5 *cùn* into the vagina], otherwise you will go past the uterus.'" The full quotation is found in the *Ishimpō* (《醫心方》 28:21).

LINE 1.7b

朴消盪胞湯治婦人立身已來全不產，及斷緒久不產三十年者方

Impure Mirabilite Uterus-Rinsing Decoction treats infertility in women who have never given birth throughout their entire adult life or who have interrupted the thread [of descendants] and have not given birth for as long as thirty years.

Impure Mirabilite Uterus-Rinsing Decoction
朴消盪胞湯 *pò xiāo dàng bāo tāng*

朴消 牡丹 當歸 大黃 桃仁（生用，各三銖） 細辛 厚朴 桔梗 赤芍藥 人參 茯苓 桂心 甘草 牛膝 橘皮（各一銖） 虻蟲（十枚） 水蛭（十枚） 附子（六銖）。

朴消	pò xiāo	Impure mirabilite	三銖 3 zhū	.375g
牡丹	mǔ dān	Bark of the root of Paeonia suffruticosa	三銖 3 zhū	.375g
當歸	dāng guī	Root of Angelica polimorpha	三銖 3 zhū	.375g
大黃	dà huáng	Root of Rheum palmatum	三銖 3 zhū	.375g
生桃仁	shēng tao rén	Fresh seed of Prunus persica	三銖 3 zhū	.375g
細辛	xì xīn	Complete plant including root of Asarum heteropoides	一銖 1 zhū	.125g
厚朴	hòu pò	Bark of Magnolia officinalis	一銖 1 zhū	.125g
桔梗	jié gěng	Root of Platycodon grandiflorum	一銖 1 zhū	.125g
赤芍藥	chì sháo yao	Root of Paeonia rubra	一銖 1 zhū	.125g
人參	rén shēn	Root of Panax ginseng	一銖 1 zhū	.125g
茯苓	fú líng	Dried fungus of Poria cocos	一銖 1 zhū	.125g
桂心	guì xīn	Shaved inner bark of Cinnamomum cassia	一銖 1 zhū	.125g
甘草	gān cǎo	Root of Glycyrrhiza uralensis	一銖 1 zhū	.125g
牛膝	niú xī	Root of Achyranthes bidentata	一銖 1 zhū	.125g
橘皮	jú pí	Peel of Citrus reticulate	一銖 1 zhū	.125g
虻蟲	méng chóng	Dried body of the female of Tabanus bivittatus	十銖 10 zhū	1.25g
水蛭	shuǐ zhì	Dried body of Whitmania pigra	十銖 10 zhū	1.25g
附子	fù zǐ	Lateral root of Aconitum carmichaeli	六銖 6 zhū	.75g

上十八味，㕮咀，以清酒五升，水五升合煮，取三升，分四服，日三夜一，每服相去三時，更服如常。覆被取少汗，汗不出，冬日著火籠之，必下積血，及冷赤膿如赤小豆汁。本為婦人子宮內有些惡物令然。或天陰臍下痛，或月水不調，為有冷血不受胎。若斟酌下盡，氣力弱，大困，不堪更服，亦可二三服即止。如大悶不堪，可食酢飯冷漿，一口即止。然恐去惡物不盡，不大得藥力。若能忍，服盡大好。一日後，仍著導藥。[1]

Pound[2] the above eighteen ingredients. Combine with five *shēng* of clear liquor and five *shēng* of water and decoct to obtain three *shēng*. Divide into four doses and take it three times a day and once at night. Wait three watches[3] between doses, then take the next one and so on.[4] Cover [the woman] with a quilt to make her sweat a little. If she does not sweat, on winter days place her over a brazier.[5] She must discharge accumulated blood and cold red pus that resembles azuki bean juice. This is caused by the fact that originally there was a malign substance within the woman's uterus.

Maybe, she felt pain in *tiān yīn*[6] or below the navel, or the menstrual flow was irregular. This indicates the presence of cold blood preventing her from receiving the fetus. If the discharge below is believed to be finished or the strength of her *qì* is so weakened and she is in such great distress that she cannot bear to consume any more doses, she may take [only] two or three doses and then stop. If she experiences such great oppression that she cannot bear [taking more of the medicine], she may eat one mouthful of vinegared rice with cold broth and then stop. However, I fear that the malign substance has not been eliminated completely and she has not received the full power of the medicine. If she can bear it, taking the entire [preparation] is best. After one day, next apply the suppository.

1. *Sòng* editors' note: "The *Qiān Jīn Yì Fāng* 千金翼方 does not use *jié gěng* 桔梗 and *gān cǎo* 甘草".
2. 㕮咀 *fǔ jǔ*: It literally means "to chew." Harper still translates it as such for the early *Hàn* period, but Sūn Sī-Miǎo specifically states in the instructions on compounding medicines in the first volume: "Whenever [compounding] medicinal decoctions, wines, or pastes, when the ancient prescriptions all state to chew [the ingredients], it means to pound them all to the size of soybeans and blow on them to remove the fine powder" (《千金方》 1:8).
3. 三時 *sān shí*: One watch equals two hours. Thus, the woman should wait six hours between doses.
4. This passage is questionable and interpreted differently in different editions. The *Sūn Zhēn Rén* edition clarifies the meaning, having a slightly different version:…三辰少時更 *sān chén shǎo shí gèng*…(…by three watches, after a short while take the next…). Thus, 更 clearly relates to the following phrase rather than being a time measurement. Given the earlier date of this edition, I adopt this meaning.
5. 火籠 *huǒ lóng*: A portable basket-shaped heater.
6. 天陰 *tiān yīn*: The meaning of this term is unclear and, to my knowledge, not attested elsewhere; it is most likely related to the reproductive organs, similar to such common expressions as 陰器 *yīn qì* (external reproductive organs), 陰戶 *yīn hù* or 陰門 *yīn mén* (entrance to the vagina), or 陰道 *yīn dào* (vagina). Alternatively, it could refer to an acupuncture point, similar to points such as 陰交 *yīn jiāo* ("Yīn Intersection," CV-7) or 石門 *shí mén* ("Stone Gate," CV-5), which are located one and two *cùn* respectively below the navel and have been recorded in texts as early as the *Zhēn Jiǔ Jiǎ Yǐ Jīng* 針灸甲乙經 to treat infertility (See 張奇文 《婦科雜病》 p. 45 for this interpretation). It could also be an alternative name for 天樞 *tiān shū* (Celestial Pivot, ST-25), located 2 *cùn* to each side of the navel and useful in the treatment of such gynecological conditions as aggregations, blood clots, leaking of red or white discharge, and untimely periods (see 《中華醫學大辭典》 p. 175).

LINE 1.8

治全不產及斷緒，服前朴消湯後，坐導藥方

For treating complete inability to give birth and interruption of the thread [of descendants to continue the family line], after first taking the above *Impure Mirabilite Decoction*, apply this suppository.

Suppository
坐導藥 *zuò dǎo yào*

皂莢 山茱萸 當歸（各一兩） 細辛 五味子 乾薑（各二兩） 大黃 礬石 戎鹽 蜀椒（各半兩）。˙

皂莢	zào jiá	Fruit of Gleditsia sinensis	一兩 1 liǎng	3g
山茱萸	shān zhū yú	Fruit of Cornus officinalis	一兩 1 liǎng	3g
當歸	dāng guī	Root of Angelica polimorpha	一兩 1 liǎng	3g
細辛	xì xīn	Complete plant including root of Asarum heteropoides	二兩 2 liǎng	6g
五味子	wǔ wèi zǐ	Fruit of Schisandra chinensis	二兩 2 liǎng	6g
乾薑	gān jiāng	Dried root of Zingiber officinale	二兩 2 liǎng	6g
大黃	dà huáng	Root of Rheum palmatum	半兩 0.5 liǎng	1.5g
礬石	fán shí	Alum	半兩 0.5 liǎng	1.5g
戎鹽	róng yán	Halite	半兩 0.5 liǎng	1.5g
蜀椒	shǔ jiāo	Seed capsules of Zanthoxylum bungeanum	半兩 0.5 liǎng	1.5g

上十味，末之，以絹袋盛，大如指長三寸，盛藥令滿，內婦人陰中。坐臥任意，勿行走急。小便時去之，更安新者。一日一度。必下青黃冷汁。汁盡止，即可幸御，自有子。若未見病出，亦可至十日安之。此藥為服朴消湯，恐去冷惡物出不盡，以導藥下之。值天陰冷不疼，不須著導藥。亦有著鹽為導藥者，然不如此藥。其服朴消湯後，即安導藥，經一日外，服紫石門冬丸。

Pulverize the above ten ingredients and put into finger-sized silk bags that are three *cùn* long. Fill the bags with the medicine to the top. Insert a bag into the woman's vagina. She may sit or lie as she wishes, but do not allow her to walk or run hastily. When she urinates, [have her] remove it and replace it once a day with a new one. She must discharge a yellow-green cold liquid. Stop [only] when the liquid is completely finished. Not until then may she be mounted [in sexual intercourse] and bear children herself. If you do not see the disease leave, she may apply [the bags] for up to ten days. This medicine functions as a precipitating suppository when [the patient] has taken *Impure Mirabilite Decoction* and one fears that the cold malign substance has not been eliminated completely. In cases where *tiān yīn* is cold but not painful, it is not necessary to apply the suppository. There are also [prescriptions] that apply salt as a suppository, but they do not equal this medicine. After [the patient] has taken *Mirabilite Decoction* and then applied the suppository, wait at least one day before taking *Fluorite and Asparagus Pills*.

*   *Sòng* editors' note: "Another text contains a variation [of this prescription] that includes 0.5 *liǎng* of *tíng lì* [*zǐ*] (葶藶[子] Seed of Lepidium apetalum) and *pī shuāng* (砒霜 Sublimed arsenic)."

LINE 1.9

紫石門冬丸治全不產及斷緒方

Fluorite and Asparagus Pills treat complete inability to give birth and interruption of the thread.

Fluorite and Asparagus Pills
紫石門冬丸 *zǐ shí mén dōng wán*[1]

紫石英 天門冬（各三兩） 當歸 芎藭 紫葳 卷柏 桂心 烏頭 乾地黃 牡蒙 禹餘糧 石斛 辛夷（各二兩） 人參 桑寄生 續斷 細辛 厚朴 乾薑 食茱萸 牡丹 牛膝（各二十銖） 柏子仁（一兩） 薯蕷 烏賊骨 甘草（各一兩半）。

紫石英	zǐ shí yīng	Fluorite	三兩 3 liǎng	9g
天門冬	tiān mén dōng	Tuber of Asparagus cochinchinensis	三兩 3 liǎng	9g
當歸	dāng guī	Root of Angelica polimorpha	二兩 2 liǎng	6g
川芎	chuān xiōng	Root of Ligusticum wallichii	二兩 2 liǎng	6g
紫葳	zǐ wēi	Flower of Campsis grandiflora	二兩 2 liǎng	6g
卷柏	juǎn bǎi	Entire plant of Selaginella tamariscina	二兩 2 liǎng	6g
桂心	guì xīn	Shaved inner bark of Cinnamomum cassia	二兩 2 liǎng	6g
烏頭	wū tóu	Main tuber of Aconitum carmichaeli	二兩 2 liǎng	6g
乾地黃	gān dì huáng	Dried root of Rehmannia glutinosa	二兩 2 liǎng	6g
牡蒙	mǔ měng	Root of Paris quadrifolia	二兩 2 liǎng	6g
禹餘糧	yǔ yú liáng	Limonite	二兩 2 liǎng	6g
石斛	shí hú	Whole plant of Dendrobium nobile	二兩 2 liǎng	6g

辛夷	xīn yí	Flower of Magnolia liliflora	二兩 2 liǎng	6g
人參	rén shēn	Root of Panax ginseng	二十銖 12 zhū	1.5g
桑寄生	sāng jì shēng	Branches and foliage of Viscum coloratum	二十銖 12 zhū	1.5g
續斷	xù duàn	Root of Dipsacus asper	二十銖 12 zhū	1.5g
細辛	xì xīn	Complete plant including root of Asarum heteropoides	二十銖 12 zhū	1.5g
厚朴	hòu pò	Bark of Magnolia officinalis	二十銖 12 zhū	1.5g
乾薑	gān jiāng	Dried root of Zingiber officinale	二十銖 12 zhū	1.5g
食茱萸	shí zhū yú	Fruit of Zanthoxylum ailanthoides	二十銖 12 zhū	1.5g
牡丹	mǔ dān	Bark of the root of Paeonia suf-fruticosa	二十銖 12 zhū	1.5g
牛膝	niú xī	Root of Achyranthes bidentata	二十銖 12 zhū	1.5g
柏子仁	bǎi zǐ rén	Seed of Platycladus orientalis	一兩 1 liǎng	3g
薯蕷	shǔ yù	Root of Dioscorea opposita	一兩半 1.5 liǎng	4.5g
烏賊骨	wū zéi gǔ	Calcified shell of Sepiella main-droni	一兩半 1.5 liǎng	4.5g
甘草	gān cǎo	Root of Glycyrrhiza uralensis	一兩半 1.5 liǎng	4.5g

上二十六味，末之，蜜和丸。酒服如梧桐子大十丸，日三，漸增至三十丸，以腹中熱為度。不禁房室，夫行不在不可服。禁如藥法。比來服者，不至盡劑即有娠。

Pulverize the above twenty-six ingredients and combine with honey to make pills. Take ten pills the size of firmiana seeds[2] in liquor, three times a day, gradually increasing the dose to a maximum of thirty pills, until there is heat in the center of the abdomen. Do not restrict sexual activity, and do not take these if the husband is away on travels. Restrictions apply as in the general methods for taking drugs. If she has recently started taking this [medicine], she will be pregnant even before she has used up the preparation.

1.   This name is an abbreviation of the names of the first two ingredients: *zǐ shí yīng* (紫石英 Fluorite) and *tiān mén dōng* (天門冬 Tuber of Asparagus cochinchinensis).
2.   梧桐子 *wú tóng zǐ*: According to the instructions on "compounding medicines" from the first volume of the *Qiān Jīn Fāng*, this measurement refers to an amount that equals two soybeans or four azuki beans. One square-inch spoon of powder can be mixed with honey to obtain ten pills the size of firmiana seeds (《千金方》 1:8).

LINE 1.10

白薇丸主令婦人有子方

Black Swallowwort Pills are the governing prescription[1] for causing a woman to bear children.

Black Swallowwort Pills
白薇丸 *bái wéi wán*

白薇 細辛 防風 人參 秦椒 白蘝 桂心 牛膝 秦艽 蕪荑 沙參 芍藥 五味子 白殭蠶 牡丹 蠐螬（各一兩）乾漆 柏子仁 乾薑 卷柏 附子 芎藭（各二十銖）紫石英 桃仁（各一兩半）鍾乳 乾地黃 白石英（各二兩）鼠婦（半兩）水蛭 虻蟲（各十五枚）吳茱萸（十八銖）麻布叩複頭[2]（一尺，燒）。

白薇	bái wéi	Root of Cynanchum atratum	一兩 1 liǎng	3g
細辛	xì xīn	Complete plant including root of Asarum heteropoides	一兩 1 liǎng	3g
防風	fáng fēng	Root of Ledebouriella divaricata	一兩 1 liǎng	3g
人參	rén shēn	Root of Panax ginseng	一兩 1 liǎng	3g
秦椒	qín jiāo	Seed capsule of Zanthoxylum bungeanum	一兩 1 liǎng	3g
白蘝	bái liǎn	Root of Ampelopsis japonica	一兩 1 liǎng	3g
桂心	guì xīn	Shaved inner bark of Cinnamomum cassia	一兩 1 liǎng	3g
牛膝	niú xī	Root of Achyranthes bidentata	一兩 1 liǎng	3g
秦艽	qín jiāo	Root of Gentiana macrophylla	一兩 1 liǎng	3g
蕪荑	wú yí	Processed fruit of Ulmus macrocarpa	一兩 1 liǎng	3g
沙參	shā shēn	Root of Adenophora tetraphylla	一兩 1 liǎng	3g
芍藥	sháo yào	Root of Paeonia albiflora	一兩 1 liǎng	3g
五味子	wǔ wèi zǐ	Fruit of Schisandra chinensis	一兩 1 liǎng	3g
白殭蠶	bái jiāng cán	Dried 4th or 5th stage larva of the moth of Bombyx mori	一兩 1 liǎng	3g
牡丹	mǔ dān	Bark of the root of Paeonia suffruticosa	一兩 1 liǎng	3g
蠐螬	qí cáo	Dried larva of Holotrichia diomphalia	一兩 1 liǎng	3g
乾漆	gān qī	Dried sap of Rhus verniciflua	二十銖 20 zhū	2.5g
柏子仁	bǎi zǐ rén	Seed of Platycladus orientalis	二十銖 20 zhū	2.5g
乾薑	gān jiāng	Dried root of Zingiber officinale	二十銖 20 zhū	2.5g
卷柏	juǎn bǎi	Entire plant of Selaginella tamariscina	二十銖 20 zhū	2.5g

附子	fù zǐ	Lateral root of Aconitum carmichaeli	二十銖 20 zhū	2.5g
川芎	chuān xiōng	Root of Ligusticum wallichii	二十銖 20 zhū	2.5g
紫石英	zǐ shí yīng	Fluorite	一兩半 1.5 liǎng	4.5g
桃仁	táo rén	Seed of Prunus persica	一兩半 1.5 liǎng	4.5g
鍾乳	zhōng rǔ	Stalactite	二兩 2 liǎng	6g
乾地黃	gān dì huáng	Dried root of Rehmannia glutinosa	二兩 2 liǎng	6g
白石英	bái shí yīng	White quartz	二兩 2 liǎng	6g
鼠婦	shǔ fù	Dried body of Armadillidium vulgare	半兩 0.5 liǎng	1.5g
水蛭	shuǐ zhì	Dried body of Whitmania pigra	十五枚 15 zhū	1.875g
虻蟲	méng chóng	Dried body of the female of Tabanus bivittatus	十五枚 15 zhū	1.875g
吳茱萸	wú zhū yú	Unripe fruit of Evodia rutaecarpa	十八銖 18 zhū	2.25g
燒麻布叩複頭	shāo má bù kòu fù tóu	Charred hempen kòufùtóu	一尺 1 chǐ	30cm

上三十二味，末之，蜜和丸，酒服如梧子大十五丸，日再，稍加至三十丸。當有所去，小覺有異即停服。

Pulverize the above thirty-two ingredients and combine with honey to make pills the size of firmiana seeds. Take fifteen pills in liquor twice a day, gradually increasing the dose to a maximum of thirty pills. [The patient] should stop taking them when something is expelled and she feels a slight difference.

1. 主 zhǔ: A common term in prescription literature. When a prescription is said to "govern" a specific symptom or disease, it means that it is the most effective treatment for it.
2. 麻布叩複頭 má bù kòu fù tóu: The exact meaning of this term is unknown, but it refers here to a medicinal ingredient made out of hemp cloth, perhaps some type of padded head covering.

LINE 1.11

(一) 論曰:古者求子，多用慶雲散，承澤丸，今代人絕不用此。雖未試驗，其法可重，故述之。 (二) 慶雲散主丈夫陽氣不足，不能施化，施化無成方

(1) Essay: The ancients used mostly *Blessing Clouds Powder* and *Luster-Granting Pills* for "seeking children," but modern people have stopped and don't use them anymore. Although I have not yet tried them, their methods are worthy of our attention, thus I have recorded them.[1]

(2) *Blessing Clouds Powder* governs a husband's insufficiency of *yáng qì*, [resulting in]

his inability to transform[2] [male essence into a fetus] or in transformation without creation [of a fetus].[3]

Blessing Clouds Powder
慶雲散 *qìng yún sǎn*

覆盆子 五味子（各一升） 天雄（一兩） 石斛 白朮（各三兩） 桑寄生（四兩） 天門冬（九兩） 菟絲子（一升） 紫石英（二兩）。

覆盆子	fù pén zǐ	Fruit of Rubus chingii	一升 1 shēng	24g
五味子	wǔ wèi zǐ	Fruit of Schisandra chinensis	一升 1 shēng	24g
烏頭	wū tóu	Main tuber of Aconitum carmichaeli	一兩 1 liǎng	3g
石斛	shí hú	Whole plant of Dendrobium nobile	三兩 2 liǎng	6g
白朮	bái zhú	Rhizome of Atractylodes macrocephala	三兩 3 liǎng	9g
桑寄生	sāng jì shēng	Branches and foliage of Viscum coloratum	四兩 4 liǎng	12g
天門冬	tiān mén dōng	Tuber of Asparagus cochinchinensis	九兩 5 liǎng	15g
菟絲子	tù sī zǐ	Seed of Cuscuta chinensis	一升 1 shēng	24g
紫石英	zǐ shí yīng	Fluorite	二兩 2 liǎng	6g

上九味，治下篩。酒服方寸匕，先食，日三服。素不耐冷者，去寄生，加細辛四兩。陽氣不少而無子者，去石斛，加檳榔十五枚。

Finely pestle and sift the above nine ingredients. Take a square-inch spoon in liquor before meals,[4] three times a day. If the patient suffers from a constitutional inability to withstand cold, leave out *sāng jì shēng* 桑寄生 and add four *liǎng* of *xì xīn* (細辛 Complete plant including root of Asarum heteropoides). If the patient suffers from infertility but without a shortage of *yáng qì*, leave out *shí hú* 石斛 and add fifteen pieces of *bīng lang* (檳榔 Fruit of Areca catechu).

1. The following two prescriptions have been identified by Jender Lee to be a quotation from the fifth century text *Sēng Shén Fāng* 僧神方 (李貞德《漢唐之間醫書中的生產之道》 p. 301).
2. 施化 *shī huà*: This is an abbreviation of the common phrase 陽施陰化 "*yáng* bestows and *yīn* transforms," describing the process of conception. My translation is informed by Elisabeth Hsu's study of the terms 變 *biàn* and 化 *huà* in the *Nèi Jīng* 內經. She points out that "Hua-changes take place inside the body, invisible to the observer, whereby the result of the change can be seen by what is put outside (e.g. 'fluids,' 'things') (Elisabeth Hsu, "Change in Chinese Medicine: Bian and Hua," p.56)." In the context of reproduction, this term refers to the transformation of male essence (and female blood) into a fetus.
3. This refers to the ability of the woman to carry a pregnancy to terms.
4. See the first volume of the *Qiān Jīn Fāng*, in the chapter on taking medicine (《千金

方》 1:8): "When the illness is in the chest or above the diaphragm, eat first and then take the medicine afterwards. When the illness is below the heart and abdomen, take the medicine first and then eat afterwards. When the illness is in the four limbs and blood channels, it is recommended to take it on an empty stomach and at dawn. When the illness is in the bones and marrow, it is recommended to take it on a full stomach and at night."

LINE 1.12

承澤丸主婦人下焦三十六疾，不孕絕產方

Luster-Granting Pills are the governing prescription for women's thirty-six diseases of the lower burner,[1] [resulting in] failure to become pregnant and interruption of childbearing.[2]

Luster-Granting Pills
承澤丸 *chéng zé wán*

梅核仁 辛夷（各一升） 葛上亭長（七枚） 澤蘭子（五合） 溲疏（二兩）
藁本（一兩）。

梅核仁	méi hé rén	Seed of Prunus mume	一升 1 shēng	24g
辛夷	xīn yí	Flower of Magnolia liliflora	一升 1 shēng	24g
葛上亭長	gé shàng tíng cháng	Dried body of Epicauta Gorhami	七枚 7 zhū	.875g
澤蘭子	zé lán zǐ	Seed of Lycopus lucidus	五合 5 gě	35ml
溲疏	sōu shū	Fruit of Deutzia scabra	二兩 2 liǎng	6g
藁本	gāo běn	Rhizome and root of Ligusticum sinense	一兩 1 liǎng	3g

上六味，末之，蜜和丸，先食，服如大豆二丸，日三，不知稍增。若腹中無
堅癖積聚者，去亭長，加通草一兩。惡甘者，和藥先以苦酒搜散，乃內少蜜
和為丸。

Pulverize the above six ingredients and combine with honey to make pills. Before meals, take two pills the size of soybeans three times a day. If no effect is noticed, increase [the dose] gradually. In cases where no hardenings, aggregations, and gatherings are present in the abdomen, leave out *gé shàng tíng cháng* 葛上亭長 and add one *liǎng* of *tōng cǎo* (通草 Pith in the stalk of Tetrapanax papyriferus); if the patient is averse to sweet [flavors], mix the medicine by first scattering the powdered drugs into bitter liquor and then adding a little honey to combine them to make pills.

1.　　下焦三十六疾 *xià jiāo sān shí liù jí*: This is a technical term in Chinese gynecology, more precisely called "the thirty-six diseases of vaginal discharge" (帶下三十六疾 *dài xià sān shí liù jí*). The *Bìng Yuán Lùn* defines them this way: "The thirty-six diseases spoken of in the various prescription collections are the twelve concretions, nine pains, seven injuries, five damages, and three intractable diseases" (《病源論》38:50). This list is quoted literally and explained by Sūn Sī-Miǎo below in the third chapter of volume four on pp. 466-467. See in particular the footnote on this topic on p. 467. (《千金方》4:3). They refer to gynecological diseases like vaginal discharge, menstrual problems, and abdominal masses. According to the *Nàn Jīng* 難經 , "The lower burner governs separating the clear from the turbid, and it governs discharge but not intake, thereby transmitting and guiding [the food]. Its treatment [should focus on the area] one *cùn* below the navel." (《難經》31) translated in the Chinese Medicine Database (www.cm-db.com). In this context, it is used as a location in a sense similar to the term 帶下 *dài xià* (below the girdle) for which, see the discussion in note 1 in the following formula, on p. 73 below.

2.   This literal translation is slightly awkward but covers the double meaning of the Chinese term 絕產 *jué chǎn*, which could mean both infertility in general as well as miscarriage specifically.

LINE 1.13

大黃丸主帶下百病，無子，服藥十日下血，二十日下長蟲及清黃汁，三十日病除，五十日肥白方

Rhubarb Pills are the governing prescription for the hundred diseases below the girdle[1] and infertility. After the medicine is taken for ten days, the patient will discharge blood; after twenty days, she will discharge long worms and a clear yellow[2] liquid; after thirty days, the illness will be eliminated; after fifty days, she will be fat and white.[3]

Rhubarb Pills
大黃丸 *dà huáng wán*

大黃（破如米豆、熬令黑）柴胡 朴消（各一升）芎藭（五兩）乾薑（一升）蜀椒（二兩）茯苓（如雞子大一枚）。

大黃,破如米豆、熬令黑	dà huáng, pò rú mǐ dòu, āo lìng hēi	Root of Rheum palmatum that has been broken into pieces the size of grains or beans and simmered until black	一升	1 shēng	24g
柴胡	chái hú	Root of Bupleurum chinense	一升	1 shēng	24g
朴消	pò xiāo	Impure mirabilite	一升	1 shēng	24g
川芎	chuān xiōng	Root of Ligusticum wallichii	五兩	5 liǎng	15g
乾薑	gān jiāng	Dried root of Zingiber officinale	一升	1 shēng	24g
蜀椒	shǔ jiāo	Seed capsules of Zanthoxylum bungeanum	二兩	2 liǎng	6g

茯苓	fú líng	Dried fungus of Poria cocos	如雞子大一枚 rú jī zǐ dà 1 méi	1 pc the size of an egg

上七味，末之，蜜和丸如梧桐子大，先食，服七丸，米飲下，加至十丸，以知為度，五日微下。

Pulverize the above seven ingredients and combine with honey to make pills the size of firmiana seeds. Take seven pills before meals, drinking them down with rice water.[4] Increase the dose to a maximum of ten pills, until an effect is noticed. After five days, there will be a slight discharge.

1. 帶下 *dài xià*: This term is highly evocative and can convey a range of meanings from the most general "women's diseases" in the sense of a medical specialization to the anatomical location of the internal organs "below the girdle," more narrowly to the reproductive organs, or in the narrowest technical sense, to the pathological condition of vaginal discharge. While Sūn Sī-Miǎo does use the term in this restricted sense elsewhere, it was especially in the early medical literature often used to refer to conglomerations (瘕 *jiǎ*, here used in the general sense of abdominal masses) and menstrual irregularities as well. The history of the term is discussed above in the Prolegomena, the chapter on "Menstrual Irregularities and Vaginal Discharge," 3c., especially p. 38.
2. 清黃汁 *qīng huáng zhī*: Several other editions have 青黃汁 (green-yellow liquid) instead.
3. 肥白 *féi bái*: A sign of great health. 肥 carries the connotation of fertility; 白 refers to the woman's complexion being glistening white.
4. 米飲下 *mǐ yǐn xià*: Similar to the term 米湯 *mǐ tāng*, this refers to the water in which rice has been cooked.

LINE 1.14

治女人積年不孕，吉祥丸方

Auspicious Fortune Pills treat women's chronic lack of pregnancy.

Auspicious Fortune Pills
吉祥丸 *jí xiáng wán*

天麻（一兩）五味子（二兩）覆盆子（一升）桃花（二兩）柳絮（一兩）白朮（二兩）芎藭（二兩）牡丹（一兩）桃仁（一百枚）菟絲子（一升）茯苓（一兩）楮實子（一升）乾地黃（一兩）桂心（一兩）。

天麻	tiān má	Rhizome of Gastrodia elata	一兩 1 liǎng	3g
五味子	wǔ wèi zǐ	Fruit of Schisandra chinensis	二兩 2 liǎng	6g
覆盆子	fù pén zǐ	Fruit of Rubus chingii	一升 1 shēng	24g
桃花	táo huā	Flower of Prunus persica	二兩 2 liǎng	6g
柳絮	liǔ xù	Seed of Salix babylonica	一兩 1 liǎng	3g
白朮	bái zhú	Rhizome of Atractylodes macro-cephala	二兩 2 liǎng	6g
川芎	chuān xiōng	Root of Ligusticum wallichii	二兩 2 liǎng	6g
牡丹	mǔ dān	Bark of the root of Paeonia suffruti-cosa	一兩 1 liǎng	3g
桃仁	tao rén	Seed of Prunus persica	一百枚 100 méi	100 pcs
菟絲子	tù sī zǐ	Seed of Cuscuta chinensis	一升 1 shēng	24g
茯苓	fú líng	Dried fungus of Poria cocos	一兩 1 liǎng	3g
楮實子	chǔ shí zǐ	Fruit of Broussonetia papyrifera	一升 1 shēng	24g
乾地黃	gān dì huáng	Dried root of Rehmannia glutinosa	一兩 1 liǎng	3g
桂心	guì xīn	Shaved inner bark of Cinnamomum cassia	一兩 1 liǎng	3g

上十四味，末之，蜜和丸如豆大，每服空心飲若酒下五丸，日中一服，晚一服。

Pulverize the above fourteen ingredients and combine with honey to make pills the size of soybeans. Take five pills per dose in fluid such as liquor* on an empty stomach, one dose in the middle of the day, one in the evening.

* 飲若酒 yǐn ruò jiǔ: My translation is based on the *Rén Mín* and *Huá Xià* editions. The *Dào Zāng* edition has 飲黃酒 yǐn huáng jiǔ (drink in rice wine).

LINE 1.15

消石大黃丸治十二癥癖，及婦人帶下，絕產無子，並服寒食藥而腹中有癖者，當先服大丸下之，乃服寒食藥耳。大丸不下水穀，但下病耳，不令人虛極。方在第十一卷中。

Niter and Rhubarb Pills treat the twelve conglomerations and aggregations,[1] the gynecological conditions of vaginal discharge, interruption of childbearing, and infertility, as well as cases where the patient is also taking medicine that is to be taken cold[2] while suffering from aggregations in the abdomen. The patient should first take the *Rhubarb Pills* to precipitate [the aggregation] before taking the medicine that is to be taken cold. *Rhubarb Pills* do not precipitate water and grain; they only precipitate the illness and therefore do not cause extreme vacuity in the patient. The prescription is found in volume 11.[3]

1.　　瘕癖 *jiǎ pǐ*: This term could be interpreted as referring to the "twelve concretions" (*shí èr zhēng* 十二癥), a standard expression for the twelve varieties of women's vaginal discharge, cited in such texts as the *Bìng Yuán Lùn* and in volume 4, section 3 of the *Qiān Jīn Fāng* below. However, I interpret it here as referring to two types of non-gendered pathological abdominal lumps. As the *Bìng Yuán Lùn* explains in volume 19 on "symptoms of concretion and aggregation diseases," *jiǎ* "conglomerations" refers to movable abdominal masses that are due to unseasonal cold or heat weakening visceral *qì* and causing non-transformation of food and drink. These are juxtaposed with *zhēng* "concretions," which are solid hard lumps caused by a similar etiology (《病源論》 19:2). In contrast, *pǐ* "aggregations" refers to solid, sometimes painful accumulations of food in the rib-side, caused by food stagnation due to an impaired movement in the intestines and stomach compounded by the presence of cold *qì* (《病源論》 20:1 and in the gynecological context, 38:46). The *Sūn Zhēn Rén* edition has 癥瘕 *zhēng jiǎ* (concretions and aggregations) here instead of 瘕癖 *jiǎ pǐ*. I read this term here as a non-gendered pathology of abdominal lumps for two reasons: First, the following pathology of vaginal discharge specifies that it is a women's condition and secondly, the prescription is found in the non-gendered volume 11 on liver diseases.

2.　　寒食藥 *hán shí yào*: This is noted specifically here because most medicines are taken as heated decoctions or in heated liquids, in particular for conditions of cold accumulations. Another citation of this prescription in the *Qiān Jīn Fāng* has "powder that is to be taken cold" instead.

3.　　不下水穀 *bù xià shuǐ gǔ*: This means that they do not act as purgatives, which are often contraindicated because of their debilitating effect on a patient's general health.

4.　　Volume 11 covers liver conditions. The prescription is found in section five on "hardenings, concretions and accumulations and gatherings" (堅癥積聚 *jiān zhèng jī jù*). Here, Sūn Sī-Miǎo repeats the pathologies above, but specifies that this prescription is for cases where you want a powder that is to be taken cold, while suffering from masses, aggregations, and fullness in the abdomen.

LINE 1.16

治月水不利閉塞，絕產十八年，服此藥二十八日有子，金城太守白薇丸方

Governor of Jīn-Chéng's[1] Black Swallowwort Pills treat inhibited and blocked menstrual flow and interruption of childbearing for eighteen years. Taking this medicine for twenty-eight days will [cause the patient] to be with child.

Governor of Jīn-Chéng's Black Swallowwort Pills
金城太守白薇丸 *jīn chéng tài shǒu bái wēi wán*

白薇（三十銖）人參 杜蘅 牡蒙（各十八銖）牛膝（半兩）細辛（三十銖）厚朴 半夏（各十八銖）沙參 乾薑（各半兩）白殭蠶（十八銖）秦

芁（半兩） 蜀椒（一兩半） 當歸（十八銖） 附子（一兩半） 防風（一兩半） 紫菀（十八銖）。[2]

白薇	bái wéi	Root of Cynanchum atratum	三十銖 30 zhū	3.75g
人參	rén shēn	Root of Panax ginseng	十八銖 18 zhū	2.25g
杜蘅	dù héng	Rhizome and root, or whole plant of Asarum forbesii	十八銖 18 zhū	2.25g
牡蒙	mǔ měng	Root of Paris quadrifolia	十八銖 18 zhū	2.25g
牛膝	niú xī	Root of Achyranthes bidentata	半兩 0.5 liǎng	1.5g
細辛	xì xīn	Complete plant including root of Asarum heteropoides	三十銖 30 zhū	3.75g
厚朴	hòu pò	Bark of Magnolia officinalis	十八銖 18 zhū	2.25g
半夏	bàn xià	Rhizome of Pinellia ternata	十八銖 18 zhū	2.25g
沙參	shā shēn	Root of Adenophora tetraphylla	半兩 0.5 liǎng	1.5g
乾薑	gān jiāng	Dried root of Zingiber officinale	半兩 0.5 liǎng	1.5g
白殭蠶	bái jiāng cán	Dried 4th or 5th stage larva of the moth of Bombyx mori	十八銖 18 zhū	2.25g
秦艽	qín jiāo	Root of Gentiana macrophylla	半兩 0.5 liǎng	1.5g
蜀椒	shǔ jiāo	Seed capsules of Zanthoxylum bungeanum	一兩半 1.5 liǎng	4.5g
當歸	dāng guī	Root of Angelica polimorpha	十八銖 18 zhū	2.25g
附子	fù zǐ	Lateral root of Aconitum carmi-chaelii	一兩半 1.5 liǎng	4.5g
防風	fáng fēng	Root of Ledebouriella divaricata	一兩半 1.5 liǎng	4.5g
紫菀	zǐ wǎn	Root and rhizome of Aster tatari-cus	十八銖 18 zhū	2.25g

上十七味，末之，蜜和，先食服如梧子三大丸，不知，稍增至四五丸。此藥不長將服，覺有妊娠則止，用之大驗。

Pulverize the above seventeen ingredients and mix with honey to make pills the size of firmiana seeds. Take three pills before meals. If no effect is noticed, gradually increase the dosage to a maximum of four or five pills. This medicine may not be taken over a long period of time. Stop as soon as she senses the presence of a pregnancy. Its use achieves great results.[3]

1. Name of a commandery during the *Jìn* 晉 period that is located in modern Gān Sù Province 甘肅省, Gāo Lán County 皋蘭縣.
2. *Sòng* editors' note: "The *Cuī Shì* 崔氏 includes eighteen *zhū* each of *jié gěng* (桔梗 Root of Platycodon grandiflorum) and *dān shā* (丹砂 Cinnabaris)."
3. The *Wài Tái Mì Yào* adds here a list of dietary restrictions against sweets, pork and beef, cold water, raw scallion, and raw vegetables.

LINE 1.17

白薇丸主久無子或斷緒，上熱下冷，百病皆治之方

Black Swallowwort Pills are the governing prescription for chronic infertility or interruption of the line of descent, heat above and cold below, and all the myriad diseases.

Black Swallowwort Pills
白薇丸 *bái wēi wán*

白薇（十八銖） 紫石英（三十銖） 澤蘭 太一餘糧（各二兩） 當歸（一兩） 赤石脂（一兩） 白芷（一兩半） 芎藭（一兩） 藁本 石膏 菴閭子 卷柏（各二十銖） 蛇床子（一兩） 桂心（二兩半） 細辛（三兩） 覆盆子 桃仁（各二兩半） 乾地黃 乾薑 蜀椒 車前子（各十八銖） 蒲黃（二兩半） 人參（一兩半） 白龍骨 遠志 麥門冬 茯苓（各二兩） 橘皮（半兩）。

白薇	bái wéi	Root of Cynanchum atratum	十八銖 18 zhū	2.25g
紫石英	zǐ shí yīng	Fluorite	三十銖 30 zhū	3.75g
澤蘭	zé lán	Foliage and stalk of Lycopus lucidus	二兩 2 liǎng	6g
太一餘糧	tài yī yú liáng	Limonite	二兩 2 liǎng	6g
當歸	dāng guī	Root of Angelica polimorpha	一兩 1 liǎng	3g
赤石脂	chì shí zhī	Halloysite	一兩 1 liǎng	3g
白芷	bái zhǐ	Root of Angelica dahurica	一兩半 1.5 liǎng	4.5g
川芎	chuān xiōng	Root of Ligusticum wallichii	一兩 1 liǎng	3g
藁本	gāo běn	Rhizome and root of Ligusticum sinense	二十銖 20 zhū	2.5g
石膏	shí gāo	Gypsum	二十銖 20 zhū	2.5g
菴閭子	ān lǘ zǐ	Fruit of Artemisia keiskeana	二十銖 20 zhū	2.5g
卷柏	juǎn bǎi	Entire plant of Selaginella tamariscina	二十銖 20 zhū	2.5g
蛇床子	shé chuáng zǐ	Fruit of Cnidium monnieri	一兩 1 liǎng	3g
桂心	guì xīn	Shaved inner bark of Cinnamomum cassia	二兩半 2.5 liǎng	7.5g
細辛	xì xīn	Complete plant including root of Asarum heteropoides	三兩 3 liǎng	9g
覆盆子	fù pén zǐ	Fruit of Rubus chingii	二兩半 2.5 liǎng	7.5g
桃仁	táo rén	Seed of Prunus persica	二兩半 2.5 liǎng	7.5g

乾地黃	gān dì huáng	Dried root of Rehmannia glutinosa	十八銖 18 zhū	2.25g
乾薑	gān jiāng	Dried root of Zingiber officinale	十八銖 18 zhū	2.25g
蜀椒	shǔ jiāo	Seed capsules of Zanthoxylum bungeanum	十八銖 18 zhū	2.25g
車前子	chē qián zǐ	Seed of Plantago asiatica	十八銖 18 zhū	2.25g
蒲黃	pú huáng	Pollen of Typha angustata	二兩半 2.5 liǎng	7.5g
人參	rén shēn	Root of Panax ginseng	一兩半 1.5 liǎng	4.5g
白龍骨	bái lóng gǔ	Bleached fossilized vertebra and bone of mammals	二兩 2 liǎng	6g
遠志	yuǎn zhì	Root of Polygala tenuifolia	二兩 2 liǎng	6g
麥門冬	mài mén dōng	Tuber of Ophiopogon japonicus	二兩 2 liǎng	6g
茯苓	fú líng	Dried fungus of Poria cocos	二兩 2 liǎng	6g
橘皮	jú pí	Peel of Citrus reticulate	半兩 0.5 liǎng	1.5g

上二十八味，末之，蜜和，酒服十五丸如梧子大，日再，漸增，以知為度，亦可至五十丸。慎豬，雞，生，冷，酢，滑，魚，蒜，驢，馬，牛肉等。覺有妊娠即停。三月正擇食時，可食牛肝及心，至四月五月不須，不可故殺，令子短壽，遇得者大良。

Pulverize the above twenty-eight ingredients and mix with honey to make pills the size of firmiana seeds. Take fifteen pills in liquor twice a day, gradually increasing the dosage until an effect is noticed. [The patient] may take up to fifty pills [per dose]. Beware of such food as pork, poultry, raw or cold foods, vinegary or slippery foods, fish, garlic, donkey or horse meat, and beef.[1] Stop as soon as she senses the presence of a pregnancy. The [first] three months[2] are a time [when a pregnant woman must] properly select her food, but she may eat beef liver and heart. Arriving at the fourth and fifth month, there is no longer any need [to observe the restrictions]. But she may not kill [animals?] intentionally [because] it will shorten the child's lifespan. If she is able to do this, it is very good.

1. See the list of dietary restrictions when taking medicine in the eighth chapter of the first volume of the *Qiān Jīn Fāng* (《千金方》 1:8): "When taking medicine, always interrupt [the consumption of] such food as raw and cold foods, vinegary and slippery foods, pork, dog, poultry, and fish, oily noodles, garlic, and fruit." The following sentences list restrictions specific to certain drugs, such as beef for *niú xī* (牛膝 Root of Achyranthes bidentata) or pork for *huáng lián* (黃連 Rhizome of Coptis chinensis) and *jié gěng* (桔梗 Root of Platycodon grandiflorum).

2. 三月 *sān yuè*: While this could be read also as "the third month," I interpret it as "the first three months [i.e., of pregnancy]" based on the context. In medieval China, the conception of the fetus (受胎 *shòu tāi*) was seen as a gradual process of which the first three months were the most critical. See, for example, the list of prohibitions and instructions for "fetal education" (胎教 *tāi jiào*) found in the third chapter of this volume (《千金方》 2:3) on "nurturing the fetus," translated in the third chapter of volume two on pp.

98-100 below. There, Sūn Sī-Miǎo states specifically that "during the first three months, [the fetus] will transform according to things, and its disposition and character are not yet fixed."

LINE 1.18

治婦人絕產，生來未產，盪滌腑藏，使玉門受子精，秦椒丸方

Shǎn-Xī Zanthoxylum Pills are a treatment for women whose childbearing has been interrupted or who have never given birth at all, by scouring and flushing the viscera and bowels and causing the jade gate[1] to receive the essence of the fetus.

Shǎn-Xī Zanthoxylum Pills
秦椒丸 *qín jiāo wán*

秦椒 天雄（各十八銖） 玄參 人參 白蘞 鼠婦 白芷 黃芪 桔梗 露蜂房 白殭蠶 桃仁 蠐螬 白薇 細辛 蕪荑（各一兩） 牡蒙 沙參 防風 甘草 牡丹皮 牛膝 卷柏 五味子 芍藥 桂心 大黃 石斛 白朮（各二十銖） 柏子仁 茯苓 當歸 乾薑（各一兩半） 澤蘭 乾地黃 芎藭（各一兩十八銖） 乾漆 白石英 紫石英 附子（各二兩） 鍾乳（二兩半） 水蛭（七十枚） 虻蟲（百枚） 麻布叩複頭（七寸，燒）。

秦椒	qín jiāo	Seed capsule of Zanthoxylum bungeanum	十八銖 18 zhū	2.25g
烏頭	wū tóu	Main tuber of Aconitum carmichaeli	十八銖 18 zhū	2.25g
玄參	xuán shēn	Root of Scrophularia ningpoensis	一兩 1 liǎng	3g
人參	rén shēn	Root of Panax ginseng	一兩 1 liǎng	3g
白蘞	bái liǎn	Root of Ampelopsis japonica	一兩 1 liǎng	3g
鼠婦	shǔ fù	Dried body of Armadillidium vulgare	一兩 1 liǎng	3g
白芷	bái zhǐ	Root of Angelica dahurica	一兩 1 liǎng	3g
黃芪	huáng qí	Root of Astragalus membranaceus	一兩 1 liǎng	3g
桔梗	jié gěng	Root of Platycodon grandiflorum	一兩 1 liǎng	3g
露蜂房	lù fēng fáng	Nest of Polistes mandarinus	一兩 1 liǎng	3g
白殭蠶	bái jiāng cán	Dried 4th or 5th stage larva of the moth of Bombyx mori	一兩 1 liǎng	3g
桃仁	táo rén	Seed of Prunus persica	一兩 1 liǎng	3g
蠐螬	qí cáo	Dried larva of Holotrichia diomphalia	一兩 1 liǎng	3g
白薇	bái wēi	Root of Cynanchum atratum	一兩 1 liǎng	3g
細辛	xì xīn	Complete plant including root of Asarum heteropoides	一兩 1 liǎng	3g

蕪荑	wú yí	Processed fruit of Ulmus macrocarpa	一兩 1 liǎng	3g
牡蒙	mǔ méng	Root of Paris quadrifolia	二十銖 20 zhū	2.5g
沙參	shā shēn	Root of Adenophora tetraphylla	二十銖 20 zhū	2.5g
防風	fáng fēng	Root of Ledebouriella divaricata	二十銖 20 zhū	2.5g
甘草	gān cǎo	Root of Glycyrrhiza uralensis	二十銖 20 zhū	2.5g
牡丹皮	mǔ dān	Bark of the root of Paeonia suffruti-cosa	二十銖 20 zhū	2.5g
牛膝	niú xī	Root of Achyranthes bidentata	二十銖 20 zhū	2.5g
卷柏	juǎn bǎi	Entire plant of Selaginella tama-riscina	二十銖 20 zhū	2.5g
五味子	wǔ wèi zǐ	Fruit of Schisandra chinensis	二十銖 20 zhū	2.5g
芍藥	sháo yào	Root of Paeonia albiflora	二十銖 20 zhū	2.5g
桂心	guì xīn	Shaved inner bark of Cinnamomum cassia	二十銖 20 zhū	2.5g
大黃	dà huáng	Root of Rheum palmatum	二十銖 20 zhū	2.5g
石斛	shí hú	Whole plant of Dendrobium nobile	二十銖 20 zhū	2.5g
白朮	bái zhú	Rhizome of Atractylodes macro-cephala	二十銖 20 zhū	2.5g
柏子仁	bǎi zǐ rén	Seed of Platycladus orientalis	一兩半 1.5 liǎng	4.5g
茯苓	fú líng	Dried fungus of Poria cocos	一兩半 1.5 liǎng	4.5g
當歸	dāng guī	Root of Angelica polimorpha	一兩半 1.5 liǎng	4.5g
乾薑	gān jiāng	Dried root of Zingiber officinale	一兩半 1.5 liǎng	4.5g
澤蘭	zé lán	Foliage and stalk of Lycopus lucidus	一兩十八銖 1 liǎng 18 zhū	5.25g
乾地黃	gān dì huáng	Dried root of Rehmannia glutinosa	一兩十八銖 1 liǎng 18 zhū	5.25g
川芎	chuān xiōng	Root of Ligusticum wallichii	一兩十八銖 1 liǎng 18 zhū	5.25g
乾漆	gān qī	Dried sap of Rhus verniciflua	二兩 2 liǎng	6g
白石英	bái shí yīng	White quartz	二兩 2 liǎng	6g
紫石英	zǐ shí yīng	Fluorite	二兩 2 liǎng	6g
附子	fù zǐ	Lateral root of Aconitum carmichaeli	二兩 2 liǎng	6g
鍾乳	zhōng rǔ	Stalactite	二兩半 2.5 liǎng	7.5g
水蛭	shuǐ zhì	Dried body of Whitmania pigra	七十枚 70 méi	70 pieces
虻蟲	méng chóng	Dried body of the female of Tabanus bivittatus	百枚 100 méi	100 pieces

麻布叩 複頭, 燒	má bù kòu fù tóu, shāo	Hempen kòufùtóu, charred	七寸 7 cùn	21cm

上四十四味，末之，蜜丸，酒服十丸如梧子，日再，稍加至二十丸。若有所去如豆汁鼻涕，此是病出，覺有異即停。

Pulverize the above forty-four ingredients and combine with honey to make pills the size of firmiana seeds. Take ten pills in liquor twice a day, gradually increasing the dosage to twenty pills. When [the patient] eliminates a substance like bean juice[2] or snivel, this is the disease coming out. Stop as soon as she senses a difference [in her condition].

1. 玉門 *yù mén*: Here, it is used as a synonym for 產門 *chǎn mén*, the "birth gate" or vagina. Sūn Sī-Miǎo also uses this term elsewhere to refer more specifically to the front part of the vagina, while the cervix and inner part of the vagina are called uterine gate (胞門 *bāo mén* — see moxibustion prescriptions below). Lastly in its most restricted sense, *yù mén* is used to refer to the vagina of virgins, as opposed to *bāo mén*, used for women who have already given birth, and 龍門 *lóng mén* ("dragon gate"), used for married women who have not yet given birth (see 《病源論》 37:24). In the context of reproduction, the entrance to the uterus is also referred to as 子門 *zǐ mén* (infant's gate). See several references in the eighth chapter of volume three (《千金方》 3:8), translated below on pp. 375-378.
2. 豆汁 *dòu zhī*: This could refer either to the liquid in which beans have been simmered, to soy milk, or to a fermented drink made from soy beans.

LINE 1.19

Moxibustion Methods for Seeking Children
求子灸法 *qiú zǐ jiǔ fǎ*[1]

(一) 婦人絕子：灸然谷五十壯，在內踝前直下一寸。 (二) 婦人絕嗣不生，胞門閉塞：灸關元三十壯，報之。 (三) 婦人妊子不成，若墮落，腹痛，漏見赤：灸胞門五十壯，在關元左邊二寸是也。右邊二寸名子戶。 (四) 婦人絕嗣不生：灸氣門穴，在關元傍三寸，各百壯。 (五) 婦人子藏閉塞，不受精，疼：灸胞門五十壯。 (六) 婦人絕嗣不生，漏赤白：灸泉門十壯，三報之，穴在橫骨當陰上際。

(1) For [the treatment of] women with infertility: Burn 50 moxa cones at Scorching Valley (KI-2),[2] in front of the inner ankle, straight down 1 *cùn*.

(2) For [the treatment of] women whose line of descent has been interrupted by a failure to bear children because of a blocked uterine gate (KI-13)[3] : Burn 30 moxa cones at Pass Head (CV-4).[4] Repeat [this treatment].

(3) For [the treatment of] women who are unable to carry a pregnancy to terms, in cases of miscarriage with abdominal pain and visible red spotting: Burn 50 moxa cones at Uterine Gate (KI-13),[5] 2 *cùn* to the left of Pass Head (CV-4). [The point] 2 *cùn* to the right is called Infant's Door.

(4) For [the treatment of] women whose line of descent has been interrupted by a failure to bear children: Burn 100 moxa cones at each Qì Gate,[6] 3 *cùn* to either side of Pass Head (CV-4).

(5) For [the treatment of] women with a blocked uterus, failure to receive [male] essence,[7] and pain: Burn 50 moxa cones at Uterine Gate (KI-13).

(6) For [the treatment of] women whose line of descent is cut off because of their inability to bear children, [presenting with] red and white spotting: Burn 10 moxa cones at Spring Gate,[8] at the upper edge of where the pubic bone meets the genitalia. Repeat three times.

1. This heading is not found in the *Huá Xià* or *Rén Mín* editons, but only in the *Sūn Zhēn Rén* editon. Since it clarifies the organization of the text, I have included it, even though it is questionable whether it was found in Sūn Sī-Miǎo's original text. The *Dào Zàng* editon states "moxibustion methods" (灸法 *jiǔ fǎ*).
2. 然谷 *rán gǔ*: KI-2. For acupoint classifications, I follow Nigel Wiseman's terminology and identification. See Nigel Wiseman and Féng Yè, *A Practical Dictionary of Chinese Medicine*, Appendix IV, "A Classified List of Acupuncture Points," pp. 746-749.
3. 胞門 *bāo mén*: While here used as a reference to the vagina in general, it is elsewhere used in conjunction with the term 子戶 *zǐ hù* (infant's door) to describe the left and right parts of the kidney, as in the expression: 腎名胞門子戶 "The kidneys are called uterine gate and infant's door," (《千金方》 2:2, translated below in the second chapter of volume two, in the introductory essay to the following chapter on "Malign obstruction in pregnancy" p. 88). In modern TCM practice, it is paired with *zǐ hù* to constitute one of the extraordinary points (奇穴 *qí xué*), still commonly used for the treatment of infertility, abnormal bleeding, abdominal pain, diarrhea, and constipation (木下晴都《中國經絡學》, p. 123). These two points are already used in this way by Sūn Sī-Miǎo, as evidenced by their occurence on the next page. Both points are also used as alternate names for KI-13.
4. 關元 *guān yuán*: CV-4, located 3 *cùn* below the navel. It is still one of the most important points in TCM practice for the treatment of reproductive problems.
5. 胞門 *bāo mén*: Here used as a name for a moxibustion point. In modern practice, it is an alternate name for KI-13 (paired with Infant's Door).
6. 氣門 *qì mén*: A pair of extraordinary points still commonly used in the treatment of infertility, uterine bleeding, and red and white postpartum discharge (see 木下晴都《中國經絡學》 p. 60).
7. This refers to the father's sperm.
8. 泉門 *quán mén*: This term is, to my knowledge, not attested elsewhere. See 李經緯, 主編.《中醫大辭典》《針灸，推拿，氣功，養生分冊》 p. 153.

LINE 1.20

論曰：陰陽調和，二氣相感，陽施陰化，是以有娠。而三陰所會則多生女，但妊娠二月名曰始膏，精氣成於胞裡。至於三月名曰始胎，血脈不流，象形而變，未有定儀，見物而化，是時男女未分，故未滿三月者，可服藥，方術轉之，令生男也。

Essay: *Yīn* and *yáng* blend in harmony, the two *qì* respond to each other, *yáng* bestows and *yīn* transforms. Because of this, pregnancy occurs. And when there is a meeting of three *yīn*,[1] it will mostly engender females. However, in the second month of pregnancy [the fetus] is called "beginning paste."[2] Essence and *qì* are brought to completion within the uterus. When reaching the third month, it is called "beginning fetus." The blood does not yet flow in the channels and [the fetus] is changed by patterning itself after outside shapes. Not yet having a fixed form, it is transformed by [the mother's] seeing things. At this time, male and female are not yet differentiated.[3] It is therefore possible, when the third month has not yet been completed, to take medicine and convert [the gender] with the art of prescriptions, causing the birth of a male.[4]

1.　三陰所會 *sān yīn suǒ huì*: The term "three *yīn*" is commonly used in medical literature to refer to the three *yīn* foot channels 足三陰經 (i.e., greater *yīn* 太陰, lesser *yīn* 少陰, and reverting *yīn* 厥陰), or more specifically to the "third *yin*," i.e., the foot greater *yīn* spleen channel 足太陰脾經. However, the term 三陰交 *sān yīn jiāo* ("three *yīn* intersection") is the name of an acupuncture point on the spleen channel (SP-6), three *cùn* above the inner ankle where the three *yīn* channels meet, mentioned already in the *Sù Wèn* (《素文》61, see also 《中華醫學大辭典》p. 46). Based on context, it is unlikely that the term here refers to the *yīn* channels. In a less technical sense, procreation is a process of extreme *yīn* characteristics, since it happens inside the female body, is related to the kidneys and water, is nourished by blood, and is located in the genitals all of which are associated with *yīn*. In that case, one could even interpret the whole phrase in a causative sense: "Since it is a meeting of triple *yīn*, it mostly engenders females."

2.　膏 *gāo*: Usually translated as "lard," that is, the soft fat from animals without horns, most often pigs. See entry on "*gāo*" in the Materia Medica Appendix B, p. 572.

3.　This contradicts the notion that the gender of the fetus is fixed from the moment of conception, as is reflected, for example, in the reference to a "male fetus" during the second month of pregnancy in the third chapter in this volume on "Nurturing the Fetus" (《千金方》2:3) (translated below in the third chapter of volume two, p. 104), as well as the methods for determining the fetus' gender in the third month by pulse diagnosis below. Sūn Sī-Miǎo apparently thought that the fetus acquired a gender at conception, but that this could be transformed until the end of the third month. Charlotte Furth points out that by the *Sòng* period, sexual differentiation had become identified with conception in medical literature and instructions on changing the fetus' gender were therefore eliminated from gynecological prescription literature. On the other hand, instructions for influencing the gender during the act of sexual intercourse, such as through the timing in relationship to the woman's menstrual cycle, became more important (Furth, *A Flourishing Yin*, p. 210).

4.　This paragraph is remarkably similar to a section in the *Tāi Chǎn Shū* 胎產書. Here the art of changing the gender of the fetus is called 內象成子 *nèi xiàng chéng zǐ* (inner imaging to complete the child) and is also recommended for the first three months. See Harper, *Early Chinese Medical Literature*, pp. 378-379, and 馬繼興, 主編《馬王堆古醫書考釋》pp.780-791). Parts of this passage are also found below in section 3 on "nurturing the fetus" in the third month (chapter three of volume two in line 3.10 on pp. 106 - 107). It is, moreover, quoted literally in the *Bìng Yuán Lùn* (《病源論》 41:3) on "converting a female into a male in pregnancy" (妊娠轉女為男 *rèn shēn zhuǎn nǔ wéi nán*).

LINE 1.21

治婦人始覺有娠，養胎並轉女為男，丹參丸方

Sage Pills are a treatment for women when they begin to sense the presence of a pregnancy, nourishing the fetus and simultaneously converting a female fetus into a male.

Sage Pills
丹參丸 *dān shēn wán*

丹參 續斷 芍藥 白膠 白朮 柏子仁（各二兩） 人參 芎藭 乾薑（各三十銖）當歸 橘皮 吳茱萸（各一兩十八銖） 白芷 冠纓（燒灰，各一兩） 蕪黃（十八銖） 乾地黃（一兩半） 甘草（二兩） 犬卵（一具，乾） 東門上雄雞頭（一枚）。

丹參	dān shēn	Root of Salvia miltiorrhiza	二兩 2 liǎng	6g
續斷	xù duàn	Root of Dipsacus asper	二兩 2 liǎng	6g
芍藥	sháo yào	Root of Paeonia albiflora	二兩 2 liǎng	6g
白膠	bái jiāo	Glue produced from Cervus nippon	二兩 2 liǎng	6g
白朮	bái zhú	Rhizome of Atractylodes macrocephala	二兩 2 liǎng	6g
柏子仁	bǎi zǐ rén	Seed of Platycladus orientalis	二兩 2 liǎng	6g
人參	rén shēn	Root of Panax ginseng	三十銖 30 zhū	3.75g
川芎	chuān xiōng	Root of Ligusticum wallichii	三十銖 30 zhū	3.75g
乾薑	gān jiāng	Dried root of Zingiber officinale	三十銖 30 zhū	3.75g
當歸	dāng guī	Root of Angelica polimorpha	一兩十八銖 1 liǎng 18 zhū	5.25g
橘皮	jú pí	Peel of Citrus reticulate	一兩十八銖 1 liǎng 18 zhū	5.25g
吳茱萸	wú zhū yú	Unripe fruit of Evodia rutaecarpa	一兩十八銖 1 liǎng 18 zhū	5.25g
白芷	bái zhǐ	Root of Angelica dahurica	一兩 1 liǎng	3g
冠纓, 燒灰	guān yīng, shāo huī	Cap tassel, charred into ashes	一兩 1 liǎng	3g

蕪荑	wú yí	Processed fruit of Ulmus macro-carpa	十八銖 18 zhū	2.25g
乾地黃	gān dì huáng	Dried root of Rehmannia gluti-nosa	一兩半 1.5 liǎng	4.5g
甘草	gān cǎo	Root of Glycyrrhiza uralensis	二兩 2 liǎng	6g
乾犬卵	gān quǎn luǎn	Dried testicles of Canis familiaris	一具 1 jù	1 set
東門上雄雞頭	dōng mén shàng xióng jī tóu	Head of a rooster from above the eastern gate	一枚 1 méi	1 pc

上十九味，末之，蜜和丸，酒服十丸，日再，稍加至二十丸，如梧子大。

Pulverize the above nineteen ingredients and combine with honey to make pills. Take ten pills in liquor twice a day, gradually increasing the dosage to twenty pills, sized like firmiana seeds.

LINE 1.23

又方

Another prescription:

取原蠶矢一枚，井花水服之，日三。

Take one piece of silk worm excrement and take it in well-flower water*, three times a day.

* 井花水 jǐng huā shuǐ: The first bucket of water drawn from an undisturbed well at dawn.

LINE 1.24

又方

Another prescription:

取弓弩弦一枚，縫囊盛，帶婦人左臂。一法以繫腰下，滿百日去之。

Take one string from a crossbow, place it in a crimson bag, and have the woman carry it on her left arm. Another method is to tie it below the girdle and remove it after a full hundred days.

LINE 1.25

又方

Another prescription:

取雄黃一兩，縫囊盛，帶之。要女者，帶雌黃。

Take one *liǎng* of *xióng huáng* (雄黃 realgar), place it in a crimson bag, and carry it around the waist. If one wants a daughter, carry *cī huáng* (雌黃 orpiment)*.

*   The sexual connotations of *xióng huáng* and *cī huáng* are obvious in the Chinese names, since 雄 *xióng* and 雌 *cí* literally refer to male and female birds respectively.

LINE 1.26

又方

Another prescription:

以斧一柄，於產婦臥牀下置之，仍繫刃向下，勿令人知。如不信者，待雞抱卵時，依此置於窠下，一窠兒子盡為雄也。

Take one axe and place it under the bed which the pregnant woman is sleeping on. Moreover, tie it with the blade pointing down. Do not let others know. If you do not trust this, wait until a chicken is about to lay eggs. Following this method, place [the axe] under the nest. The chicks in this nest will all be male.

2. Malign Obstruction in Pregnancy 妊娠惡阻

LINE 2.1

(一) 論曰：何以知婦人妊娠，脈平而虛者，乳子法也。 (二) 經云：陰搏陽別，謂之有子。此是血氣和調，陽施陰化也。 (三) 診其手少陰脈動甚者，妊子也。少陰心脈也，心主血脈。 (四) 又腎名胞門子戶，尺中腎脈也。尺中之脈，按之不絕，法妊娠也。 (五) 三部脈沈浮正等，按之無絕者，有娠也。

(1) Essay: How do you known whether a woman is pregnant? If her pulse is calm and vacuous, this is the method for [recognizing] that she is with child.

(2) The Classic states: "When the *yīn* [pulse] beats in a way that can be differentiated from the *yáng* [pulse], this is what is called being with child."[1] This means that blood and *qì* blend in harmony and that *yáng* bestows and *yīn* transforms.

(3) If you diagnose extreme movement in [a woman's] hand lesser *yīn* vessel, she is with child. The lesser *yīn* is the vessel of the heart, and the heart governs the movement of blood in the vessels.

(4) Also, the kidneys are called "uterine gate" and "infant's door."[2] The cubit pulse [indicates] the kidney vessel. If the pulse at the cubit position cannot be interrupted when pressed, this is a method for [diagnosing] pregnancy.

(5) When the pulse in the three positions is equally regular on the surface and deep levels[3] and is not interrupted when pressed, this means pregnancy.

1.   This is a quotation from the *Sù Wèn* (Plain Questions) section of the *Huáng Dì Nèi Jīng* (《素文》7). The most widely accepted interpretation of this passage explains *yīn* as referring to the cubit pulse and *yáng* as referring to the inch pulse, while *bó* refers to the movement of the pulse. The cubit position (尺 *chǐ*) is one of the three positions where the pulse is taken on the wrist. Located closest to the elbow in front of the inch (寸 *cùn*) and bar (關 *guān*) sections, it is used to diagnose the kidney channel and conditions of the lower part of the body.

2.   For these terms, see explanation above, p. 82.

3.   This is a reference to the "three positions and nine indicators" (三部九候 *sān bù jiǔ hòu*) system of pulse diagnosis, in which the pulse is taken at the superficial, middle, and deep level in each of the three positions on the wrist. For an elaboration on this system, see the eighth difficult issue in the *Nàn Jīng* (《難經》18), as translated in the Chinese Medicine Database (www.cm-db.com), especially *Xú Dà-Chūn's* 徐大椿 comparison of the *Sù*

Wèn 素問 and *Nàn Jīng* 難經 understanding of the "three positions and nine indicators". In the slightly earlier *Sù Wèn*, this phrase refers to three pulse-taking points in each of the three areas of head, upper limbs, and lower limbs, but by Sūn Sī-miǎo's time, it had become more common to diagnose the different pulses at the positions of the wrist.

LINE 2.2

(一) 妊娠初時寸微小，呼吸五至，三月而尺數也。 (二) 妊娠四月，欲知男女者，左疾為男，右疾為女；左右俱疾，為產二子。 (三) 又法，左手沈實為男，右手浮大為女；左右手俱沈實，猥生二男；俱浮大猥生二女。 (四) 尺脈若左偏大為男，右偏大為女；左右俱大，產二子。大者如實狀。 (五) 又法，左手尺中浮大者男，右手尺中沈細者女；若來而斷絕者，月水不利。 (六) 又法，左右尺俱浮為產二男，不然女作男生；俱沈為產二女，不爾男作女生。 (七) 又法，得太陰脈為男，得太陽脈為女；太陰脈沈，太陽脈浮。

(1) At the beginning of pregnancy, the inch pulse is faint and slight and arrives five times during one circle of breathing, but in the third month the cubit pulse is rapid.

(2) If, by the fourth month of pregnancy, you want to know the gender of the fetus, a racing pulse on the left side means a male; a racing pulse on the right, a female. A racing pulse on both sides means that she is carrying twins.

(3) Another method: A sunken replete pulse on the left hand means a male; a floating large pulse on the right hand, a female; a sunken replete pulse on both hands means that she will give birth to two sons; a floating large pulse on both sides, to two daughters.

(4) If the cubit pulse is large on the left side, it means a son; if it is large on the right side, a daughter; if it is large on both the right and left sides, she will give birth to twins. A large pulse appears like a replete pulse.

(5) Another method: A floating large cubit pulse on the left hand means a male [fetus], a sunken fine cubit pulse on the right hand, a female [fetus]. If [the pulse] comes but then is interrupted, it means menstrual inhibition.[1]

(6) Another method: If both the left and right cubit pulses are floating, it means the birth of two sons, or otherwise the birth of a son from a female fetus who has been turned into a male. If both [cubit pulses] are sunken, it means the birth of two daughters, or otherwise the birth of a daughter from a male fetus who has been changed into a female.

(7) Another method: Obtaining a greater *yīn* pulse[2] means a male [fetus], obtaining a greater *yáng* pulse,[3] a female. A greater *yīn* pulse is sunken, a greater *yáng* pulse is floating.[4]

1.　　This means that it is a symptom of menstrual disease, rather than a sign of pregnancy.
2.　　I.e the pulse of the hand greater *yīn* lung channel (手太陰肺經 *shǒu tài yīn fèi jīng*) and foot greater *yīn* spleen channel (足太陰脾經 *zú tài yīn pí jīng*).

3.   I.e the pulse of the hand greater *yáng* small intestine channel (手太陽小腸經 *shǒu tài yáng xiǎo cháng jīng*) and foot greater *yáng* bladder channel (足太陽膀胱經 *zú tài yáng páng guāng jīng*).

4.   This method seems to contradict the previously mentioned method where a floating pulse signifies a male fetus and a sunken pulse a female fetus. Given the association of *yīn* with female and interior, and of *yáng* with male and exterior, one might expect a scribal error. This phrase is, however, quoted literally also in *Bìng Yuán Lùn* (《病源論》 41:1). Thus, it seems to just be an alternative method of pulse diagnosis.

LINE 2.3

(一) 又，遣妊娠人面南行，還復呼之，左迴首者是男，右迴首者是女。(二) 又，看上圊時，夫從後急呼之，左迴首者是男，右迴首者是女。(三) 又，婦人妊娠，其夫左乳房有核是男，右乳房有核是女。

(1) Another: Follow a pregnant woman who is walking towards the south and call her back. If she turns her head to the left, it means a male [fetus]; if she turns it to the right, a female.

(2) Another: Watch when she is going to the privy, then call her urgently from behind. If she turns her head to the left, it means a male [fetus]; if she turns it to the right, a female.

(3) Another: If the wife is pregnant and her husband has lumps in his left breast, it means a male [fetus]; if he has lumps in the right breast, a female.*

*   This entire essay is also found in an almost literal quotation in *Bìng Yuán Lùn* (《病源論》 41:1) on the "symptoms of pregnancy" (妊娠候 *rèn shēn hòu*).

LINE 2.4

(一) 妊娠欲知將產者，懷妊離經其脈浮，設腹痛引腰脊為今出也。但離經者，不病也。(二) 又法，欲生，其脈離經，半夜覺痛，日中則生也。

(1) In cases of pregnancy, if you want to know whether [the woman] is about to give birth, when the pregnant woman's pulse becomes anomalous and floating and she begins to suffer from abdominal pain that stretches to the lumbus and spine, this means that [the fetus] is now [ready to] emerge. Nevertheless, irregularity [of the pulse] is not a sign of disease.

(2) Another method: If she is ready to give birth, when her pulse becomes anomalous and she feels pain in the middle of the night, she will give birth at midday.

LINE 2.5

(一) 論曰凡婦人虛羸，血氣不足，腎氣又弱，或當風飲冷太過，心下有淡水者，欲有胎而喜病阻。 (二) 所謂欲有胎者，其人月水尚來，顏色肌膚如常，但苦沈重憒悶，不欲食飲，又不知其患所在，脈理順時平和，則是欲有娠也。如此經二月日後，便覺不通，則結胎也。

(1) Essay: Whenever women suffer from vacuity emaciation, insuffiency of *qì* and blood, and an additional weakness of kidney *qì*, perhaps [complicated by] an excessive exposure to wind or consumption of cold drinks, and when phlegm* and fluids are present below the heart, then they tend to suffer from pathological obstruction, if they are on the verge of pregnancy.

(2) What I mean by "being on the verge of pregnancy" is that in such a patient the menstrual flow might still come and her complexion and skin are as usual, but she is troubled by deep-seated heaviness, confusion, and oppression, and is not interested in food or drink. Furthermore, she does not know where her trouble is at and her pulse pattern is smooth and timely, calm and harmonious. This [indicates] that she is on the verge of pregnancy. After she passes two months like this and then feels that [her menses] are stopped, then she is binding the fetus.

*   Based on content and parallel citations in other sources, I read 淡 *dàn* (bland/thin) as 痰 *tán* (phlegm). See *Huá Xià* edition p. 17, n.4.

LINE 2.6

(一) 阻病者，患心中憒憒，頭重眼眩，四肢沈重，懈墮不欲執作，惡聞食氣，欲噉鹹酸果實，多臥少起，世謂惡食。 (二) 其至三四月日已上，皆大劇吐逆，不能自勝舉也。 (三) 此由經血既閉，水漬於藏，藏氣不宣通，故心煩憒悶，氣逆而嘔吐也。 (四) 血脈不通，經絡否澀，則四肢沈重；挾風，則頭目眩也。

(1) A patient with obstruction disease is troubled by severe fretting in the heart, heaviness of the head and a dizzy vision, heaviness of the four limbs, fatigue, inertia, and unwillingness to exert herself in action, aversion to the smell of food, cravings for salty tasting and sour foods as well as fruit, and lying down more and being up less. This is commonly called "aversion to food."

(2) If this lasts beyond the third or fourth month, it will invariably lead to extremely severe counterflow vomiting, which the woman is unable to control and overcome by herself.

(3) This is caused by the fact that channel blood has been blocked, that water has soaked into the viscera, and that visceral *qì* is not flowing freely. This causes heart vexation with confusion and oppression, and *qì* counterflow with retching and vomiting.

(4) If the flow of blood in the vessels is stopped and the channels and network vessels are blocked and inhibited, it results in heaviness of the four limbs. If the condition is complicated by wind, it results in dizziness of the head and eyes.

LINE 2.7

(一) 覺如此候者，便宜服半夏茯苓湯，數劑後將茯苓丸，淡水消除，更欲食也。(二) 既得食力，體強氣盛，力足養胎，母便健矣。(三) 古今治阻病方有十數首，不問虛實冷熱長少，殆死者活於此方

(1) If a woman experiences these kinds of symptoms, she should take several preparations of *Pinellia and Poria Decoction* and afterwards *Poria Pills*. This will cause her phlegm and fluids to be dispersed and eliminated, and then she will want to eat again.

(2) As soon as she has the power to eat, her body will be strong and her *qì* abundant. Her strength will be sufficient for nourishing the fetus, and the mother will return to good health herself.

(3) There are dozens of prescriptions from the past and present for treating obstruction disease, but no matter whether it is a condition of vacuity or repletion, cold or heat,* long-term or short-term, [even] a person on the verge of death will survive with these prescriptions.

---

* 冷熱 *lěng rè*: Conditions characterized by either an aversion to cold and chills or by heat effusion and fever. The context makes clear that this term here does not refer to the symptom called 寒熱 *hán rè* ([aversion to] cold and heat [effusion]).

LINE 2.8

半夏茯苓湯治妊娠阻病，心中憒悶，空煩吐逆，惡聞食氣，頭眩重，四肢百節疼煩沈重，多臥少起，惡寒汗出，疲極黃瘦方

Pinellia and Poria Decoction treats obstruction disease in pregnancy with confusion and oppression in the heart, empty vexation and counterflow vomiting, aversion to the smell of food, dizziness and heaviness of the head, pain, vexation, and heaviness in the four limbs and hundred joints, lying down more and being up less, aversion to cold with sweating, and extreme tiredness and yellow emaciation.

Pinellia and Poria Decoction
半夏茯苓湯 *bàn xià fú líng tāng*

半夏 (三十銖) 茯苓 乾地黃 (各十八銖) 橘皮 細辛 人參 芍藥 旋復花 芎藭 桔梗 甘草 (各十二銖) 生薑 (三十銖)。

半夏	bàn xià	Rhizome of Pinellia ternata	三十銖 30 zhū	3.75g
茯苓	fú líng	Dried fungus of Poria cocos	十八銖 18 zhū	2.25g
乾地黃	gān dì huáng	Dried root of Rehmannia glutinosa	十八銖 18 zhū	2.25g
橘皮	jú pí	Peel of Citrus reticulate	十二銖 12 zhū	1.5g
細辛	xì xīn	Complete plant including root of Asarum heteropoides	十二銖 12 zhū	1.5g
人參	rén shēn	Root of Panax ginseng	十二銖 12 zhū	1.5g
芍藥	sháo yào	Root of Paeonia albiflora	十二銖 12 zhū	1.5g
旋復花	xuán fù huā	Flowerhead of Inula britannica	十二銖 12 zhū	1.5g
川芎	chuān xiōng	Root of Ligusticum wallichii	十二銖 12 zhū	1.5g
桔梗	jié gěng	Root of Platycodon grandiflorum	十二銖 12 zhū	1.5g
甘草	gān cǎo	Root of Glycyrrhiza uralensis	十二銖 12 zhū	1.5g
生薑	shēng jiāng	Fresh root of Zingiber officinale	三十銖 30 zhū	3.75g

上十二味，㕮咀，以水一斗煮取三升，分三服。若病阻積月日不得治，及服藥冷熱失候，病變客熱煩渴，口生瘡者，去橘皮，細辛，加前胡，知母各十二銖；若變冷下痢者，去乾地黃，入桂心十二銖；若食少，胃中虛生熱，大便閟塞，小便赤少者，宜加大黃十八銖，去地黃，加黃芩六銖。餘依方服一劑得下後，消息看氣力冷熱增損，方調定，更服一劑湯，便急服茯苓丸，令能食，便強健也。忌生，冷，醋，滑，油，膩，菘菜，海藻。

Pound the above twelve ingredients and decoct in one *dǒu* of water to obtain three *shēng*. Divide into three doses. If the obstruction has already lasted for several months without successful treatment, if after taking the medicine, the patient has experienced untimely [aversion to] cold and heat [effusion], if the illness has transformed into visiting heat* and vexing thirst, and if sores have formed in her mouth, then leave out the *jǔ pí* 橘皮 and *xì xīn* 細辛 and add twelve *zhū* each of *qián hú* (前胡 Root of Peucedanum praeruptorum) and *zhī mǔ* (知母 Root of Anemarrhena asphodeloides). If it has transformed into a cold [condition] with diarrhea, leave out the *gān dì huáng* 乾地黃 and add twelve *zhū* of *guì xīn* (桂心 Shaved inner bark of Cinnamomum cassia). In cases of reduced eating, vacuity in the stomach generating heat, constipation, and red and scanty urine, it is suitable to add eighteen *zhū* of *dà huáng* (大黃 Root of Rheum palmatum), leave out the *gān dì huáng* 乾地黃 and add six *zhū* of *huáng qín* (黃芩 Root of Scutellaria baicalensis). After taking one preparation according to the prescription and inducing discharge, stop and rest to observe the strength of her *qì*, and whether cold or heat increases or decreases. Adjust the prescription, take another preparation of the decoction, and then quickly follow up with *Poria Pills*. This will allow her to eat and thereby strengthen her health. Avoid raw, cold, vinegary, slippery, oily, and greasy foods, pakchoi, and sargassum.

---

*   客熱 *kè rè*: *kè* "visiting" refers to the termporary or seasonal nature of a condition.

LINE 2.9

(一) 茯苓丸治妊娠阻病，患心中煩悶，頭眩重，憎聞飲食氣，便嘔逆吐悶顛倒，四肢垂弱，不自勝持，服之即效。 (二) 要先服半夏茯苓湯兩劑，後可將服此方

(1) *Poria Pills* treat obstruction disease in pregnancy with complaints of vexing oppression in the heart, dizziness and heaviness of the head, loathing of the smells of food and drink, subsequent retching, counterflow vomiting, oppression, and topsy-turviness,[1] and drooping and weakness of the four limbs, [all of] which the patient cannot overcome by herself. Taking these [pills] will promptly have an effect.

(2) She should first take two preparations of *Pinellia and Poria Decoction* and then follow up with this prescription.

Poria Pills
茯苓丸 *fú líng wán*

茯苓 人參 桂心（熬） 乾薑 半夏 橘皮（各一兩） 白朮 葛根 甘草 枳實（各二兩）。[2]

茯苓	fú líng	Dried fungus of Poria cocos	一兩 1 liǎng	3g
人參	rén shēn	Root of Panax ginseng	一兩 1 liǎng	3g
桂心, 熬	guì xīn, āo	Shaved inner bark of Cinnamomum cassia, boiled	一兩 1 liǎng	3g
乾薑	gān jiāng	Dried root of Zingiber officinale	一兩 1 liǎng	3g
半夏	bàn xià	Rhizome of Pinellia ternata	一兩 1 liǎng	3g
橘皮	jú pí	Peel of Citrus reticulate	一兩 1 liǎng	3g
白朮	bái zhú	Rhizome of Atractylodes macrocephala	二兩 2 liǎng	6g
葛根	gé gēn	Root of Pueraria lobata	二兩 2 liǎng	6g
甘草	gān cǎo	Root of Glycyrrhiza uralensis	二兩 2 liǎng	6g
枳實	zhǐ shí	Unripe fruit of Poncirus trifoliata	二兩 2 liǎng	6g

上十味，末之，蜜和為丸如梧子，飲服二十丸，漸加至三十丸，日三。

Pulverize the above ten ingredients and combine with honey to make pills the size of firmiana seeds. Take twenty pills in liquid, gradually increasing the dosage to thirty pills, three times a day.[3]

---

1. 顛倒 *diān dǎo*: *diān* can be used interchangeably with 癲 *diān*, translated by Wiseman and Fēng as "withdrawal," as for example in the compound 顛狂疾 *diān kuáng jí* (mania

and withdrawal disease). In the *Sù Wèn*, 顛 is explained as a condition where vacuity below and repletion above cause a person to topple (《素文》49). The compound *diān dǎo* can refer to severe insanity, as in the *Líng Shū*: "When there is great wind in the body... [the patient] does not know east from west, south from north, now going up, now down, now turning this way, now back this way, in an abnormal state of topsy-turviness (《靈樞》75)." Féng, Mitchell, and Wiseman offer a third option by translating it as "tossing and turning" in their translation of the *Shāng Hán Lùn* (*Shāng Hán Lùn* On Cold Damage, p. 680).

2. *Sòng* editors' note: "The *Zhǒu Hòu Fāng* 肘后方 does not use *gān jiāng* 乾薑, *bàn xià* 半夏, *jú pí* 橘皮, *bái zhú* 白朮, and *gé gēn* 葛根, only including five ingredients. Furthermore, it states that '*guì xīn* 桂心 is contraindicated in pregnancy and therefore must be boiled.'"

3. The *Wài Tái Mì Yào* ends this prescription with a list of dietary restrictions against sargassum, pakchoi, sheep or goat's meat, candy, peach, plum, swallow meat, vinegar etc. Given the frequency and similarity of these notes on dietary restrictions, I ignore them in the remainder of this translation. They are cited consistently in the footnotes of the *Huá Xià* edition.

LINE 2.10

治妊娠惡阻嘔吐，不下食方

A prescription for treating malign obstruction in pregnancy with retching and vomiting and failure to get food down.

青竹茹 橘皮（各十八銖） 茯苓 生薑（各一兩） 半夏（三十銖）。

青竹茹	qīng zhú rú	Shavings of Phyllostachys nigra	十八銖 18 zhū	2.25g
橘皮	jú pí	Peel of Citrus reticulate	十八銖 18 zhū	2.25g
茯苓	fú líng	Dried fungus of Poria cocos	一兩 1 liǎng	3g
生薑	gān jiāng	Dried root of Zingiber officinale	一兩 1 liǎng	3g
半夏	bàn xià	Rhizome of Pinellia ternata	三十銖 30 zhū	3.75g

上五味，咬咀，以水六升煮取三升半，分三服，不瘥頻作。

Pound the above five ingredients and decoct in six *shēng* of water to obtain three and a half *shēng*. Divide into three doses. If the patient fails to recover, make it frequently.

LINE 2.11

治妊娠嘔吐不下食，橘皮湯方

Tangerine Peel Decoction treats retching and vomiting in pregnancy with failure to get food down.

Tangerine Peel Decoction
橘皮湯 *jú pí tāng*

橘皮 竹茹 人參 白朮（各十八銖） 生薑（一兩） 厚朴（十二銖）。

橘皮	jú pí	Peel of Citrus reticulata	十八銖 18 zhū	2.25g
竹茹	zhú rú	Shavings of the stripped core Phyllostachys stalks	十八銖 18 zhū	2.25g
人參	rén shēn	Root of Panax ginseng	十八銖 18 zhū	2.25g
白朮	bái zhú	Rhizome of Atractylodes macro-cephala	十八銖 18 zhū	2.25g
生薑	shēng jiāng	Fresh root of Zingiber officinale	一兩 1 liǎng	3g
厚朴	hòu pò	Bark of Magnolia officinalis	十二銖 12 zhū	1.5g

上六味，咬咀，以水七升煮取二升半，分三服，不瘥重作。

Pound the above six ingredients and decoct in seven *shēng* of water to obtain two and a half *shēng*. Divide into three doses. If she fails to recover, make it again.

3. Nurturing the Fetus 養胎

LINE 3.1

(一) 論曰：舊說凡受胎三月，逐物變化，稟質未定。(二) 故妊娠三月，欲得觀犀象猛獸珠玉寶物。(三) 欲得見賢人君子盛德大師，觀禮樂鍾鼓俎豆軍旅陳設。(四) 焚燒名香，口誦詩書古今箴誡。(五) 居處簡靜，割不正不食，席不正不坐。(六) 彈琴瑟，調心神，和情性，節嗜慾，庶事清淨。(七) 生子皆良，長壽忠孝，仁義聰惠，無疾。(八) 斯蓋文王胎教者也。

(1) Essay: The ancient theories all agree that during the three months of receiving the fetus,[1] it will transform according to things and its disposition and character are not yet fixed.

(2) Therefore, in the [first] three months of pregnancy, [the pregnant woman] should be able to inspect rhinoceri, elephants, and other wild beasts, as well as gems and jade and other precious objects.

(3) She should be able to observe sages, gentlemen, and eminent teachers of abundant virtue, and she should inspect ritual and music, bells and drums, sacrificial trays and vessels, and the lining up and arranging of military troops.

(4) She should burn rare incense and recite the Book of Poetry and the Book of History, as well as ancient and modern commandments and admonishings.

(5) She should live in simple and quiet surroundings and not eat improperly cut meat or sit on incorrectly laid-out mats.

(6) She should play the *qín* and *sè*[2] zithers, balance her heart and spirit, harmonize her affects and temperament, and moderate her desires and predilections. In all affairs, she should be pure and composed.

(7) [If she follows these instructions,] she will bear children who will all be good, long-lived, loyal and filial, humane, righteous, intelligent, and wise, and free of illness.

(8) Such must have been the fetal education of King Wén.[3]

1. 受胎三月 *shòu tāi sān yuè*: The first three months of pregnancy. This expression suggests that the creation of the fetus was perceived as a gradual process that took place for the duration of three months, rather than at the initial single act of sexual intercourse. While

it is clear that medieval Chinese thought of conception as occurring at a single decisive moment — hence the various methods and taboos regarding the time and position of intercourse with regards to astrology, the woman's menstrual cycle, the parents' mental state, etc,— even such basic characteristics of the fetus as its gender, appearance, intelligence, and morality were believed to remain fluid for the first three months.

2. 琴瑟 *qín sè*: Two kinds of fretted string instruments, the first with five or seven strings, the second with fifty or later twenty-five strings and movable bridges.

3. 文王 Wén Wáng: The father of the founder of the *Zhōu* dynasty, namely 武王 Wǔ Wáng (King Wǔ). King Wén's mother, Tài Rén 太任, was renowned throughout Chinese history for her perfectly upright behavior in general, but in particular for her practice of 胎教 *tāi jiào* (fetal education), as a result of which "King Wén was born an enlightened sage" (文王生而明聖 *wén wáng shēng ér míng shèng*). See (《列女傳》 1:3).

LINE 3.2

(一) 論曰：兒在胎，日月未滿，陰陽未備，腑藏骨節皆未成足。(二) 故自初訖于將產，飲食居處，皆有禁忌。

(1) Essay: When the child is in the uterus, before the days and months [to carry a pregnancy to term] are filled, *yīn* and *yáng* are not yet fully developed and the bowels and viscera, bones and joints are not yet completely formed.

(2) Therefore, prohibitions and avoidances exist, all the way from the very beginning to when she is about to deliver, with regard to food and drink and residence and surroundings.

LINE 3.3

(一) 妊娠食羊肝，令子多危。(二) 妊娠食山羊肉，令子多病。(三) 妊娠食驢馬肉，延月。(四) 妊娠食騾肉，產難。(五) 妊娠食兔肉犬肉，令子無音聲並缺脣。(六) 妊娠食雞子及乾鯉魚，令子多瘡。(七) 妊娠食雞肉糯米，令子多寸白蟲。(八) 妊娠食椹並鴨子，令子倒出心寒。(九) 妊娠食雀肉並豆醬，令子滿面多䵟䵳[1] 黑子。(十) 妊娠食雀肉飲酒，令子心淫情亂，不畏羞恥。(十一) 妊娠食鼈，令子項短。(十二) 妊娠食冰漿，絕胎。(十三) 妊娠勿向非常地大小便，必半產殺人。

(1) Eating sheep's or goat's liver during pregnancy causes many perils for the child.

(2) Eating mountain goat[2] meat during pregnancy causes many diseases for the child.

(3) Eating donkey or horse meat during pregnancy extends the months.

(4) Eating mule meat during pregnancy causes birthing difficulties.

(5) Eating rabbit meat or dog meat during pregnancy causes deafness and harelip in the child.[3]

(6) Eating chicken eggs or dried carp during pregnancy causes the child to have many skin sores.

(7) Eating chicken and glutinous rice during pregnancy causes the child to have many inch whiteworms.[4]

(8) Eating mulberries and duck eggs during pregnancy causes the child to emerge upside down[5] and have coldness in the heart.

(9) Eating sparrow meat with soy sauce during pregnancy causes the child to have many freckles and moles all over the face.[6]

(10) Eating sparrow meat and drinking liquor during pregnancy causes the child to have a licentious heart and deranged affects and not to fear shame and disgrace.

(11) Eating turtles during pregnancy causes the child to have a short neck.

(12) Drinking chilled fermented millet drink[7] during pregnancy aborts the fetus.

(13) During pregnancy, never use uncommon locations to urinate or defecate since it is bound to cause miscarriage or death.[8]

1. These are rare characters for types of black spots and moles in the face.
2. 山羊 *shān yáng*: In the *Zhōng Yī Dà Cí Diǎn,* it is equated with 山驢 *shān lǘ* (lit. mountain donkey). This is identified there as Capricornis sumatraensis (《中藥大辭典》 #0500), known in English as serow. See entry on *shān lǘ jiao* 山驢角, Materia Medica Appendix B, p. 606.
3. Abstaining from rabbit meat during pregnancy is a common proscription, already stated in the *Tāi Chǎn Shū* (MSV.3, lower half, CC 1-13). Donald Harper quotes the *Bó Wù Zhì* 博物志, a third century text by *Zhāng Huá* 張華: "A pregnant woman can neither eat rabbit nor look at a rabbit, for it causes the infant to have a split lip;..." (Harper, *Early Chinese Medical Literature*, p. 379, n. 3, and 《博物志》 2.1b).
4. 寸白蟲 *cùn bái chóng*: One of the nine worm diseases. In modern TCM equated with tape worm infestation.
5. 倒出 *dào chū*: This refers to the child being born in breech presentation with the head first.
6. This association is probably related to the fact that freckles are also referred to as 雀斑 *què bān* (sparrow spots).
7. 漿 *jiāng*: A sour alcoholic beverage, made by soaking and fermenting millet in water, more commonly known as 截漿 *cai jiāng* (but written with liquor radical). See 《中國飲食辭典》 pp. 270 and 619.
8. 半產殺人 *bàn chǎn shā rén*: Alternatively, this could be read literally as "kill the person midway through giving birth," but *bàn chǎn* is a common technical term for miscarriage. It is thus more likely that the phrase here refers to miscarriage or death [of the mother and/or child] after birth.

Xú Zhī-Cái's Month-by-Month Prescriptions
for Nurturing the Fetus
徐之才逐月養胎方

Translator's note: *Xú Zhī-Cái* was a physician in the Northern *Qí* period (550-577) who supposedly lived from 493-572. Well-versed in the medical arts, he specialized in medicinal prescriptions, in particular for women and children. He is the author of several lost texts, such as the *Duì Yào* 藥對 (*A Comparison of Medicinals*), *Jiā Chuán Mì Fāng* 家傳秘方 (*Secret Prescriptions Handed Down in the Family*), *Xiǎo Ér Fāng* 小兒方 (*Pediatric Prescriptions*), etc., none of which have survived except as quotations in other texts.

LINE 3.4

(一) 妊娠一月名始胚，飲食精熟酸美，受御，宜食大麥，無食腥辛，是謂才正。(二) 妊娠一月，足厥陰脈養，不可針灸其經。足厥陰內屬於肝，肝主筋及血。(三) 一月之時，血行否澀，不為力事，寢必安靜，無令恐畏。(四) 妊娠一月，陰陽新合為胎。

(1) The first month of pregnancy is called "beginning embryo."[2] [The mother] should eat and drink exquisite and thoroughly cooked things and fancy sour broths.[3] She should be mounted [in sexual intercourse].[4] She should eat barley, but may not eat rancid or acrid things.[5] This is what is called perfectly correct.

(2) In the first month of pregnancy, the foot reverting *yīn* vessel nourishes [the fetus].[6] You must not needle or burn moxa on this channel. The foot reverting *yīn* is associated with the liver, which governs the sinews and the blood.

(3) During the period of the first month, the blood flow is blocked and inhibited and [the pregnant woman] should not engage in strenuous activities. Her sleeping place must be peaceful and quiet and she must not be exposed to fear or alarm.

(4) In the first month of pregnancy, *yīn* and *yáng* have newly combined to constitute the fetus.

1. The parallel quotation of this text in the *Tāi Chǎn Shū* has 流形 *liú xíng* (flowing into form) instead.
2. Based on other occurrences of this text, most notably the *Tāi Chǎn Shū*, I read 美 *měi* as 羹 *gēng* (fancy broth). For more evidence on this phrase, see 馬繼興, 主編《馬王堆古醫書考釋》 p.781-3.
3. 受御 *shòu yù*: The meaning of this phrase is questionable. The editors of modern Chinese editions seem to interpret this as further instructions on the mother "receiving imperial-quality" foods or perhaps as "being waited on," by including these characters in the preceding phrase. Based on the original meaning of 御, i.e., to drive a chariot, and its frequent use in sexual cultivation literature to refer to a man's action of mounting a woman in sexual intercourse, I read 御 here in this sense. This is supported by the longer variation of this phrase in the *Ishimpô*: 無御丈夫 *wú yù zhàng fū* "Do not engage in sexual

intercourse with the husband." 無 seems to be a scribal error for 受 as both the *Qiān Jīn Fāng* and *Bìng Yuán Lùn* have 受. See (《醫心方》 22:1) and (《病源論》 41:1). The phrase is unfortunately missing in the *Tāi Chǎn Shū*.

4.   This section is almost literally identical to the *Tāi Chǎn Shū*. See Harper, *Early Chinese Medical Literature*, pp. 378-381, and 馬繼興, 主編《馬王堆古醫書考釋》pp. 781-802. The same is true for the parallel introductory sections in the following paragraphs for each month.

5.   For a beautiful visual representation of the channels and points relevant in the course of a woman's pregnancy, see *Ishimpô* (《醫心方》 23:1), 妊婦脈圖月禁法 (*Channel Charts and Monthly Restrictions for Pregnant Women*), *Huá Xià* edition pp. 441-446. See Sabine Wilms, "The Transmission of Medical Knowledge on 'Nurturing the Fetus' in Early China." Asian Medicine: Tradition and Modernity 2, 2005.

LINE 3.5

寒多為痛，熱多卒驚，舉重腰痛腹滿胞急，卒有所下，當預安之，宜服烏雌雞湯方

[During the first month of pregnancy,] for cases of pain due to increased cold; sudden panic due to increased heat; lumbar pain, abdominal fullness, and tightness in the uterus from heavy lifting; and the sudden appearance of vaginal discharge, the patient should take *Black Hen Decoction* to stabilize her as a precaution.

Black Hen Decoction
烏雌雞湯 *wū cí jī tāng*

烏雌雞（一隻，治如食法）茯苓（二兩）吳茱萸（一升）芍藥 白朮（各三兩）麥門冬（五合）人參（三兩）阿膠（二兩）甘草（一兩）生薑（一兩）。

烏雌雞, 治如食法	wū cí jī, zhì rú shí fǎ	Complete body of black female Gallus gallus domesticus, prepared as for cooking	一隻 1 zhī	one bird
茯苓	fú líng	Dried fungus of Poria cocos	二兩 2 liǎng	6g
吳茱萸	wú zhū yú	Unripe fruit of Evodia rutaecarpa	一升 1 shēng	24g
芍藥	sháo yào	Root of Paeonia albiflora	三兩 3 liǎng	9g
白朮	bái zhú	Rhizome of Atractylodes macrocephala	三兩 3 liǎng	9g
麥門冬	tiān mén dōng	Tuber of Asparagus cochinchinensis	五合 5 gě	35ml
人參	rén shēn	Root of Panax ginseng	三兩 3 liǎng	9g
阿膠	ē jiāo	Gelatinous glue produced from Equus asinus	二兩 2 liǎng	6g
甘草	gān cǎo	Root of Glycyrrhiza uralensis	一兩 1 liǎng	3g

生薑	shēng jiāng	Fresh root of Zingiber officinale	一兩 1 liǎng	3g

上十味，㕮咀，以水一斗二升煮雞，取汁六升，去雞下藥，煎取三升，內酒三升，並膠烊盡取三升，放溫，每服一升，日三。

Pound the above ten ingredients. Cook the chicken in one *dǒu* and two *shēng* of water to obtain six *shēng* of liquid. Take out the chicken, add the drugs, and simmer to obtain three *shēng*. Add three *shēng* of liquor. Mix in the *ē jiāo* 阿膠 until completely dissolved. Reduce to three *shēng*, leave it until warm* and take one *shēng* at a time, three times a day.

*　　放溫 *fàng wēn*: This means to let it cool off a little. Alternatively, it could mean to "keep it warm."

LINE 3.6

若曾傷一月胎者，當預服補胎湯方

In cases of any damage to the fetus during the first month, [the patient] should take *Fetus-Supplementing Decoction* as a precaution.

Fetus-Supplementing Decoction
補胎湯 *bǔ tāi tāng*

細辛（一兩）乾地黃 白朮（各三兩）生薑（四兩）大麥 吳茱萸（各五合）烏梅（一升）防風（二兩）。

細辛	xì xīn	Complete plant including root of Asarum heteropoides	一兩 1 liǎng	3g
乾地黃	gān dì huáng	Dried root of Rehmannia glutinosa	三兩 3 liǎng	9g
白朮	bái zhú	Rhizome of Atractylodes macrocephala	三兩 3 liǎng	9g
生薑	shēng jiāng	Fresh root of Zingiber officinale	四兩 4 liǎng	12g
大麥	dà mài	Seed of Hordeum vulgare	五合 5 gě	35ml
吳茱萸	wú zhū yú	Unripe fruit of Evodia rutaecarpa	五合 5 gě	35ml
烏梅	wū méi	Unripe fruit of Prunus mume	一升 1 shēng	24g
防風	fáng fēng	Root of Ledebouriella divaricata	二兩 2 liǎng	6g

上八味，㕮咀，以水七升煮取二升半，分三服，先食服。寒多者，倍細辛，茱萸。若熱多渴者，去細辛，茱萸，加栝樓根二兩。若有所思，去大麥，加柏子仁三合。

Pound the above eight ingredients and decoct in seven *shēng* of water to obtain two and a half *shēng*. Divide into three doses and take before meals. In cases of increased cold, double the *xì xīn* 細辛 and *wú zhū yú* 吳茱萸. In cases of increased heat and thirst, take out the *xì xīn* 細辛 and *wú zhū yú* 吳茱萸 and add two *liǎng* of *guā lóu gēn* (栝蔞根 Root of Trichosanthes kirilowii). In cases of [excessive] thought, take out the *dà mài* 大麥 and add three *gě* of *bǎi zǐ rén* (柏子仁 Seed of Platycladus orientalis).

*   *Sòng* editors' note: "Another [version of this] prescription includes one *liǎng* of *rén shēn* (人參 Root of Panax ginseng)."

LINE 3.7

(一) 妊娠二月名始膏，無食辛臊，居必靜處，男子勿勞，百節皆痛，是為胎始結。(二) 妊娠二月，足少陽脈養，不可針灸其經。足少陽內屬於膽，主精。(三) 二月之時，兒精成於胞裡，當慎護驚動也。(四) 妊娠二月，始陰陽鋸經。

(1) The second month of pregnancy is called "beginning paste."[1] [The mother] must not eat acrid or foul-smelling food. Her dwellings must be in a quiet location and in the case of a male child, she must avoid taxation.[2] All the myriad joints are painful. This is the fetus beginning to bind.[3]

(2) In the second month of pregnancy, the foot lesser *yáng* vessel nourishes [the fetus]. You must not needle or burn moxa on this channel. The foot lesser *yáng* is associated with the gallbladder, which governs essence.

(3) During the period of the second month, the child's essence is being formed inside the uterus, and [the pregnant woman] must beware of and protect herself against being alarmed.

(4) In the second month of pregnancy, *yīn* and *yáng* are beginning to occupy the channels.

1.   膏 *gāo*: Lard, specifically the soft fat from animals without horns.
2.   男子勿勞 *nán zǐ wù láo*: It is a common notion in many cultures that a male fetus is more taxing on the mother's body than a female one.
3.   結 *jié*: A common term in medical Chinese, lit. "to tie/knot." It usually "denotes a concentration of evils in a specific location, that causes hardness," such as heat, phlegm, or dampness (see Wiseman and Féng, *Practical Dictionary*, p. 18). In the context of the formation of the fetus, it refers to the process by which male essence and female blood cohere together, congeal, and harden in the woman's uterus, forming the fetus.

LINE 3.8

有寒多壞不成，有熱即萎悴，中風寒有所動搖，心滿，臍下懸急，腰背強痛，卒有所下，乍寒乍熱，艾葉湯主之方

For cases of decaying [fetus] and failure to complete [the pregnancy] due to increased cold, withered [fetus] due to heat, [fetal] stirring and agitation due to being struck by wind or cold, fullness in the heart, suspension and tension below the navel, rigidity and pain in the lumbus and back, suddenly appearing vaginal discharge, and abruptly alternating [aversion to] cold and heat [effusion], *Mugwort Decoction* is the governing prescription.

Mugwort Decoction
艾葉湯 *ài yè tāng*

艾葉 丹參 當歸 麻黃（各二兩） 人參 阿膠（各三兩） 甘草（一兩） 生薑（六兩） 大棗（十二枚）。

艾葉	ài yè	Dry-roasted foliage of Artemisia argyi	二兩 2 liǎng	6g
丹參	dān shēn	Root of Salvia miltiorrhiza	二兩 2 liǎng	6g
當歸	dāng guī	Root of Angelica polimorpha	二兩 2 liǎng	6g
麻黃	má huáng	Stalk of Ephedra sinica	二兩 2 liǎng	6g
人參	rén shēn	Root of Panax ginseng	三兩 3 liǎng	9g
阿膠	ē jiāo	Gelatinous glue produced from Equus asinus	三兩 3 liǎng	9g
甘草	gān cǎo	Root of Glycyrrhiza uralensis	一兩 1 liǎng	3g
生薑	shēng jiāng	Fresh root of Zingiber officinale	六兩 6 liǎng	18g
大棗	dà zǎo	Mature fruit of Ziziphus jujuba	十二枚 12 méi	12 pcs

上九味，㕮咀，以酒三升，水一斗煮減半，去滓內膠，煎取三升，分三服。

Pound the above nine ingredients and decoct in three *shēng* of liquor and one *dǒu* of water until reduced by half. Discard the dregs, add the *ē jiāo* 阿膠, and simmer to obtain three *shēng*. Divide into three doses.˙

---

*   *Sòng* editors' note: "Another [version of this] prescription uses one black hen, fattened up nicely, that is prepared as for cooking. Chop off the head, take the blood, and mix it with three *shēng* of liquor until well-blended. Cook the chicken in one *dǒu* and two *shēng* of water, save the liquid and take out the chicken. Add the drugs and simmer to obtain three *shēng*. Add the blood and liquor together with the *ē jiāo* 阿膠 and simmer to obtain three *shēng*. Divide and take heated in three doses."

LINE 3.9

若曾傷二月胎者，當預服黃連湯方

In cases of any damage to the fetus during the second month, [the patient] should take *Coptis Decoction* as a precaution.

Coptis Decoction
黃連湯 *huáng lián tāng*

黃連 人參（各一兩） 吳茱萸（五合） 生薑（三兩） 生地黃（五兩）。*

黃連	huáng lián	Rhizome of Coptis chinensis	一兩 1 liǎng	3g
人參	rén shēn	Root of Panax ginseng	一兩 1 liǎng	3g
吳茱萸	wú zhū yú	Unripe fruit of Evodia rutaecarpa	五合 5 gě	35ml
生薑	shēng jiāng	Fresh root of Zingiber officinale	三兩 3 liǎng	9g
生地黃	shēng dì huáng	Fresh root of Rehmannia glutinosa	五兩 5 liǎng	15g

上五味，㕮咀，以酢漿七升煮取三升，分四服，日三夜一，十日一作。若顏覺不安，加烏梅一升。加烏梅者，不用漿，直用水耳。

Pound the above five ingredients and decoct in seven *shēng* of fermented millet drink to obtain three *shēng*. Divide into four doses and take three times during the day and once at night. Make it once every ten days. If [the mother] feels slightly disquieted, add one *shēng* of *wū méi* (烏梅 Unripe fruit of Prunus mume). If you add *wū méi* 烏梅, do not use fermented millet drink, but use plain water instead.

---

*   *Sòng* editors' note: "Another [version of this] prescription uses *ē jiāo* (阿膠 Gelatinous glue produced from Equus asinus) instead of *shēng dì huáng* 生地黃. Another [version of this] prescription includes half a *liǎng* of *dāng guī* (當歸 Root of Angelica polimorpha)."

LINE 3.10

(一) 妊娠三月名始胎。當此之時，未有定儀，見物而化。(二) 欲生男者，操弓矢；欲生女者，弄珠璣；欲子美好，數視璧玉；欲子賢良，端坐清虛。(三)是謂外象而內感者也。(四) 妊娠三月，手心主脈養，不可針灸其經，手心主內屬於，心無悲哀思慮驚動。(五) 妊娠三月，為定形。

(1) The third month of pregnancy is called "beginning fetus."[1] During this time period, it does not yet have a fixed form and is transformed by [the mother's] seeing things.

(2) If you want to give birth to a son, practice with bow and arrow; if you want to give birth to a daughter, handle pearls; if you want your child to be beautiful, often look at jades; if you want your child to be virtuous and talented, seat yourself properly and be pure and

empty.[2]

(3) This is what is called "internally responding to external images."[3]

(4) In the third month of pregnancy, the hand heart-governing vessel nourishes [the fetus], and you must not needle or burn moxa on this channel. The hand heart-governor is associated with the heart. Avoid feelings of sorrow and grief, thought and preoccupation, fright and commotion.

(5) In the third month of pregnancy, the shape is being stabilized.

1.   The *Tāi Chǎn Shū* differs here and has 始脂 *shǐ zhī* (beginning hard fat). See 馬繼興, 主編《馬王堆古醫書考釋》, p. 787.
2.   清虛 *qīng xū*: In the Buddhist sense of being free from desires and distracting thoughts. This might even be a reference to practicing meditation.
3.   This paragraph is again very similar to the *Tāi Chǎn Shū*. For comparisons, see Donald Harper, *Early Chinese Medical Literature*, p. 379, and 馬繼興, 主編《馬王堆古醫書考釋》, p. 786). Compared to the previous months of gestation where Sūn Sī-miǎo's text is almost literally identical with the *Mǎ-Wáng-Duī* material, differences in the notion of fetal education (胎教 *tāi jiào*) are noteworthy: While the *Tāi Chǎn Shū* offers such simple advice as avoiding ginger and rabbit, observing male wild animals for a boy, and wearing female accessories for a girl, by Sūn Sī-miǎo's time the focus seems to have shifted to a more moral content.

LINE 3.11

有寒大便青，有熱小便難，不赤即黃，卒驚恐憂愁嗔怒，喜頓仆，動於經脈，腹滿，繞臍苦痛，或腰背痛，卒有所下，雄雞湯方

For cases of cold conditions with blue-green feces,[1] heat conditions with difficult urination of red or yellow urine, sudden fright and fear, anxiety and worrying, flights of temper and rage, a tendency to stumble and fall, stirring in the vessels, abdominal fullness, bitter pain around the navel or in the lumbus and back, and sudden presence of vaginal discharge, *Rooster Decoction* [is the governing] prescription.

Rooster Decoction
雄雞湯 *xióng jī tāng*

雄雞一隻（治如食法）甘草 人參 茯苓 阿膠（各二兩）黃芩 白朮（各一兩）麥門冬（五合）芍藥（四兩）大棗（十二枚，擘）生薑（一兩）。[2]

雄雞, 治 如食法	xióng jī, zhì rú shí fǎ	Complete body of male Gallus gallus domesticus prepared as for cooking	一隻 1 zhī	One Bird
甘草	gān cǎo	Root of Glycyrrhiza uralensis	二兩 2 liǎng	6g

人參	rén shēn	Root of Panax ginseng	二兩 2 liǎng	6g
茯苓	fú líng	Dried fungus of Poria cocos	二兩 2 liǎng	6g
阿膠	ē jiāo	Gelatinous glue produced from Equus asinus	二兩 2 liǎng	6g
黃芩	huáng qín	Root of Scutellaria baicalensis	一兩 1 liǎng	3g
白朮	bái zhú	Rhizome of Atractylodes macro-cephala	一兩 1 liǎng	3g
麥門冬	mài mén dōng	Tuber of Ophiopogon japonicus	五合 5 gě	35ml
芍藥	sháo yào	Root of Paeonia albiflora	四兩 4 liǎng	12g
大棗, 擘	dà zǎo, bò	Mature fruit of Ziziphus jujuba, broken up	十二枚 12 méi	12 pcs
生薑	shēng jiāng	Fresh root of Zingiber officinale	一兩 1 liǎng	3g

上十一味，㕮咀，以水一斗五升煮雞減半，出雞內藥煮取半，內清酒三升並膠，煎取三升，分三服，一日盡之，當溫臥。

Pound the above eleven ingredients. Cook the chicken in one *dǒu* and five *shēng* of water until [the liquid is] reduced by half. Take out the chicken, add the drugs, and simmer until reduced by half. Add three *shēng* of clear liquor together with the *ē jiāo* 阿膠 and decoct it to obtain three *shēng*. Divide it into three doses and use it all up in one day. [The patient] should be kept warm and in bed [after she has finished the medicine].[3]

1. 大便青 *dà biàn qīng*: In the *Wǔ Shí Èr Bìng Fāng* 五十二病方, blue-green feces that have not been transformed [i.e., eliminated] are associated with infant convulsions. The editors paraphrase *qīng* as 藍黑色 *lán hēi sè* (of blue-black color). See 馬繼興, 主編《馬王堆古醫書考釋》, pp. 374-6, and Donald Harper, *Early Chinese Medical Literature*, p. 233. Dark feces are a common symptom in cold-related conditions.
2. *Sòng* editors' note: "Another [version of this prescription] uses two *liǎng* each of *dāng guī* (當歸 Root of Angelica polimorpha) and *xiōng qióng* (芎藭 Root of Ligusticum wallichii), but does not use *huáng qín* 黃芩 and *shēng jiāng* 生薑."
3. 當溫臥 *dāng wēn wò*: The *Sūn Zhēn Rén* edition adds 訖 *qì* "when finished" before this phrase, which clarifies the meaning of the sentence. Otherwise, *wēn* could also refer to the medicine in the following sense: "[The medicine] should [be taken] heated and when lying down."

LINE 3.12

若曾傷三月胎者，當預服茯神湯方

In cases of any damage to the fetus during the third month, [the patient] should take *Root Poria Decoction* as a precaution.[1]

Root Poria Decoction
茯神湯 *fú shén tāng*

茯神 丹參 龍骨（各一兩） 阿膠 當歸 甘草 人參（各二兩） 赤小豆（二十一粒） 大棗（二十一枚）。²

茯神	fú shén	Dried fungus of Poria cocos	一兩 1 liǎng	3g
丹參	dān shēn	Root of Salvia miltiorrhiza	一兩 1 liǎng	3g
龍骨	lóng gǔ	Os Draconis	一兩 1 liǎng	3g
阿膠	ē jiāo	Gelatinous glue produced from Equus asinus	二兩 2 liǎng	6g
當歸	dāng guī	Root of Angelica polimorpha	二兩 2 liǎng	6g
甘草	gān cǎo	Root of Glycyrrhiza uralensis	二兩 2 liǎng	6g
人參	rén shēn	Root of Panax ginseng	二兩 2 liǎng	6g
赤小豆	chì xiǎo dòu	Fruit of Phaseolus calcaratus	二十一粒 21 lì	21 grains
大棗	dà zǎo	Mature fruit of Ziziphus jujuba	二十一枚 21 méi	21 pcs

上九味，㕮咀，以酥漿一斗煮取三升，分四服，先食服，七日後服一劑。腰痛者，加桑寄生二兩。深師有薤白二兩，麻子一升。

Pound the above nine ingredients and decoct in one *dǒu* of fermented millet drink to obtain three *shēng*. Divide into four doses and take before meals. After seven days, take another preparation. In cases of lumbar pain, add two *liǎng* of *sāng jì shēng* (桑寄生 Branches and foliage of Viscum coloratum).

1. The *Sūn Zhēn Rén* edition differs here by calling this prescription 茯苓神湯 *(Poria and Root Poria Decoction)*, an additional character that could have easily been lost in copying. Moreover, the actual prescription includes as the first ingredient 3 *liǎng* of *fú líng* (茯苓 Dried fungus of Poria cocos).
2. *Sòng* editors' note: "The *Shēn Shī*³ includes two *liǎng* of *cōng bái* (蔥白 Stalk of Allium fistulosum) and one *shēng* of *má zǐ rén* (麻子仁 Seed of Cannabis sativa)."
3. 深師 *Shēn Shī (Profound Teacher)* is a text of unknown identity, not recorded in 丹波元胤《中國醫籍考》.

LINE 3.13

(一) 妊娠四月，始受水精以成血脈。(二) 食宜稻粳，羹宜魚鴈。(三) 是謂盛血氣以通耳目，而行經絡。(四) 妊娠四月，手少陽脈養，不可針灸其經。手少陽內輸三焦。(五) 四月之時，兒六腑順成，當靜形體和心志節飲食。

(1) In the fourth month of pregnancy, [the fetus] begins to receive the essence of water and uses it to develop the blood and vessels.

(2) [The pregnant woman] should eat meals of glutinous and non-glutinous rice and should drink broths made from fish and wild goose.

(3) This is what is called making blood and *qì* exuberant so that they will penetrate to the ears and eyes and flow in the channels and network vessels.

(4) In the fourth month of pregnancy the hand lesser *yáng* vessel nourishes [the fetus], and you must not needle or burn moxa on this channel. The hand lesser *yáng* is associated with the triple burner.

(5) During the fourth month, the child's six bowels [should be allowed to] develop smoothly. [The woman] must quiet her body, harmonize her heart and will, and moderate her drink and food.

LINE 3.14

妊娠四月，有寒心下慍慍欲嘔，胸膈滿，不欲食；有熱小便難，數數如淋狀，臍下苦急；卒風寒，頸項強痛，寒熱；或驚動，身軀腰背腹痛，往來有時，胎上迫胸，心煩不得安，卒有所下，菊花湯方

In the fourth month of pregnancy,[1] for seething below the heart and desire to retch, fullness in the chest and diaphragm, and lack of appetite, all of which are related to the presence of cold; for urinary difficulties, urinating very frequently like a dribble, and bitter tension below the navel, which are related to the presence of heat; and for sudden wind-cold, rigidity and pain in the nape and neck, and [aversion to] cold and heat [effusion], [fetal] stirring, perhaps from fright, with intermittent and occasional pain in the lumbus, back, and abdomen, for the fetus ascending and distressing the chest, for heart vexation and inability to get rest, and for the sudden presence of vaginal discharge, take *Chrysanthemum Decoction*.

Chrysanthemum Decoction
菊花湯 *jú huā tāng*

菊花（如雞子大一枚） 麥門冬（一升） 麻黃 阿膠（各三兩） 人參（一兩半） 甘草 當歸（各二兩） 生薑（五兩） 半夏（四兩） 大棗（十二枚）。

菊花	jú huā	Flower of Chrysanthemum morafolii	如雞子大一枚 rú jī zǐ dà 1 méi	1 pc the size of an egg
麥門冬	mài mén dōng	Tuber of Ophiopogon japonicus	一升 1 shēng	24g
麻黃	má huáng	Stalk of Ephedra sinica	三兩 3 liǎng	9g
阿膠	ē jiāo	Gelatinous glue produced from Equus asinus	三兩 3 liǎng	9g

人參	rén shēn	Root of Panax ginseng	一兩半 1.5 liǎng	4.5g
甘草	gān cǎo	Root of Glycyrrhiza uralensis	二兩 2 liǎng	6g
當歸	dāng guī	Root of Angelica polimorpha	二兩 2 liǎng	6g
生薑	shēng jiāng	Fresh root of Zingiber officinale	五兩 5 liǎng	15g
半夏	bàn xià	Rhizome of Pinellia ternata	四兩 4 liǎng	12g
大棗	dà zǎo	Mature fruit of Ziziphus jujuba	十二枚 12 méi	12 pcs

上十味，㕮咀，以水八升煮減半，內清酒三升並阿膠，煎取三升，分三服，溫臥，當汗，以粉粉之，護風寒四五日。

Pound the above ten ingredients and decoct in eight *shēng* of water until reduced by half. Add three *shēng* of clear liquor together with the *ē jiāo* 阿膠 and simmer to obtain three shēng. Divide into three doses, [and have the patient stay] warm and in bed. You should make her sweat, dust her with powder, and protect her from wind and cold for four or five days.[2]

1.   Several parallel versions of this text, such as the *Sūn Zhēn Rén* edition and *Wài Tái Mì Yào* insert here the phrase 「為離經」 *wéi lí jīng* (…the channels are being separated).
2.   *Sòng* editors' note: "Another [version of this] prescription: Cook one rooster in water and simmer the drugs [in the liquid]."

LINE 3.15

若曾傷四月胎者，當預服調中湯方

In cases of any damage to the fetus during the fourth month, [the patient] should take *Center-Regulating Decoction* as a precaution.

Center-Regulating Decoction
調中湯 *tiáo zhōng tāng*

白芍藥（四兩）續斷 芎藭 甘草（各一兩）白朮 柴胡（各三兩）當歸（一兩半）烏梅（一升）生薑（四兩）厚朴 枳實 生李根白皮（各三兩）。

白芍藥	bái sháo yào	Root of Paeonia albiflora	四兩 4 liǎng	12g
續斷	xù duàn	Root of Dipsacus asper	一兩 1 liǎng	3g
川芎	chuān xiōng	Root of Ligusticum wallichii	一兩 1 liǎng	3g
甘草	gān cǎo	Root of Glycyrrhiza uralensis	一兩 1 liǎng	3g

白术	bái zhú	Rhizome of Atractylodes macrocephala	三兩 3 liǎng	9g
柴胡	chái hú	Root of Bupleurum chinense	三兩 3 liǎng	9g
當歸	dāng guī	Root of Angelica polimorpha	一兩半 1.5 liǎng	4.5g
烏梅	wū méi	Unripe fruit of Prunus mume	一升 1 shēng	24g
生薑	shēng jiāng	Fresh root of Zingiber officinale	四兩 4 liǎng	12g
厚朴	hòu pò	Bark of Magnolia officinalis	三兩 3 liǎng	9g
枳實	zhǐ shí	Unripe fruit of Poncirus trifoliata	三兩 3 liǎng	9g
生李根白皮	shēng lǐ gēn bái pí	Fresh White bark of the root of Prunus salicina	三兩 3 liǎng	9g

上十二味，㕮咀，以水一斗煮取三升，分四服，日三夜一，八日後復服一劑。

Pound the above twelve ingredients and decoct in one *dǒu* of water to obtain three *shēng*. Divide into four doses and take three times during the day and once at night. After eight days, take a second preparation.

LINE 3.16

(一) 妊娠五月始受火精以成其氣。(二) 臥必晏起，沐浴浣衣，深其居處，厚其衣裳。(三) 朝吸天光以避寒殃。(四) 其食稻麥，其羹牛羊，和以茱萸，調以五味。(五) 是謂養氣以定五藏。(六) 妊娠五月，足太陰脈養，不可針灸其經。足太陰內輸於脾。(七) 五月之時，見四肢皆成，無大飢，無甚飽，無食乾燥，無自炙熱，無勞倦。

(1) In the fifth month of pregnancy, [the fetus] begins to receive the essence of fire and uses it to develop its *qì*.

(2) [The pregnant woman] must rise late from her sleep; she must wash her hair thoroughly, bathe herself, and wash her clothes; deepen her dwelling;[1] and wear thick clothing.

(3) In the morning, she must inhale the rays from heaven in order to avert cold disaster.

(4) [The pregnant woman] should eat meals of glutinous rice and wheat and should drink beef and sheep or goat's meat broth, combined with *wú zhū yú* (吳茱萸 Unripe fruit of Evodia rutaecarpa) and balanced in the five flavors.

(5) This is what is called nurturing *qì* to stabilize the five viscera.

(6) In the fifth month of pregnancy, the foot greater *yīn* vessel nourishes [the fetus], and you must not needle or burn moxa on this channel. The foot greater *yīn* is associated with

the spleen.

(7) During the fifth month, the child's four limbs are all being developed. [The woman] must avoid both great hunger and overeating; she must not eat dried food, get overheated, or become taxed and fatigued.

1.   深其居處 *shēn qí jū chù*: While this expression could be understood in a larger sense as withdrawing to a remote location away from her regular residence, it is more likely to mean specifically to "withdraw deep inside the house." This is similar to what the *Tāi Chǎn Shū* recommends in a parallel paragraph: 厚衣居堂 *hòu yí jū táng* (wear thick clothes and remain inside the house). See 馬繼興, 主編《馬王堆古醫書考釋》, p. 793.

LINE 3.17

妊娠五月，有熱苦頭眩，心亂嘔吐，有寒苦腹滿痛，小便數，卒有恐怖，四肢疼痛，寒熱，胎動無常處，腹痛，悶頓欲仆，卒有所下，阿膠湯主之方

In the fifth month of pregnancy,[1] for dizziness in the head, a deranged heart, and retching and vomiting, which are related to the presence of heat; for abdominal fullness and pain, which are related to the presence of cold; and for frequent urination, sudden fear and panic, pain in the four limbs, [aversion to] cold and heat [effusion], stirring of the fetus in unusual places, abdominal pain, oppression that suddenly puts the patient on the verge of collapse, and sudden presence of vaginal discharge, *Ass Hide Glue Decoction* is the governing prescription.

Ass Hide Glue Decoction
阿膠湯 *ē jiāo tāng*

阿膠（四兩）旋復花（二合）麥門冬（一升）人參（一兩）吳茱萸（七合）生薑（六兩）當歸 芍藥 甘草 黃芩（各二兩）。

阿膠	ē jiāo	Gelatinous glue produced from Equus asinus	四兩 4 liǎng	12g
旋復花	xuán fù huā	Flowerhead of Inula britannica	二合 2 gě	14ml
麥門冬	mài mén dōng	Tuber of Ophiopogon japonicus	一升 1 shēng	24g
人參	rén shēn	Root of Panax ginseng	一兩 1 liǎng	3g
吳茱萸	wú zhū yú	Unripe fruit of Evodia rutaecarpa	七合 7 gě	49ml
生薑	shēng jiāng	Fresh root of Zingiber officinale	六兩 6 liǎng	18g
當歸	dāng guī	Root of Angelica polimorpha	二兩 2 liǎng	6g
芍藥	sháo yào	Root of Paeonia albiflora	二兩 2 liǎng	6g
甘草	gān cǎo	Root of Glycyrrhiza uralensis	二兩 2 liǎng	6g

黃芩	huáng qín	Root of Scutellaria baicalensis	二兩 2 liǎng	6g

上十味，㕮咀，以水九升煮藥減半，內清酒三升並膠，微火煎取三升半，
分四服，日三夜一，先食服便愈，不瘥再服。

Pound the above ten ingredients and decoct the drugs in nine *shēng* of water until
reduced by half. Add three *shēng* of clear liquor as well as the *ē jiāo* 阿膠 and simmer
over a small flame to obtain three and a half *shēng*. Divide into four doses and take three
times during the day and once at night, before meals. After this, [she should] recover. If
there is no difference [in her condition], take another [preparation].[2]

1. Several parallel versions of this text, such as the *Sūn Zhēn Rén* edition and *Wài Tái Mì Yào* insert here the phrase 「毛髮初生」 *máo fà chū shēng* (…the hair begins to grow) .
2. *Sòng* editors' note: "Another [version of this prescription]: Butcher one black hen, take the blood from its throat and put it in the liquor. Cook the chicken in the water and then simmer the drugs in this until reduced by half. Add the liquor and *ē jiāo* 阿膠 and simmer it to obtain three and a half *shēng*. Divide into four doses."

LINE 3.18

曾傷五月胎者，當預服安中湯方

In cases of any damage to the fetus during the fifth month, [the patient] should take
Center-Quieting Decoction as a precaution.

Center-Quieting Decoction
安中湯 *ān zhōng tāng*

黃芩（一兩） 當歸 芎藭 人參 乾地黃（各二兩） 甘草 芍藥（各三兩） 生薑
（六兩） 麥門冬（一升） 五味子（五合） 大棗（三十五枚） 大麻仁（五
合）。

黃芩	huáng qín	Root of Scutellaria baicalensis	一兩 1 liǎng	3g
當歸	dāng guī	Root of Angelica polimorpha	二兩 2 liǎng	6g
川芎	chuān xiōng	Root of Ligusticum wallichii	二兩 2 liǎng	6g
人參	rén shēn	Root of Panax ginseng	二兩 2 liǎng	6g
乾地黃	gān dì huáng	Dried root of Rehmannia glutinosa	二兩 2 liǎng	6g
甘草	gān cǎo	Root of Glycyrrhiza uralensis	三兩 3 liǎng	9g
芍藥	sháo yào	Root of Paeonia albiflora	三兩 3 liǎng	9g
生薑	shēng jiāng	Fresh root of Zingiber officinale	六兩 6 liǎng	18g

麥門冬	mài mén dōng	Tuber of Ophiopogon japonicus	一升 1 shēng	24g
五味子	wǔ wèi zǐ	Fruit of Schisandra chinensis	五合 5 gě	35ml
大棗	dà zǎo	Mature fruit of Ziziphus jujuba	三十五枚 35 méi	35 pcs
大麻仁	dà má rén	Seed of Cannabis sativa	五合 5 gě	35ml

上十二味，㕮咀，以水七升，清酒五升煮取三升半，分四服，日三夜一，七日復服一劑。

Pound the above twelve ingredients and decoct in seven *shēng* of water and five *shēng* of clear liquor to obtain three and a half *shēng*. Divide into four doses and take three times during the day and once at night. After seven days, take a second preparation.

LINE 3.19

(一) 妊娠六月，始受金精以成其筋。(二) 身欲微勞，無得靜處，出遊於野，數觀走犬，及視走馬。(三) 食宜鷙鳥猛獸之肉。(四) 是謂變腠理紉筋，以養其力，以堅背膂。(五) 妊娠六月，足陽明脈養，不可針灸其經。足陽明內屬於胃，主其口目。(六) 六月之時，兒口目皆成，調五味，食甘美，無大飽。

(1) In the sixth month of pregnancy, [the fetus] begins to receive the essence of metal and uses it to develop its sinews.

(2) The [pregnant woman's] body tends to feel slightly taxed. Do not retreat to quiet places, but roam outside in the wild; often watch running dogs and galloping horses.

(3) [The pregnant woman] should eat the meat of birds of prey and wild beasts.

(4) This is what is called forming the interstices and stitching together the sinews to nourish their strength and harden the back and spinal column.

(5) In the sixth month of pregnancy, the foot *yáng* brightness vessel nourishes [the fetus], and you must not needle or burn moxa on this channel. The foot *yáng* brightness is associated with the stomach and governs [the fetus'] mouth and eyes.

(6) During the sixth month, the child's mouth and eyes are developing. Balance the five flavors and eat sweets and delicacies, but do not overeat.

LINE 3.20

妊娠六月，卒有所動不安，寒熱往來，腹內脹滿，身體腫，驚怖，忽有所下，腹痛如欲產，手足煩疼，宜服麥門冬湯方

In the sixth month of pregnancy, for sudden stirring [of the fetus], alternating [aversion to] cold and heat [effusion], intestinal fullness in the abdomen, swelling of the body, fright and fear, sudden presence of vaginal discharge, abdominal pain as if she was going into labor; and vexation and pain in the extremities, [the patient] should take *Ophiopogon Decoction*.

Ophiopogon Decoction
麥門冬湯 *mài mén dōng tāng*

麥門冬（一升） 人參 甘草 黃芩（各二兩） 乾地黃（三兩） 阿膠（四兩）
生薑（六兩） 大棗（十五枚）。

麥門冬	mài mén dōng	Tuber of Ophiopogon japonicus	一升 1 shēng	24g
人參	rén shēn	Root of Panax ginseng	二兩 2 liǎng	6g
甘草	gān cǎo	Root of Glycyrrhiza uralensis	二兩 2 liǎng	6g
黃芩	huáng qín	Root of Scutellaria baicalensis	二兩 2 liǎng	6g
乾地黃	gān dì huáng	Dried root of Rehmannia glutinosa	三兩 3 liǎng	9g
阿膠	ē jiāo	Gelatinous glue produced from Equus asinus	四兩 4 liǎng	12g
生薑	shēng jiāng	Fresh root of Zingiber officinale	六兩 6 liǎng	18g
大棗	dà zǎo	Mature fruit of Ziziphus jujuba	十五枚 15 méi	15 pcs

上八味，咬咀，以水七升煮減半，內清酒二升並膠，煎取三升，分三服，
中間進糜粥。

Pound the above eight ingredients and decoct in seven *shēng* of water until reduced by half. Add two *shēng* of clear liquor as well as the *ē jiāo* 阿膠 and simmer to obtain three *shēng*. Divide into three doses. In between doses, eat some rice gruel.*

---

*   *Sòng* editors' note: "Another [version of this prescription]: Cook one black hen in the water and simmer the drugs in [the liquid]."

LINE 3.21

若曾傷六月胎者，當預服柴胡湯方

In cases of any damage to the fetus in the sixth month, [the patient] should take *Bupleurum Decoction* as a precaution.

Bupleurum Decoction
柴胡湯 *chái hú tāng*

柴胡（四兩） 白朮 芍藥 甘草（各二兩） 蓯蓉（一兩） 芎藭（二兩） 麥門冬（二兩） 乾地黃（五兩） 大棗（三十枚） 生薑（六兩）。 *

柴胡	chái hú	Root of Bupleurum chinense	四兩 4 liǎng	12g
白朮	bái zhú	Rhizome of Atractylodes macro-cephala	二兩 2 liǎng	6g
芍藥	sháo yào	Root of Paeonia albiflora	二兩 2 liǎng	6g
甘草	gān cǎo	Root of Glycyrrhiza uralensis	二兩 2 liǎng	6g
蓯蓉	cōng róng	Stalk of Cistanche salsa	一兩 1 liǎng	3g
川芎	chuān xiōng	Root of Ligusticum wallichii	二兩 2 liǎng	6g
麥門冬	mài mén dōng	Tuber of Ophiopogon japonicus	二兩 2 liǎng	6g
乾地黃	gān dì huáng	Dried root of Rehmannia glutinosa	五兩 5 liǎng	15g
大棗	dà zǎo	Mature fruit of Ziziphus jujuba	三十枚 13 méi	13 pcs
生薑	shēng jiāng	Fresh root of Zingiber officinale	六兩 6 liǎng	18g

上十味，㕮咀，以水一斗煮取三升，分四服，日三夜一，中間進糜粥，勿食生冷及堅硬之物，七日更服一劑。

Pound the above ten ingredients and decoct in one *dǒu* of water to obtain three *shēng*. Divide into four doses and take three times during the day and once at night. In between doses, eat some rice gruel. Do not eat raw, cold, or hard substances. After seven days, take another preparation.

*   *Sòng* editors' note: "Another [version of this prescription] has *zǐ wēi* (紫葳 Flower of Campsis grandiflora) instead of *sháo yào* 芍藥."

LINE 3.22

(一) 妊娠七月，始受木精以成其骨。(二) 勞身搖肢，無使定止，動作屈伸，以運血氣。(三) 居處必燥，飲食避寒，常食稻粳，以密腠理。(四) 是謂養骨而堅齒。(五) 妊娠七月，手太陰脈養，不可針灸其經。手太陰內屬於肺，主皮毛。(六) 七月之時，兒皮毛已成，無大言，無號器，無薄衣，無洗浴，無寒飲。

(1) In the seventh month of pregnancy, [the fetus] begins to receive the essence of wood and uses it to develop its bones.

(2) Tax the body and shake the limbs; do not let it be solid and motionless; move around and bend and stretch, all in order to make the blood and *qì* flow.

(3) The dwelling must be dry; avoid cold drink and food; and regularly eat glutinous and non-glutinous rice, all in order to seal the interstices.

(4) This is what is called nourishing the bones and hardening the teeth.

(5) In the seventh month of pregnancy, the hand greater *yīn* vessel nourishes [the fetus], and you must not needle or burn moxa on this channel. The hand greater *yīn* is associated with the lung and governs the skin and hair.

(6) During the seventh month, the child's skin and hair are already developed. Do not speak loudly; do not wail or cry; do not wear thin clothes; do not bathe; and do not consume cold drinks.

LINE 3.23

妊娠七月，忽驚恐搖動，腹痛，卒有所下，手足厥冷，脈若傷寒，煩熱，腹滿，短氣，常苦頸項及腰背強，蔥白湯主之方

In the seventh month of pregnancy, for sudden fright and fear [causing the fetus to] shake and stir, abdominal pain, sudden presence of vaginal discharge, reversal cold in the hands and feet, a pulse as if she was suffering from cold damage, vexing heat, abdominal fullness, shortness of breath, and constant complaints of rigidity in the nape and neck as well as lumbus and back, *Scallion White Decoction* is the governing prescription.

Scallion White Decoction
蔥白湯 *cōng bái tāng*

蔥白（長三四寸，十四莖）半夏（一升）生薑（八兩）甘草 當歸 黃芪（各三兩）麥門冬（一升）阿膠（四兩）人參（一兩半）黃芩（一兩）旋復花（一合）。

蔥白	cōng bái	Stalk of Allium fistulosum	長三四寸，十四莖 3-4 cùn	14 stalks, 3-4 inches long
半夏	bàn xià	Rhizome of Pinellia ternata	一升 1 shēng	24g
生薑	shēng jiāng	Fresh root of Zingiber officinale	八兩 8 liǎng	24g
甘草	gān cǎo	Root of Glycyrrhiza uralensis	三兩 3 liǎng	9g
當歸	dāng guī	Root of Angelica polimorpha	三兩 3 liǎng	9g
黃芪	huáng qí	Root of Astragalus membranaceus	三兩 3 liǎng	9g

麥門冬	mài mén dōng	Tuber of Ophiopogon japonicus	一升 1 shēng	24g
阿膠	ē jiāo	Gelatinous glue produced from Equus asinus	四兩 4 liǎng	12g
人參	rén shēn	Root of Panax ginseng	一兩半 1.5 liǎng	4.5g
黃芩	huáng qín	Root of Scutellaria baicalensis	一兩 1 liǎng	3g
旋復花	xuán fù huā	Flowerhead of Inula britannica	一合 1 gě	7ml

上十一味，㕮咀，以水八升煮減半，內清酒三升及及膠，煎取四升，服一升，日三夜一，溫臥，當汗出。若不出者，加麻黃二兩，煮服如前法。若秋後，勿強責汗。

Pound the above eleven ingredients and decoct in eight *shēng* of water until reduced by half. Add three *shēng* of clear liquor as well as the *ē jiāo* 阿膠 and simmer to obtain four *shēng*. Take one *shēng* three times a day and once at night. Keep [the patient] warm and in bed. She should sweat. If she fails to do so, add two *liǎng* of *má huáng* (麻黃 Stalk of Ephedra sinica), decoct it and take it as in the method above. If [the time of year] is past autumn, do not insist on forcing her to sweat.*

*   *Sòng* editors' note: "Another [version of this prescription]: Butcher one yellow hen by cutting its throat. Take the blood and put it in the liquor. Cook the yellow hen and take the liquid to simmer the drugs in it."

LINE 3.24

若曾傷七月胎者，當預服杏仁湯方

In cases of any damage to the fetus in the seventh month, [the patient] should take *Apricot Kernel Decoction* as a precaution.

Apricot Kernel Decoction
杏仁湯 *xìng rén tāng*

杏仁 甘草（各二兩） 麥門冬 吳茱萸（各一升） 鍾乳 乾薑（各二兩） 五味子（五合） 紫菀（一兩） 粳米（五合）。

杏仁	xìng rén	Dried seed of Prunus armeniaca	二兩 2 liǎng	6g
甘草	gān cǎo	Root of Glycyrrhiza uralensis	二兩 2 liǎng	6g
麥門冬	mài mén dōng	Tuber of Ophiopogon japonicus	一升 1 shēng	24g
吳茱萸	wú zhū yú	Unripe fruit of Evodia rutaecarpa	一升 1 shēng	24g

鍾乳	zhōng rǔ	Stalactite	二兩 2 liǎng	6g
乾薑	gān jiāng	Dried root of Zingiber officinale	二兩 2 liǎng	6g
五味子	wǔ wèi zǐ	Fruit of Schisandra chinensis	五合 5 gě	35ml
紫菀	zǐ wǎn	Root and rhizome of Aster tataricus	一兩 1 liǎng	3g
粳米	jīng mǐ	Grain of the non-glutinous variety of Oryza sativa	五合 5 gě	35ml

上九味，哎咀，以水八升煮取三升半，分四服，日三夜一，中間進食，七日服一劑。

Pound the above nine ingredients and decoct in eight *shēng* of water to obtain three and a half *shēng*. Divide into four doses and take three times during the day and once at night. In between [doses], eat some food, and after seven days take another preparation.*

*   *Sòng* editors' note: "Another [version of this] prescription: Cook one white chicken and simmer the drugs in the liquid."

LINE 3.25

(一) 妊娠八月，始受土精，以成膚革。(二) 和心靜息，無使氣極。(三) 是謂密腠理而光澤顏色。(四) 妊娠八月，手陽明脈養，不可針灸其經。手陽明內屬於大腸，主九竅。(五) 八月之時，兒九竅皆成，無食燥物，無輒失食，無忍大起。

(1) In the eighth month of pregnancy, [the fetus] begins to receive the essence of earth and uses it to develop the inner and outer layers of the skin.[1]

(2) Harmonize the heart and quiet the breathing; avoid any causes of extreme *qì* damage.[2]

(3) This is what is called sealing the interstices while enhancing the sheen of the facial complexion.

(4) In the eighth month of pregnancy, the hand *yáng* brightness vessel nourishes [the fetus], and you must not needle or burn moxa on this channel. The hand *yáng* brightness is associated with the large intestine and governs the nine orifices.[3]

(5) During the eighth month, the child's nine orifices are all developing. Do not eat dry substances; do not abruptly stop eating; and avoid exposure to great arousal.

1.   膚革 *fū gé*: In a comment on the parallel section of this text in the *Tāi Chǎn Shū*, *Mǎ Jì-Xíng* 馬繼興 explains 革, literally "animal hide," as the thick layer on the inside of the skin. See 馬繼興, 主編《馬王堆古醫書考釋》, p. 800, n. 2).

2. 無使氣極 *wú shǐ qì jí. Qì* extreme is a technical term, referring to one of the six extremes (六極 *liù jí*), the six pathological conditions of extreme damage to the blood, sinews, flesh, qì, bone, and essence, found in such standard texts as the *Bìng Yuán Lùn, Qiān Jīn Fāng*, and *Jīn Guì Yào Luè. Qì* extreme, caused by vacuity detriment to the lung, causes extreme shortage of *qì* and breath, distention of the chest and ribs, inability to speak, and rage (《中華醫學大辭典》, p. 246).

3. 九竅 *jiǔ qiào*: This expression can be understood either as referring to the seven upper orifices of the ears, eyes, nostrils, and mouth, in conjunction with the lower orifices of the posterior and anterior *yīn* (urethra and anus) or only to the orifices in the head, that is, the ears, eyes, nostrils, mouth, tongue, and throat. This is how the term seems to have been understood in the *Nàn Jīng*: As the thirty-seventh issue states, "The five viscera are above gated by the nine orifices" (五臟者當上關於九竅也, my translation). See the translation in the Chinese Medicine Database (www.cm-db.com), as well as in the translation in Paul U. Unschuld, *Nan-ching*, p. 387, and the discussion of the phrase by various commentators on pp. 388-390. Sūn Sī-miǎo's usage of the term in a prescription for "lubricating the fetus" below, however, strongly suggests that he intended to include the lower orifices as well. See below, line 3.32, p. 126.

LINE 3.26

妊娠八月，中風寒，有所犯觸，身體盡痛，乍寒乍熱，胎動不安，常苦頭眩痛，繞臍下寒，時時小便白如米汁，或青或黃，或使寒慄，腰背苦冷而痛，目𥆧𥆧，芍藥湯主之方

In the eighth month of pregnancy, for wind or cold strike, offenses against prohibitions, pain all over the body, abruptly alternating [aversion to] cold and heat [effusion], stirring fetus, constant problems with dizziness and headaches, coldness below and around the navel, frequent urination of a white substance like rice juice[1] or a green or yellow substance, or accompanied by cold shivering, bitter cold and pain in the lumbus and back, or blurred vision, *White Peony Decoction* is the governing prescription.

Peony Decoction
芍藥湯 *sháo yào tāng*

芍藥 生薑（各四兩）厚朴（二兩）甘草 當歸 白朮 人參（各三兩）薤白（切，一升）。

芍藥	sháo yào	Root of Paeonia albiflora	四兩 4 liǎng	12g
生薑	shēng jiāng	Fresh root of Zingiber officinale	四兩 4 liǎng	12g
厚朴	hòu pò	Bark of Magnolia officinalis	二兩 2 liǎng	6g
甘草	gān cǎo	Root of Glycyrrhiza uralensis	三兩 3 liǎng	9g
當歸	dāng guī	Root of Angelica polimorpha	三兩 3 liǎng	9g
白朮	bái zhú	Rhizome of Atractylodes macrocephala	三兩 3 liǎng	9g

| 人參 | rén shēn | Root of Panax ginseng | 三兩 3 liǎng | 9g |
| 薤白,切 | xiè bái, qiē | Stalk of Allium macrostemon, minced | 一升 1 shēng | 24g |

上八味，㕮咀，以水五升，清酒四升合煮取三升，分三服，日再夜一。

Pound the above eight ingredients and decoct in a mixture of nine *shēng* of water and four *shēng* of clear liquor, to obtain three *shēng*. Divide into three doses and take twice during the day and once at night. [2]

1. *Mǐ zhī* 米汁: The liquid obtained by grinding rice in water.
2. *Sòng* editors' note: "Another [version of this] prescription: Cook a black hen and use the liquid to simmer the drugs."

LINE 3.27

若曾傷八月胎者，當預服葵子湯方

In cases of any damage to the fetus in the eighth month, [the patient] should take *Mallow Seed Decoction* as a precaution.

Mallow Seed Decoction
葵子湯 *kuí zǐ tāng*

葵子（二升）生薑（六兩）甘草（二兩）芍藥（四兩）白朮 柴胡（各三兩）大棗（二十枚）厚朴（二兩）。

葵子	kuí zǐ	Seeds of Malva verticillata	二升 2 shēng	48g
生薑	shēng jiāng	Fresh root of Zingiber officinale	六兩 6 liǎng	18g
甘草	gān cǎo	Root of Glycyrrhiza uralensis	二兩 2 liǎng	6g
芍藥	sháo yào	Root of Paeonia albiflora	四兩 4 liǎng	12g
白朮	bái zhú	Rhizome of Atractylodes macro-cephala	三兩 3 liǎng	9g
柴胡	chái hú	Root of Bupleurum chinense	三兩 3 liǎng	9g
大棗	dà zǎo	Mature fruit of Ziziphus jujuba	二十枚 20 méi	20 pcs
厚朴	hòu pò	Bark of Magnolia officinalis	二兩 2 liǎng	6g

上八味，㕮咀，以水九升煮取三升，分三服，日三，十日一劑。

Pound the above eight ingredients and decoct in nine *shēng* of water to obtain three *shēng*. Divide into three doses and take three times during the day. After ten days, take another preparation.*

* *Sòng* editors' note: "Another [version of this] prescription: Cook one black hen in water and simmer the drugs [in the liquid]."

LINE 3.28

(一) 妊娠九月，始受石精，以成皮毛。(二) 六腑百節莫不畢備，飲醴食甘，緩帶自持而待之。(三) 是謂養皮毛，致才力。(四) 妊娠九月，足少陰脈養，不可針灸其經。足少陰內屬於腎，腎主續縷。(五) 九月之時，兒脈續縷皆成，無處濕冷，無著炙衣。

(1) In the ninth month of pregnancy, [the fetus] begins to receive the essence of stone and uses it to develop its body hair.[1]

(2) Of the six bowels and hundred joints, all are completed and prepared [for birth]. Allow [the mother] to drink sweet wine and eat sweets, and to loosen her girdle and act aloof.[2] Wait on her.[3]

(3) This is what is called nourishing the hair[4] and perfecting talents and capabilities.

(4) In the ninth month of pregnancy, the foot lesser *yīn* vessel nourishes [the fetus] and you must not needle or burn moxa on this channel. The foot lesser *yīn* is associated with the kidney, which controls childbearing.

(5) During the ninth month, the child's vessels and reproductive functions are all developing. Do not abide in damp and cool places; do not wear roasting-hot clothes.

1. 皮毛 *pí máo*: While this could also mean "skin and hair," I interpret it as "hair on the skin" because the skin has already developed in the eighth month. Moreover, the textual parallel in the *Tāi Chǎn Shū* has 豪毛 *háo máo*, which Harper translates as "filament hairs." See Harper, *Early Chinese Medical Literature*, p. 381 and 馬繼興, 主編《馬王堆古醫書考釋》, p. 801.
2. This means that she should relax and follow her whims, in contrast to the modesty and restraint she was instructed to maintain earlier in pregnancy.
3. 而待之 *ér dài zhī*: This phrase is missing in the *Sūn Zhēn Rén* edition.
4. On both body and head.

LINE 3.29

妊娠九月，若卒得下痢，腹滿懸急，胎上衝心，腰背痛不可轉側，短氣，半夏湯方

In the ninth month of pregnancy, for suddenly contracted diarrhea, abdominal fullness with a sensation of suspension and fullness, fetus surging up against the heart, lumbar and back pain with inability to turn or bend, and shortness of breath, *Pinellia Decoction* [is the governing prescription].

Pinellia Decoction
半夏湯 *bàn xià tāng*

半夏 麥門冬（各五兩） 吳茱萸 當歸 阿膠（各三兩） 乾薑（一兩） 大棗（十二枚）。

半夏	bàn xià	Rhizome of Pinellia ternata	五兩 5 liǎng	15g
麥門冬	mài mén dōng	Tuber of Ophiopogon japonicus	五兩 5 liǎng	15g
吳茱萸	wú zhū yú	Unripe fruit of Evodia rutaecarpa	三兩 3 liǎng	9g
當歸	dāng guī	Root of Angelica polimorpha	三兩 3 liǎng	9g
阿膠	ē jiāo	Gelatinous glue produced from Equus asinus	三兩 3 liǎng	9g
乾薑	gān jiāng	Dried root of Zingiber officinale	一兩 1 liǎng	3g
大棗	dà zǎo	Mature fruit of Ziziphus jujuba	十二枚 12 méi	12 pcs

上七味，㕮咀，以水九升煮取三升，去滓，內白蜜八合，微火上溫，分四服，痢即止。

Pound the above seven ingredients and decoct in nine *shēng* of water to obtain three *shēng*. Discard the dregs, add eight *gě* of white honey, and warm it over a small flame. Divide into four doses. Stop as soon as [the medicine induces] diarrhea.*

*   *Sòng* editors' note: "Another [version of this] prescription: Cook one black hen and simmer the drugs in the liquid."

LINE 3.30

若曾傷九月胎者，當預服豬腎湯方

In cases of any damage to the fetus in the ninth month, [the patient] should take *Pig's Kidney Decoction* as a precaution.

Pig's Kidney Decoction
豬腎湯 *zhū shèn tāng*

豬腎（一具） 白朮（四兩） 茯苓 桑寄生 乾薑 乾地黃 芎藭（各三兩） 麥門

冬（一升）附子（中者一枚）大豆（三合）。

豬腎	zhū shèn	Kidneys of Sus scrofa domestica	一具 1 jù	1 set
白朮	bái zhú	Rhizome of Atractylodes macro-cephala	四兩 4 liǎng	12g
茯苓	fú líng	Dried fungus of Poria cocos	三兩 3 liǎng	9g
桑寄生	sāng jì shēng	Branches and foliage of Viscum coloratum	三兩 3 liǎng	9g
乾薑	gān jiāng	Dried root of Zingiber officinale	三兩 3 liǎng	9g
乾地黃	gān dì huáng	Dried root of Rehmannia glutinosa	三兩 3 liǎng	9g
川芎	chuān xiōng	Root of Ligusticum wallichii	三兩 3 liǎng	9g
麥門冬	mài mén dōng	Tuber of Ophiopogon japonicus	一升 1 shēng	24g
附子	fù zǐ	Lateral root of Aconitum carmi-chaeli	中者一枚 zhōng zhě 1 méi	one piece from the center
大豆	dà dòu	Seed of Glycine max	三合 3 gě	21ml

上十味，㕮咀，以水一斗煮腎令熟，去腎，內諸藥，煎取三升半，分四服，日三夜一，十日更一劑。

Pound the above ten ingredients. Cook the kidney in one *dǒu* of water until done, then take it out and add all the drugs. Simmer to obtain three and a half *shēng*. Divide into four doses and take three times during the day and once at night. After ten days, take another preparation.

LINE 3.31

妊娠十月，五藏俱備，六腑齊通，納天地氣於丹田，故使關節人神皆備，但俟時而生。

In the tenth month of pregnancy, the five viscera are all completed, the six bowels are equally connected, and [the fetus] has absorbed the *qì* of heaven and earth in the cinnabar field, thereby allowing for the completion of all the joints and the human spirits.[*] It merely awaits its time and then is born.

---

*　　神 *shén* is purposely rendered in plural based on the phrase 諸神 *zhū shén* (the various spirits) in the next section. This reflects the notion that the bodily spirits only begin inhabiting the fetus immediately before birth.

LINE 3.32

(一) 妊娠一月始胚，二月始膏，三月始胞，四月形體成，五月能動，六月筋骨立，七月毛髮生，八月藏腑具，九月穀氣入胃，十月諸神備，日滿即產矣。(二) 宜服滑胎藥，入月即服。

(1) In the first month of pregnancy, it is "beginning embryo;" in the second month "beginning paste;" in the third month "beginning fetus;" [1] in the fourth month, the form is completed; in the fifth month, it is able to stir; in the sixth month; the sinews and bones develop; in the seventh month, the hair grows; in the eighth month, the viscera and bowels are complete; in the ninth month, grain *qì* enters the stomach; in the tenth month, the various spirits are complete and [the fetus] will be born as soon as the days are fulfilled.

(2) [The mother] should take "fetus-lubricating medicines," [2] but only after she has entered the month [of childbirth]. [3]

1. 始胞 *shǐ bāo*. This differs from the earlier term used for the third month, 始胎 *shǐ tāi*, but their meaning is interchangeable. In either case, the name suggests that the third month was an important turning point, when a woman's pregnancy and the presence of a fetus in her uterus was recognized medically. This must have been significant also in ethical questions regarding the difference between menstrual regulation and a conscious and intentional abortion.
2. 滑胎藥 *huá tāi yào*. This term covers an entire category of medicines, intended to prepare for and ease delivery. Since many of these drugs would induce miscarriage if taken too early, it was essential to wait until the last month of pregnancy. See 李貞德《漢唐之間醫書中的生產之道》 pp. 539-42. The following prescriptions in the remainder of this section all fall into this category. The term 滑胎 is used more commonly in contemporary TCM to refer to the pathology of "habitual miscarriage."
3. 入月 *rù yuè*: This is a technical term indicating the final stage of pregnancy, when a woman had reached the month of delivery and the household needed to make preparations for the birth, such as setting up the birthing chamber, preparing special medicines, and ritually cleansing the delivery area. While earlier texts show a greater range for when such medicines as *Salvia Paste* were recommended in the course of a woman's pregnancy, by the time in which the *Qiān Jīn Fāng* was composed, this had been standardized to be limited only to the tenth month. See 李貞德《漢唐之間醫書中的生產之道》 pp. 539-42.

LINE 3.33

養胎臨月服，令滑易產，丹參膏方

Salvia Paste is a prescription for nourishing the fetus, to be taken in the month of delivery, lubricating the fetus and easing childbirth.

Salvia Paste
丹參膏 *dān shēn gāo*

丹參（半斤） 芎藭 當歸（各三兩） 蜀椒（五合）。

丹參	dān shēn	Root of Salvia miltiorrhiza	半斤 0.5 jīn	24g
川芎	chuān xiōng	Root of Ligusticum wallichii	三兩 3 liǎng	9g
當歸	dāng guī	Root of Angelica polimorpha	三兩 3 liǎng	9g
蜀椒*	shǔ jiāo	Seed capsules of Zanthoxylum bungeanum	五合 5 gě	35ml

上四味，㕮咀，以清酒溲濕，停一宿，以成煎豬膏四升，微火煎，膏色赤如血膏成，新布絞去滓。每日取如棗許，內酒中服之，不可逆服，至臨月可服。舊用常驗。

Pound the above four ingredients and let them steep in clear liquor overnight. To complete [the prescription], simmer the drugs in four *shēng* of pork lard over a small flame until the paste becomes red. When it looks like blood, the paste is done. Squeeze it through a new cloth and discard the dregs. Every day, take an amount the size of a jujube, put it in liquor and drink it. You must not take this [medicine] contrary to these instructions, and you can only take it when the month [of childbirth] has arrived. The ancients have used it with constant results.

*   *Sòng* editors' note: "For heat conditions, use *dà má rén* (大麻仁 Seed of Cannabis sativa) instead of *shǔ jiāo* 蜀椒."

LINE 3.34

甘草散令易生，母無疾病，未生一月日預服，過三十日行步動作如故，兒生墮地皆不自覺方

Licorice Powder eases childbirth and prevents [postpartum] disease for the mother. Take it daily for one month prior to the birth as a precaution. After thirty days of moving about and engaging in activities as usual, the child will be born by dropping to the ground, all without the mother herself feeling it.

Licorice Powder
甘草散 *gān cǎo sǎn*

甘草（二兩） 大豆黃卷 黃芩 乾薑 桂心 麻子仁 大麥蘗 吳茱萸（各三兩）
。

甘草	gān cǎo	Root of Glycyrrhiza uralensis	二兩 2 liǎng	6g
大豆黃卷	dà dòu huáng juǎn	Sprouted seed of Glycine max	三兩 3 liǎng	9g
黃芩[1]	huáng qín	Root of Scutellaria baicalensis	三兩 3 liǎng	9g
乾薑	gān jiāng	Dried root of Zingiber officinale	三兩 3 liǎng	9g
桂心	guì xīn	Shaved inner bark of Cinnamomum cassia	三兩 3 liǎng	9g
麻子仁	má zǐ rén	Seed of Cannabis sativa	三兩 3 liǎng	9g
大麥蘖[2]	dà mài niè	Seed of Hordeum vulgare	三兩 3 liǎng	9g
吳茱萸	wú zhū yú	Unripe fruit of Evodia rutaecarpa	三兩 3 liǎng	9g

上八味，治下篩，酒服方寸匕，日三。煖水服亦得。

Finely pestle the above eight ingredients and sift them. Take a square-inch spoon in liquor, three times a day. You may also take it in warm water.

1.　*Sòng* editors' note: "Another [version] has *fú líng* (茯苓 Dried fungus of Poria cocos) instead of *huáng qín* 黃芩."

2.　*Sòng* editors' note: "Another [version] has *jīng mǐ* (粳米 Grain of the non-glutinous variety of Oryza sativa) instead of *dà mài niè* 大麥蘖."

LINE 3.35

千金丸主養胎，及產難，顛倒，胞不出，服一丸。傷毀不下，產餘病汗不出，煩滿不止，氣逆滿，以酒服一丸。良。一名保生丸方

Thousand Gold Pills are the governing prescription for nourishing the fetus; as well as for the treatment of birthing difficulties, upside down [presentation], and for a retained placenta, by taking [just] one pill. For the treatment of a damaged or destroyed fetus that will not descend, and for such residual conditions as inability to sweat, incessant vexing fullness, and qì counterflow and fullness, take one pill in liquor. [This treatment] is good. An alternate name is *Life-Saving Pills*.

Thousand Gold Pills
千金丸 *qiān jīn wán*

甘草 貝母 秦椒 乾薑 桂心 黃芩 石斛 石膏 粳米 大豆黃卷（各六銖）當歸（十三銖）麻子（三合）。[1]

| 甘草 | gān cǎo | Root of Glycyrrhiza uralensis | 六銖 6 zhū | .75g |
| 貝母 | bèi mǔ | Bulb of Fritillaria cirrhosa | 六銖 6 zhū | .75g |

秦椒	qín jiāo	Seed capsule of Zanthoxylum bungeanum	六銖 6 zhū	.75g
乾薑	gān jiāng	Dried root of Zingiber officinale	六銖 6 zhū	.75g
桂心	guì xīn	Shaved inner bark of Cinnamomum cassia	六銖 6 zhū	.75g
黃芩	huáng qín	Root of Scutellaria baicalensis	六銖 6 zhū	.75g
石斛	shí hú	Whole plant of Dendrobium nobile	六銖 6 zhū	.75g
石膏	shí gāo	Gypsum	六銖 6 zhū	.75g
粳米[2]	jīng mǐ	Grain of the non-glutinous variety of Oryza sativa	六銖 6 zhū	.75g
大豆黃卷	dà dòu huáng juǎn	Sprouted seed of Glycine max	六銖 6 zhū	.75g
當歸	dāng guī	Root of Angelica polimorpha	十三銖 13 zhū	1.625g
麻子	fù zǐ	Lateral root of Aconitum carmichaeli	三合 3 gě	21ml

上十二味，末之，蜜和丸如彈子大，每服一丸，日三，用棗湯下。

Pulverize the above twelve ingredients and combine with honey to make pellet-sized pills. Take one pill as a dose, three times a day. Use *jujube decoction* to get it down.

1.   *Sòng* editors' note: "Another [version of this prescription] includes one *liǎng* of *pú huáng* (蒲黃 Pollen of Typha angustata)."
2.   *Sòng* editors' note: "Another [version] has *nuò mǐ* (糯米 Grain of Oryza glutinosa) instead of *jīng mǐ* 粳米."

LINE 3.36

治妊娠養胎令易產，蒸大黃丸方

Steamed Rhubarb Pills are a treatment for nourishing the fetus during pregnancy and easing childbirth.

Steamed Rhubarb Pills
蒸大黃丸 *zhēng dà huáng wán*

大黃（三十銖，蒸）枳實 芎藭 白朮 杏仁（各十八銖）芍藥 乾薑 厚朴（各十二銖）吳茱萸（一兩）。

大黃, 蒸	dà huáng, zhēng	Root of Rheum palmatum, steamed	三十銖 30 zhū	3.75g
枳實	zhǐ shí	Unripe fruit of Poncirus trifoliata	十八銖 18 zhū	2.25g
川芎	chuān xiōng	Root of Ligusticum wallichii	十八銖 18 zhū	2.25g
白朮	bái zhú	Rhizome of Atractylodes macro-cephala	十八銖 18 zhū	2.25g
杏仁	xìng rén	Dried seed of Prunus armeniaca	十八銖 18 zhū	2.25g
芍藥	sháo yào	Root of Paeonia albiflora	十二銖 12 zhū	1.5g
乾薑	gān jiāng	Dried root of Zingiber officinale	十二銖 12 zhū	1.5g
厚朴	hòu pò	Bark of Magnolia officinalis	十二銖 12 zhū	1.5g
吳茱萸	wú zhū yú	Unripe fruit of Evodia rutaecarpa	一兩 1 liǎng	3g

上九味，末之，蜜丸如梧桐子大，空腹酒下二丸，日三，不知稍加之。

Pulverize the above nine ingredients and combine with honey into pills the size of firmiana seeds. On an empty stomach, down two pills in liquor, three times a day. If no effect is noticed, increase the amount gradually.

LINE 3.37

滑胎令易產方

A prescription for lubricating the fetus and easing childbirth:

Formula

車前子（一升）阿膠（八兩）滑石（二兩）。

車前子	chē qián zǐ	Plantago asiatica	一升 1 shēng	24g
阿膠	ē jiāo	Gelatinous glue produced from Equus asinus	八兩 8 liǎng	24g
滑石	huá shí	Talcum	二兩 2 liǎng	6g

上三味，治下篩，飲服方寸匕，日再。至生月乃服，藥利九竅，不可先服。

Finely pestle the above three ingredients and sift them. Take a square-inch spoon in liquid, twice a day. Only take this after reaching the month of childbirth. This medicine disinhibits the nine openings and you [therefore] cannot take it any earlier.

4. The Various Diseases of Pregnancy 妊娠諸病

4a Stirring Fetus and Repeated Miscarriages
胎動及數墮胎

LINE 4a.1

治妊娠二三月，上至八九月，胎動不安，腰痛，已有所見方

A prescription for treating stirring fetus with lumbar pain, when there are already visible [symptoms],[1] from the second or third month of pregnancy all the way to the eighth or ninth month.

Formula

艾葉 阿膠 芎藭 當歸（各三兩）甘草（一兩）。

艾葉	ài yè	Dry-roasted foliage of Artemisia argyi	三兩 3 liǎng	9g
阿膠	ē jiāo	Gelatinous glue produced from Equus asinus	三兩 3 liǎng	9g
川芎[2]	chuān xiōng	Root of Ligusticum wallichii	三兩 3 liǎng	9g
當歸	dāng guī	Root of Angelica polimorpha	三兩 3 liǎng	9g
甘草	gān cǎo	Root of Glycyrrhiza uralensis	一兩 1 liǎng	3g

上五味，咬咀，以水八升煮取三升，去滓，內膠令消，分三服，日三。

Pound the above five ingredients and decoct in eight *shēng* of water to obtain three *shēng*. Discard the dregs, add the *ē jiāo* 阿膠, and let it disperse. Divide into three doses and take it three times a day.[3]

1. 已有所見 *yǐ yǒu suǒ jiàn*: The meaning of this phrase is unclear. It could refer either to visible symptoms in general, to the fetus beginning to appear during delivery, or to any vaginal discharge as a result of stirring fetus. In the last case, it would mean that this formula is effective even for cases that are so advanced that the woman is about to miscarry.
2. *Sòng* editors' note: "The *Zhǒu Hòu Fāng* does not use *chuān xiōng* 川芎."
3. This prescription, as well as the prescription for treating stirring fetus, shouting and

screaming day and night, clenched jaw and stretched lips (see line 4a.4, p. 134 below) are cited literally in the *Ishimpô*. However, they are credited not to the *Qiān Jīn Fāng*, but to the *Jí Yàn Fāng*. See (《醫心方》 22:7).

LINE 4a.2

治妊娠胎動，去血，腰腹痛方

A prescription for treating stirring fetus with [vaginal] bleeding and lumbar and abdominal pain during pregnancy:

Formula

芎藭 當歸 青竹筎（各三兩） 阿膠（二兩）。 *

川芎	chuān xiōng	Root of Ligusticum wallichii	三兩 3 liǎng	9g
當歸	dāng guī	Root of Angelica polimorpha	三兩 3 liǎng	9g
青竹筎	qīng zhú rú	Shavings of Phyllostachys nigra	三兩 3 liǎng	9g
阿膠	ē jiāo	Gelatinous glue produced from Equus asinus	二兩 2 liǎng	6g

上四味，㕮咀，以水一斗半煮銀二斤，取六升，去銀，內藥煎取二升半，內膠令烊，分三服，不瘥重作。

Pound the above four ingredients. Boil two *jīn* of silver in one and a half *dǒu* of water to obtain six *shēng*. Take out the silver and add the drugs. Simmer to obtain two and a half *shēng*. Add the *ē jiāo* 阿膠 and let it melt. Divide into three doses. If [the patient] does not recover, make it again.

*   *Sòng* editors' note: "Another [version of this prescription] includes two *liǎng* of *gān cǎo* (甘草 Root of Glycyrrhiza uralensis)."

LINE 4a.3

治妊娠胎動不安，腹痛，蔥白湯方

Scallion White Decoction treats stirring fetus with abdominal pain during pregnancy.

Scallion White Decoction
蔥白湯 *cōng bái tāng*

蔥白（切，一升） 阿膠（二兩） 當歸 續斷 芎藭（各三兩）。

蔥白,切	cōng bái, qiē	Stalk of Allium fistulosum, sliced	一升 1 shēng	24g
阿膠	ē jiāo	Gelatinous glue produced from Equus asinus	二兩 2 liǎng	6g
當歸	dāng guī	Root of Angelica polimorpha	三兩 3 liǎng	9g
續斷	xù duàn	Root of Dipsacus asper	三兩 3 liǎng	9g
川芎	chuān xiōng	Root of Ligusticum wallichii	三兩 3 liǎng	9g

上五味，㕮咀，以水一斗先煮銀六七兩，取七升，去銀，內藥煎取二升半，下膠令烊，分三服，不瘥重作。

Pound the above five ingredients. Boil six or seven *liǎng* of silver in one *dǒu* of water to obtain seven *shēng*. Take out the silver and add the drugs. Simmer to obtain two and a half *shēng*. Drop in the *ē jiāo* 阿膠 and let it melt. Divide into three doses. If [the patient] fails to recover, make it again.

LINE 4a.4

治妊娠胎動，晝夜叫呼，口噤脣搴塞，及下重痢不息方

This prescription treats stirring fetus with shouting and screaming day and night, clenched jaw and pulled lips,[1] as well as heaviness below and incessant diarrhea during pregnancy:

艾葉㕮咀，以好酒五升煮取四升，去滓，更煎取一升服。口閉者，格口灌之，藥下即瘥。亦治妊娠腰痛及妊娠熱病，並妊娠卒下血。

Pound *ài yè* (艾葉 Dry-roasted foliage of Artemisia argyi) and decoct it in five *shēng* of good liquor to obtain four *shēng*. Discard the dregs and simmer [the liquid] again to obtain one *shēng*. Drink it. If her mouth is shut, force it open and pour it in. She will recover as soon as she has downed the medicine. [This prescription] also treats lumbar pain in pregnancy and heat disease in pregnancy as well as sudden descent of blood in pregnancy.

1.   脣搴 *chún qiān*: Some versions of the text, such as the *Sūn Zhēn Rén* edition, have 脣塞 *chún sài* "sealed lips" instead. Either way, the meaning is similar.
2.   下重痢不止 *xià zhòng/chóng lì bù zhǐ*: An alternative translation could be "repeated diarrhea that will not stop." An interpretation of 重 as *chóng* "repeated" is supported by an otherwise literal quotation of this prescription in the *Ishimpô* where the character is missing completely. See (《醫心方》22:7). Grammatically, however, a reading as "heaviness" is more likely. In any case, the meaning is not significantly affected by this lack of clarity.

LINE 4a.5

治妊娠六七月，胎不安，常服旋復花湯方

To treat disquieted fetus in the sixth and seventh month of pregnancy, regularly take *Inula Decoction*.

Inula Decoction
旋覆花湯 *xuán fù huā tāng*

旋復花（一兩）厚朴 白朮 黃芩 茯苓 枳實（各三兩）半夏 芍藥 生薑（各二兩）。

旋復花	xuán fù huā	Flowerhead of Inula britannica	一兩 1 liǎng	3g
厚朴	hòu pò	Bark of Magnolia officinalis	三兩 3 liǎng	9g
白朮	bái zhú	Rhizome of Atractylodes macrocephala	三兩 3 liǎng	9g
黃芩	huáng qín	Root of Scutellaria baicalensis	三兩 3 liǎng	9g
茯苓	fú líng	Dried fungus of Poria cocos	三兩 3 liǎng	9g
枳實	zhǐ shí	Unripe fruit of Poncirus trifoliata	三兩 3 liǎng	9g
半夏	bàn xià	Rhizome of Pinellia ternata	二兩 2 liǎng	6g
芍藥	sháo yào	Root of Paeonia albiflora	二兩 2 liǎng	6g
生薑	shēng jiāng	Fresh root of Zingiber officinale	二兩 2 liǎng	6g

上九味，咬咀，以水一斗煮取二升半，分五服，日三夜二，先食服。

Pound the above nine ingredients and decoct in one *dǒu* of water to obtain two and a half *shēng*. Divide into five doses and take three times during the day and twice at night, before meals.

LINE 4a.6

治妊娠數墮胎方

A prescription for treating repeated miscarriage in pregnancy:

赤小豆末，米酒服方寸，日二。亦治妊娠數月，月水尚來者。

Pulverize *chì xiǎo dòu* (赤小豆 Fruit of Phaseolus calcaratus) and take a square-inch spoon in rice liquor, twice a day. [This formula] also treats cases where the menstrual flow comes even though a pregnancy has [already lasted for] several months.

LINE 4a.7

又

Another [treatment]:

Moxibustion Treatment

妊娠三月，灸膝下一寸，七壯。

In the third month of pregnancy, burn seven cones of moxa one *cùn* below the knee.

4b Uterine Spotting　漏胞

LINE 4b.1

治妊娠下血如故，名曰漏胞，胞乾便死方

A prescription for treating descent of blood during pregnancy [that occurs at the same monthly time] as prior [to the pregnancy].[1] It is called "uterine spotting."[2] If the uterus dries out, [the patient] will die.[3]

生地黃半斤㕮咀，以清酒二升煮三沸，絞去滓，服之無時，能多服佳。

Pound half a *jīn* of *shēng dì huáng* (生地黃 Fresh root of Rehmannia glutinosa) and cook it in two *shēng* of clear liquor, bringing it to a boil three times. Wring out and discard the dregs. Take it constantly. The more she can take the better.[4]

1.　漏胞 *lòu bāo*: In modern TCM, this condition is more commonly referred to as 胎漏 *tāi lòu*, translated by Wiseman and Fēng as "fetal spotting." See also 李經緯, 主編.《中醫大辭典》, entry on 胎漏, p. 1291. See note 3 below for more information on the early medieval understanding of this disease.
2.　下血如故 *xià xuè rǔ gù*: This means bleeding at the regular time when the woman's menstrual period would have occurred if she were not pregnant.
3.　This reading is supported by the statement in the *Bìng Yuán Lùn* 病源論: "Uterine spotting refers to the condition when the menstrual period comes at the usual time after several months of pregnancy" (漏胞者謂妊娠數月而經水時). See (《病源論》41:8). To paraphrase the following discussion there, it is caused by vacuity in the thoroughfare and controlling vessels, leading to their inability to contain the menstrual blood in the greater *yáng* and lesser *yīn* channels. It is a serious and potentially fatal condition. In contrast, bleeding in pregnancy at irregular times and accompanied by stirring fetus falls under the category of "stirring fetus in pregnancy" (妊娠胎動候 *rèn shēn tāi dòng hòu*). This is discussed in the following chapter in the *Bìng Yuán Lùn*: It is caused by exhaustion of strength and *qì* due to contracting cold or heat, or an inappropriate diet or residence. In mild cases, it is curable; in severe cases, it leads to miscarriage. For quotations from other gynecological texts to clarify the difference between these two conditions, including theory, treatment, and case histories, see (張奇文, 主編《胎產病証》 pp. 30-47).
　　It is unclear both in the *Qiān Jīn Fāng* and the *Bìng Yuán Lùn* whether a dried uterus or exhausted blood is fatal only to the fetus or to the mother also. The following prescription which specifies that it is fatal to the child would suggest the former, but incessant hemorrhaging during pregnancy is obviously also a life-threatening condition for the mother.
4.　*Sòng* editors' note: "Physician Yáo adds one head from a yellow hen, prepared as for cooking; Master Cuī uses chicken blood, combined with the drugs and taken together."

LINE 4b.2

治妊娠血下不止，名曰漏胞，血盡子死方

A prescription for treating incessant bleeding during pregnancy. This is called "uterine spotting." When the [mother's] blood is exhausted, the child dies.

乾地黃擣末，以三指撮酒服，不過三服。

Grind *gān dì huáng* (乾地黃 Dried root of Rehmannia glutinosa) into a powder. Take an amount the size of a three-finger pinch in liquor. Do not exceed three doses.

LINE 4b.3

又方

Another prescription:

生地黃汁一升，以清酒四合煮三四沸，頓服之。不止頻服。

Use one *shēng* of *shēng dì huáng zhī* (生地黃汁 Fresh root of Rehmannia glutinosa juice). Decoct it with four *gě* of clear liquor, bringing it to a boil three or four times. Quaff in a single dose. If [the bleeding] will not stop, take it continuously.

LINE 4b.4

又方

Another prescription:

Formula

乾地黃（四兩）乾薑（二兩）。

| 乾地黃 | gān dì huáng | Dried root of Rehmannia glutinosa | 四兩 4 liǎng | 12g |
| 乾薑 | gān jiāng | Dried root of Zingiber officinale | 二兩 2 liǎng | 6g |

上二味，治下篩以酒服方寸匕，日再，三服。

Finely pestle the above two ingredients and sift them. Take a square-inch spoon in liquor, two to three doses a day.

4c Child Vexation 子煩

LINE 4c.1

治妊娠常苦煩悶，此是子煩，竹瀝湯方

Bamboo Sap Decoction treats constant suffering from vexation and oppression during pregnancy. This is child vexation.

Bamboo Sap Decoction
竹瀝湯 *zhú lì tāng*

竹瀝（一升）防風 黃芩 麥門冬（各三兩）茯苓（四兩）。

竹瀝	zhú lì	Sap of Phyllostachys	一升 1 shēng	24g
防風	fáng fēng	Root of Ledebouriella divaricata	三兩 3 liǎng	9g
黃芩	huáng qín	Root of Scutellaria baicalensis	三兩 3 liǎng	9g
麥門冬	mài mén dōng	Tuber of Ophiopogon japonicus	三兩 3 liǎng	9g
茯苓	fú líng	Dried fungus of Poria cocos	四兩 4 liǎng	12g

上五味，㕮咀，以水四升合竹瀝煮取二升，分三服，不瘥再作。

Pound the above five ingredients. Decoct them in four *shēng* of water together with the bamboo sap to obtain two *shēng*. Divide into three doses. If she fails to recover, make it again.

LINE 4c.2

又方

Another prescription:

時時服竹瀝，隨多少，取瘥止。

Constantly take *zhú lì* (竹瀝 Sap of Phyllostachys) in any desired amount. Stop when she recovers.

4d Heart, Abdominal, and Lumbar Pain and Abdominal Fullness
心腹腰痛及脹滿

* Translator's note: The *Sūn Zhēn Rén* edition titles this section 妊娠忽心腹痛方 *rèn shēn hū xīn fù tòng fāng* (Prescriptions for Sudden Heart and Abdominal Pain in Pregnancy) instead. Assuming that this version is likely to reflect an earlier wording that preceded the *Sòng* revisions, this change might indicate an increasing sophistication within the medical field of gynecology, requiring a greater amount of specificity with regards to locating the pain. Accordingly, the *Bìng Yuán Lùn* divides this category into five different symptoms, namely heart pain, heart and abdominal pain, lumbar pain, lumbar and abdominal pain, and lower abdominal pain, which are each explained with different etiologies (see 《病源論》 41:12-16). The editions of the *Qiān Jīn Fāng* that have undergone the *Sòng* revisions do distinguish clearly between the different locations of pain in the following prescriptions, dividing this section into groups of prescriptions for heart pain, abdominal pain, heart and abdominal pain, lumbar pain, and intestinal fullness. It is significant, however, that this order of prescriptions and their categorization according to symptoms is not replicated in the *Sūn Zhēn Rén* edition where the prescriptions are listed in a completely different order and without any apparent organizational scheme. This suggests that the sophisticated treatment of localized discomfort in pregnancy by medicinal prescriptions tailored to very specific etiologies was a development of gynecology that occured around the time of the composition of the *Qiān Jīn Fāng* (as evidenced by the advanced differentiation in the *Bìng Yuán Lùn*) or was perhaps even stimulated by the *Qiān Jīn Fāng*. This is also reflected in the small number and nature of ingredients in the prescriptions of this section, suggesting more a repertoire of simple household recipes than the complicated prescriptions of an elite scholar-physician.

LINE 4d.1

治妊娠心痛方

A prescription for treating heart pain in pregnancy:

青竹皮一升以酒二升煮三兩沸，頓服之。

Decoct one *shēng* of *qīng zhú pí* (青竹皮 Bark of Phyllostachys) in two *shēng* of liquor, bringing it to a boil two or three times. Quaff in a single dose.

LINE 4d.2

又方

Another prescription:

破生雞子一枚，和酒服之。

Break open one raw chicken egg and take it mixed in liquor.

LINE 4d.3

又方

Another prescription:

Formula

青竹筎（一升）羊脂（八兩）白蜜（三兩）。

青竹筎	qīng zhú rú	Shavings of Phyllostachys nigra	一升 1 shēng	24g
羊脂	yáng zhī	Unrendered fat of Capra hircus	八兩 8 liǎng	24g
白蜜	bái mì	Honey of Apis cerana	三兩 3 liǎng	9g

上三味，合煎，食頃服如棗核大三枚，日三。

Blend the above three ingredients and simmer them. Shortly after meals, take three pieces the size of jujube pits, three times a day.

LINE 4d.4

又方

Another prescription:

蜜一升和井底泥，泥心下。

Mix one *shēng* of honey with mud from the bottom of a well and spread it on the area below the heart.

LINE 4d.5

又方

Another prescription:

燒棗二七枚末，尿服之立愈。

Char two times seven *dà zǎo* (大棗 Mature fruit of Ziziphus jujuba),and pulverize them. Taking them with urine will bring immediate recovery.

LINE 4d.6

治妊娠腹中痛方

A prescription for treating pain in the abdomen during pregnancy:

生地黃三斤擣絞取汁，用清酒一升合煎減半，頓服。

Pound three *jīn* of *shēng dì huáng* (生地黃 Fresh root of Rehmannia glutinosa) and wring it out to obtain the juice. Combine with one *shēng* of clear liquor and simmer until reduced by half. Quaff in a single dose.

LINE 4d.7

又方

Another prescription:

燒車缸脂，內酒中服。亦治妊娠欬嗽，並難產三日不出。

Another prescription: Char cart axle grease and take it with liquor. It also treats coughing in pregnancy, as well as difficult delivery [when the baby has not emerged] for three days.

LINE 4d.8

又方

Another prescription:

頓服一升蜜，良。

Quaffing one *shēng* of honey in a single dose is good.

LINE 4d.9

治妊娠腹中滿痛入心，不得飲食方

A prescription for treating fullness and pain in the center of the abdomen and entering the heart,* with inability to eat or drink, during pregnancy:

Formula

白朮（六兩） 芍藥（四兩） 黃芩（三兩）。

白朮	bái zhú	Rhizome of Atractylodes macrocephala	六兩 6 liǎng	18g
芍藥	sháo yào	Root of Paeonia albiflora	四兩 4 liǎng	12g
黃芩	huáng qín	Root of Scutellaria baicalensis	三兩 3 liǎng	9g

上三味，㕮咀，以水六升煮取三升，分三服。半日令藥盡。微下水，令易生，月飲一劑為善。

Pound the above three ingredients and decoct in six *shēng* of water to obtain three *shēng*. Divide into three doses and use up the medicine within half a day. [It will produce] a slight vaginal discharge of water. [The medicine] causes an easy childbirth. It is good to drink one preparation every month.

---

*   入心 *rù xīn*: Other versions of the text have slight alternatives, such as 又心中厭厭 *yòu xīn zhōng yàn yàn* (great loathing in the heart) in the *Sūn Zhēn Rén* edition ; 又心 *chá xīn* (jamming up the heart) in the *Dào Zàng* edition; or 又惡心 *yòu è xīn* (together with nausea) in a later text. See *Huá Xià* edition, p. 55, n. 1.

LINE 4d.10

治妊娠忽苦心腹痛方

A prescription for treating sudden discomfort from heart and abdominal pain during pregnancy:

燒鹽令赤熱，三指撮，酒服之，立產。

Char salt until it is glowing red. Take an amount the size of a three-finger pinch in liquor. This will induce the birth.

LINE 4d.11

治妊娠傷胎結血，心腹痛方

A prescription for treating a damaged fetus and bound blood with heart and abdominal pain during pregnancy:

服小兒尿二升，頓服之，立瘥，大良。

Drink two *shēng* of urine from a small child, quaffing it in a single dose. It will cause recovery. [This prescription is] very good.

LINE 4d.12

治妊娠中惡心腹痛方

A prescription for treating malignity strike* with heart and abdominal pain, during pregnancy:

新生雞子二枚，破著杯中，以糯米粉和如粥，頓服。亦治妊娠卒胎動不安，或但腰痛，或胎轉搶心，或下血不止。

Break two recently laid chicken eggs into a cup and mix with glutinous rice flour to a gruel-like consistency. Quaff in a single dose. It also treats a suddenly stirring fetus in pregnancy, sometimes resulting only in lumbar pain, sometimes in the fetus turning around and prodding the heart, sometimes in incessant descent of blood.

---

*   中惡 *zhòng è*: In the context of pregnancy and this particular prescription, it is most likely that 惡 refers to 惡阻 *è zǔ* (malignity obstruction), one of the most common pathologies of pregnancy that is similar to the modern concept of morning sickness.

LINE 4d.13

又方

Another prescription:

水三升洗夫靴，剔汁溫服。

Wash the husband's leather boots in three *shēng* of water. Scrape off the liquid and take it heated.

LINE 4d.14

治妊娠中蠱，心腹痛方

A prescription for treating being struck by *gǔ* venom[1] with heart and abdominal pain during pregnancy:

燒敗鼓皮，酒服方寸匕，須臾自呼蠱主姓名。

Char a rotten drum skin and take a square-inch spoon [of the ashes] in liquor. Instantly have [the woman] herself call out the *gǔ* ruler[2] by the first and last name.

1.　　　蠱 *gǔ*: An ancient magical ailment first attested in *Shāng* inscriptions. Originally, it referred to a toxic potion, prepared intentionally by placing several venomous insects in a vessel (as represented by the character) and waiting until all but one of the creatures had died. According to Donald Harper, "demonic bugs or female witchcraft are likely factors in the identity of the ailment" in the *Mǎ-Wáng-Duī* material (see Donald Harper, *Early Chinese Medical Literature*, pp. 300-301). See also 《病源論》 25:1 and Paul U. Unschuld, *Medicine in China. A History of Ideas*, pp. 46-50.

2.　　　This refers to the person who manufactured the poison and accursed her.

LINE 4d.15

治妊娠腰痛方

A prescription for treating lumbar pain during pregnancy:

大豆二升，以酒三升煮取二升，頓服之。亦治常人卒腰痛。

Cook two *shēng* of *dà dòu* (大豆 Seed of Glycine Max) in three *shēng* of liquor to obtain two *shēng*. Quaff it in a single dose. It also treats sudden lumbar pain in non-pregnant patients.

LINE 4d.16

又方

Another prescription:

麻子三升，以水五升煮取汁三升，分五服。亦治心痛。

Cook three *shēng* of *má zǐ rén* (麻子仁 Seed of Cannabis sativa) in five *shēng* of water to obtain three *shēng* of liquid. Divide into five doses. It also treats heart pain.

LINE 4d.17

又方

Another prescription:

Formula

榆白皮（三兩）豉（二兩）。

| 榆白皮 | yú bái pí | The fibrous inner bark of the root or trunk of Ulmus pumila | 三兩 3 liǎng | 9g |
| [豆]豉 | [dòu] chǐ | Preparation of Glycine max | 二兩 2 liǎng | 6g |

上二味，熟擣，蜜丸如梧桐子大，服二七丸。亦治心痛。

Thoroughly grind the above two ingredients and mix with honey into pills the size of firmiana seeds. Take two times seven pills [per dose]. It also treats heart pain.

LINE 4d.18

又方

Another prescription:

燒牛屎焦末，水服方寸匕，日三服。

Char cow excrement until scorched and pulverize it. Take a square-inch spoon in water, three times a day.

LINE 4d.19

又方

Another prescription:

地黃汁八合，酒五合合煎，分溫服。

Mix eight *gě* of *dì huáng* (地黃 Rehmannia glutinosa) juice with five *gě* of liquor and simmer together. Divide [into three doses] and take it warm.

LINE 4d.20

治妊娠脹滿方

A prescription for treating abdominal fullness during pregnancy:

服秤鎚酒良，燒之淬酒中服。亦治妊娠卒下血。

Drinking Steelyard weight liquor is good. Char [the steelyard weight], temper it by dipping it into liquor, and drink [the heated liquor]. It also treats sudden descent of blood in pregnancy.

4e Cold Damage 傷寒

LINE 4e.1

治妊娠傷寒，頭痛，壯熱，肢節煩疼方

This prescription treats cold damage in pregnancy with headache, high fever, and vexing pain in the limbs and joints.

Formula

石膏（八兩） 前胡 梔子仁 知母（各四兩） 大青 黃芩（各三兩） 蔥白（一升）。

石膏	shí gāo	Gypsum	八兩 8 liǎng	24g
前胡	qián hú	Root of Peucedanum praeruptorum	四兩 4 liǎng	12g
梔子仁	zhī zǐ rén	Fruit of Gardenia jasminoides	四兩 4 liǎng	12g
知母	zhī mǔ	Root of Anemarrhena asphodeloides	四兩 4 liǎng	12g
大青	dà qīng	Indigo-colored foliage of Isatis tinctoria	三兩 3 liǎng	9g
黃芩	huáng qín	Root of Scutellaria baicalensis	三兩 3 liǎng	9g
蔥白, 切	cōng bái, qiē	Stalk of Allium fistulosum, Chopped	一升 1 shēng	24g

上七味，㕮咀，以水七升煮取二升半，去滓，分五服，別相去如人行七八里再服。不利。

Pound the above seven ingredients and decoct in seven *shēng* of water to obtain two and a half *shēng*. Discard the dregs and divide into five doses. Separating doses by as long as it takes a person to walk seven or eight *lǐ*, take another one. [This medicine] does not disinhibit.*

---

*   不利 *bù lì*: The interpretation of *lì* as "disinhibit," — instead of reading the phrase as "[otherwise] it will not benefit"— is suggested by the fact that it was a central criterion for drugs during pregnancy that they must not disinhibit the flow of blood, an action that could potentially induce a miscarriage. Since this prescription addresses a cold condition, that is, an exterior disease which is usually treated by expelling the pathogenic agent, this note is meant to reassure the cautious practitioner that it would not be dangerous to take this prescription during pregnancy.

LINE 4e.2

治妊娠頭痛，壯熱，心煩，嘔吐，不下食方

A prescription for treating headache, vigorous heat [effusion], heart vexation, retching and vomiting, and inability to get food down, during pregnancy:

Formula

生蘆根（一升）知母（四兩）青竹筎（三兩）粳米（五合）。

生蘆根，切	shēng lú gēn, qiē	Fresh Rhizome of Phragmites communis, chopped	一升 1 shēng	24g
知母	zhī mǔ	Root of Anemarrhena asphodeloides	四兩 4 liǎng	12g
青竹筎	qīng zhú rú	Shavings of Phyllostachys nigra	三兩 3 liǎng	9g
粳米	jīng mǐ	Seed of the non-glutinous variety of Oryza sativa	五合 5 gě	35ml

上四味，㕮咀，以水五升煮取二升半，稍稍飲之，盡更作，瘥止。

Pound the above four ingredients and decoct in five *shēng* of water to obtain two and a half *shēng*. Sip it little by little and when used up, make it again. Stop when she has recovered.

LINE 4e.3

治妊娠傷寒，服湯後頭痛，壯熱不歇，宜用此拭湯方

For the treatment of cold damage in pregnancy, after taking the decoction [above], the patient should use this wiping decoction for headaches and high unremitting fever.

Wiping Decoction
拭湯 *shì tāng*

麻黃（半斤）竹葉（切，一升）石膏末（三升）。

麻黃	má huáng	Stalk of Ephedra sinica	半斤 0.5 jīn	24g
竹葉, 切	zhú yè, qiē	Leaves of Phyllostachys, chopped	一升 1 shēng	24g
石膏, 末	shí gāo, mò	Gypsum, powdered	三升 3 shēng	72g

上三味，以水五升煮取一升，去滓，冷用以拭身體，又以故布擒頭額胸心，燥則易之。患瘧者，加恆山五兩。

Decoct the above three ingredients in five *shēng* of water to obtain one *shēng* and discard the dregs. When cooled, rub it on her body. Also, use an old cloth [soaked in the decoction] and place it on her head, forehead, chest, and heart. When it is dry, change it. If she suffers from malaria,[2] add five *liǎng* of *héng shān* (恒山 Root of Dichroa febrifuga).

1.　Its meaning here is also somewhat unclear and could range from slapping the body with the soaked cloth to rubbing it on in the manner of an ink rubbing, as in the character 搨 *tà*. My translation is based on context since its most likely use would be as a cooling compress.

2.　瘧 *nüè*: The oldest Chinese character dictionary explains it as "intermittent chills and fevers" (《說文解字》7b). See also Harper, *Early Chinese Medical Literature*, p. 205, n. 4, where it is translated as "cold and hot syndrome." Wiseman and Féng explain it as "a recurrent disease characterized by shivering, vigorous heat [effusion], and sweating and classically attributed to contraction of summerheat during the hot season, contact with mountain forest miasma, or contraction of cold-damp" (*Practical Dictionary*, p. 383).

LINE 4e.4

治妊娠傷寒方

A prescription for treating cold damage in pregnancy:

Formula

蔥白（十莖）生薑（二兩，切）。

| 蔥白 | cōng bái | Stalk of Allium fistulosum | 十莖 10 jīng | 10 stalks |
| 生薑, 切 | shēng jiāng, qiē | Fresh root of Zingiber officinale, chopped | 二兩 2 liǎng | 6g |

上二味，以水三升煮取一升半，頓服取汗。

Decoct the above two ingredients in three *shēng* of water to obtain one and a half *shēng*.

Quaff in a single dose to induce sweating.

LINE 4e.5

治妊娠中風，寒熱，腹中絞痛，不可針灸方

A prescription for treating wind strike with [aversion to] cold and heat [effusion] and gripping pain in the abdomen during pregnancy, when she may not be treated with acupuncture or moxibustion:

鯽魚一頭燒作灰，擣末，酒服方寸匕，取汁。

Char one golden carp into ashes and grind into a powder. Take a square-inch spoon in liquor to induce sweating.

LINE 4e.6

治妊娠遭時疾，令子不落方

A prescription for treating [a woman who] has contracted a seasonal condition in pregnancy, which is preventing the child from descending:

取竈中黃土，水和塗臍，乾復塗之。

Take dirt from the inside of a stove,[1] mix it with water, and spread it on her the navel. When it has dried, repeat the application.[2]

1. This is the earth taken from an earthen stove and called 灶心土 *zào xīn tǔ* in modern TCM. It is also called 伏龍肝 *fú lóng gān* (lit. "crouching dragon liver") and is translated by Wiseman and Fēng as "oven earth."
2. *Sòng* editors' note: "In another [version of this] prescription, mix it with liquor and spread [on her navel] in a five-*cùn* square. Alternatively, mix it with rice water and spread it on. All these [methods] are excellent."

LINE 4e.7

又方

Another prescription:

犬尿泥塗腹，勿令乾。

Take mud on which a dog has urinated and spread it on the abdomen. Do not allow it to dry out.

LINE 4e.8

治妊娠熱病方

A prescription for treating heat disease in pregnancy:

車轄脂酒服，大良。

Take cart linchpin grease in liquor. Very good.

LINE 4e.9

又方

Another prescription:

Formula

蔥白（五兩）頭豉（二升）。

蔥白	cōng bái	Stalk of Allium fistulosum	五兩 5 liǎng	15g
頭豉	dòu chǐ	Preparation of Glycine max	二升 2 shēng	48g

上二味，以水六升煮取二升，分二服，取汗。

Decoct the above two ingredients in six *shēng* of water to obtain two *shēng*. Divide into two doses and induce sweating.

LINE 4e.10

又方

Another prescription:

蔥白一把，以水三升煮令熟，服之取汗，食蔥令盡。亦主安胎。若胎已死者，須臾即出。

Decoct one handful of *cōng bái* (蔥白 Stalk of Allium fistulosum) in three *shēng* of water until thoroughly cooked. Drink [the liquid] and induce sweating. Eat the *cōng bái* 蔥白 up completely. [This prescription] also governs calming the fetus. If the fetus has already died, [the medicine] will make it emerge instantly.

LINE 4e.11

又方

Another prescription:

水服伏龍肝一雞子大。

Take a piece of *fú lóng gān* (伏龍肝 stove earth) the size of a chicken egg in water.

LINE 4e.12

又方

Another prescription:

井底泥泥心下三寸，立愈。

Spread mud from the bottom of a well [on the area] three *cùn* below the heart. She will immediately recover.

LINE 4e.13

又方

Another prescription:

青羊屎塗腹上。

Spread dung from a young sheep or goat on the [pregnant woman's] abdomen.

LINE 4e.14

治大熱煩悶者方

A prescription for treating great fever with vexing oppression:

葛根汁二升，分三服。如人行五里進一服。

[Prepare] two *shēng* of *gé gēn* (葛根 Root of Pueraria lobata) juice and divide into three doses. Drink one dose in the amount of time it takes a person to walk five *lǐ*.

LINE 4e.15

又方

Another prescription:

槐實燒灰，服方寸匕，酒和服。

Char *huái shí* (槐實 Fruit of Sophora japonica) into ashes. Take a square-inch spoon, mixed into liquor.

LINE 4e.16

又方

Another prescription:

燒大棗七枚，末，酒和服。

Char seven *dà zǎo* (大棗 Mature fruit of Ziziphus jujuba), pulverize, and take mixed into liquor.

4f Malaria 瘧病

LINE 4f.1

治妊娠患瘧湯方

A decoction for treating patients who suffer from malaria in pregnancy:

Formula

柏山（二兩） 甘草（一兩） 黃芩（三兩） 烏梅（十四枚） 石膏（八兩）
。

柏山	héng shān	Root of Dichroa febrifuga	二兩 2 liǎng	6g
甘草	gān cǎo	Root of Glycyrrhiza uralensis	一兩 1 liǎng	3g
黃芩	huáng qín	Root of Scutellaria baicalensis	三兩 3 liǎng	9g
烏梅	wū méi	Unripe fruit of Prunus mume	十四枚 14 méi	14 pieces
石膏	shí gāo	Gypsum	八兩 8 liǎng	24g

上五味，㕮咀，以酒水各一升半合清藥一宿，煮三四沸，去滓，初服六
合，次服四合，後服二合，凡三服。

Pound the above five ingredients. Combine one and a half *shēng* each of liquor and water, and soak the drugs in this over night. Then decoct it, bringing it to a boil three or four
times, and discard the dregs. First take six *gě*, for the next dose take four *gě*, and then
two, taking a total of three doses.

LINE 4f.2

又方

Another prescription:

Formula

怕山 竹葉（各三兩） 石膏（八兩） 粳米（一百粒。崔氏，外臺作糯米；集

驗，救急作秫米）。

恒山	héng shān	Root of Dichroa febrifuga	三兩 3 liǎng	9g
竹葉	zhú yè	Leaves of Phyllostachys	三兩 3 liǎng	9g
石膏	shí gāo	Gypsum	八兩 8 liǎng	24g
粳米	jīng mǐ[1]	Seed of the non-glutinous variety of Oryza sativa	一百粒 100 lì	100 grains

上四味，㕮咀，以水六升煮取二升半，去滓，分三服：第一服取未發前一食頃服之；第二服取臨欲發服之；餘一服用以塗頭額及胸前五心。藥滓置頭邊。當一日勿近水及進飲食，過發後乃進粥食。

Pound the above four ingredients and decoct in six *shēng* of water to obtain two and a half *shēng*. Discard the dregs and divide into three doses: Take the first dose shortly before an attack.[2] Take the second dose immediately prior to the attack. Use the remaining dose to rub on the head and forehead, in front of the chest, and in the "five hearts."[3] Place the dregs of the medicine next to the head. Wait one day before approaching any water and eating and drinking. Only after the attack has passed may the patient eat a meal of gruel.

1.   *Sòng* editors' note: "*Cuī Shì* and *Wài Tái Mì Yào* use glutinous rice; *Jí Yàn Fāng* and *Jiù Jí Fāng* use glutinous millet."
2.   未發前一食頃服之 *wèi fā qián yī shí qǐng fú zhī*: This translation assumes that the attacks come at predictable times. This is supported by the explanation of malaria in the *Bìng Yuán Lùn* 病源論 (《病源論》 11:1). It is stressed here that malaria attacks are related to the regular cyles of protective *qì* and the progression of malign *qì* from the interstices into the channels and the rest of the body. They therefore occur in predictable intervals and at predictable times of the day.
3.   五心 *wǔ xīn*: A technical term referring to the soles of the feet, palms of the hands, and the center of the chest.

4g Descent of Blood 下血

LINE 4g.1

治妊娠忽暴下血數升，胎燥不動方

A prescription for treating sudden and fulminant descent of blood during pregnancy with the loss of several *shēng* [of blood], and a dried fetus that is not moving:

Formula

榆白皮（三兩）當歸 生薑（各二兩）乾地黃（四兩）葵子（一升，《肘後》不用）。

榆白皮	yú bái pí	The fibrous inner bark of the root or trunk of Ulmus pumila	三兩 3 liǎng	9g
當歸	dāng guī	Root of Angelica polimorpha	二兩 2 liǎng	6g
生薑	shēng jiāng	Fresh root of Zingiber officinale	二兩 2 liǎng	6g
乾地黃	gān dì huáng	Dried root of Rehmannia glutinosa	四兩 4 liǎng	12g
葵子	kuí zǐ*	Seeds of Malva verticillata	一升 1 shēng	24g

上五味，㕮咀，以水五升煮取二升半，分三服，不瘥便作。服之甚良。

Pound the above five ingredients and decoct in five *shēng* of water to obtain two and a half *shēng*. Divide into three doses. If she fails to recover, make it again. Taking this is most excellent.

*   *Sòng* editors' note: "The *Zhǒu Hòu Fāng* leaves out *kuí zǐ* 葵子."

LINE 4g.2

治妊娠卒驚奔走，或從高墮下，暴出血數升，馬通湯方

Horse Dung Decoction treats fulminant bleeding of several *shēng* during pregnancy, after fleeing and running from a sudden scare or falling down from a high place:

Horse Dung Decoction
馬通湯 mǎ tǒng tāng

馬通汁（一升）乾地黃（四兩）當歸（三兩）阿膠（四兩）艾葉（三兩）。

馬通汁	mǎ tōng zhī	Dung juice of Equus caballus	一升 1 shēng	70ml
乾地黃	gān dì huáng	Dried root of Rehmannia glutinosa	四兩 4 liǎng	12g
當歸	dāng guī	Root of Angelica polimorpha	三兩 3 liǎng	9g
阿膠	ē jiāo	Gelatinous glue produced from Equus asinus	四兩 4 liǎng	12g
艾葉	ài yè	Dry-roasted foliage of Artemisia argyi	三兩 3 liǎng	9g

上五味，㕮咀，以水五升煮取二升半，去滓，內馬通汁及膠令烊，分三服，不瘥重作。

Pound the above five ingredients. Decoct [the drugs] in five *shēng* of water to obtain two and a half *shēng*. Discard the dregs and add the *mǎ tōng zhī* 馬通汁 and *ē jiāo* 阿膠, letting it melt. Divide into three doses. If she fails to recover, make it again.

LINE 4g.3

治妊娠二三月，上至七八月，其人頓仆失踞，胎動不下，傷損，腰腹痛欲死，若有所見，及胎奔上搶心，短氣，膠艾湯方

Ass Hide Glue and Mugwort Decoction is a treatment for women from the second and third months of pregnancy up to the seventh and eighth months who have stumbled and fallen or lost [their balance] when kneeling, resulting in stirring fetus,[1] injury,[2] lumbar and abdominal pain so intense that [the patient] wants to die, if she shows visible symptoms, to the point of the fetus racing upwards and prodding the heart, and shortness of breath.

Ass Hide Glue and Mugwort Decoction
膠艾湯 jiāo ài tāng

阿膠（二兩）艾葉（三兩）芎藭 芍藥 甘草 當歸（各二兩）乾地黃（四兩）。

阿膠	ē jiāo	Gelatinous glue produced from Equus asinus	二兩 2 liǎng	6g
艾葉	ài yè	Dry-roasted foliage of Artemisia argyi	三兩 3 liǎng	9g
川芎	chuān xiōng	Root of Ligusticum wallichii	二兩 2 liǎng	6g
芍藥	sháo yào	Root of Paeonia albiflora	二兩 2 liǎng	6g

甘草	gān cǎo	Root of Glycyrrhiza uralensis	二兩 2 liǎng	6g
當歸	dāng guī	Root of Angelica polimorpha	二兩 2 liǎng	6g
乾地黃	gān dì huáng	Dried root of Rehmannia glutinosa	四兩 4 liǎng	12g

上七味，㕮咀，以水五升，好酒三升合煮取三升，去滓內膠，更上火令消盡，分三服，日三，不瘥更作。

Pound the above seven ingredients. Mix five *shēng* of water with three *shēng* of good liquor and simmer [the drugs] in this to obtain three *shēng*. Discard the dregs and add the *ē jiāo* 阿膠. Return to the flame and let it melt completely. Divide into three doses and take three times a day. If she fails to recover, make it again.

1. 胎動不下 *tāi dòng bù xià*: Literally translated, "stirring fetus failing to descend." The *Sūn Zhēn Rén* edition has 不安 *bù ān* (disquieted) instead of 不下. Based on the fact that the prescription applies to women in the early as well as late stages of pregnancy, I interpret 不下 as a scribal error and have adopted 不安 as the much more likely version. Furthermore, 胎動不安 is a common expression that is found very frequently in this text.
2. 傷損 *shāng sǔn*: It is unclear here whether this refers to the fetus or the mother, as the original was not punctuated. Modern Chinese editions vary in their punctuation.

LINE 4g.4

治妊娠卒下血方

A prescription for treating sudden descent of blood in pregnancy:

葵子一升，以水五升煮取二升，分三服，瘥止。

Decoct one *shēng* of *kuí zǐ* (葵子 Seeds of Malva verticillata) in five *shēng* of water to obtain two *shēng*. Divide into three doses. Stop when she has recovered.

LINE 4g.5

又方

Another prescription:

生地黃切一升，以酒五升煮取三升，分三服。亦治落身後血。

Another prescription: Chop one *shēng* of *shēng dì huáng* (生地黃 Fresh root of Rehmannia glutinosa) and decoct it in five *shēng* of liquor to obtain three *shēng*. Divide into three doses. It also treats bleeding after a fall.

LINE 4g.6

又方

Another prescription:

葵根莖燒作灰，以酒服方寸匕，日三。

Char *kuí gēn* (葵根 Root of Malva verticillata) into ashes and take a square-inch spoon in liquor three times a day.

LINE 4g.7

治妊娠僵仆失踞，胎動轉上搶心，甚者血從口出，逆不得息，或注下血一斗五升，胎不出，子死則寒，熨人腹中，急如產狀，虛乏少氣，困頓欲死，煩悶反覆，服藥母即得安，下血亦止，其當產者立生，蟹爪湯方

Crab's Claw Decoction is a treatment for pregnant women who have fallen over or lost [their balance] when kneeling, [resulting in] the fetus stirring, turning and prodding the heart, in serious cases with bleeding from the mouth, counterflow and inability to breathe, and perhaps downpouring bleeding of [as much as] one *dǒu* and five *shēng*, failure of the fetus to emerge, [aversion to] cold if the fetus has died, [heat] as if another person were applying a heat compress in the center of her abdomen, tension as if in labor, vacuity and lack of *qì*, exhaustion and fatigue to the point of near-death, and alternating vexation and oppression. As soon as she has taken this medicine, the mother will find peace, her bleeding will stop, and if she is ready to deliver, it will induce the birth.

Crab's Claw Decoction
蟹爪湯 *xiè zhǎo tāng*

蟹爪（一升）甘草桂心（各二尺）阿膠（二兩）。

蟹爪	xiè zhǎo	Claw of Eriocheir sinensis	一升 1 shēng	24g
甘草	gān cǎo	Root of Glycyrrhiza uralensis	二尺 2 chǐ	60cm
桂心	guì xīn	Shaved inner bark of Cinnamomum cassia	二尺 2 chǐ	60cm
阿膠	ē jiāo	Gelatinous glue produced from Equus asinus	二兩 2 liǎng	6g

上四味，㕮咀以東流水一斗煮取三升，去滓，內膠烊盡，能為一服佳。不能者，食頓再服之。若口急不能飲者，格口灌之，藥下便活也，與母俱生。

若胎已死，獨母活也。若不僵仆，平安妊娠無有所見，下血，服此湯即止。
或云桂不安胎，亦未必爾。

Pound the above four ingredients. Decoct in one *dǒu* of water from an east-flowing source to obtain three *shēng*. Discard the dregs, add the *ē jiāo* 阿膠 and let it melt completely. It is best if [the patient] is able to take it in a single dose. If unable to do so, drink some more in a short while. If her mouth is clenched and she is unable to take in fluids, force it open and pour in [the medicine]. If she can get the medicine down, it means life. Both [the fetus] and the mother will survive. If the fetus has already died, only the mother will survive. If she has not fallen and has had a calm and stable pregnancy without visible symptoms [so far], but now is bleeding, taking this medicine will stop it. Some people say that *guì xīn* 桂心 does not quiet the fetus, but that is not necessarily so.

LINE 4g.8

治妊娠胎墮下血不止方

A prescription for treating miscarriage and incessant descent of blood during pregnancy:

丹參十二兩㕮咀，以清酒五升煮取三升，溫服一升，日三。

Pound twelve *liǎng* of *dān shēn* (丹參 Root of Salvia miltiorrhiza) and decoct in five *shēng* of clear liquor to obtain three *shēng*. Take one *shēng* heated, three times a day.

LINE 4g.9

又方

Another prescription:

地黃汁和代赭末，服方寸匕。

Take a square-inch spoon of *dì huáng* (地黃 Rehmannia glutinosa) juice mixed with pulverized *dài zhě* (代赭 Hematite).

LINE 4g.10

又方

Another prescription:

桑蠍蟲矢燒灰，酒服方寸匕。

Char *sāng xiē chóng shǐ* (桑蝎蟲矢 Mulberry worm excrement) into ashes and take a square-inch spoon in liquor.

LINE 4g.11

治半產下血不盡，苦來去煩滿欲死，香豉湯方

Fermented Soybean Decoction treats cases of miscarriage when the precipitated blood is not eliminated completely,* with recurring discomfort and vexing fullness to the point of near-death.

Fermented Soybean Decoction
香豉湯 *xiāng chǐ tāng*

香豉一升半，以水三升煮三沸，漉去滓，內成末鹿角一方匕，頓服之，須臾血自下。鹿角燒亦得。

Cook one and a half *shēng* of *xiāng chǐ* (香豉 Preparation of Fermented Glycine max) in three *shēng* of water, bringing it to a boil three times. Filter it and discard the dregs. Add one square-inch spoon of pulverized *lù jiǎo* 鹿角 and quaff it in a single dose. The [remaining] blood will naturally descend in an instant. Charring the *lù jiǎo* (鹿角 Ossified antler or antler base of Cervus nippon) is also possible.

---

* 　　下血不盡 *xià xuè bù jìn*: I interpret this as referring to an incomplete miscarriage where some of the blood has remained in the uterus. Alternatively, *bù jìn* can also be read as "endlessly." While the two translations seem quite opposite in English, their meaning is actually quite similar in the framework of medieval medical thinking: It was of great concern to medical writers that the blood remaining in a woman's uterus after childbirth or miscarriage would be eliminated and purged completely because it was seen as a highly pathogenic substance, commonly referred to as 惡露 *è lù* ("malign dew," that is, lochia). See for example the introductions to chapter one of volume three, on "Vacuity Detriment" (p. 234 below) and chapter five of volume three on "Malign Dew," p. 318 below or the essay on "incomplete elimination of malign dew after birth with abdominal pain" in the *Bìng Yuán Lùn*: "If she contracts wind-cold before the malign dew has been eliminated completely, this causes wind-cold to contend with the blood, the blood will become blocked and stagnate instead of flowing freely and dispersing. It will accumulate inside.... In severe cases, it transforms into blood accumulations and may also cause amenorrhea" (《病源論》43:3:2). The intended action of this prescription to complete the elimination of the fetus after miscarriage is also suggested by the effect described below that "the blood will descend naturally" (血自下 *xuè zì xià*).

4h Urinary Diseases　小便病

LINE 4h.1

治妊娠小便不利方

A prescription for treating inhibited urination in pregnancy:

Formula

葵子（一升）榆白皮（一把，切）。

葵子	kuí zǐ	Seeds of Malva verticil-lata	一升 1 shēng	24g
榆白皮, 切	yú bái pí, qiē	Fibrous inner bark of the root or trunk of Ulmus pumila, chopped	一把 1 bǎ	1 handful

上二味，以水五升煮五沸，服一升，日三。

Cook the above two ingredients in five *shēng* of water, bringing them to a boil five times. Take one *shēng* three times a day.

LINE 4h.2

又方

Another prescription:

Formula

葵子 茯苓（各一兩）。

葵子	kuí zǐ	Seeds of Malva verticillata	一兩 1 liǎng	3g
茯苓	fú líng	Dried fungus of Poria cocos	一兩 1 liǎng	3g

上二味，末之，以水服方寸匕，日三，小便利則止。

Pulverize the above two ingredients and take a square-inch spoon in water three times a day. Stop when urination is disinhibited.[1]

1.   *Sòng* editors' note: "[Zhāng] Zhòng-Jǐng states: "Cases of water *qì*[2] in pregnancy [present with] heaviness of the body, inhibited urination, aversion to cold as if being sprayed with water, and dizziness in the head upon rising."

2.   水氣 *shuǐ qì*: Defined by Wiseman and Féng as "pathological excesses of water in the body and, specifically, water swelling provoked by it. The main cause is impairment of movement and transformation of water due to spleen-kidney yáng vacuity" (*Practical Dictionary*, p. 668).

LINE 4h.3

治妊娠患子淋方

A prescription for treating strangury of pregnancy:[*]

葵子一升，以水三升煮取二升，分再服。

Decoct one *shēng* of *kuí zǐ* (葵子 Seeds of Malva verticillata) in three *shēng* of water to obtain two *shēng*. Divide into two doses.

*   妊娠子淋 *rèn shēn zǐ lín*: Literally "child dribbling in pregnancy." According to the *Bìng Yuán Lùn* 病源論, this pathology is due to kidney vacuity causing heat in the bladder (《病源論》 42:41). *Lín* is described in the *Jīn Guì Yào Luè* as 小便如粟狀小腹弦急痛引臍中 (millet-grain-like urination (i.e., small amounts), bowstring tension in the lower abdomen, and pain stretching to the center of the navel) (quoted in 《中華醫學大辭典》 p. 1203). It is frequently associated with 渴 *kě* (thirst). Occasionally, Sūn Sī-Miǎo uses the character also to refer to menstrual problems. Wiseman and Féng define it as "a disease pattern characterized by urinary urgency, frequent short painful rough voidings, and dribbling incontinence" (*Practical Dictionary*, p. 583).

LINE 4h.4

又方

Another prescription:

葵根一把，以水三升煮取二升，分再服。

Decoct one handful of *kuí gēn* (葵根 Root of Malva verticillata) in three *shēng* of water to obtain two *shēng*. Divide into two doses.

LINE 4h.5

治妊娠小便不通利方

A prescription for treating blocked and inhibited urination:

蕪菁子十合為末，水和服方寸匕，日三服。

Pulverize ten *gě* of *wú jīng zǐ* (蕪菁子 Seeds of Brassica rapa) and take a square-inch spoon mixed in water three times a day.

LINE 4h.6

治妊娠尿血方

A prescription for treating bloody urine in pregnancy:

黍穰燒灰，酒服方寸匕，日三服。

Char millet stalks into ashes and take a square-inch spoon in liquor, three doses a day.

LINE 4h.7

治婦人無故尿血方

A prescription for treating bloody urine without a cause in [pregnant] women:[*]

龍骨五兩治下篩，酒服方寸匕，空腹服，日三。久者，二十服愈。

Finely pestle and sift five *liǎng* of *lóng gǔ* (龍骨 Os draconis). Take a square-inch spoon in liquor on an empty stomach three times a day. In chronic cases, twenty doses will bring recovery.

---

[*]   Unlike most of the other prescriptions in this chapter, this one is addressed to women in general. On the one hand, this could be a scribal error since the *Qiān Jīn Fāng* has a separate section on "strangury and thirst" (unrelated to pregnancy) in the third volume. On the other hand, though, several other prescriptions addressed to women in general below conclude with the statement: 亦治丈夫 *yì zhì zhàng fū* (it also treats the husband). See Line 4h.12, p. 167 below.

LINE 4h.8

又方

Another prescription:

Formula

瓜甲 亂髮。

瓜甲	zhǎo jiǎ	finger nails of homo sapiens
亂髮	luàn fà	matted hair of homo sapiens

上二味，並燒末等分，酒服方寸匕，日三。飲服亦得。

Char equal amounts of the above two ingredients and pulverize them. Take a square-inch spoon in liquor three times a day. Taking it in [any other] liquid is also possible.

LINE 4h.9

又方

Another prescription:

Formula

麋角屑 大豆黃卷 桂心（各一兩）。

屑麋角	xiè lù jiǎo	Chips of Ossified antler or ant-ler base of Cervus nippon	一兩 1 liǎng	3g
大豆黃卷	dà dòu huáng juǎn	Dried sprouts of Glycine max	一兩 1 liǎng	3g
桂心	guì xīn	Shaved inner bark of Cinnamo-mum cassia	一兩 1 liǎng	3g

上三味，治下篩，酒服方寸匕，日三服。

Finely pestle and sift the above three ingredients. Take a square-inch spoon in liquor three times a day.

LINE 4h.10

又方

Another prescription:

取夫爪甲燒作灰，酒服之。

Take the husband's finger nails and char into ashes. Take in liquor.

LINE 4h.11

又方

Another prescription:

取故舡上竹茹暴乾，擣末，酒服方寸匕，日三。亦主遺尿。

Take rotten bamboo shavings* that have been dried in the sun and pulverized. Take a square-inch spoon in liquor three times a day. It also governs urinary incontinence.

*   故舡上竹茹 *gù chuán shàng zhú rú*: More often called 敗船茹 *bài chuán rú*, these are shavings of entangled bamboo roots used to fix leaks in boats.

LINE 4h.12

治婦人遺尿不知出時方

A prescription for treating women's urinary incontinence and inability to predict the time of discharge:

Formula

白薇 芍藥（各一兩）。

白薇	bái wēi	Root of Cynanchum atratum	一兩	1 liǎng	3g
芍藥	sháo yào	Root of Paeonia albiflora	一兩	1 liǎng	3g

上二味，治下篩，酒服方寸匕，日三。

Finely pestle and sift the above two ingredients. Take a square-inch spoon in liquor three times a day.

LINE 4h.13

又方

Another prescription:

胡鷰窠中草燒末，酒服半錢匕。亦治丈夫。

Char and pulverize straw from a swallow's nest. Take a half-*qián* spoon in liquor. It also treats the husband.

LINE 4h.14

又方

Another prescription:

Formula

礬石 牡蠣（各二兩）。

礬石	fán shí	Alum	二兩	2 liǎng	6g
牡蠣	mǔ lì	Shell of Ostrea rivularis	二兩	2 liǎng	6g

上二味，治下篩，酒服方寸匕。亦治丈夫。

Finely pestle and sift the above two ingredients. Take a square-inch spoon in liquor. It also treats the husband.

LINE 4h.15

又方

Another prescription:

燒遺尿人薦草灰，服之瘥。

Char the straw bedding from a person with urinary incontinence into ashes. Taking it will cause recovery.

LINE 4h.16

又

Another :

Moxibustion Method

灸橫骨當陰門七壯。

Burn seven cones of moxa on the point where the pubic bone meets the vagina.

4i Diarrhea 下痢

*   Translator's note: 痢 *lì*: A disease term referring to dysfunctional bowel movements that are caused by vacuity in the spleen and stomach and often associated with wind damage contracted in the spring. The term is etymologically related to the concept of 利 *lì*, un-inhibited [bowel movements]. See almost the entire volume 17 of the *Bìng Yuán Lùn* for a detailed etiology and differentiation of the different types. Sūn Sī-Miǎo distinguishes broadly between two types, 赤痢 *chì lì* (red diarrhea), which refers to diarrhea with blood in the stool, and 白痢 *bái lì* (white diarrhea), which refers to diarrhea with pus in the stool.

LINE 4i.1

治妊娠下痢方

A prescription for treating diarrhea in pregnancy:

Formula

酸石榴皮 黃芩 人參（各三兩） 欅皮（四兩） 粳米（三合）。

酸石榴皮	suān shí liú pí	Sour rind of the fruit of Punica granatum	三兩 3 liǎng	9g
黃芩	huáng qín	Root of Scutellaria baicalensis	三兩 3 liǎng	9g
人參	rén shēn	Root of Panax ginseng	三兩 3 liǎng	9g
欅皮	jǔ pí	Bark of Zelkova schneideriana	四兩 4 liǎng	12g
粳米	jīng mǐ	Seed of the non-glutinous variety of Oryza sativa	三合 3 gě	21ml

上五味，㕮咀，以水七升煮取二升半，分三服。

Pound the above five ingredients and decoct in seven *shēng* of water to obtain two and a half *shēng*. Divide into three doses.

LINE 4i.2

治妊娠患膿血赤滯，魚腦白滯，臍腹絞痛不可忍者方

A prescription for treating women in pregnancy who are suffering from red diarrhea with pus and blood [in the stool] or [fish brain-like] white diarrhea, in conjunction with unbearable gripping pain in the navel and abdomen:

Formula

薤白（切，一升）酸石榴皮（二兩）阿膠（二兩）黃蘗（三兩，《產寶》作黃連）地榆（四兩）。

薤白, 切	xiè bái, qiē	Stalk of Allium macrostemon, chopped	一升 1 shēng	24g
酸石榴皮	suān shí liú pí	Sour rind of the fruit of Punica granatum	二兩 2 liǎng	6g
阿膠	ē jiāo	Gelatinous glue produced from Equus asinus	二兩 2 liǎng	6g
黃蘗*	huáng bò	Bark of Phellodendron amurense	三兩 3 liǎng	9g
地榆	dì yú	Root of Sanguisorba officinalis	四兩 4 liǎng	12g

上五味，㕮咀，以水七升煮取二升半，分三服，不瘥更作。

Pound the above five ingredients and decoct in seven *shēng* of water to obtain two and a half *shēng*. Divide into three doses. If she fails to recover, make it again.

---

* *Sòng* editors' note: "The *Chǎn Bǎo* uses *huáng lián* (黃連 Rhizome of Coptis chinensis) instead."

LINE 4i.3

治妊娠下痢方

A prescription for treating diarrhea in pregnancy:

白楊皮一斤㕮咀，以水一大升*煮取二小升，分三服。

Pound one *jīn* of *bái yáng pí* (白楊皮 Bark of Populus davidiana) and decoct in one large *shēng* of water to obtain two small *shēng*. Divide into three doses.

* 大升 *dà shēng*: The equivalent of three regular *shēng*.

LINE 4i.4

又方

Another prescription:

燒中衣帶三寸 ， 末 ， 服之 。

Char three *cùn* of the girdle of an undergarment. Pulverize and take it.

LINE 4i.5

又方

Another prescription:

羊脂如棋子大十枚 ， 溫酒一升 ， 投中頓服之 ， 日三 。

Take ten pieces of *yáng zhī* (羊脂 Unrendered fat of Capra hircus) the size of chess pieces and put them in one *shēng* of heated liquor. Quaff in a single dose, three times a day.

LINE 4i.6

治妊娠注下不止方

A prescription for treating incessant downpour diarrhea during pregnancy:

Formula

阿膠 艾葉 酸石榴皮 （ 各二兩 ） 。

阿膠	ē jiāo	Gelatinous glue produced from Equus asinus	二兩	2 liǎng	6g
艾葉	ài yè	Dry-roasted foliage of Artemisia argyi	二兩	2 liǎng	6g
酸石榴皮	suān shí liú pí	Sour rind of the fruit of Punica granatum	二兩	2 liǎng	6g

上三味 ， 㕮咀 ， 以水七升煮取二升 ， 去滓 ， 內膠令烊 ， 分三服 。

Pound the above three ingredients and decoct in seven *shēng* of water to obtain two *shēng*. Discard the dregs, add the *ē jiāo* 阿膠 and let it melt. Divide into three doses.

LINE 4i.7

治妊娠及產已寒熱下痢方

A prescription for treating diarrhea with [aversion to] cold and heat [effusion] during pregnancy or after delivery:

Formula

黃連（一升）梔子（二十枚）黃蘗（一斤）。

黃連	huáng lián	Rhizome of Coptis chinensis	一升 1 shēng	24g
梔子	zhī zǐ	Fruit of Gardenia jasminoides	二十枚 20 méi	20 pieces
黃蘗	huáng bò	Bark of Phellodendron amurense	一斤 1 jīn	48g

上三味，哎咀，以水五升漬一宿，煮三沸，服一升，一日一夜令盡。嘔者，加橘皮一兩，生薑二兩。亦治丈夫常痢。

Pound the above three ingredients. Soak them overnight in five *shēng* of water, then bring them to a boil three times. Take one *shēng*, once during the day and once at night, to use it up. In cases of retching, add one *liǎng* of *jú pí* (橘皮 Peel of Citrus reticulata) and two *liǎng* of *shēng jiāng* (生薑 Fresh root of Zingiber officinale). It also treats a husband's persistent diarrhea.

LINE 4i.8

治婦人痢，欲痢輒先心痛腹脹滿，日夜五六十行方

A prescription for treating women's diarrhea, with heart pain and abdominal and intestinal fullness right before bowel movements, and with fifty or sixty [bowel] movements throughout the day and night:

Formula

麴[1] 石榴皮 黃蘗 烏梅 黃連 艾（各一兩）防已（二兩）阿膠 乾薑（各三兩）附子（五兩）。

陳麴	chén qū	Medicated leaven	一兩 1 liǎng	3g
石榴皮	shí liú pí	Rind of the fruit of Punica granatum	一兩 1 liǎng	3g
黃蘗²	huáng bò	Bark of Phellodendron amurense	一兩 1 liǎng	3g
烏梅	wū méi	Unripe fruit of Prunus mume	一兩 1 liǎng	3g
黃連	huáng lián	Rhizome of Coptis chinensis	一兩 1 liǎng	3g
艾葉	ài yè	Dry-roasted foliage of Artemisia argyi	一兩 1 liǎng	3g
防已	fáng jǐ	Root of Aristolochia fangchi	二兩 2 liǎng	6g
阿膠	ē jiāo	Gelatinous glue produced from Equus asinus	三兩 3 liǎng	9g
乾薑	gān jiāng	Dried root of Zingiber officinale	三兩 3 liǎng	9g
附子	fù zǐ	Lateral root of Aconitum carmichaeli	五兩 5 liǎng	15g

上十味，末之，蜜和丸，飲服如梧子大二十丸，日三，漸加至三十四十丸。

Pulverize the above ten ingredients and combine with honey into pills the size of firmiana seeds. Take twenty pills in fluid, three times a day, gradually increasing the dose to thirty or forty pills.

1. 麴 qū: Usually referred to as 陳麴 chén qū (aged leaven) or 神麴 shén qū (medicated leaven).
2. Sòng editors' note: "Another [version of this prescription] uses mài niè (麥蘗 Shoots of Hordeum vulgare)."

LINE 4i.9

Moxibustion Treatment

婦人水洩痢，灸氣海百壯，三報。

For [the treatment of] women with watery diarrhea, burn 100 cones of moxa at the Sea of Qì (氣海 qì hǎi: CV-6). Repeat [the treatment] three times.

4j Water Swelling 水腫

Translator's note: A pathology explained by Wiseman and Féng as "swelling of the flesh arising when organ dysfunction (spleen, kidney, lung) due to internal or external causes allows water to accumulate" (*Practical Dictionary*, p. 668).

LINE 4j.1

治妊娠體腫有水氣，心腹急滿湯方

This decoction treats swelling of the body and presence of water *qì*, with tension and fullness in the heart and abdomen, during pregnancy:

Formula

茯苓 白朮（各四兩，《崔氏》無朮）黃芩（三兩）旋復花（二兩）杏仁（三兩）。

茯苓	fú líng	Dried fungus of Poria cocos	四兩 4 liang	12g
白朮*	bái zhú	Rhizome of Atractylodes macrocephala	四兩 4 liang	12g
黃芩	huáng qín	Root of Scutellaria baicalensis	三兩 3 liǎng	9g
旋復花	xuán fù huā	Flowerhead of Inula britannica	二兩 2 liǎng	6g
杏仁	xìng rén	Dried seed of Prunus armeniaca	三兩 3 liǎng	9g

上五味，㕮咀，以水六升煮取二升半，分三服。

Pound the above five ingredients and decoct in six *shēng* of water to obtain two and a half *shēng*. Divide into three doses.

*   *Sòng* editors' note: "The *Cuī Shì* lacks *bái zhú* 白朮."

LINE 4j.2

治妊娠腹大，胎間有水氣，鯉魚湯方

Carp Decoction treats an enlarged abdomen and water *qì* in the space for the fetus, during pregnancy.

Carp Decoction
鯉魚湯 *lǐ yú tāng*

鯉魚（一頭，重二斤）白朮（五兩）生薑（三兩）芍藥 當歸（各三兩）茯苓（四兩）。

鯉魚	lǐ yú	Meat or whole body of Cyprinus carpio	二斤 2 jīn	96g
白朮	bái zhú	Rhizome of Atractylodes macrocephala	五兩 5 liǎng	15g
生薑	shēng jiāng	Fresh root of Zingiber officinale	三兩 3 liǎng	9g
芍藥	sháo yào	Root of Paeonia albiflora	三兩 3 liǎng	9g
當歸	dāng guī	Root of Angelica polimorpha	三兩 3 liǎng	9g
茯苓	fú líng	Dried fungus of Poria cocos	四兩 4 liǎng	12g

上六味，㕮咀，以水一斗二升先煮魚熟，澄清，取八升，內藥煎取三升，分五服。

Pound the above six ingredients. First cook the fish in one *dǒu* and two *shēng* of water until done. Clarify the liquid by letting the impurities settle to the bottom. Take eight *shēng*, add the drugs, and simmer to obtain three *shēng*. Divide into five doses.

LINE 4j.3

治妊娠毒腫方

A prescription for treating toxic swelling[1] in pregnancy:[2]

蕪菁根淨洗去皮，擣，酢和如薄泥，勿令有汁，猛火煮之二沸，適性薄腫，以帛急裹之，日再易，寒時溫覆。非根時，用子。若腫在咽中，取汁含咽之。

Clean and wash *wú jīng gēn* (蕪菁根 Root of Brassica rapa), remove the peel, pound, and mix with vinegar to the consistency of fine mud. Make sure there is no liquid [left]. Cook over a fierce flame, bringing it to a boil twice. Thinly spread it on the swelling according to her liking[3] and wrap it tightly with a silk cloth. Change it twice a day. In the winter, keep her warm under covers. In seasons when the root is unavailable, use the seed. If the swelling is located in the throat, drink the juice and hold it in the throat.

1.   毒腫 *dú zhǒng*: According to Wiseman and Féng, "swelling due to the presence of toxin" (*Practical Dictionary*, p. 621). This roughly corresponds to the biomedical diseases of toxemia or preeclampsia, characterized by hypertension, proteinuria, and edema, as well as, in severe cases, disturbed liver functions.

2.   Instead of this heading, the *Sūn Zhēn Rén* states: 妊娠及男女毒腫 *rèn shēn jí nán nǚ dú zhǒng* (toxin swelling in pregnancy or in men or women [in general]).

3.   適性 *shì xìng*: Most likely, this is a reference to the temperature of the mix.

LINE 4j.4

又方

Another prescription:

燒憖牛屎，酢和傅之，乾則易。亦可服方寸匕，日三。

Char *qín niú shǐ* (憖牛屎 Qín buffalo dung). Mix it with vinegar and spread it on [the swelling]. Change it, when it dries out. It is also possible to internally take a square-inch spoon three times a day.

*   A rare character. It refers to a type of buffalo that is smaller than the water buffalo and prevalent in the North. See 《本草綱目》 50:1779 (entry on 牛 *niú*).

LINE 4j.5

治妊娠手腳皆腫攣急方

A prescription for treating swelling and hypertonicity in all the extremities during pregnancy:

Formula

赤小豆（五升）商陸根（一斤，切）。*

赤小豆	chì xiǎo dòu	Fruit of Phaseolus calcaratus	五升 5 shēng	120g
商陸根，切	shāng lù gēn, qiē	Root of Phytolacca acinosa, chopped	一斤 1 jīn	48g

上二味，以水三斗煮取一斗，稍稍飲之，盡更作。

Cook the above two ingredients in three *dǒu* water to obtain one *dǒu*. Sip it slowly. When it is used up, make it again.

*   *Sòng* editors' note: Another [version of this prescription] includes one *jīn* of *zé lán* (澤蘭 Foliage and stalk of Lycopus lucidus).

5. Birthing Difficulties 產難

LINE 5.1

(一) 論曰：產婦雖是穢惡，然將痛之時，及未產已產，並不得令死喪污穢家人來視之，則生難。若已產者，則傷兒也。(二) 婦人產乳，忌友支月。若值此月，當在牛皮上，若灰上。(三) 勿令水血惡物著地，則殺人。及浣濯衣水皆以器盛，過此忌月乃止。

(1) Essay: Although a woman in childbirth is herself in a filthy and malign condition, nevertheless, from the time when her labor pains begin and when she has not yet given birth to the point when she has already given birth, all this time you must not allow people from homes polluted by the filth of death or mourning to come and see her. [If that happens,] it will result in complications during delivery. If she has already given birth, it will then damage the child.

(2) Women in childbirth must avoid the opposite branch month.[1] If [the birth] does fall directly on this month, she must [deliver] on top of a cow hide or otherwise on top of ashes.

(3) Do not let any fluids, blood, or malign substances touch the ground. [If that happens], it will kill someone. Moreover, the water used for washing and rinsing her clothes must all be contained in a vessel.[2] You may only stop [following these rules] after the prohibited month has passed.[3]

1. 反支月 *fǎn zhī yuè*: Determining the opposite branch month is based on a variety of calendrical and hemerological calculations that is explained in iatromantic literature. In the context of childbirth, the *Ishimpô*, quoting the *Chǎn Jīng*, lists several different aspects in its chapter on "monthly taboos for the opposite branch" (反支月忌): "The opposite branch hurts people when it comes around, thus it is called opposite branch. If the woman in childbirth violates it, there will be certain death, so she must absolutely beware..." It then lists details on how to determine taboo months based on the mother's birth year, her age, the taboo days for the lunar quarters, etc (《醫心方》 23:2). Sūn Sī-Miǎo's abbreviated reference to the calendrical and hemerological calculations seems to suggest that, as a sophisticated physician, he might have disproved of some aspects of iatromancy, but that these methods were too popular and generally accepted to be completely ignored. However, it is also possible that he simply expected these technicalities to be covered in specialized texts on iatromantic techniques. According to Jender Lee, *Táng* doctors maintained the practice of "taboos on days and directions" (日遊反支 *rì yóu fǎn zhī*) to calm down overanxious women in delivery (Jender Lee, "*Gender and*

Medicine in Tang China," p. 4).

2.   The blood of childbirth was considered highly offensive to the spirits and therefore had to be contained carefully so that it would not offend the earth spirits by touching the ground. As a late *Táng* Daoist text explains: "Childbirth causes various predicaments. During women's monthly flow, when they clean dirty clothes, or when they bear children, their blood dirties the earth gods. Dirty fluids pour out into streams, rivers, ponds, and wells. Without knowledge and awareness, people draw water for drink and food and offer it as sacrifice to the spirits. Thus they violently offend the Three Luminaries." (元始天尊濟度血湖真經, translated in Jender Lee, "*Gender and Medicine in Tang China,*" p. 18).

3.   The paragraph is also found in the *Ishimpô* where it is identified as a quotation from the *Chǎn Jīng* (《醫心方》 23:2).

LINE 5.2

(一) 凡生產不依產圖，脫有犯觸，於後母子皆死。(二) 若不至死，即母子俱病，庶事皆不稱心。(三) 若能依圖無所犯觸，母即無病，子亦易養。

(1) Whenever childbirth is not done according to the birth charts,* offenses and violations might occur that later cause the death of both mother and child.

(2) If they do not lead to death, the mother and child will both fall ill and none of your affairs will proceed according to your wishes.

(3) Nevertheless, if you are able to accord with the charts and avoid offenses and violations, the mother will be free from illness and the child will also be easy to raise.

*   產圖 *chǎn tú*: This term originally included three different types of charts, for setting up the birth hut (outdoors) or screen (indoors), for the position of the woman during labor, and for the burial of the placenta. For detailed information on each of these categories as well as the process of synthesis and standardization that occured in the early medieval period, see 李貞德 《漢唐之間醫書中的生產之道》 pp. 542-545.

LINE 5.3

(一) 凡欲產時，特忌多人瞻視，惟得三二人在傍待揔，產訖乃可告語諸人也。若人眾看之，無不難產耳。(二)凡產婦第一不得忽忽忙怕。傍人極須穩審，皆不得預緩預急，及憂悒，憂悒則難產。(三) 若腹痛，眼中火生，此兒迴轉，未即生也。(四) 兒出訖，一切人及母皆忌問是男是女。

(1) Whenever the time of delivery arrives, it is particularly prohibited to have many people watch and stare. Only allow three or two people by her side to attend and support her. When the birth is over, you can then inform all the others. If crowds of people observe it, it is bound to cause a difficult delivery.

(2) Always, the first priority is that the woman in labor must not be rushed or frightened. It is also of extreme importance that her attendants be stable, judicious and never too leisurely nor too urgent in their preparations, nor overly concerned. If they are overly concerned, this will result in a difficult delivery.

(3) When the abdomen is painful and fire is engendered in her eyes,* this means that the child is turning around, but not yet that the birth is imminent.

(4) After the child has emerged, nobody, not even the mother, may ask its gender.

---

*　　眼中火生 *yǎn zhōng huǒ shēng*: This appears to be a reference to red eyes, caused by the exertion of pushing during the final stage of labor.

LINE 5.4

(一) 兒始落地，與新汲井水五咽，忌與暖湯物。(二) 勿令母看視穢污。(三) 凡產婦慎食熱藥熱麵，食常識此，飲食當如人肌溫溫也。(四) 凡欲臨產時，必先脫尋常所著衣以籠竈頭及竈口，令至密，即易產也。(五) 凡產難及子死腹中，並逆生與胞胎不出，諸篇方可通檢，用之。

(1) When the child has just dropped to the ground, give it five mouthfuls of freshly-drawn well water. You must not give it warm soups or solids.

(2) Do not let the mother look at the filth and pollution.

(3) In all cases, a woman in childbirth must beware of eating hot medicines or hot noodle meals. Keep this in mind at all times. Food and drink should be slightly warmed to skin temperature.

(4) Always, when the time of delivery has arrived, you must first take off [the woman's?] ordinarily worn clothes and use them to cover the top and the mouth of the stove, sealing it tightly.[2] This will cause an easy delivery.

(5) In all cases of birthing difficulties, including death of the child in the abdomen as well as breech birth[3] and retained placenta, the various prescriptions can all be consulted. Make use of them.

1.　　At this point, the *Sūn Zhēn Rén* inserts a prescription for "Four [Ingredients] Center-Normalizing and -Rectifying Pills" 四順理中丸 *sì shùn lǐ zhōng wán*, consisting of honey pills made from *gān cǎo* (甘草 Root of Glycyrrhiza uralensis), *rén shēn* (人參 Root of Panax ginseng), *bái zhú* (白朮 Rhizome of Atractylodes macrocephala), and *gān jiāng* (乾薑 Dried Zingiber officinale) and taken in liquor to nourish organ *qì* that has been depleted in the birth. In the *Huá Xià* and *Rén Mín* editions, this prescription is found in Volume 3, chapter 1, right after the introduction, translated in Line 1.5 of that volume, on pp. 220 below. In general, the order of prescriptions in this section varies considerably between the different editions, especially from the *Huá Xià* and *Rén Mín* editions to the *Sūn Zhēn Rén* and *Dào Zàng* editions.

2.   Like many of the restrictions above, this one is also intended to avoid offending the spirits, in this case the powerful stove god, by preventing them from any contact with the spiritually-polluting event of childbirth.

3.   逆產 *nì chǎn*: Literally "birth against the flow." Besides the narrow technical meaning of adverse or breech presentation (i.e., buttocks first), it is used here in the more general sense of any abnormal presentation, similar to the popular understanding of the term "breech birth" in English. Thus, it also includes transverse (i.e., cross) presentation (橫生 *héng shēng*), birth with hands or feet first (手足先出 *shǒu zú xiān chū*), or side-ways (i.e., face) presentation (側生 *cè shēng*). When it is used in the narrow sense of adverse presentation, I translate it as "breech presentation." For a variety of positions and prescriptions, see below, chapter 7 on "breech birth," translated in pp. 188 - 192.

LINE 5.5

治產難，或半生，或胎不下，或子死腹中，或著脊，及坐草數日不產，血氣上搶心，母面無顏色，氣欲絕者方

This prescription treats birthing difficulties, whether miscarriage, failure of the fetus to descend, death of the fetus in the abdomen, or a fetus that is attached to the spine; including cases where labor has continued* for several days without delivery of [the child], with *qì* and blood ascending and prodding the heart, lack of color in [the mother's face], and imminent *qì* expiry:

Formula

成煎豬膏（一升） 白蜜（一升） 淳酒（二升）。

成煎豬膏	chéng jiān zhū gāo	Completely cooked lard of Sus scrofa domestica	一升 1 shēng	24g
白蜜	bái mì	Honey of Apis cerana	一升 1 shēng	70ml
淳酒	chún jiǔ	pure grain spirit	二升 2 shēng	140ml

上三味，合煎取二升，分再服，不能再服，可隨所能服之。治產後惡血不除，上搶心痛煩急者，以地黃汁代醇酒。

Combine the above three ingredients and simmer to obtain two *shēng*. Divide into two doses. If she cannot take two doses, she may take as much as she can. For treating cases of painful vexation and tension due to failure to eliminate the malign blood after birth [causing it to] ascend and prod the heart, replace *chún jiǔ* 醇酒 with *dì huáng zhī* (地黃汁 Rehmannia glutinosa juice).

*   坐草 *zuò cǎo*: a standard expression in early medical literature, connoting the time spent in active labor. It is based on the custom of spreading grass on the ground underneath the laboring woman, to keep the pollution of childbirth, specifically the birth blood, from touching the ground and offending the spirits.

LINE 5.6

治難產方

A prescription for treating difficult delivery:*

Formula

槐枝（切，二升） 瞿麥 通草（各五兩） 牛膝（四兩） 榆白皮（切） 大麻仁（各一升）。

槐枝, 切	huái zhī, qiē	Tender branches of Sophora japonica, chopped	二升 2 shēng	48g
瞿麥	qú mài	Entire plant, including flowers, of Dianthus superbus	五兩 5 liǎng	15g
通草	tōng cǎo	Pith in the stalk of Tetrapanax papyriferus	五兩 5 liǎng	15g
牛膝	niú xī	Root of Achyranthes bidentata	四兩 4 liǎng	12g
榆白皮, 切	yú bái pí, qiē	The fibrous inner bark of the root or trunk of Ulmus pumila, chopped	一升 1 shēng	24g
大麻仁	dà má rén	Seed of Cannabis sativa	一升 1 shēng	24g

上六味，㕮咀，以水一斗二升煮取三升半，分五服。

Pound the above six ingredients and decoct in one *dǒu* and two *shēng* of water to obtain three and a half *shēng*. Divide into five doses.

*   難產 *nán chǎn*: I am unsure whether the reversal of the order of the characters is due to a scribal error or whether it is intentional. The term 產難 *chǎn nàn* is a technical term that refers to the specific disease category of life-threatening childbirth-related emergencies. According to the *Bìng Yuán Lùn*, it is caused by "fetal leakage and bleeding in pregnancy, a narrow uterus, offenses against the prohibitions, or premature exhaustion in labor and breaking of the water due to excitement or fright" (《病源論》 43:2:1). *Nán chǎn* refers more generally to a difficult delivery and, according to the *Bìng Yuán Lùn*, comprises the subcategories of "birthing difficulties" (*chǎn nàn*), as well as stalled or premature labor, abnormal presentation, and death of the fetus in the uterus. Sūn Sī-Miǎo's use of *nán chǎn* here might indicate that the prescription is intended for treating even mild cases of difficult labor.

LINE 5.7

治產難累日，氣力乏盡，不能得生，此是宿有病方

This prescription treats birthing difficulties that have lasted for several consecutive days, [causing] a total exhaustion of *qì* and strength, and inability to give birth. This indicates the presence of an abiding disease.*

Formula

赤小豆（二升）阿膠（二兩）。

| 赤小豆 | chì xiǎo dòu | Fruit of Phaseolus calcaratus | 二升 2 shēng | 48g |
| 阿膠 | ē jiāo | Gelatinous glue produced from Equus asinus | 二兩 2 liǎng | 6g |

上二味，以水九升煮豆令熟，去滓，內膠令烊，一服五合，不覺更服，不過三服即出。

Of the above two ingredients, cook the *chì xiǎo dòu* 赤小豆 in nine *shēng* of water until done, discard the dregs, add the *ē jiāo* 阿膠 and let it melt. Take five *gě* as one dose. If she doesn't feel any effect, take another dose. The child will emerge as soon as she has taken no more than three doses.

*   宿有病 *sù yǒu bìng*: While *sù* literally means "staying over one night," in the medical context, it refers to chronic conditions that persist over many years.

LINE 5.8

又方

Another prescription:

Formula

槐子（十四枚）蒲黃（一合）。

| 槐子 | huái zǐ | Fruit of Sophora japonica | 十四枚 14 méi | 14 pieces |
| 蒲黃 | pú huáng | Pollen of Typha angustata | 一合 1 gě | 7ml |

上二味，合內酒中，溫服，須臾不生，再服之。水服亦得。

Combine the above two ingredients and mix into liquor. Take heated. If [the child] is not born shortly, take another dose. It is also possible to take it in water.

LINE 5.8

又方

Another prescription:

Formula

生地黃汁（半升）生薑汁（半升）。

| 生地黃汁 | shēng dì huáng zhī | Fresh root of Rehmannia glutinosa juice | 半升 0.5 shēng | 35ml |
| 生薑汁 | shēng jiāng zhī | Fresh root of Zingiber officinale juice | 半升 0.5 shēng | 35ml |

上二味，合煎熟，頓服之。

Blend the above two ingredients and simmer until cooked. Quaff it in a single dose.

LINE 5.9

治產難，及日月未足而欲產者方

A prescription for treating birthing difficulties, as well as cases where she is about to give birth before the full number of days and months:

知母一兩為末，蜜丸如兔屎，服一丸，痛不止，更服一丸。

Pulverize one liǎng of zhī mǔ (知母 Root of Anemarrhena asphodeloides). Combine with honey into pills the size of rabbit feces. Take one pill per dose. If the pain does not stop, take another pill.

LINE 5.10

治產難方

A prescription for treating birthing difficulties:

吞皂莢子二枚。

Swallow two pieces of *zào jiá* (皂莢 Fruit of Gleditsia sinensis).

LINE 5.11

治產難三日不出方

A prescription for treating birthing difficulties that have lasted for three days without the child emerging:

取鼠頭燒作屑，井花水服方寸匕，日三。

Take a rat's head and char it into little pieces. Take a square-inch spoon in well-flower water three times a day.

LINE 5.12

又方

Another prescription:

車軸脂，吞大豆許兩丸。

Swallow two pills of cart axle grease about the size of soybeans.

LINE 5.13

又方

Another prescription:

燒大力鐶`，以酒一杯沃之，頓服即出。救死不分娩者。

Char a large knife ring and submerge it in one cup of liquor. Quaff in a single dose and [the child] will emerge promptly. It will rescue a woman unable to deliver from death.

*   刀環 *dāo huán*: The ring at the end of the knife. It is possible that the circular shape of the ring, as well as the cutting action of the knife, has magical connotations for making the delivery proceed.

LINE 5.14

又方

Another prescription:

燒藥杵令赤，內酒中飲之。

Char a medicine pestle until it is red and immerse it in liquor. Drink it.

LINE 5.15

治難產方

A prescription for treating difficult delivery:

取廁前已用草二七枚，燒作屑，水調服之。

Take two times seven pieces of straw from the privy that have already been used. Char them into little pieces and take this mixed with water.

LINE 5.16

又方

Another prescription:

令夫唾婦口中二七過，立出。

Make the husband blow into the wife's mouth two times seven times. It will make [the child] emerge instantly.

LINE 5.17

難產

For difficult delivery:

Acupuncture Method

針兩肩井，入一寸，寫之，須臾即分免。

Needle both *jiān jǐng* [Shoulder Well] (肩井 GB-21) points, entering one *cùn*. Drain it.* The delivery will take place momentarily.

---

*   寫 *xiè*: A technical term referring to a specific needling method which is described in the
       following way in the *Sù Wèn*: "Insert the needle during inhalation, do not cause the *qì* to
       go astray, keep it still, and leave it for a long time, not letting the evil spread. When inhal-
       ing (again), rotate the needle to obtain the *qì*. Wait until [the patient] is exhaling before
       pulling on the needle, and take it out when the exhalation is finished. The great *qì* has
       completely come out; therefore it is called 'draining' (《素文》 27).

LINE 5.18

羚羊角散治產後心悶，是血氣上衝心方

Antelope Horn Powder treats postpartum heart oppression. This indicates that the blood and *qì* are surging up against the heart:

Antelope Horn Powder
羚羊角散 *líng yáng jiǎo sǎn*

羚羊角一枚燒作灰，下篩，以東流水服方寸匕。若未瘥，須臾再服。取悶瘥乃止。

Char one piece of *líng yáng jiǎo* (羚羊角 Horn of the male Saiga tatarica) into ashes and sift it down. Take a square-inch spoon in east-flowing water. If she does not recover, take another dose shortly. Stop only after she has recovered from the oppression.*

---

*   On first sight, it seems that this and the following prescription, also for treating postpar-
       tum heart oppression, should have been placed in the section on postpartum conditions in
       the third volume. Nevertheless, Sūn Sī-Miǎo deliberately placed these prescriptions in the
       section on birthing difficulties because of the etiology of this condition: As the *Bìng Yuán
       Lùn* explains: "If the child in childbirth rises and presses against the heart, it is because
       birthing difficulties made [the mother] exert [excessive] force, causing stirring fetus and
       counterflow *qì*, [with the result that] the fetus rises and prods the heart. Whenever the
       fetus presses up against the heart, it leads to sudden oppression and expiry [of *qì*]. The
       woman revives only when the fetus descends." (《病源論》 43:2:4). The *Bìng Yuán Lùn*
       also repeatedly explains that heart oppression is caused by the fetus turning, a condition

caused by immoderate and inappropriate lifestyle or violation of the various pregnancy and childbirth taboos. Consequently, Sūn Sī-Miǎo probably included these two prescriptions here to be used preventatively during labor if the fetus rose up, in order to avoid postpartum loss of consciousness. Medieval physicians apparently did not differentiate between the upward movement of the fetus (during labor) and of *qì* and blood (postpartum) to oppress the heart, since both conditions were experienced identically by the afflicted woman.

LINE 5.19

又方

Another prescription:

羖羊角燒作灰，以溫酒服方寸匕，不瘥須臾再服。

Char *gǔ yáng jiǎo* (羖羊角 Horn of the male *Capra hircus*) into ashes. Take a square-inch spoon in warm liquor. If she does not recover, take another dose shortly.*

* *Sòng* editors' note: "The *Bèi Jí Fāng* 《備急方》 uses it to treat birthing difficulties."

LINE 5.20

治產乳運絕方

A prescription for treating fainting expiry* in childbed:

半夏一兩擣篩，丸如大豆，內鼻孔中即愈。此是扁鵲法。

Pound and sift one *liǎng* of *bàn xià* (半夏 Rhizome of *Pinellia ternata*) and make pills the size of soybeans. As soon as you insert them into her nostrils, she will recover. This is Biǎn Què's method.

* 運絕 *yùn jué*. This is the definition offered by the modern commentators of the *Rén Mín* edition who equate 運 *yùn* with 暈 *yūn* (dizziness), a technical term that it is often used as a substitute (see 張登本, 主編《內經辭典》, p. 518). They go on to explain 絕 as an abbreviation of 氣絕 *qì jué* (*qì* expiry). Alternatively, the phrase could be interpreted as revolution and upward movement of the fetus causing *qì* expiry, i.e., fainting. Interpreting 運 more literally as revolving (and moving up instead of down inside the mother's body) rather than as "dizziness" is supported by its frequent use in the *Bìng Yuán Lùn* section on birthing difficulties, most notably in the title of a section: "method for preventing [the fetus'] turning during birth" (產防運法 *chǎn fáng yùn fǎ*) (《病源論》 43:1:2). In any case, the prescription addresses a woman's loss of consciousness in childbed.

LINE 5.21

又方

Another prescription:

神麴末水服方寸匕。亦治產難。

Pulverize *shén qū* (神麴 Medicated leaven) and take a square-inch spoon in water. It also treats birthing difficulties.

LINE 5.22

又方

Another prescription:

赤小豆擣為散，東流水服方寸匕，不瘥更服。

Pound *chì xiǎo dòu* (赤小豆 Fruit of Phaseolus calcaratus) into a powder and take a square-inch spoon in east-flowing water. If she does not recover, take it again.

LINE 5.23

又方

Another prescription:

合釀醋潠面即愈。凡悶即潠之，愈。

Take concentrated vinegar into your mouth and squirt it in her face. She will promptly recover. In all cases of oppression, squirt her [with vinegar] to make her recover.

LINE 5.24

又方

Another prescription:

取釀醋，和產血如棗許大，服之。

Take concentrated vinegar and mix it with blood from the birth, an amount about the size of a jujube. Drink it.

LINE 5.25

治心悶方

A prescription for treating heart oppression:

產後心悶，眼不得開，即當頂上取髮如兩指大，強以人牽之，眼即開。

If she is unable to open her eyes due to postpartum heart oppression, grab some hair on top of her head, about as much as two fingers, and have a person yank it with great force. As a result, she will promptly open her eyes.

6. Fetal Death in the Abdomen 子死腹中

LINE 6.1

(一) 論曰：凡婦人產難死生之候：(二) 母面赤古青者，兒死母活。(三) 母脣口青，口兩邊沫出者，母子俱死。(四) 母面青舌赤，口中沫出者，母死子活。

(1) Essay: In all cases of birthing difficulties, [these are] the symptoms of death or life:

(2) If the mother's face is red and her tongue green, the child will die and the mother live.

(3) If the mother's lips and mouth are green and she is foaming at both sides of the mouth, both mother and child will die.

(4) If the mother's face is green and her tongue red, and she is foaming from the middle of the mouth, the mother will die and the child will live.*

*   This is an almost literal and slightly abbreviated quotation from an essay on birthing difficulties in the *Bìng Yuán Lùn* (《病源論》 43:2:1).

LINE 6.2

治動胎及產難子死腹中，並妊兩兒，一死一生，令死者出，生胎安，神驗方

This prescription treats stirring fetus and birthing difficulties [due to] fetal death in the abdomen, as well as simultaneously carrying two fetuses, of whom one is dead and one alive. This medicine will expel the dead one and stabilize the living one. Divine results.

Formula

蟹爪（一升） 甘草（二尺） 阿膠（三兩）。

蟹爪	xiè zhǎo	Claw of Eriocheir sinensis	一升 1 shēng	24g
甘草	gān cǎo	Root of Glycyrrhiza uralensis	二尺 2 chǐ	60cm
阿膠	ē jiāo	Gelatinous glue produced from Equus asinus	三兩 3 liǎng	9g

上三味，以東流水一斗先煮二物，得三升，去滓，內膠令烊，頓服之。不能，分再服。若人困，拗口內藥，藥入即活。煎藥作東向竈，用葦薪煮之。

Of the above three ingredients, simmer the first two ingredients in one *dǒu* of east-flowing water to obtain three *shēng*. Discard the dregs and add the *ē jiāo* 阿膠, letting it melt. Quaff in a single dose. If she is unable to [quaff it all at once], divide it into two doses. If she is encumbered, force open her mouth and pour in the medicine. If you can make the medicine, enter she will survive. For simmering the medicine, make it on an east-facing stove and use reed for firewood.

LINE 6.3

治子死腹中不出方

A prescription for treating a dead fetus in the abdomen that is failing to emerge:

以牛屎塗母腹上，立出。

Spread cow's excrement on the area above the mother's abdomen. This will make [the fetus] emerge instantly.

LINE 6.4

治子死腹中方

A prescription for treating fetal death in the abdomen:

取竈下黃土三指撮，以酒服之，立出。土當著兒頭上出。亦治逆生，及橫生不出，手足先見者。

Take a three-finger pinch of stove ashes. Take it in liquor, and [the fetus] will emerge instantly. The dirt should adhere to the top of the child's head when it emerges. [This prescription] also treats adverse and transverse presentation preventing [the child] from emerging, as well as cases where the hands and feet appear first.

LINE 6.5

治胎死腹中，真朱湯方

Pearl Decoction treats fetal death in the abdomen.

Pearl Decoction
真朱湯 *zhēn zhū tāng*

熟真朱（一兩）榆白皮（切，一升）。

真朱, 熟*	zhēn zhū, shú	Pearl, cooked	一兩 1 liǎng	3g
榆白皮, 切	yú bái pí, qiē	Fibrous inner bark of the root or trunk of Ulmus pumila, chopped	一升 1 shēng	24g

上二味，以苦酒三升煮取一升，頓服，死胎立出。

Cook the above two ingredients in three *shēng* of bitter liquor to obtain one *shēng* and quaff in a single dose. This will make the dead fetus emerge instantly.

*   *Sòng* editors' note: "According to Lǐ Shí-Zhēn, *zhēn zhū* (真珠 Pearl) need to be soaked in human breast milk for three days and then cooked before they can be used as a medicinal ingredient."

LINE 6.6

又方

Another prescription:

服水銀三兩，立出。

Take three *liǎng* of *shuǐ yín* (水銀 Mercury) and the fetus will emerge instantly.

LINE 6.7

又方

Another prescription:

三家雞卵各一枚，三家鹽各一撮，三家水各一升，合煮，令產婦東向飲之，立出。

Mix and cook together one egg each from three different households, one pinch of salt each from three different households, and one *shēng* of water each from three different households. Have the woman in labor drink this while facing east, and the fetus will emerge instantly.

LINE 6.8

又方

Another prescription:

取夫尿二升煮令沸，飲之。

Take two *shēng* of the husband's urine and simmer it, bringing it to a rolling boil. Drink it.

LINE 6.9

又方

Another prescription:

吞槐子二七枚。亦治逆生。

Swallow two times seven pieces of *huái zǐ* (槐子 Fruit of Sophora japonica). It also treats breech birth.

LINE 6.10

又方

Another prescription:

酢二升，拗口開灌之，即出。

[Take] two *shēng* of vinegar. As soon as you force her mouth open and pour it in, [the child] will emerge.

LINE 6.11

治產難子死腹中方

A prescription for treating birthing difficulties with fetal death in the abdomen:

瞿麥一斤，以水八升煮取一升，服一升，不出再服

Decoct one *jīn* of *qú mài* (瞿麥 Entire plant, including flowers, of Dianthus superbus) in eight *shēng* of water to obtain one *shēng*.* Take a dose of one *shēng*. If [the child] fails to emerge, take another dose.

* 一升 *yī shēng*: This must be a textual corruption since a prescription is typically reduced to half or at most a quarter of the original amount of liquid. Also, the following instruction to "take one *shēng* as a dose" suggests that the amount should be taken out of a larger amount, since it would otherwise advise to "quaff in a single dose" (頓服之 *dùn fú zhī*). Lastly, the next instruction to "take another dose" again suggests that there should be more than one *shēng* of medicine initially; otherwise the text would instruct to "make it again" (再作 *zào zuò*). See, for example, the following prescription.

LINE 6.12

治胎死腹中，乾燥著背方

A prescription for treating a dead fetus in the abdomen that has dried out and is adhering to the back:

Formula

葵子（一兩）阿膠（五兩）。

| 葵子 | kuí zǐ | Seeds of Malva verticillata | 一兩 1 liǎng | 3g |
| 阿膠 | ē jiāo | Gelatinous glue produced from Equus asinus | 五兩 5 liǎng | 15g |

上二味，以水五升煮取二升，頓服之，未出再煮服。

Decoct the above two ingredients in five *shēng* of water to obtain two *shēng*. Quaff in a single dose. If [the fetus] still fails to come out, cook another batch and take it.

LINE 6.13

治妊娠未足月，而胎卒死不出，其母欲死方

A prescription for treating sudden fetal death and failure to emerge before the pregnancy has reached full term, when the mother is about to die:

以苦酒濃煮大豆，一服一升，死胎立出，不能頓服，分再服。

Cook *dà dòu* (大豆 Seed of Glycine max) in bitter liquor until thickened. Take one *shēng* as one dose, and the dead fetus will emerge instantly. If she is unable to quaff it in a single dose, divide it into two doses.[*]

*   *Sòng* editors' note: "Another [version of this prescription] uses hard liquor to cook the *dà dòu* 大豆. It also treats accumulations and gatherings that have become conglomerations."

LINE 6.14

治妊娠胎死腹中，若子生胞衣不出，腹中引腰背痛方

A prescription for treating fetal death in the abdomen during pregnancy or a retained placenta after childbirth, with pain stretching from the center of the abdomen to the lumbus and back:

Formula

甘草（一尺）蒲黃（二合）筒桂（四寸）香豉（二升）雞子（一枚）。

甘草	gān cǎo	Root of Glycyrrhiza uralensis	一尺 1 chǐ	30 cm
蒲黃	pú huáng	Pollen of Typha angustata	二合 2 gě	14ml
筒桂	tǒng guì	Bark of Cinnamomum cassia	四寸 4 chǐ	120 cm
香豉	xiāng chǐ	Preparation of Fermented Glycine max	二升 2 shēng	48g
雞子	jī zǐ	Egg of Gallus gallus domesticus	一枚 1 méi	1 piece

上五味，以水六升煮取一升，頓服之，胎胞穢惡盡去，大良。

Decoct the above five ingredients in six *shēng* of water to obtain one *shēng* and quaff in a single dose. The placenta, filth, and malign [blood] will be completely removed. Very good!

LINE 6.15

治妊娠得病須去胎方

A prescription for having to abort a fetus because [the mother] has contracted a disease during pregnancy:

以雞子一枚，鹽三指撮和服，立下。

Mix one egg with a three-finger pinch of salt and take it. It will bring down the fetus immediately.*

* *Sòng* editors' note: "This is identical to the treatment of difficult delivery by *Ruǎn* from *Hé-nán*."
The *Sūn Zhēn Rén* edition is missing any prescriptions to induce abortions but cites a very similar prescription to "take one *gě* of salt together with one egg" in a group of prescriptions for expelling a dead fetus.

LINE 6.16

又方

Another prescription:

麥蘗一升末，和蜜一升，服之立下。

Pulverize one *shēng* of *mài niè* (麥蘗 Shoots of Hordeum vulgare) and mix with one *shēng* of honey. Take it, and [the fetus] will descend immediately.

LINE 6.17

又方

Another prescription:

七月七日神麴三升，酢一升煮兩沸，宿不食，且頓服即下。

Cook three *shēng* of *shén qū* (神麴 Medicated leaven), made on the seventh day of the seventh month,* with one *shēng* of vinegar, bringing it to a boil twice. After fasting overnight, quaff it at dawn in a single dose. [The fetus] will descend promptly.

* 七月七日神麴 *qī yuè qī rì shén qū*: My reading is based on instructions for making spirit

leaven from the *Běn Cǎo Gāng Mù*: "On the fifth day of the fifth month, or the sixth day of the sixth month, or during the days of *sān fú* 三伏 [i.e., the last of the three ten-day periods of the hot season], mix a hundred *jīn* of white flour with..." (《本草綱目》25:947). *Lǐ Shí-Zhēn* himself states that "you should use the day on which the various spirits gather and congregate to prepare it. For this reason, it has received the name 'spirit leaven.'" An alternative intepretation would be "on the seventh day of the seventh month (either referring to the day of the year or the duration of the pregnancy), cook three *shēng* of spirit leaven." This is suggested by the punctuation of the *Huá Xià* edition, where 七月七日 is separated from 神麴 by a comma.

LINE 6.18

又方

Another prescription:

大麥麴五升，酒一斗煮三沸，去滓，分五服，令盡，當宿勿食，其子如糜，令母肥盛無疾苦，千金不傳。

Cook five *shēng* of *dà mài qū* (大麥麴 Barley leaven) in one *dǒu* of liquor, bringing it to a boil three times. Discard the dregs and divide into five doses. Use it all up, then fast overnight. The child[1] will resemble rice gruel. [The medicine] will make the mother fat and exuberant and free her from illness and suffering. Even for a thousand pieces of gold, do not transmit this.[2]

---

1.   This refers to the fetal matter expelled during the abortion.
2.   Warnings against freely transmitting a text or prescription are common in early Chinese medical literature. The earliest reference to this phrase that I am aware of is found on bamboo slips excavated in *Gān-sù*, dating to the first century CE (cited in Nathan Sivin, "*Text and Experience in Classical Chinese Medicine*," p. 183). The prohibition here is probably related to the fact that this is a prescription for inducing an abortion.

7. Breech Birth 逆生

LINE 7.1

論曰：凡產難，或兒橫生側生，或手足先出，可以針錐刺兒手足，入一二分許，兒得痛，驚轉即縮，自當回順也。

Essay: In all cases of birthing difficulties, whether the child is born crosswise or [in a] sideways position, or with hands or feet emerging first, you can prick the child's hand or foot with a needle or awl, entering maybe one or two *fēn*. When the child feels the pain, it will shift its position in fright and contract. Thus it will naturally turn and come out smoothly.

LINE 7.2

治逆生方

A prescription for treating breech birth:

以鹽塗兒足底，又可急搔之，並以鹽摩產婦腹上，即愈。

Rub salt on the child's feet. Or you can pinch it quickly and at the same time massage the top of the laboring woman's abdomen with salt. This will remedy the situation promptly.

LINE 7.3

又方

Another prescription:

以鹽和粉塗兒足下，即順。

Rub a mixture of salt and flour on the bottom of the child's feet, and it will come out smoothly.˙

*   *Sòng* editors' note: "The *Zǐ Mǔ Mì Lù* says 'salt and *hú fěn* (胡粉 Lead carbonite).'"

LINE 7.4

又方

Another prescription:

梁上塵取如彈丸許二枚，治末，三指撮溫酒服之。

Take two balls of roofbeam dust, about the size of pellets or pills. Grind them into a powder and take a three-finger pinch in warm liquor.*

*   *Sòng* editors' note: "The *Sūn Zhēn Rén* edition has *mǐ yǐn* (米飲 Water that rice has been
cooked in) instead."

LINE 7.5

治逆生及橫生不出，手足先見者。

[A prescription] for treating cases where the child fails to emerge due to adverse and
transverse presentation, and cases where the hands or feet appear first:

燒蛇脫皮，末，服一刀圭，亦云三指撮，面向東，酒服，即順。

Char and pulverize a *shé tuì pí* (蛇蛻皮 Sloughed snake skin from Elaphe taeniurus).[1]
[Per dose,] take one knife tip, which is also referred to as a three-finger pinch.[2] As soon
as [the mother] faces east and takes it in warm liquor, the child will be born smoothly.

1.   The use of such substances as *shé tuì pí* 蛇蛻皮 or *chán tuì* (蟬蛻 Cicada moulting) for
the treatment of birthing difficulties is obviously related to magical reasoning.
2.   The explanation regarding the "knife tip" is marked in some editions as *Sòng* commentary. Since the *Sūn Zhēn Rén* only states to "take a three-finger pinch in warm liquor,"
the rest of the text might well be later additions. In the first volume of the *Qiān Jīn Fāng*,
Sūn Sī-Miǎo explains that a "knife tip" (刀圭 *dāo guī*) is the equivalent of one tenth of a
square-inch spoon.

LINE 7.6

又方

Another prescription:

以蟬殼二枚治為末，三指撮溫酒服。

Grind two *chán tuì* (蟬蛻 Cicada moultings) into powder and take a three-finger pinch in warm liquor.[*]

[*] *Sòng* editors' note: "*Cuī Shì*, the *Wài Tái Mì Yào*, and the *Zǐ Mǔ Mì Lù* instruct to make two pellet or pill-sized pieces, pulverize them, and take them in liquor."

LINE 7.7

又方

Another prescription:

取夫陰毛二七莖燒，以豬膏和丸如大豆吞之，兒子即持丸出，神驗。

Take two times seven strands of the husband's pubic hair, char and mix with pig lard into a pill the size of a soybean. As soon as [the mother] swallows it, the child will emerge with the pill in its hand. Divine results.

LINE 7.8

又方

Another prescription:

蛇蛻皮燒灰，豬膏和丸東向服。

Char a *shé tuì pí* (蛇蛻皮 Sloughed snake skin from Elaphe taeniurus) into ashes, mix with pig lard into a pill and take it facing east.

LINE 7.9

又方

Another prescription:

以手中指取釜底墨，交畫兒足下，即順生。

Use the middle finger of your hand to get soot from the bottom of a pan. Paint an x on the bottom of the child's foot, and it will promptly be born smoothly.

LINE 7.10

又方

Another prescription:

取父名書兒足下，即順生。

Write the father's name on the bottom of the child's foot, and it will promptly be born smoothly.

LINE 7.11

治橫生及足先出者方

A prescription for treating transverse presentation, as well as cases where the feet emerge first:

取梁上塵，竈突墨，酒服之。

Take roofbeam dust and stove-pipe soot. Take in liquor.

LINE 7.12

又方

Another prescription:

取車釭中脂，書兒腳下及掌中。

Take grease from inside a cart's axle and write [with it] on the bottom of the child's feet and the inside of its palms.

LINE 7.13

治縱橫生不可出者方

A prescription for treating vertical or horizontal presentation, when the child is unable to emerge:

菟絲子末，酒若米汁服方寸匕，即生。車前子亦好，服如上法。

Pulverize *tù sī zǐ* (菟絲子 Seed of Cuscuta chinensis) and take a square-inch spoon in liquor or rice juice. [The child] will be born promptly. *Chē qián zǐ* (車前子 Seed of Plantago asiatica) also works well, taken in the same manner.

LINE 7.14

又方

Another prescription:

水若酒服竈突黑塵。

Take stove-pipe soot and dust in water or liquor.

LINE 7.15

治產時子但趨穀道者方

A prescription for treating cases where the child at the time of delivery moves down the grain passage* instead:

熬鹽熨之自止。

Toast salt and apply as a hot compress, then it will stop on its own.

---

*   穀道 *gǔ dào*: This is a reference to the anus.

8. Retained Placenta 胞胎不出

Translator's comment: In the following prescriptions, the condition of retained placenta is mostly referred to as 胞衣不出 *bāo yī bù chū*. It is most likely due to a scribal error or terminological vagueness that the title refers to *bāo tāi* instead. While *tāi bāo* is sometimes used to refer literally to the fetus AND the placenta, *bāo tāi* literally translated means "that which wraps the fetus" and is therefore simply a synonym for *bāo yī* "coating of the uterus." A less likely possibility would be that the title intentionally refers to the two pathologies of retained placenta AND retained fetus, two conditions that were in any case not clearly differentiated in early Chinese medicine. The *Sūn Zhēn Rén* edition has 胞衣不出 *bāo yī bù chū*.

The order of prescriptions in this section varies considerably between the *Sòng* revision and other editions. Moreover, this category is used quite loosely and is not clearly distinguished from the section above on "fetal death in the abdomen." The *Sūn Zhēn Rén* edition even includes here a prescription for "childbirth complication lasting for several consecutive days..." that is found in chapter five of volume two on "Birthing Difficulties", line 5.7 above (p. 185). In theoretical literature, the conditions of stalled labor and retained placenta were distinguished clearly. See the classification in the *Bìng Yuán Lùn*, volume 43. There, for example, the symptom of "retained placenta" is included among "diseases [that arise] when delivery is pending" (婦人將產病 *fù rén jiāng chǎn bìng*) and is thus treated prior to, — rather than being included among, — the various symptoms of "difficult childbirth." (《病源論》 43:1:3). In the prescription literature, however, similar or identical medicines and techniques were used for expelling a dead fetus (including intentional abortion), treating stalled labor, and expelling a retained placenta. Sūn Sī-Miǎo's lack of precision in regard to the intended actions of a specific prescription might suggest a lack of familiarity on his part with this aspect of women's healthcare. This would support Jender Lee's impression that "male doctors do not, however, seem to have had many real experiences in midwifery" (Jender Lee, "*Gender and Medicine in Tang China*", p. 4).

LINE 8.1

治產兒胞衣不出 , 令胞爛 , 牛膝湯方

Achyranthes Decoction treats retained placenta in childbirth, which is causing the uterus to rot.

Achyranthes Decoction
牛膝湯 *niú xī tāng*

牛膝 瞿麥（各一兩）滑石（二兩）當歸（一兩半）通草（一兩半）葵子（半升）。

牛膝	niú xī	Root of Achyranthes bidentata	一兩 1 liǎng	3g
瞿麥	qú mài	Entire plant, including flowers, of Dianthus superbus	一兩 1 liǎng	3g
滑石*	huá shí	Talcum	二兩 2 liǎng	6g
當歸	dāng guī	Root of Angelica polimorpha	一兩半 1.5 liǎng	4.5g
通草	tōng cǎo	Pith in the stalk of Tetrapanax papyriferus	一兩半 1.5 liǎng	4.5g
葵子	kuí zǐ	Seed of Malva verticillata	半升 0.5 shēng	12g

上六味，㕮咀，以水九升煮取三升，分三服。

Pound the above six ingredients and decoct in nine *shēng* of water to obtain three *shēng*. Divide into three doses.

*   *Sòng* editors' note: "Another [version] uses *guì xīn* (桂心 Shaved inner bark of Cinnamomum cassia)."

LINE 8.2

治產難胞衣不出，橫倒者，及兒死腹中，母氣欲絕方

A prescription for treating birthing difficulties with retained placenta, as well as transverse and breech presentation, and fetal death in the abdomen, when the mother's *qì* is about to expire:

Formula

半夏 白蘞（各二兩）。

半夏	bàn xià	Rhizome of Pinellia ternata	二兩 2 liǎng	6g
白蘞	bái liǎn	Root of Ampelopsis japonica	二兩 2 liǎng	6g

上二味，治下篩，服方寸匕，小難一服，橫生二服，倒生三服，兒死四服。亦可加代赭，瞿麥各二兩，為佳。

Finely pestle and sift the above two ingredients. Take a square-inch spoon. For minor complications, take one dose; for transverse presentation, two doses; for breech presentation, three doses; for a dead child, four doses. You can also add two *liǎng* each of *dài zhě* (代赭 Hematite) and *qú mài* (瞿麥 Entire plant, including flowers, of Dianthus superbus), which is excellent.

LINE 8.3

治胎死腹中，若母病欲下之方

A prescription for treating fetal death in the abdomen or desire to abort due to maternal sickness.*

取榆白皮細切，煮汁三升，服之即下。難生者，亦佳。

Take *yú bái pí* (榆白皮 The fibrous inner bark of the root or trunk of Ulmus pumila) and chop it finely. Decoct it [to obtain] three *shēng* of liquid. As soon as [the mother] takes it, [the fetus] will be discharged. It is also excellent for difficult births.

---

*   Based on these indications, the prescription should be placed in chapter six of volume two on "Fetal death in the abdomen" (pp. 194-201). Sūn Sī-Miǎo might have placed it here since the medicinal action required for expelling a fetus is similar to that for expelling a retained placenta. It is therefore possible that this prescription was used for both conditions.

LINE 8.4

又方

Another prescription:

Formula

牛膝（三兩）葵子（一升）。

牛膝	niú xī	Root of Achyranthes bidentata	三兩 3 liǎng	9g
葵子	kuí zǐ	Seed of Malva verticillata	一升 1 shēng	24g

上二味，以水七升煮取三升，分三服。

Cook the above two ingredients in seven *shēng* of water to obtain three *shēng*. Divide into three doses.

LINE 8.5

又方

Another prescription:

生地黃汁一升，苦酒三合，令暖服之。不能頓服，分再服，亦得。

[Mix] one *shēng* of *shēng dì huáng zhī* (生地黃汁 Fresh root of Rehmannia glutinosa juice) and three *gě* of bitter liquor. Warm it up and drink it. If she is unable to quaff it in a single dose, dividing it into two doses is also possible.

LINE 8.6

又方

Another prescription:

Formula

澤蘭葉（三兩） 滑石（五合） 生麻油（二合）。

澤蘭葉	zé lán yè	Foliage of Lycopus lucidus	三兩 3 liǎng	9g
滑石	huá shí	Talcum	五合 5 gě	35ml
生麻油	shēng má yóu	Fresh oil of Sesamum indicum	二合 2 gě	14ml

上三味，以水一升半煮澤蘭，取七合，去滓，內麻油，滑石，頓服之。

Of the above three ingredients, decoct the *zé lán yè* 澤蘭葉 in one and a half *shēng* of water to obtain seven *gě*. Discard the dregs and add the *shēng má yóu* 生麻油 and *huá shí* 滑石. Quaff in a single dose.

LINE 8.7

治胞衣不出方

A prescription for treating retained placenta:

取小麥合小豆，煮令濃，飲其汁，立出。亦治橫逆生者。

Cook *xiǎo mài* (小麥 Seed or flour of Triticum aestivum) and *[chì] xiǎo dòu* ([赤]小豆 Fruit of Phaseolus calcaratus) until thickened. Drink the juice, and [the placenta] will emerge instantly. It also treats transverse and breech presentation.

LINE 8.8

治逆生胎不出方

A prescription for treating breech birth and fetus failing to emerge:*

取竈屋上墨，以酒煮一兩沸，取汁服。

Take stove top soot and simmer it in liquor, bringing it to a boil once or twice. Take the liquid and drink it.

---

* 胎不出 *tāi bù chū*: If translated literally, this prescription should more accurately be placed in the chapter five on "Birthing Difficulties" or chapter seven on "Breech Birth" above. It is, however, also possible that 胎 *tāi* is a scribal error for 胞 *bāo* (placenta), which is often called 胎胞 *tāi bāo*. Moreover, while the fetus in the context of pregnancy is referred to mostly at 胎 *tāi*, in the context of labor and delivery it is much more commonly referred to as 子 *zǐ* (child). Most likely, the lack of clarity in this aspect of women's treatment suggests that medieval Chinese physicians did not yet distinguish clearly between 胎 *tāi* (fetus), 胞 *bāo* (literally: the uterus), 胞胎 *bāo tāi* or 胞衣 *bāo yī* (the placenta), and lastly 胎胞 *tāi bāo* (strictly speaking, the fetus and the placenta).

LINE 8.9

治胞衣不出方

A prescription for treating retained placenta:

取瓜瓣二七枚，服之立出，良。

Take two times seven pieces of *guā bàn* (瓜瓣 Seed of Benincasa hispida), ingest them, and [the placenta] will emerge instantly. Good.

LINE 8.10

又方

Another prescription:

苦酒服真朱一兩。

Take one *liǎng* of *zhēn zhū* (真珠 Pearl) in bitter liquor.

LINE 8.11

又方

Another prescription:

服蒲黃如棗許，以井花水。

Take *pú huáng* (蒲黃 Pollen of Typha angustata), about the size of a jujube, in well-flower water.

LINE 8.12

又方

Another prescription:

生男，吞小豆七枚；生女者，十四枚；即出。

When having delivered a boy, swallow seven pieces of *[chì] xiǎo dòu* ([赤]小豆 Fruit of Phaseolus calcaratus); when having delivered a girl, fourteen. This medicine* will emerge promptly.

---

*   From the context, it appears most likely that this prescription is intended to be used after delivery and that it will therefore expel the placenta. But it is also possible to interpret it as a treatment for stalled labor: "When delivering a boy, swallow…when delivering a girl,…[The child] will emerge promptly.

LINE 8.13

又方

Another prescription:

取水煮弓弩弦，飲其汁五合，即出。亦可燒灰，酒和服。

Boil a crossbow string in water. [The placenta] will emerge as soon as [the mother] drinks five *gě* of the liquid. You can also char [the string] into ashes and take it with liquor.

LINE 8.14

又方

Another prescription:

雞子一枚，苦酒一合，和飲之，即出。

Mix one egg with one *gě* of bitter liquor and drink it. [The placenta] will emerge promptly.

LINE 8.15

又方

Another prescription:

墨三寸末之，酒服。

Pulverize a stick of ink, three *cùn* long. Take in liquor.

LINE 8.16

又方

Another prescription:

取宅中所埋柱掘出，取坎底當柱下土大如雞子，酒和服之，良。

Excavate a post that is buried in the center of the house. Take an egg-sized amount of dirt from the bottom of the hole under the post and take it mixed in liquor. Good.

LINE 8.17

治產後胞不時出方

A prescription for treating failure to expel the placenta in a timely manner after delivery:

井底土如雞子中黃，以井花水和服之，立出。

Take mud from the bottom of a well, an amount the size of the yolk in a chicken egg. Take it mixed into well-flower water, and [the placenta] will emerge instantly.

LINE 8.18

又方

Another prescription:

取井中黃土，丸如梧桐子，吞之，立出。又治兒不出。

Take yellow dirt from inside a well and make a pill the size of a firmiana seed. Swallow it, and [the placenta] will emerge instantly. It also treats failure of the child to emerge.

LINE 8.19

治子死腹中，若衣不出，欲上搶心方

A prescription for treating a dead child in the abdomen or a retained placenta, which are about to ascend and prod the heart:

急取蟻蛭土三升，熬之令熱，囊盛熨心下，令胎不得上搶心，甚良。

Quickly take three *shēng* of ant hill dirt and toast it until it is hot. Fill it into a bag and apply as a hot compress below the heart. It will make it impossible for the fetus to ascend and prod the heart. Very good.

LINE 8.20

又方

Another prescription:

末竈突中墨三指撮，以水若酒服之，立出。當著兒頭生。

Pulverize a three-finger pinch of stove-pipe soot and take it in water or liquor. [The child or placenta] will emerge instantly. [The soot] should cover the child's head when it is born.

LINE 8.21

又方

Another prescription:

取炊蔽當戶前燒，服之。

Take a steaming basket. You must char it in front of the door. Ingest it.

LINE 8.22

又方

Another prescription:

取夫內衣，蓋井上，立出。

Take the husband's underclothes and cover the top of the well. [The fetus or placenta] will emerge instantly.

9. Precipitating the Breast Milk 下乳

Translator's note: This section contains prescriptions to stimulate lactation. We have chosen a literal translation rather than the biomedical term agalactia because that implies the idea that the milk production is insufficient. In Chinese medical theory, however, problems related to lactation are a complicated issue since breast milk is seen as an alternate form of menstrual blood, which nourishes the fetus during pregnancy, ascends into the breasts after the delivery, and transforms into breast milk. Thus, lactation problems can be caused by a variety of underlying conditions and need to be treated accordingly: According to the 婦人大全良方 *Fù Rén Dà Quán Liáng Fāng* (composed in 1237), deficient or excessive flow of breast milk is always caused by vacuity and weakness of *qì* and blood, and by a lack of balance in the vessels. In young women who experience distended breasts after their first birth, it is due to the presence of wind or heat and must be treated with clearing and disinhibiting medicines to encourage the flow of breast milk. Women with an absence of milk after several births, by contrast, suffer from a lack of fluids and need to be treated with supplementing and boosting medicines in order to activate the flow. Women suffering from a scanty flow, lastly, must take medicines that encourage the flow in the vessels (《婦人大全良方》 23:10).

It is noteworthy that Sūn Sī-Miào does not yet distinguish between different symptoms and etiologies but merely uses the phrase 乳無汁 *rǔ wú zhī*, litterally, "absence of fluid in the breasts." This apparent lack of sophistication might indicate that issues related to breast-feeding were most often attended to by midwives or other female caregivers rather than male educated physicians, and therefore emerged later in male elite medical discourse than other areas of women's health. The *Bìng Yuán Lùn* does distinguish between the symptoms of "postpartum absence of breast milk" (產後乳無汁候 *chǎn hòu rǔ wú zhī*) and "postpartum spillage of breast milk" (產後乳汁溢 *chǎn hòu rǔ zhī yì*), but the etiology also seems noticably less sophisticated than, for example, the explanation of menstrual conditions (《病源論》 44:40-41). As evidenced by the ninth-century text *Chǎn Bǎo*, physicians' knowledge in this area had increased considerably by then (see, for example, volume 2, "discussion and prescriptions for postpartum absence of breast milk" (產後乳無汁方論 *chǎn hòu rǔ wú zhī fāng lùn*), "discussion and prescriptions for postpartum binding and abscesses in the breasts" (產後乳結癰方論 *chǎn hòu rǔ jié yōng fāng lùn*), and "discussion and prescriptions for the symptom of postpartum breast milk spillage" (產後乳汁溢出候方論 *chǎn hòu rǔ yì chū hòu fāng lùn*), all quoted in 張奇文, 主編《胎產病証》 pp. 538, 538-9, and 551, respectively). In the *Sūn Zhēn Rén* edition, this heading is missing altogether and the following prescriptions are subsumed under the previous category.

LINE 9.1

治婦人乳無汁，鍾乳湯方

Stalactite Decoction treats absence of breast milk.

Stalactite Decoction
鍾乳湯 *zhōng rǔ tāng*

石鍾乳 白石脂（各六銖）通草（十二銖）桔梗（半兩，切）消石（六銖）。

石鍾乳	shí zhōng rǔ	Stalactite	六銖 6 zhū	.75g
白石脂	bái shí zhī	Kaolin	六銖 6 zhū	.75g
通草	tōng cǎo	Pith in the stalk of Tetrapanax papyriferus	十二銖 12 zhū	1.5g
桔梗, 切	jié gěng, qiē	Root of Platycodon grandiflorum, chopped	半兩 0.5 liǎng	1.5g
消石[1]	xiāo shí	Niter	六銖 6 zhū	.75g

上五味，㕮咀，以水五升煮三沸，三上三下，去滓，內消石令烊，分服。

Pound the above five ingredients and decoct in five shēng of water, bringing them to a boil and then letting them settle three times.[2] Discard the dregs, add the *xiāo shí* 消石, and let it melt. Divide into [two?] doses.

1.   *Sòng* editors' note: "Another [version] uses *huá shí* (滑石 talcum)."
2.   三上三下 *sān shàng sān xià*: As explained in the section on "compounding medicines," in the first volume of the *Qiān Jīn Fāng*, this expression refers to preparing pastes: "When decocting pastes, one should make them rise three times and descend three times so that the drugs' potency will leak out, making it possible for the drugs' properties to come out. Raising them means to bring them to a vigorous boil, lowering them means to let the rolling boil settle down and waiting a good while..." (《千金方》1:7).

LINE 9.2

治婦人乳無汁，漏蘆湯方

Rhaponticum Decoction treats absence of breast milk.

Rhaponticum Decoction
漏蘆湯 *lòu lú tāng*

漏蘆 通草（各二兩） 石鍾乳（一兩） 黍米（一升）。

漏蘆	lòu lú	Root of Rhaponticum uniflorum	二兩 2 liǎng	6g
通草	tōng cǎo	Pith in the stalk of Tetrapanax papyriferus	二兩 2 liǎng	6g
石鍾乳	shí zhōng rǔ	Stalactite	一兩 1 liǎng	3g
黍米	shǔ mǐ	Seed of the non-glutinous variety of Panicum miliaceum	一升 1 shēng	24g

上四味，咬咀，米宿漬，揩撻取汁三升，煮藥三沸，去滓，作飲飲之，日三。

Pound the above four ingredients. Soak the *shǔ mǐ* 黍米 overnight,* then grind and smash it to obtain three *shēng* of liquid. [Use it to] decoct the drugs, bringing them to a boil three times. Discard the dregs, make a drink, and drink it three times a day.

* 　　米宿漬 *mǐ sù zì*: Several editions insert the character 泔 *gān* (rice water) here and read this phrase as "Soak [the drugs] in rice water overnight." But the following makes clear that the [other] drugs are to be added only on the second day and that 米 *mǐ* should therefore be read as an abbreviation for 黍米 *shǔ mǐ*.

LINE 9.3

治婦人乳無汁，單行石膏湯方

Single Agent Gypsum Decoction treats absence of breast milk.

Single Agent Gypsum Decoction
單行石膏湯 *dān xíng shí gāo tāng*

石膏四兩研，以水二升煮三沸，稍稍服，一日令盡。

Grind four *liǎng* of *shí gāo* (石膏 Gypsum) and decoct it in two *shēng* of water, bringing it to a boil three times. Sip it slowly, finishing it up in one day.

LINE 9.4

又方

Another prescription:[1]

Formula

通草 石鍾乳。

| 通草[2] | tōng cǎo | Pith in the stalk of Tetrapanax papyriferus |
| 石鍾乳 | shí zhōng rǔ | Stalactite |

上二味，各等分末，粥飲服方寸匕，日三。後可兼養兩兒。

Pulverize equal amounts of the above two ingredients and take one square-inch spoon in rice gruel three times a day. Afterwards, she will be able to nourish two children simultaneously.[3]

1. This prescription is called *Rice-Paper Plant Pith Powder* (通草散 *tōng cǎo sǎn*) in the *Wài Tái Mì Yào*.
2. *Sòng* editors' note: "As for *tōng cǎo* 通草, if it has horizontal [lines] in the core, this is it."
    Do not use *yáng táo gēn* 羊桃根, which has a yellow color and is of no use [here]. The similarity between Rice-paper Plant Pith and Carambola Root is mentioned neither in the *Zhōng Yào Dà Cí Diǎn* nor in the *Běn Cǎo Gāng Mù*. The *Běn Cǎo Gāng Mù* does, however, list *yáng táo gēn* only several entries behind *tōng cǎo* (通草 Pith in the stalk of Tetrapanax papyriferus), thus suggesting a relation between the two plants (《本草綱目》18:618 and 630 respectively).
3. *Sòng* editors' note: "In another [version of this prescription], you soak the two ingredients overnight in five *shēng* of liquor, and then bring them to a rolling boil the next morning, discard the dregs, and take one *shēng* three times a day. Take it cold in the summer and warm in the winter."

LINE 9.5

治婦人乳無汁，麥門冬散方

Ophiopogon Powder treats absence of breast milk:

Ophiopogon Powder
麥門冬散 *mài mén dōng sǎn*

麥門冬 石鍾乳 通草 理石。

麥門冬	mài mén dōng	Tuber of Ophiopogon japonicus
石鍾乳	shí zhōng rǔ	Stalactite
通草	tōng cǎo	Pith in the stalk of Tetrapanax papyriferus
理石	lǐ shí	Fibrous gypsum

上四味，各等分，治下篩，先食酒服方寸匕，日三。

Finely pestle and sift equal amounts of the above four ingredients. Before meals, take a square-inch spoon in liquor, three times a day.

LINE 9.6

治婦人乳無汁，漏蘆散方

Rhaponticum Powder treats absence of breast milk:

Rhaponticum Powder
漏蘆散 *lòu lú sǎn*

漏蘆（半兩）石鍾乳 栝樓根（各一兩）蠐螬（三合）。

漏蘆	lòu lú	Root of Rhaponticum uniflorum	半兩 0.5 liǎng	1.5g
石鍾乳	shí zhōng rǔ	Stalactite	一兩 1 liǎng	3g
栝樓根	guā lóu gēn	Root of Trichosanthes kirilowii	一兩 1 liǎng	3g
蠐螬	qí cáo	Dried larva of Holotrichia diomphalia	三合 3 gě	21ml

上四味，治下篩，先食糖水服方寸匕，日三。

Finely pestle and sift the above four ingredients. Before meals, take a square-inch spoon in sugar water,* three times a day.

* 糖水 *táng shuǐ*: In early times, 糖 *táng* referred to malt sugar made from wheat, but from the *Táng* period on, more commonly to sugar made from sugar cane. See 楊吉成, 編者《中國飲食辭典》 p. 414.

LINE 9.7

又方

Another prescription:

Formula

麥門冬 通草 石鍾乳 理石 土瓜根 大棗 蠐螬。

麥門冬	mài mén dōng	Tuber of Ophiopogon japonicus
通草	tōng cǎo	Pith in the stalk of Tetrapanax papyriferus
石鍾乳	shí zhōng rǔ	Stalactite
理石	lǐ shí	Fibrous gypsum
土瓜根	tǔ guā gēn	Root of Trichosanthes cucumerina
大棗	dà zǎo	Mature fruit of Ziziphus jujuba
蠐螬	qí cáo	Dried larva of Holotrichia diomphalia

上七味，等分，治下篩，食畢用酒服方寸匕，日三。

Finely pestle and sift equal amounts of the above seven ingredients. After finishing a meal, take a square-inch spoon with liquor three times a day.

LINE 9.8

治乳無汁方

A prescription for treating absence of breast milk:

Formula

石鍾乳（四兩） 甘草（二兩） 漏蘆（三兩） 通草（五兩） 栝樓根（五兩）。

石鍾乳	shí zhōng rǔ	Stalactite	四兩 4 liǎng	12g
甘草[1]	gān cǎo	Root of Glycyrrhiza uralensis	二兩 2 liǎng	6g
漏蘆	lòu lú	Root of Rhaponticum uniflorum	三兩 3 liang	9g
通草	tōng cǎo	Pith in the stalk of Tetrapanax papy-riferus	五兩 5 liǎng	15g
栝樓根[2]	guā lóu gēn	Root of Trichosanthes kirilowii	五兩 5 liǎng	15g

上五味，㕮咀，以水一升煮取三升，分三服。

Pound the above five ingredients and decoct in one *dǒu* of water to obtain three *shēng*. Divide into three doses.

1. *Sòng* editors' note: "Another [version] does not use *gān cǎo* 甘草."
2. *Sòng* editors' note: "Another [version of this prescription] uses one piece of *guā lóu shí* (栝樓實 Fruit of Trichosanthes kirilowii)."

LINE 9.9

又方

Another prescription:

母豬蹄一具，粗切，以水二升煮熟，得五六升汁，飲之。不出更作。

Thoroughly decoct one set of coarsely chopped sow hooves˙ in two *dǒu* of water to obtain five or six *shēng* of liquid. Drink it, and if [the milk] does not emerge, make it again.

˙   母豬蹄 *mǔ zhū tí*: In most medicinal uses of pig's hooves, as in the following prescription, the gender is not specified. It is quite possible that sow's hooves are used here specifically because of a magical connotation of sows with abundance, fertility, and breast milk.

LINE 9.10

又方

Another prescription:

Formula

豬蹄（二枚，熟炙，槌碎）通草（八兩，細切）。

| 豬蹄，熟炙，槌碎 | zhū tí, shú zhì, chuí suì | Hooves of Sus scrofa domestica, charred and smashed into pieces | 二枚 2 méi | 2 pieces |
| 通草，細切 | tōng cǎo, xì qiē | Pith in the stalk of Tetrapanax papyriferus, finely chopped | 八兩 8 liǎng | 24g |

上二味，以清酒一斗浸之，稍稍飲盡，不出更作。

Soak the above two ingredients in one *dǒu* of clear liquor and slowly sip it until it is all finished. If [the milk] does not emerge, make it again.˙

*   *Sòng* editors' note: "In the [version of this prescription] quoted in the *Wài Tái Mì Yào*, the pig's hooves are not charred, but decocted in one *dŏu* of water to obtain four *shēng*. This is boiled with four *shēng* of liquor and then drunk."

LINE 9.11

又方

Another prescription:

栝樓根切一升，酒四升煮三沸，去滓，分三服。

Chop one *shēng* of *guā lóu gēn* (栝蔞根 Root of Trichosanthes kirilowii) and decoct it in four *shēng* of liquor, bringing it to a boil three times. Discard the dregs and divide into four doses.

LINE 9.12

又方

Another prescription:

取栝樓子尚青色大者一枚，熟擣，以白酒一斗煮取四升，去滓，溫服一升，日三。黃色小者，用二枚，亦好。

Take one large seed of *guā lóu zǐ* (栝樓子 Seed of Trichosanthes kirilowii) that is still green, pound it thoroughly, and decoct it in one *dŏu* of white liquor to obtain four *shēng*. Discard the dregs and take a dose of one *shēng* heated, three times a day. If the seeds are small and yellow, you can use two seeds.

LINE 9.13

又方

Another prescription:

Formula

石鍾乳 通草（各一兩）漏蘆（半兩）桂心 甘草 栝樓根（各六銖）。

石鍾乳	shí zhōng rǔ	Stalactite	一兩	1 liǎng	3g
通草	tōng cǎo	Pith in the stalk of Tetrapanax papyriferus	一兩	1 liǎng	3g
漏蘆	lòu lú	Root of Rhaponticum uniflorum	半兩	0.5 liǎng	1.5g
桂心	guì xīn	Shaved inner bark of Cinnamomum cassia	六銖	6 zhū	.75g
甘草	gān cǎo	Root of Glycyrrhiza uralensis	六銖	6 zhū	.75g
栝樓根	guā lóu gēn	Root of Trichosanthes kirilowii	六銖	6 zhū	.75g

上六味，治下篩，酒服方寸匕，日三，最驗。

Finely pestle and sift the above six ingredients. Take a square-inch spoon in liquor three times a day. Best results.

LINE 9.14

又方

Another prescription:

Formula

石鍾乳 漏蘆（各二兩）。

石鍾乳	shí zhōng rǔ	Stalactite	二兩	2 liǎng	6g
漏蘆	lòu lú	Root of Rhaponticum uniflorum	二兩	2 liǎng	6g

上二味，治下篩，飲服方寸匕，即下。

Finely pestle and sift the above two ingredients. As soon as [the patient] takes a square-inch spoon in liquid, [the milk] will descend promptly.

LINE 9.15

又方

Another prescription:

燒鯉魚頭未，酒服三指撮。

Char the head of a carp. Pulverize it and take a three-finger pinch in liquor.

LINE 9.16

又方

Another prescription:

燒死鼠作屑，酒服方寸匕，日三，立下。勿令知。

Char a dead rat into little pieces and take a square-inch spoon in liquor three times a day. [The milk] will immediately descend. Do not let it be known.[*]

---

[*] 勿令知 *wù lìng zhī*: This probably means to execute the prescription secretly, that is, without the patient or her family knowing. It could also mean, however, to keep the prescription a secret.

LINE 9.17

下乳汁，鯽魚湯方

Golden Carp Decoction precipitates breast milk:

Golden Carp Decoction
鯽魚湯 *jì yú tāng*

鯽魚（長七寸）　豬肪（半斤）　漏蘆（八兩）　石鍾乳（八兩）。

鯽魚	jì yú	Meat or whole body of Carassius auratus	長七寸 seven cùn long	21 cm
豬肪[1]	zhū fáng	Lard of Sus scrofa domestica	半斤 0.5 jīn	24g
漏蘆	lòu lú	Root of Rhaponticum uniflorum	八兩 8 liǎng	24g
石鍾乳	shí zhōng rǔ	Stalactite	八兩 8 liǎng	24g

上四味，切，豬肪，魚不須洗治，清酒一斗二升合煮，魚熟藥成，絞去滓，適寒溫，分五服，即乳下。飲其間相去須臾一飲，令藥力相及。

Chop the above four ingredients. You do not have to prepare the pork lard and fish by washing.[2] Cook everything together in one *dǒu* and two *shēng* of clear liquor. When the fish is well-done, the medicine is ready. Wring out and discard the dregs. Divide [the medicine] into five doses and take it at whatever temperature you like. The milk will descend promptly. As for spacing the doses, wait [only] a little while before drinking another dose so that the power of the medicine can reach that [of the previous dose].

1. 豬肪 *zhū fáng*: Pork lard. As a medicinal ingredient, more commonly called 豬膏 *zhū gāo*.
2. 上四味切豬肪魚不須洗治 *yòu sì wèi qiē zhū fáng yú bù xū xǐ zhì*: Depending on punctuation, this phrase could also mean: "Of the above four ingredients, chop the pork lard. The fish does not need to be prepared by washing. The various modern Chinese editions differ here.

LINE 9.18

治婦人乳無汁，單行鬼箭湯方

Single Agent Winged Spindle Tree Decoction treats absence of breast milk:

Single Agent Winged Spindle Tree Decoction
單行鬼箭湯 *dān xíng guǐ jiàn tāng*

鬼箭五兩，以水六升煮取四升，一服八合，日三。亦可燒作灰，水服方寸匕，日三。

Decoct five *liǎng* of *guǐ jiàn* (鬼箭 Branch or plumes of Euonymus alatus) in six *shēng* of water to obtain four *shēng*. Take eight *gě* per dose three times a day. You may also char it into ashes and take a square-inch spoon in water three times a day.

LINE 9.19

治婦人乳無汁方

A prescription for treating absence of breast milk:

Formula

栝樓根（三兩）石鍾乳（四兩）漏蘆（三兩）白頭翁（一兩）滑石（二兩）通草（二兩）。

栝樓根	guā lóu gēn	Root of Trichosanthes kirilowii	三兩 3 liang	9g
石鍾乳	shí zhōng rǔ	Stalactite	四兩 4 liǎng	12g

漏蘆	lòu lú	Root of Rhaponticum uniflorum	三兩 3 liang	9g
白頭翁	bái tóu wēng	Root of Pulsatilla chinensis	一兩 1 liǎng	3g
滑石	huá shí	Talcum	二兩 2 liǎng	6g
通草	tōng cǎo	Pith in the stalk of Tetrapanax papyriferus	二兩 2 liǎng	6g

上六味，治下篩，以酒服方寸匕，日三。

Finely pestle and sift the above six ingredients. Take a square-inch spoon in liquor, three times a day.

LINE 9.20

治婦人乳無汁，甘草散方

Licorice Powder treats absence of breast milk:

Licorice Powder
甘草散 *gān cǎo sǎn*

甘草（一兩）通草（三十銖）石鍾乳（三十銖）雲母（二兩半）屋上散草（二把，燒成灰）。

甘草	gān cǎo	Root of Glycyrrhiza uralensis	一兩 1 liǎng	3g
通草	tōng cǎo	Pith in the stalk of Tetrapanax papyriferus	三十銖 30 zhū	3.75g
石鍾乳	shí zhōng rǔ	Stalactite	三十銖 30 zhū	3.75g
雲母	yún mǔ	Muscovite	二兩半 2.5 liǎng	7.5g
屋上散草, 燒成灰	wū shàng sǎn cǎo, shāo chéng huī	Roof top grass, charred into ashes	二把 2 bǎ	2 handfuls

上五味，治下篩，食後，溫漏蘆湯，服方寸匕，日三，乳下止。

Finely pestle and sift the above five ingredients. After meals, take a square-inch spoon in heated *Rhaponticum Decoction*˙ three times a day. Stop when the breast milk descends.

---

*   漏蘆湯 *lòu lú tāng*: Almost certainly, this prescription does not refer to the prescription for *Rhaponticum Decoction* above, but to another commonly known preparation by that name, also known as "*Rhaponticum Drink*" (漏蘆飲 *lòu lú yǐn*). This is quoted in the *Qiān Jīn Fāng* in the section on welling and flat abscesses as a treatment for abscesses, cinnabar poisoning, aversion to meat, seasonal heat toxin red swelling, and nasal abscesses that are purple, hard, and painful (《千金方》 22:2). That prescription is cited as the primary reference for *lòu lú tāng* in the *Zhōng Huá Yī Xué Dà Cí Diǎn* (《中華醫學大辭典》 pp. 1503-1504).

LINE 9.21

又方

Another prescription:

土瓜根治下篩，服半錢匕，日三，乳如流水。

Finely pestle and sift *tǔ guā gēn* (土瓜根 Root of Trichosanthes cucumerina) and take a half-*qián* spoon three times a day. The breast milk will flow like a river.

Bèi Jí Qiān Jīn Yào Fāng

備急千金要方

Volume 3

卷第三

1. Vacuity Detriment 虛損

Translator's note: In the context of women's illnesses, it is highly significant that Sūn Sī-Miǎo places this category right behind the section on childbirth: The greatest factor in the etiology of all gynecological conditions is vacuity of the body (體虛 *tǐ xū*) and taxation damage of *qì* and blood (勞傷氣血 *láo shāng qì xuè*), which are seen as caused by the strains of women's reproductive cycles, in particular the strains of pregnancy and childbirth (see for example, *Bìng Yuán Lùn* scrolls 37-8). In the context of modern TCM, Wiseman and Féng explain the condition this way: "Vacuity detriment is any form of severe chronic insufficiency of *yīn-yáng*, *qì*-blood, and bowels and viscera, arising through internal damage by the seven affects, taxation fatigue, diet, excesses of drink and sex, or enduring illness" (*Practical Dictionary*, p. 646).

LINE 1.1

(一) 論曰：凡婦人非止臨產須憂，至於產後，大須將慎，危篤之至，其在於斯。(二) 勿以產時無佗，乃縱心恣意，無所不犯。犯時微若秋毫，感病廣於嵩岱。(三)何則。產後之病，難治於餘病也。(四) 婦人產訖，五藏虛羸，惟得將補，不可轉瀉。(五) 若其有病，不須駃藥。若行駃藥，轉更增虛，就中更虛，向生路遠。

(1) Essay: In all cases, it is not only during delivery that women must worry. When they arrive at the postpartum stage, they must [also] exercise particular caution. This is where the greatest threat to their lives is found.

(2) Do not leave them without company at the time of delivery. Otherwise they might act without restraint and follow their whims, in which case they are bound to violate the prohibitions. At the time of the violation, it might be as tiny as autumn down.[1] But the contracted illness will be larger than Mt. Sòng or Mt. Dài.[2]

(3) Why is this so? Postpartum illnesses are more difficult to treat than others.

(4) After women have completed a delivery, their five organs suffer from vacuity emaciation. You may only use supporting and supplementing [treatments] and must not use shifting and draining [treatments].[3]

(5) In cases where [a new mother] suffers from an illness, you must not prepare "galloping" medicines.[4] If one employs galloping medicines, [the condition] will shift into one of an even greater vacuity, resulting in her center becoming even more vacuous. You are

[thus] distancing her from the path towards life.

1.   微若秋毫 *wēi ruò qiū háo*: The finest hair that appears in animal coats in the autumn. Thus, it refers here to a trifling, highly insignificant thing.
2.   嵩岱 *Sōng Dài*: A reference to two of the five sacred peaks (五嶽 *wǔ yuè*) in China: Mount *Sōng* (嵩山 *Sōng-Shān*) in *Hé-Nán* and Mount *Dài* (岱山 *Dài-Shān* in *Shān-Dōng*).
3.   惟得將補不可轉瀉 *wéi děi jiāng bǔ bù kě zhuǎn xiè*: 將 can be read as "to take" in a sense similar to 把 *bǎ*, but it could also be interpreted as a full verb in the sense of "to support," as in the compound 將養 *jiāng yáng*. Regarding 轉, the *Sūn Zhēn Rén* edition has 輕 *qīng* "lightly/carelessly" instead, which would also fit the context. I understand 轉 literally as "passing things through the body." In this context, the phrase 轉瀉 *zhuǎn xiè* thus refers to a treatment with strong purging and blood-moving medicinals, which were apparently quite common in this context, related to the aim of eliminating all the filth and blood that remained in the uterus after delivery. Note the similarity with medicinals in the previous section on prescriptions to make the breast milk descend. Lastly, 轉 could also refer to the notion of "turning around the flow of *qì* and blood" (i.e., directing it downward) to treat such common postpartum conditions as coughing or heart pain, caused by *qì* counterflow and ascent. For examples of this use of 轉, see the discussions in the *Bìng Yuán Lùn* under the entries for "symptoms of postpartum heart pain" (產後心痛候 *chǎn hòu xīn tòng hòu*) and "symptoms of postpartum *qì* ascent" (產後上氣候 *chǎn hòu shàng qì hòu*) (《病源論》 43:3:10 and 15 respectively), or as used in the formula title, "*Reversing Qì Decoction*" (轉氣湯 *zhuǎn qì tāng*), a prescription to treat postpartum coughing caused by *qì* counterflow (cited in 《中華醫學大辭典》 p. 819).
4.   駃藥 *kuài yào*: This refers to harsh purgatives.

LINE 1.2

(一) 所以婦人產後百日已來，極須慇懃憂畏。(二) 勿縱心犯觸，及即便行房。(三) 若有所犯，必身反強直，猶如角弓反張，名曰蓐風，則是其犯候也。(四) 若似角弓，命同轉燭，凡百女人，宜好思之。(五) 苟或在微不慎，戲笑作病，一朝困臥，控告無所。(六) 縱多出財寶，遍處求醫，醫者未必解此。縱得醫來，大命已去，何處追尋。

(1) Therefore, until the first hundred days postpartum have passed, women must be extremely diligent and attentive, worried and cautious.

(2) Do not [allow them to] indulge in their whims and thereby violate [the prohibitions] and offend [the spirits]. This includes even [the prohibition against] bedchamber matters.[1]

(3) If a violation has occurred, it is inevitable that her body will become rigid and arched backwards, resembling arched-back rigidity."[2] This condition is called "childbed wind"[3] and is exactly the symptom related to a violation of the prohibitions.[4]

(4) If [a woman's body] resembles a crossbow [arched backwards], her fate is like a flickering candle. All the myriads of women should heed this well.

(5) If there is even the slightest lack of caution on occasion and an illness is born out of play and laughter, she will lie encumbered in bed by the next morning and there will be no one else to blame.[5]

(6) Even if you were to expend great riches and treasures, and search everywhere for [the best] physicians, they would not necessarily be able to resolve this [condition]. And even if you did manage to have [the best] physicians come, the essence of her life will have already been lost. So where are you going to look for it?

1. Apparently, Sūn Sī-Miǎo deemed it unnecessary to repeat the numerous postpartum prohibitions that restricted a new mother's range of activities, referred to in contemporary China as 坐月子 *zuò yuè zǐ* (sitting out the month). He might have chosen not to discuss them because he considered them common knowledge or in the domain of other specialists such as ritualists and mothers-in-law.

2. 角弓反張 *jiǎo gōng fǎn zhāng*: This refers to postpartum convulsions with only head and feet on the ground. It is equivalent to the modern biomedical term "opisthotonos".

3. 蓐風 *rù fēng*: This dreaded disease is similar to the biomedical condition of puerperal or childbed fever, a type of lockjaw or tetanus infection to occur within the first ten days postpartum. In spite of the similarity of the symptoms, I have chosen not to translate it as such since the etiology differs greatly: As the name implies, this deathly condition is, in medieval Chinese medical theory, caused by Wind (風 *fēng*), which is able to invade the body due to childbirth-related injuries, stirring of blood and *qì*, and taxation damage of the internal organs that have caused a general vacuity of *qì*. The *Bìng Yuán Lùn* distinguishes carefully between different types of "postpartum wind strike" (產後中風 *chǎn hòu zhòng fēng*), based on which organ is invaded by the wind evil. This determines the symptoms as well as the acupuncture treatment methods and prognosis (See 《病源論》 43:3:25, as well as 26-29, the following entries on wind-inflicted postpartum conditions).

4. It is highly significant that Sūn Sī-Miǎo chose here to blame a violation of postpartum taboos, rather than the more strictly medical explanation offered by Cháo Yuán-Fāng in the *Bìng Yuán Lùn* that the body is exhausted and depleted after childbirth and therefore more vulnerable to wind invasion.

5. 控告 *kòng gào*: A legal term meaning "to sue in court." Thus, Sūn Sī-Miǎo is explicitly placing responsibility for this condition with the woman or the caregivers responsible for enforcing the prohibitions.

LINE 1.3

(一) 學者於此一方，大須精熟，不得同於常方耳。特忌上廁便利，宜室中盆上佳。(二) 凡產後滿百日，乃可合會。不爾，至死虛羸，百病滋長，慎之。(三) 凡婦人皆患風氣，臍下虛冷，莫不由此早行房故也。(四)凡產後七日內，惡血未盡，不可服湯，候臍下塊散，乃進羊肉湯。(五) 有痛甚切者，不在此例。後三兩日消息，可服澤蘭丸。比至滿月，丸盡為佳。不爾，虛損不可平復也。(六) 全極消瘦不可救者，服五石澤蘭丸。(七) 凡在蓐，必須服澤蘭丸補之。服法必七日外，不得早服也。

(1) For students [of this text], it is of utmost importance that you familiarize yourselves with this one [section of] prescriptions¹ thoroughly. You must not equate these with ordinary prescriptions! It is particularly prohibited [for new mothers] to use the privy² to empty her bowels. She should do it inside on a chamber pot.

(2) In all cases, she may only engage in sexual intercourse after the full one hundred days [of postpartum prohibitions] are over. Otherwise, [she will suffer from] vacuity emaciation for the rest of her life and the myriad illnesses will flourish and grow. Beware of this!

(3) In all cases, whenever women suffer from wind *qì* and vacuity cold below the navel, there is no other reason for this than that she has engaged in sexual intercourse too soon.

(4) In all cases, for the duration of the first seven days after delivery, the malign blood³ is not yet eliminated completely and she may not take any [medicinal] decoctions. Wait until the lumps below her navel have dissipated and only then introduce *Sheep or Goat's Meat Decoction*.⁴

(5) In cases of severe and sharp pain, this rule does not apply. After the vicissitudes of the first two or three days, she may take *Lycopus Pills*.⁵ It is excellent if she waits until the end of the [postpartum] month before she stops [taking] the pills. Otherwise, she will not be able to recover from vacuity detriment.

(6) In cases of extreme emaciation that she is unable to recover from, she should take *Five Stone Lycopus Pills*.⁶

(7) In all cases, women absolutely must take *Lycopus Pills* during the lying-in period as a supplement. As for taking it, as a rule it must be outside the [first] seven days. They may not take it any earlier!

1. 方 *fāng*: In this context, the term *fāng* clearly refers not only to the narrow meaning of medicinal formulas and acupuncture prescriptions, but to its broader meaning of the various types of technical advice, such as ritual instructions, astrological rules, alchemical secrets, and household recipes.
2. 厠 *cè*: An outdoor structure, the use of which would make her susceptible to an invasion of wind from below.
3. 惡血 *è xuè*: This refers to postpartum vaginal discharge or lochia. It is also referred to as 惡露 *è lù* (malign dew) or 惡物 *è wù* (malign substance).
4. 羊肉湯 *yáng ròu tāng*: For the prescription, see line 1.10 (p. 243) below.
5. 澤蘭丸 *zé lán wán*: No prescription with this name is found in this section. From the following sentences it is obvious that it was a standard preparation that women should take continuously during the first month postpartum, after the first seven days had passed. Thus, Sūn Sī-Miǎo might be referring literally to simple pills made from lycopus. Prescriptions for *Lycopus Decoction* are found below in chapter five volume 3, line 5.3 (p. 320) and chapter six volume three, line 6.11 (pp. 345 - 347).
6. 五石澤蘭丸 *wǔ shí zé lán wán*: While Sūn Sī-Miǎo does cite two prescriptions with "Five Stones" in the title, none of them is called precisely "Five Stone Lycopus Pills."

Therefore, I again assume that he is referring to pills made with "five stones" and lycopus. Based on the prescription for "*Five Stones Decoction*" below in line 1.19 (pp. 251 - 252), I assume that "Five Stones" refers to *zǐ shí yīng* (紫石英 fluorite), *shí zhōng rǔ* (石鐘乳 stalactite), *bái shí yīng* (白石英 white quartz), *chì shí zhī* (赤石脂 Halloysite), and *shí gāo* (石膏 gypsum).

LINE 1.4

(一) 凡婦人因暑月產乳取涼太多得風冷，腹中積聚，百病競起，迄至於老。百方治不能瘥。(二) 桃仁煎主之，出蓐後服之。婦人縱令無病，每至秋冬須服一兩劑，以至年內常將服之佳。

(1) In all cases when women, because they gave birth during the months of summer heat, have cooled themselves off too much and have contracted wind-cold, it causes accumulations and gatherings in the abdomen and the myriad illnesses, which arise unexpectedly and will last all the way until their old age. They will be unable to recover even if treated with a myriad prescriptions.

(2) *Peach Pit Brew* ˙ is the governing prescription for this condition. Take it after coming out of the lying-in period. Even if women are not suffering from any illness, they should take one or two preparations every fall and winter. Taking it often throughout the year is excellent.

˙   The prescription is in line 1.6 (p. 239) below. While I translate the term 煎 *jiān* more generally as "brew," it refers most specifically to the process of boiling down substances, usually in sugar or lard, to make a concentrated paste.

LINE 1.5

亦產訖可服四順理中丸方。

After the delivery is over, she may take *Four [Ingredients] Center-Normalizing and Rectifying Pills*.

Four [Ingredients] Center-Normalizing and Rectifying Pills
四順理中丸 *sì shùn lǐ zhōng wán*

甘草（二兩）人參 白朮 乾薑（各一兩）。

| 甘草 | gān cǎo | Root of Glycyrrhiza uralensis | 二兩 2 liǎng | 6g |
| 人參 | rén shēn | Root of Panax ginseng | 一兩 1 liǎng | 3g |

| 白朮 | bái zhú | Rhizome of Atractylodes macrocephala | 一兩 1 liǎng | 3g |
| 乾薑 | gān jiāng | Dried root of Zingiber officinale | 一兩 1 liǎng | 3g |

上四味，末之，蜜和丸如梧子，服十丸，稍增至二十丸。新生藏虛，此所以養藏氣也。

Make a powder with the above four ingredients and mix with honey into pills the size of firmiana seeds. Take ten pills [per dose], gradually increasing the amount to twenty pills. Right after delivery, the viscera are depleted. For this reason, you must [use this medicine] to nourish visceral *qì*.

LINE 1.6

桃仁煎治婦人產後百疾，諸氣補益，悅澤方。

Peach Pit Brew treats the myriad diseases of women after childbirth, by supplementing and boosting all her *qì*, making her happy and radiant.

Peach Pit Brew
桃仁煎 *táo rén jiān*

桃仁一千二百枚，擣令細熟，以上好酒一斗五升研濾三四遍，如作麥粥法，以極細為佳。內長項瓷瓶中，密塞以麵封之，內湯中煮一伏時，不停火，亦勿令火猛，使瓶口常出在湯上，無令沒之，熟訖出。溫酒服一合，日再服。丈夫亦可服之。

Pound 1200 pieces of *táo rén* (桃仁 Seed of Prunus persica) to a very fine consistency. In one *dǒu* and five *shēng* of highest grade liquor, grind them and strain them three or four times, as if you were making wheat gruel, the finer the consistency the better. Fill it into a long-necked porcelain jug and plug it tightly, sealing it with dough. Simmer in hot water for twenty-four hours. Do not let the fire go out, but do not let the flames get too high either. Make sure that the mouth of the jar is always above the hot liquid, and do not let it get immersed. When it is done cooking, take it out. Take one *gě* in warm liquor twice a day. The husband may also take this.*

---

*   丈夫亦可服之 *zhàng fū yì kě fú zhī*: This means that this prescription can also be beneficial for supplementing men's *qì*. A different meaning is suggested in the *Sūn Zhēn Rén* edition, which replaces 可 *kě* with 須 *xū* (must). This suggests that the husband needs to take these pills simultaneously with his wife for maximum efficacy.

LINE 1.7

治婦人虛羸，短氣，胸逆滿悶，風氣，石斛地黃煎方。

Dendrobium and Rehmannia Brew treats women's vacuity emaciation, with shortness of breath, counterflow, fullness, and oppression in the chest, and wind *qì*.

Dendrobium and Rehmannia Brew
石斛地黃煎 *shí hú dì huáng jiān*

石斛（四兩） 生地黃汁（八升） 桃仁（半升） 桂心（二兩） 甘草（四兩） 大黃（八兩） 紫菀（四兩） 麥門冬（二升） 茯苓（一斤） 淳酒（八升）。

石斛	shí hú	Whole plant of Dendrobium nobile	四兩 4 liǎng	12g
生地黃汁	shēng dì huáng zhī	Juice from the fresh root of Rehmannia glutinosa	八升 8 shēng	560ml
桃仁	táo rén	Seed of Prunus persica	半升 0.5 shēng	12g
桂心	guì xīn	Shaved inner bark of Cinnamomum cassia	二兩 2 liǎng	6g
甘草	gān cǎo	Root of Glycyrrhiza uralensis	四兩 4 liǎng	12g
大黃	dà huáng	Root of Rheum palmatum	八兩 8 liǎng	24g
紫菀	zǐ wǎn	Root and rhizome of Aster tataricus	四兩 4 liǎng	12g
麥門冬	mài mén dōng	Tuber of Ophiopogon japonicus	二升 2 shēng	48g
茯苓	fú líng	Dried fungus of Poria cocos	一斤 1 jīn	48g
淳酒	chún jiǔ	Pure grain spirit	八升 8 shēng	560ml

上十味，為末，於銅器中炭火上熬，內鹿角膠一斤，耗得一斗。次內飴三斤，白蜜三升和調，更於銅器中釜上煎微耗，以生竹攪，無令著，耗令相得藥成，先食酒服如彈子一丸，日三，不知稍加至二丸。

Pulverize the above ten ingredients. Place them in a copper pot and stew over a charcoal fire. Add one *jīn* of *lù jiǎo jiāo* (鹿角膠 Gelatinous glue produced from ossified antler or antler base of Cervus nippon) and reduce to obtain one *dǒu*. Then add three *jīn* of malt syrup[1] and three *shēng* of honey. Stir to mix it and simmer it again in the copper pot, placed on top of a cauldron, until reduced slightly. Stir it with [a stick of] fresh bamboo and do not let it burn. Reduce it until everything is mixed together and the medicine is done. Before meals, take one pellet-sized pill in liquor three times a day. If no effect is noticed, gradually increase the dosage to a maximum of two pills.[2]

1. 飴 *yí*: A thick jelly-like paste made from sprouted wheat or other grains, in the *Běn Cǎo Gāng Mù* described as a "moist sugar of a consistency like thick honey or soft candy" (《本草綱目》 25:950). In a harder consistency, it is called 膠飴 *jiāo yí*, which I translate as "malt candy."

2. *Sòng* editors' note: "Another [version of this] prescription includes three *liǎng* of *rén shēn* (人參 Root of Panax ginseng)."

LINE 1.8

治婦人產後欲令肥白，飲食平調，地黃羊脂煎方。

Rehmannia and Sheep or Goat Fat Brew is a treatment for women after childbirth, making them plump and white by calming and regulating their [digestion of] food and drink.

Rehmannia and Sheep or Goat Fat Brew
地黃羊脂煎 *dì huáng yáng zhī jiān*

生地黃汁（一斗）生薑汁（五升）羊脂（二斤）白蜜（五升）。

生地黃汁	shēng dì huáng zhī	Juice from the fresh root of Rehmannia glutinosa	一斗 1 dǒu	700ml
生薑汁	shēng jiāng zhī	Juice from the fresh root of Zingiber officinale	五升 5 shēng	350ml
羊脂	yáng zhī	Unrendered fat of Capra hircus or Ovis aries	二斤 2 jīn	96g
白蜜	bái mì	Honey of Apis cerana	五升 5 shēng	350ml

上四味，先煎地黃令得五升，次內羊脂合煎減半，內薑汁復煎令減，合蜜著銅器中，煎如飴，取雞子大一枚，投熱酒中服，日三。

Of the above four ingredients, first simmer the *shēng dì huáng zhī* (生地黃汁 Juice from the fresh root of Rehmannia glutinosa) to obtain five *shēng*. Next, add the sheep or goat fat, mix it in, and simmer everything together until reduced to half. Add the ginger juice and again simmer it to reduce it. Blend it with the honey, place it in a copper pot, and boil it down to the consistency of malt syrup. Take an egg-sized amount, put it in hot liquor, and take it three times a day.

LINE 1.9

地黃酒治產後百病，未產前一月當預釀之，產訖蓐中服之方。

Rehmannia Wine treats the hundred postpartum diseases. It should be brewed in advance, one month before delivery, and taken when the birth is over during the lying-in period.

Rehmannia Wine
地黃酒 *dì huáng jiǔ*

地黃汁（一升）好麴（一斗）好米（二升）。

地黃汁	dì huáng zhī	Rehmannia glutinosa juice	一升 1 shēng	70ml
好麴	hǎo qū	Good leaven	一斗 1 dǒu	700ml
好米	hǎo mǐ	Good rice	二升 2 shēng	48g

上三味，先以地黃汁漬麴令發，準家去醞之至熟，封七日，取清服之。常使酒氣相接，勿令斷絕。慎蒜，生，冷，酢，滑，豬，雞，魚。一切婦人皆須服之。但夏三月熱不可合，春秋冬並得合服。地黃並滓內米中，炊合用之，一石十石一準此一升為率。先服羊肉當歸湯三劑，乃服之，佳。

Of the above three ingredients, first soak the leaven[1] in the rehmannia juice until it rises. According to the standard household method, ferment it until done. Seal it for seven days, then take the clear [liquid] to drink it [as medicine]. Make sure that the *qì* of the wine is always connected and do not allow it to get interrupted.[2] Beware of garlic, raw and cold foods, vinegary and slippery foods, pork, chicken, and fish. All women must take[3] this without exception. It is only in the heat of the three months of summer that you must not combine [the medicine with the foods listed above]. In the spring, fall, and winter, you can take it together with these. Use [the medicine] by adding the [leavened] rehmannia[4] and the dregs to [uncooked] rice and cooking them together. Make the proportions one *shí* [of *rehmannia wine*] to ten *shí* [of rice] to prepare one *shēng* as a rule. Consume three preparations of *Sheep or Goat's Meat and Chinese Angelica Decoction*[5] first and take this only afterwards for best results.

1. 麴 *qū*: As explained in the *Běn Cǎo Gāng Mù*, *qū* refers specifically to a yeast starter for making liquor, which is why it is also called 酒母 *jiǔ mǔ*. For medicinal purposes, it can be made from wheat berries, wheat flour, or rice, and is best made in the sixth month (《本草綱目》 25:946). The following entry on 神麴 *shén qū* (divine leaven) explains that the ancients used wine-making yeast for their medicines, but later physicians started preparing a special, more powerful leaven specifically for use in medicine, which is called *shén qū* (《本草綱目》 25:947).

2. The meaning of this phrase is unclear to me.

3. The *Sūn Zhēn Rén* edition has 忌 *jì* (avoid) instead, which appears much more likely in the context of this prescription. This list of dietary restrictions is quite common and found in many of the other formulas in this text.

4. This apparently refers to the rehmannia juice that has been prepared in the manner described above.

5. 羊肉當歸湯 *yáng ròu dāng guī tāng*: This most likely refers to the following prescrip-

tion for *Sheep or Goat's Meat Decoction*. Alternatively, it could refer to the prescription for *Sheep or Goat's Meat and Chinese Angelica Decoction* found in chapter four volume three, line 4.7 on p. 301.

LINE 1.10

治產後虛羸，喘乏，白汗出，腹中絞痛，羊肉湯方。

Sheep or Goat's Meat Decoction treats postpartum vacuity emaciation, with panting and lack of breath, perspiration of white sweat,[1] and gripping pain in the center of the abdomen.

Sheep or Goat's Meat Decoction
羊肉湯 *yáng ròu tāng*

肥羊肉（三斤，去脂）當歸（一兩）桂心（二兩）芍藥（四兩）甘草（二兩）生薑（四兩）芎藭（三兩）乾地黃（五兩）。

肥羊肉,去脂	féi yáng ròu, qù zhī	Fat Capra hircus or Ovis aries meat, with the fat removed	三斤 3 jīn	144g
當歸[2]	dāng guī	Root of Angelica polimorpha	一兩 1 liǎng	3g
桂心	guì xīn	Shaved inner bark of Cinnamomum cassia	二兩 2 liǎng	6g
芍藥[3]	sháo yào	Root of Paeonia albiflora	四兩 4 liǎng	12g
甘草	gān cǎo	Root of Glycyrrhiza uralensis	二兩 2 liǎng	6g
生薑	shēng jiāng	Fresh root of Zingiber officinale	四兩 4 liǎng	12g
川芎[4]	chuān xiōng	Root of Ligusticum wallichii	三兩 3 liǎng	9g
乾地黃	gān dì huáng	Dried root of Rehmannia glutinosa	五兩 5 liǎng	15g

上八味，㕮咀，以水一斗半先煮肉，取七升，去肉內餘藥，煮取三升，去滓。分三服，不瘥重作。

Pound the above eight ingredients. First cook the meat in one and a half *dǒu* of water to obtain seven *shēng*. Take out the meat and add the remaining drugs. Decoct them to obtain three *shēng* and discard the dregs. Divide into three doses. If she fails to recover, make it again.[5]

1.　　　白汗出 *bái hàn chū*: Sweat is associated with the heart and occurs when *qì* fails to contain the fluids. White sweat is sweat that is not related to the presence of heat and, according to the *Sù Wèn*, a sign of "true vacuity, discomfort in the heart, *qì* reversal, and chronic distress." (《素文》21).

2.   *Sòng* editors' note: "Mr. Yao uses *cōng bái* (蔥白 Stalk of Allium fistulosum)."
3.   *Sòng* editors' note: "The *Zǐ Mǔ Mì Lù* uses *cōng bái* (蔥白 Stalk of Allium fistulosum)."
4.   *Sòng* editors' note: "The *Zǐ Mǔ Mì Lù* uses *[dòu] chǐ* ([豆]豉 Preparation of Glycine max)."
5.   *Sòng* editors' note: "The *Qiān Jīn Yì Fāng* includes one *jīn* of *cōng bái* (蔥白 Stalk of Allium fistulosum). The *Zǐ Mǔ Mì Lù* states: "For slight heat in the chest, add one *liǎng* each of *huáng qín* (黃芩 Root of Scutellaria baicalensis) and *mài mén dōng* (麥門冬 Tuber of Ophiopogon japonicus). For headache, add one *liǎng* of *shí gāo* (石膏 Gypsum). For wind strike, add one *liǎng* of *fáng fēng* (防風 Root of Ledebouriella divaricata). For constipation, add one *liǎng* of *dà huáng* (大黃 Root of Rheum palmatum). For urinary problems, add one *liǎng* of *kuí zǐ* (葵子 Seed of Malva verticillata). For *qì* ascent and counterflow cough, add one *liǎng* of *wǔ wèi zǐ* (五味子 Fruit of Schisandra chinensis)."

LINE 1.11

治產後虛羸，喘乏，乍寒乍熱，病如瘧狀，名為蓐勞，豬腎湯方。

Pig's Kidney Decoction treats postpartum vacuity emaciation with panting, lack of breath, and abruptly alternating [aversion to] cold and heat [effusion]. This condition resembles malaria and is called "childbed taxation."

Pig's Kidney Decoction
豬腎湯 *zhū shèn tāng*

豬腎（一具，去脂，四破，無則用羊腎代）香豉（綿裡）白粳米 蔥白（各一斗）。

豬腎, 去脂 , 四破, 無則用羊腎代	zhū shèn, qù zhī, sì pò, wú zé yòng yáng shèn dài	Kidneys of Sus scrofa domestica, fat removed, and quartered, if unavailable, substitute goat's or sheep's kidneys.	一具 1 jù	1 set
香豉, 綿裡	xiāng chǐ, mián lǐ	Preparation of Glycine max, wrapped in thin silk cloth	一斗 1 dǒu	700ml
白粳米	bái jīng mǐ	White seed of the non-gluti-nous variety of Oryza sativa	一斗 1 dǒu	700ml
蔥白	cōng bái	Stalk of Allium fistulosum	一斗 1 dǒu	700ml

上四味，以水三斗煮取五升，去滓，任情服之，不瘥更作。

Decoct the above four ingredients in three *dǒu* of water to obtain five *shēng*. Discard the dregs. Take it however you like to. If she fails to recover, make it again.˙

*   *Sòng* editors' note: "The *Guǎng Jì Fāng* includes 2 *liǎng* each of *rén shēn* (人參 Root of Panax ginseng) and *dāng guī* (當歸 Root of Angelica polimorpha), using a total of six ingredients.)"

LINE 1.12

羊肉黃芪湯治產後虛乏，補益方。

Sheep or Goat's Meat and Astragalus Decoction treats postpartum vacuity by supplementing and boosting:

Sheep or Goat's Meat and Astragalus Decoction
羊肉黃芪湯 *yáng ròu huáng qí tāng*

羊肉（三斤） 黃芪（三兩） 大棗（三十枚） 茯苓 甘草 當歸 桂心 芍藥 麥門冬 乾地黃（各一兩）。

羊肉	yáng ròu	Unrendered fat of Capra hircus or Ovis aries	三斤 3 jīn	144g
黃芪	huáng qí	Root of Astragalus membranaceus	三兩 3 liǎng	9g
大棗	dà zǎo	Mature fruit of Ziziphus jujuba	三十枚 30 méi	30 pcs
茯苓	fú líng	Dried fungus of Poria cocos	一兩 1 liǎng	3g
甘草	gān cǎo	Root of Glycyrrhiza uralensis	一兩 1 liǎng	3g
當歸	dāng guī	Root of Angelica polimorpha	一兩 1 liǎng	3g
桂心	guì xīn	Shaved inner bark of Cinnamomum cassia	一兩 1 liǎng	3g
芍藥	sháo yào	Root of Paeonia albiflora	一兩 1 liǎng	3g
麥門冬	mài mén dōng	Tuber of Ophiopogon japonicus	一兩 1 liǎng	3g
乾地黃	gān dì huáng	Dried root of Rehmannia glutinosa	一兩 1 liǎng	3g

上十味，㕮咀，以水二斗煮羊肉，取一斗，去肉內諸藥，煎取三升，去滓。分三服，日三。

Pound the above ten ingredients. Cook the sheep or goat's meat in two *dǒu* of water to obtain one *dǒu*. Take out the meat and add the various drugs, simmer to obtain three *shēng* and discard the dregs. Divide into three doses and take three times a day.

LINE 1.13

鹿肉湯治產後虛羸，勞損，補乏方。

Venison Decoction treats postpartum vacuity emaciation and taxation detriment, by supplementing the lack.

Venison Decoction
鹿肉湯 *lù ròu tāng*

鹿肉（四斤） 乾地黃 甘草 芎藭（各三兩） 人參 當歸（各二兩） 黃芪 芍藥 麥門冬 茯苓（各二兩） 半夏（一升） 大棗（二十枚） 生薑（二兩）。

鹿肉	lù ròu	Meat of Cervus nippon	四斤 4 jīn	192g
乾地黃	gān dì huáng	Dried root of Rehmannia gluti- nosa	三兩 3 liǎng	9g
甘草	gān cǎo	Root of Glycyrrhiza uralensis	三兩 3 liǎng	9g
川芎	chuān xiōng	Root of Ligusticum wallichii	三兩 3 liǎng	9g
人參	rén shēn	Root of Panax ginseng	二兩 2 liǎng	6g
當歸	dāng guī	Root of Angelica polimorpha	二兩 2 liǎng	6g
黃芪	huáng qí	Root of Astragalus membranaceus	二兩 2 liǎng	6g
芍藥	sháo yào	Root of Paeonia albiflora	二兩 2 liǎng	6g
麥門冬	mài mén dōng	Tuber of Ophiopogon japonicus	二兩 2 liǎng	6g
茯苓	fú líng	Dried fungus of Poria cocos	二兩 2 liǎng	6g
半夏	bàn xià	Rhizome of Pinellia ternata	一升 1 shēng	24g
大棗	dà zǎo	Mature fruit of Ziziphus jujuba	二十枚 20 méi	20 pcs
生薑	shēng jiāng	Fresh root of Zingiber officinale	二兩 2 liǎng	6g

上十三味，㕮咀，以水二斗五升煮肉，取一斗三升，去肉內藥，煎取五升，去滓。分四服，日三夜一。

Pound the above thirteen ingredients. Cook the meat in two *dǒu* and five *shēng* of water to obtain one *dǒu* and three *shēng*. Take out the meat and add the drugs. Simmer to obtain five *shēng*. Discard the dregs, divide into four doses, and take three times during the day and once at night.

LINE 1.14

治產後虛乏，五勞七傷，虛損不足，藏腑冷熱不調，獐骨湯方。

Water Deer's Bone Decoction treats postpartum vacuity, the five taxations and seven damages, vacuity detriment and insufficiency, and failure to regulate cold and heat in the viscera and bowels.

Water Deer's Bone Decoction
獐骨湯 *zhāng gǔ tāng*

獐骨（一具） 遠志 黃芪 芍藥 乾薑 防風 茯苓 厚朴（各三兩） 當歸 橘皮 甘草 獨活 芎藭（各二兩） 桂心 生薑（各四兩）。

獐骨	zhāng gǔ	Bones of Hydropotes inermis	一具	1 set
遠志	yuǎn zhì	Root of Polygala tenuifolia	三兩 3 liǎng	9g
黃芪	huáng qí	Root of Astragalus membranaceus	三兩 3 liǎng	9g
芍藥	sháo yào	Root of Paeonia albiflora	三兩 3 liǎng	9g
乾薑	gān jiāng	Dried root of Zingiber officinale	三兩 3 liǎng	9g
防風	fáng fēng	Root of Ledebouriella divaricata	三兩 3 liǎng	9g
茯苓*	fú líng	Dried fungus of Poria cocos	三兩 3 liǎng	9g
厚朴	hòu pò	Bark of Magnolia officinalis	三兩 3 liǎng	9g
當歸	dāng guī	Root of Angelica polimorpha	二兩 2 liǎng	6g
橘皮	jú pí	Peel of Citrus reticulata	二兩 2 liǎng	6g
甘草	gān cǎo	Root of Glycyrrhiza uralensis	二兩 2 liǎng	6g
獨活	dú huó	Root and rhizome of Angelica pubescens	二兩 2 liǎng	6g
川芎	chuān xiōng	Root of Ligusticum wallichii	二兩 2 liǎng	6g
桂心	guì xīn	Shaved inner bark of Cinnamomum cassia	四兩 4 liǎng	12g
生薑	shēng jiāng	Fresh root of Zingiber officinale	四兩 4 liǎng	12g

上十五味，㕮咀，以水三斗煮獐骨，取二斗，去骨內藥，煎取五升，去滓，分五服。

Pound the above fifteen ingredients. Cook the deer bones in three *dǒu* of water to obtain two *dǒu*. Take out the bones and add the drugs. Simmer to obtain five *shēng*, discard the dregs, and divide into five doses.

*   *Sòng* editors' note: "Another [version] uses *fú shén* (茯神 Dried fungus of Poria cocos)."

LINE 1.15

當歸芍藥湯治產後虛損，逆害飲食方。

Chinese Angelica and Peony Decoction treats postpartum vacuity detriment with counterflow, which is harming the [digestion of] food and drink.

Chinese Angelica and Peony Decoction
當歸芍藥湯 *dāng guī sháo yào tāng*

當歸（一兩半） 芍藥 人參 桂心 生薑 甘草（各一兩） 大棗（二十枚） 乾地黃（一兩）。

當歸	dāng guī	Root of Angelica polimorpha	一兩半 1.5 liǎng	4.5g
芍藥	sháo yào	Root of Paeonia albiflora	一兩 1 liǎng	3g
人參	rén shēn	Root of Panax ginseng	一兩 1 liǎng	3g
桂心	guì xīn	Shaved inner bark of Cinnamomum cassia	一兩 1 liǎng	3g
生薑	shēng jiāng	Fresh root of Zingiber officinale	一兩 1 liǎng	3g
甘草	gān cǎo	Root of Glycyrrhiza uralensis	一兩 1 liǎng	3g
大棗	dà zǎo	Mature fruit of Ziziphus jujuba	二十枚 20 méi	20 pcs
乾地黃	gān dì huáng	Dried root of Rehmannia glutinosa	一兩 1 liǎng	3g

上八味，㕮咀，以水七升煮取三升，去滓。分三服，日三。

Pound the above eight ingredients and decoct in seven *shēng* of water to obtain three *shēng*. Discard the dregs and divide into three doses, [to take] three times a day.

LINE 1.16

治產後虛氣，杏仁湯方。

Apricot Kernel Decoction treats postpartum vacuity of *qì*.

Apricot Kernel Decoction
杏仁湯 *xìng rén tāng*

杏仁 橘皮 白前 人參（三兩） 桂心（四兩） 蘇葉（一升） 半夏（一升） 生薑（十兩） 麥門冬（一兩）。

杏仁	xìng rén	Dried seed of Prunus armeniaca	三兩 3 liǎng	9g
橘皮	jú pí	Peel of Citrus reticulata	三兩 3 liǎng	9g
白前	bái qián	Root and rhizome of Cynanchum stauntoni	三兩 3 liǎng	9g
人參	rén shēn	Root of Panax ginseng	三兩 3 liǎng	9g

桂心	guì xīn	Shaved inner bark of Cinnamomum cassia	四兩 4 liǎng	12g
蘇葉	sū yè	Foliage of Perilla frutescens	一升 1 shēng	24g
半夏	bàn xià	Rhizome of Pinellia ternata	一升 1 shēng	24g
生薑	shēng jiāng	Fresh root of Zingiber officinale	十兩 10 liǎng	30g
麥門冬	mài mén dōng	Tuber of Ophiopogon japonicus	一兩 1 liǎng	3g

上九味，㕮咀，以水一斗二升煮取三升半，去滓，分五服。

Pound the above nine ingredients and decoct in one *dǒu* and two *shēng* of water to obtain three and a half *shēng*. Discard the dregs and divide into five doses.

LINE 1.17

治產後上氣，及婦人賁豚氣，積勞藏氣不足，胸中煩躁，關元以下如懷五千錢狀方。

This prescription treats postpartum ascent of *qì*, as well as women's running piglet *qì*,[1] accumulation taxation and insufficiency of visceral *qì*, vexation and agitation in the chest, and the feeling that she was pregnant with [the weight of] five thousand gold pieces below Pass Head.[2]

Formula

厚朴 桂心 當歸 細辛 芍藥 石膏（各三兩）甘草 黃芩 澤瀉（各二兩）吳茱萸（五兩，（《千金翼》作大黃）乾地黃（四兩）桔梗（三兩）乾薑（一兩）。

厚朴	hòu pò	Bark of Magnolia officinalis	三兩 3 liǎng	9g
桂心	guì xīn	Shaved inner bark of Cinnamomum cassia	三兩 3 liǎng	9g
當歸	dāng guī	Root of Angelica polimorpha	三兩 3 liǎng	9g
細辛	xì xīn	Complete plant including root of Asarum heteropoides	三兩 3 liǎng	9g
芍藥	sháo yào	Root of Paeonia albiflora	三兩 3 liǎng	9g
石膏	shí gāo	Gypsum	三兩 3 liǎng	9g
甘草	gān cǎo	Root of Glycyrrhiza uralensis	二兩 2 liǎng	6g
黃芩	huáng qín	Root of Scutellaria baicalensis	二兩 2 liǎng	6g
澤瀉	zé xiè	Rhizome of Alisma plantago-aquatica	二兩 2 liǎng	6g
吳茱萸[3]	wú zhū yú	Unripe fruit of Evodia rutaecarpa	五兩 5 liǎng	15g

乾地黃	gān dì huáng	Dried root of Rehmannia glutinosa	四兩 4 liǎng	12g
桔梗	jié gěng	Root of Platycodon grandiflorum	三兩 3 liǎng	9g
乾薑	gān jiāng	Dried root of Zingiber officinale	一兩 1 liǎng	3g

上十三味，哎咀，以水一斗二升煮取三升，去滓，分三服，服三劑，佳。

Pound the above thirteen ingredients and decoct in one *dǒu* and two *shēng* of water to obtain three *shēng*. Discard the dregs and divide into three doses. Taking three preparations is excellent.

1. 奔豚氣 *bēn tún qì*: According to the *Bìng Yuán Lùn*, an accumulation of *qì* in the kidneys caused by fright or worrying. Fright damages the spirit, which is stored in the heart. Excessive worrying damages the will, which is stored in the kidneys. When the spirit and will are damaged and stirred, *qì* accumulates in the kidneys and roams up and down like a running piglet" (《病源論》 13:6). In modern TCM, Wiseman and Féng describe it as a type of kidney acculumation characterized by upsurge from the lower abdomen to the chest and throat, accompanied by gripping abdominal pain, oppression in the chest, rapid breathing, dizziness, heart palpitations, and heart vexation (*Practical Dictionary*, p. 510). See also *Zhōng Huá Yī Xué Dà Cí Diǎn*, p. 815.
2. 關元 *guān yuán*: CV-4. On the controlling vessel, 3 *cùn* below the navel.
3. *Sòng* editors' note: "The *Qiān Jīn Yì Fāng* has *dà huáng* (大黃 Root of Rheum palmatum)."

LINE 1.18

治產後七傷虛損，少氣不足，並主腎勞寒冷，補益氣，乳蜜湯方。

Milk and Honey Decoction is a postpartum treatment for the seven damages and vacuity detriment, for shortage and insufficiency of *qì*, and is the governing prescription for kidney taxation and coldness, by supplementing and boosting *qì*.

Milk and Honey Decoction
乳蜜湯 *rǔ mì tāng*

牛乳（七升） 白蜜（一升半） 當歸 人參 獨活（各三兩） 大棗（二十枚） 甘草 桂心（各二兩）。

牛乳[1]	niú rǔ	Milk of Bos taurus domesticus	七升 7 shēng	490ml
白蜜	bái mì	Honey of Apis cerana	一兩半 1.5 liǎng	4.5g
當歸	dāng guī	Root of Angelica polimorpha	三兩 3 liǎng	9g
人參	rén shēn	Root of Panax ginseng	三兩 3 liǎng	9g

獨活	dú huó	Root and rhizome of Angelica pubescens	三兩 3 liǎng	9g
大棗	dà zǎo	Mature fruit of Ziziphus jujuba	二十枚 20 méi	20 pcs
甘草	gān cǎo	Root of Glycyrrhiza uralensis	二兩 2 liǎng	6g
桂心	guì xīn	Shaved inner bark of Cinnamomum cassia	二兩 2 liǎng	6g

上八味，㕮咀，諸藥以乳蜜中煮取三升，去滓，分四服。

Pound the above eight ingredients. Decoct all the drugs in the milk and honey to obtain three *shēng*, discard the dregs, and divide into four doses.[2]

1.   *Sòng* editors' note: "If *niú rǔ* 牛乳 is unavailable, then use *yáng rǔ* (羊乳 Milk of Capra hircus)."
2.   In the *Sūn Zhēn Rén* edition, this prescription and the two following prescriptions for "Five Stones Decoction" and "Three Stones Decoction" are found later in chapter three of volume three on "wind strike," (translated here in Lines 1.19 and 20 (p. 251 - 253) below). This shows the close connection and overlap between the etiologies of childbirth-related vacuity and externally contracted wind strike during the postpartum period.

LINE 1.19

治產後虛冷七傷，時寒熱，體痛乏力，補腎並治百病，五石湯方。

Five Stones Decoction treats postpartum vacuity cold and the seven damages, with periodic [aversion to] cold and heat [effusion], generalized pain, and lack of strength, by supplementing the kidneys and also treating the myriad diseases.

Five Stones Decoction
五石湯 *wǔ shí tāng*

紫石英 鍾乳 白石英 赤石脂 石膏 茯苓 白朮 桂心 芎藭 甘草（各二兩）薤白（六兩）人參 當歸（各三兩）生薑（八兩）大棗（二十枚）。

紫石英	zǐ shí yīng	Fluorite	二兩 2 liǎng	6g
鐘乳	zhōng rǔ	Stalactite	二兩 2 liǎng	6g
白石英	bái shí yīng	White quartz	二兩 2 liǎng	6g
楮實子	chǔ shí zǐ	Fruit of Broussonetia papyrifera	二兩 2 liǎng	6g
石膏	shí gāo	Gypsum	二兩 2 liǎng	6g
茯苓	fú líng	Dried fungus of Poria cocos	二兩 2 liǎng	6g
白朮	bái zhú	Rhizome of Atractylodes macrocephala	二兩 2 liǎng	6g

桂心	guì xīn	Shaved inner bark of Cinnamomum cassia	二兩 2 liǎng	6g
川芎	chuān xiōng	Root of Ligusticum wallichii	二兩 2 liǎng	6g
甘草	gān cǎo	Root of Glycyrrhiza uralensis	二兩 2 liǎng	6g
薤白	xiè bái	Stalk of Allium macrostemon	六兩 6 liǎng	18g
人參	rén shēn	Root of Panax ginseng	三兩 3 liǎng	9g
當歸	dāng guī	Root of Angelica polimorpha	三兩 3 liǎng	9g
生薑	shēng jiāng	Fresh root of Zingiber officinale	八兩 8 liǎng	24g
大棗	dà zǎo	Mature fruit of Ziziphus jujuba	二十枚 20 méi	20 pcs

上十五味，五石並末之，諸藥各㕮咀，以水一斗二升煮取三升六合，去
滓，分六服。若中風，加葛根，獨活各二兩；下痢，加龍骨一兩。

Of the fifteen ingredients above, pulverize the five stones together and pound each of the various drugs. Decoct in one *dǒu* and two *shēng* of water to obtain three *shēng* and six *gě*. Discard the dregs and divide into six doses. In cases of wind strike, add two *liǎng* each of *gé gēn* (葛根 Root of Pueraria lobata) and *dú huó* (獨活 Root and rhizome of Angelica pubescens). In cases of diarrhea, add one *liǎng* of *lóng gǔ* (龍骨 Os draconis).

LINE 1.20

三石湯主病如前方。

Three Stones Decoction governs the same conditions as above.

Three Stones Decoction
三石湯 *sān shí tāng*

紫石英（二兩）白石英（二兩半）鍾乳（二兩半）生薑 當歸 人參 甘草（
各二兩）茯苓 乾地黃 桂心（各三兩）半夏（五兩）大棗（十五枚）。

紫石英	zǐ shí yīng	Fluorite	二兩 2 liǎng	6g
白石英	bái shí yīng	White quartz	二兩半 2.5 liǎng	7.5g
鐘乳	zhōng rǔ	Stalactite	二兩半 2.5 liǎng	7.5g
生薑	shēng jiāng	Fresh root of Zingiber officinale	二兩 2 liǎng	6g
當歸	dāng guī	Root of Angelica polimorpha	二兩 2 liǎng	6g
人參	rén shēn	Root of Panax ginseng	二兩 2 liǎng	6g
甘草	gān cǎo	Root of Glycyrrhiza uralensis	二兩 2 liǎng	6g

茯苓	fú líng	Dried fungus of Poria cocos	三兩 3 liǎng	9g
乾地黃	gān dì huáng	Dried root of Rehmannia glutinosa	三兩 3 liǎng	9g
桂心	guì xīn	Shaved inner bark of Cinnamomum cassia	三兩 3 liǎng	9g
半夏	bàn xià	Rhizome of Pinellia ternata	五兩 5 liǎng	15g
大棗	dà zǎo	Mature fruit of Ziziphus jujuba	十五枚 15 méi	15 pcs

上十二味，三石末之，㕮咀諸藥，以水一斗二升煮取三升，去滓，分四服。若中風，加葛根四兩。

Of the twelve ingredients above, pulverize the three stones and pound the various drugs. Decoct in one *dǒu* and two *shēng* of water to obtain three *shēng*. Discard the dregs and divide into four doses. In cases of wind strike, add four *liǎng* of *gé gēn* (葛根 Root of Pueraria lobata).

LINE 1.21

內補黃芪湯主婦人七傷，身體疼痛，小腹急滿，面目黃黑，不能食飲，並諸虛乏不足少氣，心悸不安方。

Internally Supplementing Astragalus Decoction is the governing prescription for women's seven damages, pain in the body, tension and fullness in the lower abdomen, yellow or black face and eyes, inability to eat or drink, as well as the various [conditions of] vacuity, insufficiency, and shortage of *qì* with heart palpitations and disquietude.

Internally Supplementing Astragalus Decoction
內補黃芪湯 *nèi bǔ huáng qí tāng*

黃芪 當歸 芍藥 乾地黃 半夏（各三兩）茯苓 人參 桂心 遠志 麥門冬 甘草 五味子 白朮 澤瀉（各二兩）乾薑（四兩）大棗（三十枚）。

黃芪	huáng qí	Root of Astragalus membranaceus	三兩 3 liǎng	9g
當歸	dāng guī	Root of Angelica polimorpha	三兩 3 liǎng	9g
芍藥	sháo yào	Root of Paeonia albiflora	三兩 3 liǎng	9g
乾地黃	gān dì huáng	Dried root of Rehmannia glutinosa	三兩 3 liǎng	9g
半夏	bàn xià	Rhizome of Pinellia ternata	三兩 3 liǎng	9g
茯苓	fú líng	Dried fungus of Poria cocos	二兩 2 liǎng	6g
人參	rén shēn	Root of Panax ginseng	二兩 2 liǎng	6g
桂心	guì xīn	Shaved inner bark of Cinnamomum cassia	二兩 2 liǎng	6g

遠志	yuǎn zhì	Root of Polygala tenuifolia	二兩 2 liǎng	6g
麥門冬	mài mén dōng	Tuber of Ophiopogon japonicus	二兩 2 liǎng	6g
甘草	gān cǎo	Root of Glycyrrhiza uralensis	二兩 2 liǎng	6g
五味子	wǔ wèi zǐ	Fruit of Schisandra chinensis	二兩 2 liǎng	6g
白朮	bái zhú	Rhizome of Atractylodes macro-cephala	二兩 2 liǎng	6g
澤瀉	zé xiè	Rhizome of Alisma plantago-aquat-ica	二兩 2 liǎng	6g
乾薑	gān jiāng	Dried root of Zingiber officinale	四兩 4 liǎng	12g
大棗	dà zǎo	Mature fruit of Ziziphus jujuba	三十枚 30 méi	30 pcs

上十六味，㕮咀，以水一斗半煮取三升，去滓。一服五合，日三夜一服。

Pound the above sixteen ingredients and decoct in one and a half *dǒu* of water to obtain three *shēng*. Discard the dregs and take five *gě* per dose three times during the day and once at night.

LINE 1.22

治產後虛羸，盜汗，濇濇惡寒，吳茱萸湯方。

Evodia Decoction treats postpartum vacuity emaciation with nightsweats and huddled aversion to cold.

Evodia Decoction
吳茱萸湯 *wú zhū yú tāng*

吳茱萸三兩以清酒三升漬一宿，煮如蟻鼻沸，減得二升許，中分之，頓服一升，日再，間日再作服。亦治產後腹中疾痛。

Soak three *liǎng* of *wú zhū yú* (吳茱萸 Unripe fruit of Evodia rutaecarpa) overnight in three *shēng* of clear liquor. Boil it until it resembles bubbling ant noses,ˆ reducing it to obtain about two *shēng*. Divide it in half and quaff one *shēng* as a single dose twice a day. On alternate days, prepare and take it again. It also treats postpartum abdominal sickness and pain.

---

* 煮如蟻鼻沸 *zhǔ rú yǐ bí fèi*: This means that it should be simmered in such a way that the tiniest bubbles rise to the surface of the liquid. "Ant nose" is an expression indicating tiny size. Alternatively, the *Sūn Zhēn Rén* edition has 魚目 *yú mù* (fish eyes) instead, in which case the phrase would mean "cook it like bubbling fish eyes."

LINE 1.23

治產後體虛，寒熱，自汗出，豬膏煎方。

Pork Lard Brew treats postpartum generalized vacuity with [aversion to] cold and heat [effusion] and spontaneous sweating.

Pork Lard Brew
豬膏煎 *zhū gāo jiān**

豬膏（一升）清酒（五合）生薑汁（一升）白蜜（一升）。

豬膏	zhū gāo	Lard of Sus scrofa domestica	一升 1 shēng	24g
清酒	qīng jiǔ	Clear liquor	五合 5 gě	35ml
生薑汁	shēng jiāng zhī	Juice from the fresh root of Zingiber officinale	一升 1 shēng	70ml
白蜜	bái mì	Honey of Apis cerana	一升 1 shēng	70ml

上四味，煎令調和，五上五下，膏成。隨意以酒服方寸匕。當炭火上熬。

Simmer the above four ingredients, blending them together. Bring [the mixture] to a boil and then let it settle five times to make a paste. Whenever you like, take a square-inch spoon in liquor. It must be stewed over a charcoal fire.

*   In the *Sūn Zhēn Rén* edition, this prescription is found in chapter 3 of this volume on "wind strike."

LINE 1.24

鯉魚湯主婦人體虛，流汗不止，或時盜汗方。

Carp Decoction is the governing prescription for women's generalized vacuity with incessant flowing of sweat and occasional nightsweats.

Carp Decoction
鯉魚湯 *lǐ yú tāng*

鯉魚（二升）蔥白（切，一升）豉（一升）乾薑（二兩）桂心（二兩）
。

鯉魚	lǐ yú	Meat or whole body of Cyprinus carpio	二升 2 shēng	48g
蔥白，切	cōng bái, qiē	Stalk of Allium fistulosum, chopped	一升 1 shēng	24g
[豆]豉	[dòu] chǐ	Preparation of Glycine max	一升 1 shēng	24g
乾薑	gān jiāng	Dried root of Zingiber officinale	二兩 2 liǎng	6g
桂枝	guì zhī	Twigs of Cinnamonum cassia	二兩 2 liǎng	6g

上五味，㕮咀四物，以水一斗煮魚，取六升，去魚內諸藥，微火煮取二升，去滓，分再服，取微汗即愈。勿用生魚。

Of the five ingredients above, pound the four [medicinal] substances. Cook the fish in one *dǒu* of water to obtain six *shēng*. Take out the fish and add the various drugs. Decoct them on a small flame to obtain two *shēng*. Discard the dregs and divide into two doses. As soon as she begins to sweat lightly, she will recover. Do not use fresh fish.

LINE 1.25

治產後風虛，汗出不止，小便難，四肢微急難以屈伸者，桂枝加附子湯方。

Cinnamon Twig Decoction Plus Aconite treats postpartum wind vacuity with incessant sweating, difficult urination, and slight tension and difficulty to bend and stretch the four limbs.

Cinnamon Twig Decoction Plus Aconite
桂枝加附子湯 *guì zhī jiā fù zǐ tāng*

桂枝 芍藥（各三兩）甘草（一兩半）附子（二枚）生薑（三兩）大棗（十二枚）。

桂枝	guì zhī	Twigs of Cinnamonum cassia	三兩 3 liǎng	9g
芍藥	sháo yào	Root of Paeonia albiflora	三兩 3 liǎng	9g
甘草	gān cǎo	Root of Glycyrrhiza uralensis	一兩半 1.5 liǎng	4.5g
附子	fù zǐ	Lateral root of Aconitum carmichaeli	二枚 2 méi	2 pcs
生薑	shēng jiāng	Fresh root of Zingiber officinale	三兩 3 liǎng	9g
大棗	dà zǎo	Mature fruit of Ziziphus jujuba	十二枚 12 méi	12 pcs

上六味，㕮咀，以水七升煎取三升，分為三服。

Pound the above six ingredients and simmer in seven *shēng* of water to obtain three *shēng*. Divide into three doses.

2. Vacuity Vexation 虛煩

LINE 2.1

薤白湯治產後胸中煩熱逆氣方。

Chinese Chive Decoction treats postpartum vexing heat in the chest and counterflow *qì*.

Chinese Chive Decoction
薤白湯 *xiè bái tāng*

薤白 半夏 甘草 人參 知母（二兩） 石膏（四兩） 栝樓根（三兩） 麥門冬（半斤）。

薤白	xiè bái	Stalk of Allium macrostemon	二兩 2 liǎng	6g
半夏	bàn xià	Rhizome of Pinellia ternata	二兩 2 liǎng	6g
甘草	gān cǎo	Root of Glycyrrhiza uralensis	二兩 2 liǎng	6g
人參	rén shēn	Root of Panax ginseng	二兩 2 liǎng	6g
知母	zhī mǔ	Root of Anemarrhena asphodeloides	二兩 2 liǎng	6g
石膏	shí gāo	Gypsum	四兩 4 liǎng	12g
栝蔞根	guā lóu gēn	Root of Trichosanthes kirilowii	三兩 3 liǎng	9g
麥門冬	mài mén dōng	Tuber of Ophiopogon japonicus	半斤 0.5 jīn	24g

上八味，㕮咀，以水一斗三升煮取四升，去滓，分五服，日三夜二。熱甚，即加石膏，知母各一兩。

Pound the above eight ingredients and decoct in one *dǒu* and three *shēng* of water to obtain four *shēng*. Discard the dregs, divide into five doses, and take three times during the day and twice at night. In cases of extreme heat, add an extra *liǎng* each of *shí gāo* 石膏 and *zhī mǔ* 知母.

LINE 2.2

竹根湯治產後虛煩方。

Bamboo Root Decoction treats postpartum vacuity vexation.

Bamboo Root Decoction
竹根湯 *zhú gēn tāng*

甘竹根細切一斗五升，以水二斗煮取七升，去滓，內小麥二升，大棗二十枚，復煮麥熟三四沸，內甘草一兩，麥門冬一升，湯成去滓。服五合，不瘥更服取瘥。短氣，亦服之。

Finely chop one *dǒu* and five *shēng* of *gān zhú gēn* (甘竹根 Roots of sweet Phyllostachys) and decoct it in two *dǒu* of water to obtain seven *shēng*. Discard the dregs. Add two *shēng* of *xiǎo mài* (小麥 Seed of Triticum aestivum) and twenty pieces of *dà zǎo* (大棗 Mature fruit of Ziziphus jujuba). Boil it again until the wheat is cooked, bringing it to a rolling boil three or four times. Add one *liǎng* of *gān cǎo* (甘草 Root of Glycyrrhiza uralensis) and one *shēng* of *mài mén dōng* (麥門冬 Tuber of Ophiopogon japonicus). When the decoction is done, discard the dregs. Take five *gě*. If she fails to recover, take another dose to gain recovery. [You may] also take [this prescription in cases of] shortness of breath.

LINE 2.3

人參當歸湯治產後煩悶不安方。

Ginseng and Chinese Angelica Decoction treats postpartum vexation, oppression, and disquietude.

Ginseng and Chinese Angelica Decoction
人參當歸湯 *rén shēn dāng guī tāng*

人參 當歸 麥門冬 桂心 乾地黃（各一兩） 大棗（二十個） 粳米（一升） 淡竹葉（三升） 芍藥（四兩）。

人參	rén shēn	Root of Panax ginseng	一兩 1 liǎng	3g
當歸	dāng guī	Root of Angelica polimorpha	一兩 1 liǎng	3g
麥門冬	mài mén dōng	Tuber of Ophiopogon japonicus	一兩 1 liǎng	3g
桂心	guì xīn	Shaved inner bark of Cinnamomum cassia	一兩 1 liǎng	3g

乾地黃	gān dì huáng	Dried root of Rehmannia glutinosa	一兩 1 liǎng	3g
大棗	dà zǎo	Mature fruit of Ziziphus jujuba	二十個 20 gè	20 pcs
粳米*	jīng mǐ	Seed of the non-glutinous variety of Oryza sativa	一升 1 shēng	24g
淡竹葉	dàn zhú yè	Leaves of Lopatherum gracile	三升 3 shēng	72g
芍藥	sháo yào	Root of Paeonia albiflora	四兩 4 liǎng	12g

上九味，㕮咀，以水一斗二升先煮竹葉及米，取八升，去滓，內藥煮取三升，去滓，分三服。若煩悶不安者，當取豉一升，以水三升煮取一升，盡服之，甚良。

Pound the above nine ingredients. First decoct the bamboo leaves and rice in one *dǒu* and two *shēng* of water to obtain eight *shēng*. Discard the dregs and add the drugs. Decoct to obtain three *shēng*, discard the dregs, and divide into three doses. In cases of vexation oppression and disquietude, one should take one *shēng* of [dòu] chǐ ([豆]豉 Preparation of Glycine max) and decoct it in three *shēng* of water to obtain one *shēng*. Consuming it all is excellent.

*   *Sòng* editors' note: "The *Sūn Zhēn Rén* editon has 生米 *shēng mǐ* (fresh rice)."

LINE 2.4

甘竹筎湯治產後內虛，煩熱短氣方。

Sweet Bamboo Shavings Decoction treats postpartum internal vacuity with vexation heat and shortness of breath.

Sweet Bamboo Shavings Decoction
甘竹筎湯 *gān zhú rú tāng*

甘竹筎（一升）人參 茯苓 甘草（各一兩）黃芩（三兩）。

甘竹筎	gān zhú rú	Shavings of sweet Phyllostachys	一升 1 shēng	24g
人參	rén shēn	Root of Panax ginseng	一兩 1 liǎng	3g
茯苓	fú líng	Dried fungus of Poria cocos	一兩 1 liǎng	3g
甘草	gān cǎo	Root of Glycyrrhiza uralensis	一兩 1 liǎng	3g
黃芩	huáng qín	Root of Scutellaria baicalensis	三兩 3 liǎng	9g

上五味，㕮咀，以水六升煮取二升，去滓，分三服，日三。

Pound the above five ingredients and decoct in six *shēng* of water to obtain two *shēng*. Discard the dregs and divide into three doses. Take three times a day.

LINE 2.5

知母湯治產後乍寒乍熱，通身溫壯，胸心煩悶方。

Anemarrhena Decoction treats abruptly alternating [aversion to] cold and heat [effusion] postpartum with vigorous warmth[1] throughout the whole body and vexation and oppression in the chest and heart.

Anemarrhena Decoction
知母湯 *zhī mǔ tāng*

知母（三兩） 芍藥 黃芩（各二兩） 桂心 甘草（各一兩）。

知母	zhī mǔ	Root of Anemarrhena asphodeloides	三兩 3 liǎng	9g
芍藥	sháo yào	Root of Paeonia albiflora	二兩 2 liǎng	6g
黃芩	huáng qín	Root of Scutellaria baicalensis	二兩 2 liǎng	6g
桂心[2]	guì xīn	Shaved inner bark of Cinnamomum cassia	一兩 1 liǎng	3g
甘草	gān cǎo	Root of Glycyrrhiza uralensis	一兩 1 liǎng	3g

上五味，㕮咀，以水五升煮取二升半，分三服。

Pound the above five ingredients and decoct in five *shēng* of water to obtain two and a half *shēng*. Divide into three doses.

---

1. 溫壯 *wēn zhuàng*: A symptom similar to a high fever (壯熱 *zhuàng rè*), but of lesser intensity. It is probably similar to the modern expression 溫壯熱 *wēn zhuàng rè*, which is described as "similar to a high fever... warm throughout but not severe,... which mostly affects small children." See 《中華醫學大辭典》 p. 1323.
2. *Sòng* editors' note: "Another [version of this] prescription does not use *guì xīn* 桂心, but includes *shēng dì huáng* (生地黃 Fresh root of Rehmannia glutinosa)."

LINE 2.6

竹葉湯治產後心中煩悶不解方。

Bamboo Leaves Decoction treats postpartum vexation and oppression in the heart that fails to be resolved.

Bamboo Leaves Decoction
竹葉湯 *zhú yè tāng*

生淡竹葉 麥門冬（各一升） 甘草（二兩） 生薑 茯苓（各三兩） 大棗（十四個） 小麥（五合）。

生淡竹葉	shēng dàn zhú yè	Fresh leaves of Lopatherum gracile	一升 1 shēng	24g
麥門冬	mài mén dōng	Tuber of Ophiopogon japonicus	一升 1 shēng	24g
甘草	gān cǎo	Root of Glycyrrhiza uralensis	二兩 2 liǎng	6g
生薑	shēng jiāng	Fresh root of Zingiber officinale	三兩 3 liǎng	9g
茯苓	fú líng	Dried fungus of Poria cocos	三兩 3 liǎng	9g
大棗	dà zǎo	Mature fruit of Ziziphus jujuba	十四個 14 gè	14 pcs
小麥	xiǎo mài	Seed or flour of Triticum aestivum	五合 5 gě	35ml

上七味，㕮咀，以水一斗先煮竹葉，小麥，取八升，內諸藥，煮取三升，去滓，分三服。若心中虛悸者，加人參二兩；其人食少無穀氣者，加粳米五合；氣逆者，加半夏二兩。

Pound the above seven ingredients. First decoct the *dàn zhú yè* 淡竹葉 and *xiǎo mài* 小麥[1] in one *dǒu* of water to obtain eight *shēng*. Add the various drugs and decoct to obtain three *shēng*. Discard the dregs and divide into three doses. In cases of vacuity palpitations in the heart, add two *liǎng* of *rén shēn* (人參 Root of Panax ginseng).[2] In cases of reduced eating and lack of grain *qì*,[3] add five *gě* of *jīng mǐ* (粳米 Seed of the non-glutinous variety of Oryza sativa). In cases of *qì* counterflow, add two *liǎng* of *bàn xià* (半夏 Rhizome of Pinellia ternata).[4]

1. The *Sūn Zhēn Rén* editon adds *mài mén dōng* 麥門冬 here instead of *xiǎo mài* 小麥.
2. Instead of this sentence, the *Sūn Zhēn Rén* editon has: 若有人參，可入一二兩為善 (If you have *rén shēn* 人參, it is good to add 1-2 *liǎng*).
3. 穀氣 *gǔ qì*: This is a reference to *yáng qì*, derived from the consumption of food.
4. *Sòng* editors' note: "The *Sūn Zhēn Rén* editon does not include *xiǎo mài* 小麥, thus using only six ingredients. The version of this prescription in the *Wài Tái Mì Yào* (in the chapter on postpartum thirst) adds *rén shēn* (人參 Root of Panax ginseng) and *bàn xià* (半夏 Rhizome of Pinellia ternata), thus using a total of nine ingredients (《外台秘要》34)."

LINE 2.7

淡竹茹湯治產後虛煩，頭痛，短氣欲絕，心中悶亂不解，必效方。

Bamboo Shavings Decoction is a treatment of unfailing efficacy for postpartum vacuity vexation with headache, shortness of breath verging on *qì* expiry, and oppression and turmoil in the center of the heart that fails to be resolved.

Bamboo Shavings Decoction
淡竹茹湯 *dàn zhú rú tāng*

生淡竹筎（一升）　麥門冬（五合）　甘草（一兩）　小麥（五合）　生薑（三兩）　大棗（十四枚）。

生淡竹筎	shēng dàn zhú rú	Fresh shavings of Lopatherum gracile	一升 1 shēng	24g
麥門冬	mài mén dōng	Tuber of Ophiopogon japonicus	五合 5 gě	35ml
甘草	gān cǎo	Root of Glycyrrhiza uralensis	一兩 1 liǎng	3g
小麥	xiǎo mài	Seed or flour of Triticum aestivum	五合 5 gě	35ml
生薑[1]	shēng jiāng	Fresh root of Zingiber officinale	三兩 3 liǎng	9g
大棗[2]	dà zǎo	Mature fruit of Ziziphus jujuba	十四枚 14 méi	14 pcs

上六味，㕮咀，以水一斗煮竹筎，小麥，取八升，去滓，乃內諸藥，煮取一升，去滓。分二服，羸人分作三服。若有人參，入一兩；若無人參，內茯苓一兩半亦佳；人參，茯苓皆治心煩悶及心虛驚悸，安定精神。有，則為良；無，自依方服一劑，不瘥更作。若氣逆者，加半夏二兩。

Pound the above six ingredients. Decoct the *dàn zhú rú* 淡竹筎 and *xiǎo mài* 小麥 in one *dǒu* of water to obtain eight *shēng*. Discard the dregs and then add the various drugs. Decoct to obtain one *shēng*. Discard the dregs and divide into two doses. For a markedly emaciated patient, divide it into three doses. If you have *rén shēn* (人參 Root of Panax ginseng), add one *liǎng*. If you don't have *rén shēn* 人參, adding one and a half *liǎng* of *fú líng* (茯苓 Dried fungus of Poria cocos) is also excellent. The *rén shēn* 人參 and *fú líng* 茯苓 both treat heart vexation and oppression as well as heart vacuity fright palpitations, by calming the essence spirit. If you have them, it is good. If not, simply take one preparation according to the formula and make another one, if she fails to recover. In cases of *qì* counterflow, add two *liǎng* of *bàn xià* (半夏 Rhizome of Pinellia ternata).

.

1.　*Sòng* editors' note: "The *Chǎn Bǎo* uses *gān gé gēn* (乾葛根 Dried root of Pueraria lobata)."
2.　*Sòng* editors' note: "The *Chǎn Bǎo* also uses 3 *liǎng* of *shí gāo* (石膏 Gypsum)."

LINE 2.8

赤小豆散治產後煩悶，不能食，虛滿方。

Azuki Bean Powder treats postpartum vexation and oppression with inability to eat and vacuity fullness.

Azuki Bean Powder
赤小豆散 *chì xiǎo dòu sǎn*

赤小豆三七枚，燒作末，以冷水和，頓服之。

Char and pulverize three times seven pieces of *chì xiǎo dòu* (赤小豆 Fruit of Phaseolus calcaratus). Mix with cool water and quaff in a single dose.

LINE 2.9

治產後煩悶，蒲黃散方。

Typha Pollen Powder treats postpartum vexation and oppression.

Typha Pollen Powder
蒲黃散 *pú huáng sǎn*

蒲黃以東流水和方寸匕服，極良。

Take a square-inch spoon of *pú huáng* (蒲黃 Pollen of Typha angustata) mixed into east-flowing water. Extremely good.

LINE 2.10

蜀漆湯治產後虛熱往來，心胸煩滿，骨節疼痛，及頭痛壯熱，晡時輒甚，又如微瘧方。

Dichroa Leaf Decoction treats postpartum cases of intermittent vacuity heat, vexing fullness in the heart and chest, pain in the bones and joints, as well as headache and vigorous heat that are always worst in the afternoon, and furthermore conditions that resemble mild malaria.[1]

Dichroa Leaf Decoction
蜀漆湯 *shǔ qī tāng*

蜀漆葉（一兩）黃芪（五兩）桂心 甘草 黃芩（各一兩）知母 芍藥（各二兩）生地黃（一斤）。

蜀漆葉	shǔ qī yè	Foliage of Dichroa febrifuga	一兩 1 liǎng	3g
黃芪	huáng qí	Root of Astragalus membranaceus	五兩 5 liǎng	15g
桂心	guì xīn	Shaved inner bark of Cinnamomum cassia	一兩 1 liǎng	3g
甘草	gān cǎo	Root of Glycyrrhiza uralensis	一兩 1 liǎng	3g
黃芩	huáng qín	Root of Scutellaria baicalensis	一兩 1 liǎng	3g
知母	zhī mǔ	Root of Anemarrhena asphodeloides	二兩 2 liǎng	6g
芍藥	sháo yào	Root of Paeonia albiflora	二兩 2 liǎng	6g
生地黃	shēng dì huáng	Fresh root of Rehmannia glutinosa	一斤 1 jīn	48g

上八味，㕮咀，以水一斗煮取三升，分三服。此湯治寒熱，不傷人。²

Pound the above eight ingredients and decoct them in one *dǒu* of water to obtain three *shēng*. Divide into three doses. This decoction treats [aversion to] cold and heat [effusion] without injuring the patient.

1. This prescription and the following one are not found in the *Sūn Zhēn Rén* editon. Instead, that edition has a prescription for treating miscarriage with incessant bleeding and discomforting vexation, which is completely unrelated in function or ingredients to the prescriptions found in the other editions.
2. 不傷人 *bù shāng rén*: This means that it is safe to use even in the postpartum period since it has no iatrogenic side effects. In a similar vain, the introductory essay to the next section on wind strike explains that due to the special vulnerabilities of women during the immediate postpartum period, extra care must be taken to avoid unbalancing and weakening the woman's body even further.

LINE 2.11

芍藥湯治產後虛熱頭痛方。

Peony Decoction treats postpartum vacuity heat with headache.

Peony Decoction
芍藥湯 *sháo yào tāng*

白芍藥 乾地黃 牡蠣 (各五兩) 桂心 (三兩) 。

白芍藥	bái sháo yào	Paeonia lactiflora	五兩 5 liǎng	15g
乾地黃	gān dì huáng	Dried root of Rehmannia glutinosa	五兩 5 liǎng	15g
牡蠣	mǔ lì	Shell of Ostrea rivularis	五兩 5 liǎng	15g
桂心	guì xīn	Shaved inner bark of Cinnamomum cassia	三兩 3 liǎng	9g

上四味，㕮咀，以水一斗煮取二升半，去滓，分三服，日三。此湯不傷損人，無毒。亦治腹中拘急痛。若通身發熱，加黃芩二兩。

Pound the above four ingredients and decoct in one *dǒu* of water to obtain two and a half *shēng*. Discard the dregs and divide into three doses, to take three times a day. This decoction does not injure the patient and is non-toxic. It also treats acute hypertonicity and pain in the center of the abdomen. In cases of heat effusion throughout the body, add two *liǎng* of *huáng qín* (黃芩 Root of Scutellaria baicalensis).

3. Wind Strike 中風

LINE 3.1

論曰凡產後角弓反張，及諸風病，不得用毒藥，惟宜單行一兩味。亦不得大發汗。特忌轉瀉吐利，必死無疑。

Essay: In all cases of postpartum arched-back rigidity and the various wind diseases, you must not use toxic medicines. It is only appropriate to use singly acting [medicinals and prescriptions with] one or two ingredients.[1] You must also not induce great sweating and must particularly avoid shifting and draining,[2] vomiting and disinhibiting [therapies]. This will invariably cause [the patient's] certain death.[3]

1.   This requirements contradicts most of the prescriptions below, which except for the first three consist of prescriptions with numerous ingredients. This contradiction would support a suspicion that this essay and the following three prescriptions were inserted here by the *Sòng* editors but are found elsewhere in the *Sūn Zhēn Rén* edition. Moreover, throughout the following prescriptions we can find contrasting instructions with regard to inducing or avoiding perspiration as part of her treatment (see below, for example, on line 3.8 (p. 274) especially the footnote to this formula). We thus see two opposing medical opinions and treatment methods reflected in this section. On the one hand, purging prescriptions, intended to induce sweating, vomiting, or diarrhea, were the most common treatment method in cases of wind strike, aiming at dispersing wind, 消風 *xiāo fēng*. However, this treatment was often contraindicated in the postpartum period because it aggravated the severe vacuity that the patient suffered from after childbirth. Thus, this particular essay might reflect a later, more sophisticated medical development or the opinion of a different medical school that discouraged the use of harsh drugs during the postpartum period.
2.   轉瀉 *zhuǎn xiè*: See chapter one of volume three, on line 1.1 (pp. 234 - 235) and the accompanying note 3 above, which explains the expression.
3.   This essay is missing here in the *Sūn Zhēn Rén edition* and found later, following the prescription for *Chicken's Droppings Wine.*

LINE 3.2

大豆紫湯產後大善。治產後百病，及中風痱痙，或背口噤，或但煩熱若渴，或頭身皆重，或身癢，劇者嘔逆直視，此皆因虛風冷濕，及勞傷所為，大豆紫湯方。

Soybean Purple Decoction is excellent after childbirth. It treats the myriad postpartum diseases, including wind strike with disablement[1] and tetany,[2] possibly with a rigid back and clenched mouth, or merely vexing heat or thirst, or heaviness of both head and body, or itching of the body, or in severe cases, retching counterflow and forward-staring eyes. These [symptoms] are all caused by vacuity wind [-related] cold and dampness and by taxation damage.[3]

Soybean Purple Decoction
大豆紫湯 *dà dòu zǐ tāng*

大豆（五升）清酒（一斗）。

| 大豆 | dà dòu | Seed of Glycine max | 五升 5 shēng | 120g |
| 清酒 | qīng jiǔ | Clear liquor | 一斗 1 dǒu | 700ml |

上二味，以鐵鐺猛火熬豆，令極熱焦煙出，以酒沃之，去滓。服一升，日夜數過，服之盡，更合。小汗則愈。一以去風。二則消血結。如妊娠傷折，胎死在腹中三日，服此酒即瘥。

Of the above two ingredients, roast the beans over a high fire in an iron skillet, letting them get extremely hot until they are scorched and smoking. Then use the liquor to douse them and discard the dregs. Take one *shēng* per dose, several times during the day and at night. When it is all used up, compound another [batch].[4] When she sweats lightly, recovery will follow. The first batch expels wind. The second batch disperses blood bind. In cases of injury during pregnancy and a dead fetus in the abdomen for three days, she will promptly recover after taking this liquor.

1.　　痱 *féi*: Name of a disorder characterized by flaccidity of the four limbs, inability to move, and slight turmoil in the spirit and will. It is described in *Líng Shū* as follows: "When a patient suffers from disablement, the body is without pain, the four limbs fail to contract, and the turmoil in the mind is not severe. If the [patient's] words are somewhat coherent, it is treatable. In severe cases, [the patient] is unable to speak and the condition is untreatable." (《靈樞》 23). See also the entry on "symptoms of wind disablement" (風痱候 *fēng féi hòu*) in the *Bìng Yuán Lùn*, which is almost identical to the *Líng Shū* quote (《病源論》 1:7).

2.　　痙 *jìng*: Wiseman and Féng describe this condition as "severe spasm such as rigidity of the neck, clenched jaw, convulsions of the limbs, and arched-back rigidity. Repletion patterns are attributed to wind, cold, dampness, phlegm, or fire congesting the channels, whereas vacuity patterns occur when excessive sweating, loss of blood, or constitutional vacuity causes *qì* vacuity, shortage of blood, and insufficiency of the fluids… To resolve tetany, repletion patterns are treated primarily by dispelling wind and secondarily by supporting right *qì*, whereas vacuity patterns are treated primarily by boosting *qì* and nourishing blood and secondarily by extinguishing wind…" (*Practical Dictionary*, p. 606-607). The prescriptions in this sections demonstrate how tetany in pregnancy was understood by Sūn Sī-Miǎo both in terms of vacuity and repletion.

3. In the *Sūn Zhēn Rén* edition, this and the following two prescriptions are found in the section below on "Postpartum Heart and Abdominal Pain." The prescription's action is described as "regulating *qì* and blood and treating wind strike with convulsions and *fěi* paralysis...." Instead of the prescription, it states: "*Purple Decoction* is the governing prescription for this [condition]. The prescription is found below in the chapter on 'malign dew'." However, the prescription is not found there, but in the chapter on "postpartum heart and abdominal pain." There, it is said to be the governing prescription for "the myriad postpartum diseases by regulating blood and *qì*, as well as for wind strike tetany and *fěi* paralysis by relieving pain, for a rigid back and clenched mouth, for mere vexation heat, bitter thirst, heaviness of both the head and the body, in severe cases with retching counterflow. All of these are caused by wind-cold and dampness, as well as taxation damaging the stomach."

4. 更合 *gèng hé*. Following this, the *Sūn Zhēn Rén* edition has "...*Pubescent Angelica Decoction*. The reason for this is that after childbirth, [the mother] is often depleted and suffers from wind. Use *dú huó* (獨活 Root and rhizome of Angelica pubescens) to disperse wind and remove blood. In severe cases, make ten batches."

LINE 3.3

治產後百日中風痙，口噤不開，並治血氣痛，勞傷，補腎，獨活紫湯方。

Pubescent Angelica Purple Decoction treats wind strike tetany during the first hundred days postpartum˙ with clenched mouth that cannot be opened, as well as for treating blood and *qì* pain and taxation damage, by supplementing the kidneys.

Pubescent Angelica Purple Decoction
獨活紫湯 *dú huó zǐ tāng*

獨活（一斤）大豆（五升）酒（一斗三升）。

獨活	dú huó	Root and rhizome of Angelica pubescens	一斤 1 jīn	48g
大豆	dà dòu	Seed of Glycine max	五兩 5 liǎng	15g
酒	jiǔ	Liquor	一斗，三升 1 dǒu, 3 shēng	940ml

上三味，先以酒漬獨活再宿，若急須，微火煮之，令減三升，去滓，別熬大豆極焦，使煙出，以獨活酒沃之，去豆。服一升，日三夜二。

Of the three ingredients above, first soak the *dú huó* 獨活 in the liquor for two nights. If it is urgent, decoct it [instead] over a small flame until reduced to three *shēng*. Discard the dregs. Separately, roast the *dà dòu* 大豆 until they are extremely scorched and smoking. Use the *dú huó* 獨活 wine to douse them and remove the beans. Take one *shēng* per dose three times a day and twice at night.

*   產後百日 *chǎn hòu bǎi rì*: The *Sūn Zhēn Rén* edition has 產後百病 instead. Thus, the
      whole phrase reads: "… treats the myriad postpartum diseases, with wind strike tetany…"

LINE 3.4

小獨活湯治如前狀方。

Minor Pubescent Angelica Decoction treats the same [conditions] as above.

Minor Pubescent Angelica Decoction
小獨活湯 *xiǎo dú huó tāng*

獨活（八兩） 葛根（六兩） 甘草（二兩） 生薑（六兩）。

獨活	dú huó	Root and rhizome of Angelica pubescens	八兩 8 liǎng	24g
葛根	gé gēn	Root of Pueraria lobata	六兩 6 liǎng	18g
甘草	gān cǎo	Root of Glycyrrhiza uralensis	二兩 2 liǎng	6g
生薑	shēng jiāng	Fresh root of Zingiber officinale	六兩 6 liǎng	18g

上四味，㕮咀，以水九升煮取三升，去滓，分四服，微汗，佳。

Pound the above four ingredients and decoct in nine *shēng* of water to obtain three
shēng. Discard the dregs and divide into four doses. Inducing light sweating is ideal.

LINE 3.5

甘草湯治在蓐中風，背強不得轉動，名曰風痙方。

Licorice Decoction treats wind strike in childbed with rigidity of the back and inability to
turn or move. [This condition] is called wind tetany.

Licorice Decoction
甘草湯 *gān cǎo tāng*

甘草 乾地黃 麥門冬 麻黃（各二兩） 芎藭 黃芩 栝樓根（各三兩） 杏仁（五
十枚） 葛根（半斤）。

甘草	gān cǎo	Root of Glycyrrhiza uralensis	二兩 2 liǎng	6g
乾地黃	gān dì huáng	Dried root of Rehmannia glutinosa	二兩 2 liǎng	6g
麥門冬	mài mén dōng	Tuber of Ophiopogon japonicus	二兩 2 liǎng	6g
麻黃	má huáng	Stalk of Ephedra sinica	二兩 2 liǎng	6g
川芎	chuān xiōng	Root of Ligusticum wallichii	三兩 3 liǎng	9g
黃芩	huáng qín	Root of Scutellaria baicalensis	三兩 3 liǎng	9g
栝蔞根	guā lóu gēn	Root of Trichosanthes kirilowii	三兩 3 liǎng	9g
杏仁	xìng rén	Dried seed of Prunus armeniaca	五十枚 50 méi	50 pcs
葛根	gé gēn	Root of Pueraria lobata	半斤 0.5 jīn	24g

上九味，㕮咀，以水一斗五升，酒五升合煮葛根取八升，去滓，內諸藥，煮取三升，去滓，分再服，一劑不瘥，更合良。

Pound the above nine ingredients. Decoct the *gé gēn* 葛根 in one *dǒu* and five *shēng* of water mixed with five *shēng* of liquor, to obtain eight *shēng*. Discard the dregs, add the various [other] drugs, and decoct them to obtain three *shēng*. Discard the dregs and divide into two doses. If [the patient] fails to recover after one batch, it is good to compound another one.˙

---

*   *Sòng* editors' note: "The [versions of this prescription in the] *Qiān Jīn Yì Fāng* and *Cuī Shì* also include 3 *liǎng* of *qián hú* 前胡."

LINE 3.6

獨活湯治產後中風，口噤不能言方。

Pubescent Angelica Decoction treats postpartum wind strike with clenched mouth and inability to speak.

Pubescent Angelica Decoction
獨活湯 *dú huó tāng*

獨活（五兩）防風 秦艽 桂心 白朮 甘草 當歸 附子（各二兩）葛根（三兩）生薑（五兩）防已（一兩）。

獨活	dú huó	Root and rhizome of Angelica pubescens	五兩 5 liǎng	15g
防風	fáng fēng	Root of Ledebouriella divaricata	二兩 2 liǎng	6g
秦椒	qín jiāo	Seed capsule of Zanthoxylum bungeanum	二兩 2 liǎng	6g
桂心	guì xīn	Shaved inner bark of Cinnamomum cassia	二兩 2 liǎng	6g

白朮	bái zhú	Rhizome of Atractylodes macrocephala	二兩 2 liǎng	6g
甘草	gān cǎo	Root of Glycyrrhiza uralensis	二兩 2 liǎng	6g
當歸	dāng guī	Root of Angelica polimorpha	二兩 2 liǎng	6g
附子	fù zǐ	Lateral root of Aconitum carmichaeli	二兩 2 liǎng	6g
葛根	gé gēn	Root of Pueraria lobata	三兩 3 liǎng	9g
生薑	shēng jiāng	Fresh root of Zingiber officinale	五兩 5 liǎng	15g
防己	fáng jǐ	Root of Aristolochia fangchi	一兩 1 liǎng	3g

上十一味，㕮咀，以水一斗二升煮取三升，去滓，分三服。

Pound the above eleven ingredients and decoct in one *dǒu* and two *shēng* of water to obtain three *shēng*. Discard the dregs and divide into three doses.

LINE 3.7

雞糞酒主產後中風及百病，並男子中一切風，神效方。

Chicken's Droppings Wine is the governing prescription for postpartum wind strike and the [other] myriad [postpartum] diseases, as well as for every type of wind strike in men. Divine efficacy.

Chicken's Droppings Wine
雞糞酒 *jī fèn jiǔ*

雞糞（一升，熬令黃）烏豆（一升，熬令聲絕，勿焦）。

雞糞,熬令黃	jī fèn, āo lìng huáng	Excrement of Gallus gallus domesticus, roasted until yellow	一升 1 shēng	24g
烏豆,熬令聲絕，勿焦	wū dòu, āo lìng shēng jué, wù jiāo	Black Glycine max, roasted until they stop making sounds, but not scorched	一升 1 shēng	24g

上二味，以清酒三升半先淋雞糞，次淋豆，取汁。一服一升，溫服取汗。病重者，凡四五日服之，無不愈。

Of the two ingredients above, first wet the chicken's droppings in three and a half *shēng* of clear liquor, then wet the beans, and take the liquid. Take one *shēng* per dose heated to induce sweating. For serious conditions, take it continuously for four or five days, and [the patient] is bound to recover.

LINE 3.8

治產後中風，發熱，面正赤，喘氣，頭痛，竹葉湯方。

Bamboo Leaf Decoction treats postpartum wind strike with fever, full red facial complexion, panting, and headache.

Bamboo Leaf Decoction
竹葉湯 *zhú yè tāng*

淡竹葉（一握）葛根（三兩）防風（二兩）桔梗 甘草 人參（各一兩）大附子（一枚）生薑（五兩）大棗（十五枚）桂心（一兩）。

淡竹葉	dàn zhú yè	Leaves of Lopatherum gracile	一握 1 wò	1 handful
葛根	gé gēn	Root of Pueraria lobata	三兩 3 liǎng	9g
防風	fáng fēng	Root of Ledebouriella divaricata	二兩 2 liǎng	6g
桔梗	jié gěng	Root of Platycodon grandiflorum	一兩 1 liǎng	3g
甘草	gān cǎo	Root of Glycyrrhiza uralensis	一兩 1 liǎng	3g
人參	rén shēn	Root of Panax ginseng	一兩 1 liǎng	3g
大附子	dà fù zǐ	Lateral root of Aconitum carmichaeli	一枚 1 méi	1 big pc
生薑	shēng jiāng	Fresh root of Zingiber officinale	五兩 5 liǎng	15g
大棗	dà zǎo	Mature fruit of Ziziphus jujuba	十五枚 15 méi	15 pcs
桂心	guì xīn	Shaved inner bark of Cinnamomum cassia	一兩 1 liǎng	3g

上十味，㕮咀，以水一斗煮取二升半，去滓。分三服，日三，溫覆使汗出。若頸項強者，用大附子；若嘔者，加半夏四兩。

Pound the above ten ingredients and decoct in one *dǒu* of water to obtain two and a half *shēng*. Discard the dregs, divide into three doses, and take three times a day. Keep [the patient] warm and covered to induce sweating.* In cases of rigidity of the nape and neck, use a large [piece of] *fù zǐ* 附子; In cases of retching, add four *liǎng* of *bàn xià* 半夏.

---

*   Instead of this sentence, the *Sūn Zhēn Rén* edition advises the opposite: 勿使得汗 *wù shǐ dé hàn* (do not make her sweat).

LINE 3.9

防風湯治產後中風，背急，短氣方。

Saposhnikovia Decoction treats postpartum wind strike with tension in the back and shortness of breath.*

* Sòng editors' note: "The *Qiān Jīn Yì Fāng* instead has 'internal tension and shortness of breath.'"

Saposhnikovia Decoction
防風湯 *fáng fēng tāng*

防風（五兩） 當歸 芍藥 人參 甘草 乾薑（各二兩） 獨活 葛根（各五兩）。

防風	fáng fēng	Root of Ledebouriella divaricata	五兩 5 liǎng	15g
當歸	dāng guī	Root of Angelica polimorpha	二兩 2 liǎng	6g
芍藥	sháo yào	Root of Paeonia albiflora	二兩 2 liǎng	6g
人參	rén shēn	Root of Panax ginseng	二兩 2 liǎng	6g
甘草	gān cǎo	Root of Glycyrrhiza uralensis	二兩 2 liǎng	6g
乾薑	gān jiāng	Dried root of Zingiber officinale	二兩 2 liǎng	6g
獨活	dú huó	Root and rhizome of Angelica pubescens	五兩 5 liǎng	15g
葛根	gé gēn	Root of Pueraria lobata	五兩 5 liǎng	15g

上八味，㕮咀，以水九升煮取三升，去滓。分三服，日三。

Pound the above eight ingredients and decoct in nine *shēng* of water to obtain three *shēng*. Discard the dregs and divide into three doses, to be taken three times a day.

LINE 3.10

鹿肉湯治產後風虛，頭痛，壯熱，言語邪僻方。

Venison Decoction treats postpartum wind vacuity with headache, vigorous heat [effusion], and evil and mean speech.

Venison Decoction
鹿肉湯 *lù ròu tāng*

鹿肉（三斤） 芍藥（三兩） 半夏（一升） 乾地黃（二兩） 獨活（三兩）
生薑（六兩） 桂心 芎藭（各一兩） 甘草 阿膠（各一兩） 人參 茯苓（各四
兩，《千金翼》作茯神） 秦艽 黃芩 黃芪（各三兩）。

鹿肉	lù ròu	Meat of Cervus nippon	三斤 3 jīn	144g
芍藥	sháo yào	Root of Paeonia albiflora	三兩 3 liǎng	9g
半夏	bàn xià	Rhizome of Pinellia ternata	一升 1 shēng	24g
乾地黃	gān dì huáng	Dried root of Rehmannia glutinosa	二兩 2 liǎng	6g
獨活	dú huó	Root and rhizome of Angelica pubescens	三兩 3 liǎng	9g
生薑	shēng jiāng	Fresh root of Zingiber officinale	六兩 6 liǎng	18g
桂心	guì xīn	Shaved inner bark of Cinnamomum cassia	一兩 1 liǎng	3g
川芎	chuān xiōng	Root of Ligusticum wallichii	一兩 1 liǎng	3g
甘草	gān cǎo	Root of Glycyrrhiza uralensis	一兩 1 liǎng	3g
阿膠	ē jiāo	Gelatinous glue produced from Equus asinus	一兩 1 liǎng	3g
人參	rén shēn	Root of Panax ginseng	四兩 4 liǎng	12g
茯苓*	fú líng	Dried fungus of Poria cocos	四兩 4 liǎng	12g
秦艽	qín jiāo	Root of Gentiana macrophylla	三兩 3 liǎng	9g
黃芩	huáng qín	Root of Scutellaria baicalensis	三兩 3 liǎng	9g
黃芪	huáng qí	Root of Astragalus membranaceus	三兩 3 liǎng	9g

上十五味，㕮咀，以水二斗煮肉得一斗二升，去肉內藥，煎取三升，去
滓，內膠令烊。分四服，日三夜一。

Pound the above fifteen ingredients. Cook the meat in two *dǒu* of water to obtain one *dǒu* and two *shēng*. Remove the meat, add the drugs, and simmer to obtain three *shēng*. Discard the dregs and add the gelatin, letting it melt. Divide into four doses and take three times during the day and once at night.

*   *Sòng* editors' note: "The *Qiān Jīn Yì Fāng* has *fú shén* (茯神 Sclerotium (i.e., white, hardened core in the center) of Poria cocos)."

LINE 3.11

治產後中風，獨活酒方。

Pubescent Angelica Wine treats postpartum wind strike.

Pubescent Angelica Wine
獨活酒 *dú huó jiǔ*

獨活（一斤）桂心（三兩）秦艽（五兩）。

獨活	dú huó	Root and rhizome of Angelica pubescens	一斤 1 jīn	48g
桂心	guì xīn	Shaved inner bark of Cinnamomum cassia	三兩 3 liǎng	9g
秦艽	qín jiāo	Root of Gentiana macrophylla	五兩 5 liǎng	15g

上三味，哎咀，以酒一斗半漬三日，飲五合，稍加至一升。不能多飲，隨性服。*

Pound the above three ingredients and soak in one and a half *dǒu* of liquor for three days. Drink five *gě* [per dose], gradually increasing it to a maximum of one *shēng*. She may not drink too much and take it at her will.

---

* 不能多飲隨性服 *bù néng duō yǐn suí xìng fú*: This could also be interpreted as: "If she cannot drink a lot, she can take it at her will." However, the *Sūn Zhēn Rén* edition has an abbreviated version that clarifies the meaning. It merely states: "She may not [take it] at her will." 不能隨性 *bù néng suí xìng*.

LINE 3.12

大豆湯主產後卒中風，發病倒悶不知人，及妊娠挾風，兼治在蓐諸疾方。

Soybean Decoction is the governing prescription for postpartum sudden wind strike with falling, oppression, and inability to recognize people when the condition erupts, as well as for wind complications during pregnancy, and also treats the various sicknesses when in childbed.

Soybean Decoction
大豆湯 *dà dòu tāng*

大豆（五升，炒令微焦）葛根 獨活（各八兩）防已（六兩）。

大豆, 炒令微焦	dà dòu, chǎo lìng wēi jiāo	Seed of Glycine max, fried until lightly scorched	五升 5 shēng	120g
葛根	gé gēn	Root of Pueraria lobata	八兩 8 liǎng	24g
獨活	dú huó	Root and rhizome of Angelica pubescens	八兩 8 liǎng	24g
防己	fáng jǐ	Root of Aristolochia fangchi	六兩 6 liǎng	18g

上四味，㕮咀，以酒一斗二升煮豆取八升，去滓內藥，煮取四升，去滓。分六服，日四夜二。

Pound the above four ingredients. Cook the beans in one *dǒu* and two *shēng* of liquor to obtain eight *shēng*. Discard the dregs and add the drugs, decocting them to obtain four *shēng*. Discard the dregs. Divide into six doses and take four times during the day and twice at night.

LINE 3.13

五石湯主產後卒中風，發疾口噤，倒悶吐沫，瘛瘲，眩冒，不知人，及濕痹緩弱，身體痙，妊娠百病方。

Five Stones Decoction is the governing prescription for postpartum sudden wind strike with clenched mouth, falling, oppression, and foaming at the mouth, tugging and slackening [of the channels],[1] veiling dizziness, and inability to recognize people, when the disease erupts; as well as for damp impediment[2] with flaccidity, generalized tetany, and the myriad diseases of pregnancy.

Five Stones Decoction
五石湯 *wǔ shí tāng*

白石英 鍾乳 赤石脂 石膏（各二兩） 紫石英（三兩） 牡蠣 人參 黃芩 白朮 甘草 栝樓根 芎藭 桂心 防己 當歸 乾薑（各二兩） 獨活（三兩） 葛根（四兩）。

白石英	bái shí yīng	White quartz	二兩 2 liǎng	6g
鍾乳	zhōng rǔ	Stalactite	二兩 2 liǎng	6g
赤石脂	chì shí zhī	Halloysite	二兩 2 liǎng	6g
石膏	shí gāo	Gypsum	二兩 2 liǎng	6g
紫石英	zǐ shí yīng	Fluorite	三兩 3 liǎng	9g
牡蠣	mǔ lì	Shell of Ostrea rivularis	二兩 2 liǎng	6g
人參	rén shēn	Root of Panax ginseng	二兩 2 liǎng	6g

黃芩	huáng qín	Root of Scutellaria baicalensis	二兩 2 liǎng	6g
白朮	bái zhú	Rhizome of Atractylodes macrocephala	二兩 2 liǎng	6g
甘草	gān cǎo	Root of Glycyrrhiza uralensis	二兩 2 liǎng	6g
栝蔞根	guā lóu gēn	Root of Trichosanthes kirilowii	二兩 2 liǎng	6g
川芎	chuān xiōng	Root of Ligusticum wallichii	二兩 2 liǎng	6g
桂心	guì xīn	Shaved inner bark of Cinnamomum cassia	二兩 2 liǎng	6g
防己	fáng jǐ	Root of Aristolochia fangchi	二兩 2 liǎng	6g
當歸	dāng guī	Root of Angelica polimorpha	二兩 2 liǎng	6g
乾薑	gān jiāng	Dried root of Zingiber officinale	二兩 2 liǎng	6g
獨活	dú huó	Root and rhizome of Angelica pubescens	三兩 3 liǎng	9g
葛根	gé gēn	Root of Pueraria lobata	四兩 4 liǎng	12g

上十八味，末五石，咬咀諸藥，以水一斗四升煮取三升半，分五服，日三夜二。

Of the eighteen ingredients above, pulverize the five stones and pound all the drugs. Decoct [everything] in one *dǒu* and four *shēng* of water to obtain three and a half *shēng*. Divide into five doses and take three times during the day and twice at night.[3]

1. 瘛瘲 *chì zòng*: A condition where the channels and sinews contract and relax involuntarily, identical to the more common variant 瘈瘲 *chì zòng* (as in the following prescription). According to the *Líng Shū*, it is caused by tension in the heart channel and always related to fire stirring up wind. See 《中華醫學大辭典》 p. 1541 and Wiseman and Féng, *Practical Dictionary*, p. 631.
2. 濕痺 *shī bì*: 痺 is a disease defined in *Sù Wèn* as follows: "The three *qì* of wind, cold, and dampness arrive mixed together, they combine to form impediment... Impediment means blockage (痺閉也 *bì bì yě*). Blood and *qì* are congealed and inhibited and fail to flow. Impediment can be differentiated by the three [types of] *qì* into wind, cold, and dampness. It can also be differentiated into impediment of the skin, muscles, sinews, bones, five viscera, of the outside, and mixed..." (《素文》 43). For a modern TCM explanation, see Wiseman and Féng, *Practical Dictionary*, pp. 295-296, entry on "impediment."
3. *Sòng* editors' note: "Another [version of this] prescription includes two *liǎng* each of *huá shí* (滑石 Talcum) and *hán shuǐ shí* (寒水石 Sodium calcium sulfate), and twenty pieces of *dà zǎo* (大棗 Mature fruit of Ziziphus jujuba).
   This note is found both in the editions revised during the *Sòng* period as well as the *Sūn Zhēn Rén* edition. It could therefore stem from the original text.

LINE 3.14

四石湯治產後卒中風，發疾口噤，瘈瘲，悶滿，不知人，並緩急諸風毒痺，身體痙強，及挾胎中風，婦人百病方。

Four Stones Decoction treats sudden postpartum wind strike with clenched mouth, tugging and slackening [of the channels], oppression and fullness, and inability to recognize people, when the disease erupts; as well as slackening and tensing in the various wind poison impediments, generalized tetany and rigidity, and lastly wind strike during pregnancy and the myriad diseases of women.

Four Stones Decoction
四石湯 *sì shí tāng*

紫石英 白石英 石膏 赤石脂（各三兩） 獨活 生薑（各六兩） 葛根（四兩）
桂心 芎藭 甘草 芍藥 黃芩（各二兩）。

紫石英	zǐ shí yīng	Fluorite	三兩 3 liǎng	9g
白石英	bái shí yīng	White quartz	三兩 3 liǎng	9g
石膏	shí gāo	Gypsum	三兩 3 liǎng	9g
赤石脂	chì shí zhī	Halloysite	三兩 3 liǎng	9g
獨活	dú huó	Root and rhizome of Angelica pubescens	六兩 6 liǎng	18g
生薑	shēng jiāng	Fresh root of Zingiber officinale	六兩 6 liǎng	18g
葛根	gé gēn	Root of Pueraria lobata	四兩 4 liǎng	12g
桂心	guì xīn	Shaved inner bark of Cinnamomum cassia	二兩 2 liǎng	6g
川芎	chuān xiōng	Root of Ligusticum wallichii	二兩 2 liǎng	6g
甘草	gān cǎo	Root of Glycyrrhiza uralensis	二兩 2 liǎng	6g
芍藥	sháo yào	Root of Paeonia albiflora	二兩 2 liǎng	6g
黃芩	huáng qín	Root of Scutellaria baicalensis	二兩 2 liǎng	6g

上十二味，㕮咀，以水一斗二升煮取三升半，去滓。分五服，日三夜二。

Pound the above twelve ingredients and decoct in one *dǒu* and two *shēng* of water to obtain three and a half *shēng*. Discard the dregs and divide into five doses, to take three times during the day and twice at night.

LINE 3.15

治婦人在蓐得風，蓋四肢苦煩熱，皆自發露所為。若頭痛，與小柴胡湯；頭
不痛但煩熱，與三物黃芩湯。小柴胡湯方。

A treatment for women who have contracted wind while in childbed, possibly with discomfort, vexation, and heat in the four limbs. This is always caused by the occurrence of [malign] dew.[1] In cases with headache, give *Minor Bupleurum Decoction*.[2] In cases with no headache and only vexing heat, give *Three Agents Scutellaria Decoction*.

Minor Bupleurum Decoction
小柴胡湯 *xiǎo chái hú tāng*

柴胡（半斤）黃芩 人參 甘草（各三兩）生薑（二兩）大棗（十二枚）半夏（半升）。

柴胡	chái hú	Root of Bupleurum chinense	半斤 0.5 jīn	24g
黃芩	huáng qín	Root of Scutellaria baicalensis	三兩 3 liǎng	9g
人參	rén shēn	Root of Panax ginseng	三兩 3 liǎng	9g
甘草	gān cǎo	Root of Glycyrrhiza uralensis	三兩 3 liǎng	9g
生薑	shēng jiāng	Fresh root of Zingiber officinale	二兩 2 liǎng	6g
大棗	dà zǎo	Mature fruit of Ziziphus jujuba	十二枚 12 méi	12 pcs
半夏	bàn xià	Rhizome of Pinellia ternata	半升 0.5 shēng	12g

上七味，㕮咀，以水一斗二升煮取六升，去滓。服一升，日三服。

Pound the above seven ingredients and decoct in one *dǒu* and two *shēng* of water to obtain six *shēng*. Discard the dregs and take one *shēng* per dose three times a day.

1. 發露 *fā lù*: This refers to "malign dew" (惡露 *è lù*) or lochia, the old blood and fetal matter remaining in the uterus after childbirth, which were considered highly pathogenic. See chapter five of volume three on the treatment of "Malign Dew" (pp. 318 - 336 below).
2. The following prescription for *Minor Bupleurum Decoction* is missing in the *Sūn Zhēn Rén* edition.

LINE 3.16

Three Agents Scutellaria Decoction
三物黃芩湯 *sān wù huáng qín tāng*

黃令 苦三（各二兩）乾地黃（四兩）。

黃芩	huáng qín	Root of Scutellaria baicalensis	二兩 2 liǎng	6g
苦參	kǔ shēn	Root of Sophora flavescens	二兩 2 liǎng	6g
乾地黃	gān dì huáng	Dried root of Rehmannia glutinosa	四兩 4 liǎng	12g

上㕮咀，以水八升煮取二升，去滓。適寒溫服一升，日二。多吐，下蟲。

Pound the above [ingredients] and decoct in eight *shēng* water to obtain two *shēng*. Discard the dregs. Take one *shēng* twice a day at whatever temperature you like. It will cause increased vomiting and precipitate worms.

LINE 3.17

治產後腹中傷絕，寒熱，恍惚，狂言見鬼，此病中風內絕，藏氣虛所為，甘草湯方。

Licorice Decoction treats postpartum abdominal damage and expiry with [aversion to] cold and heat [effusion], abstraction, and manic speech and visions of ghosts. This condition is caused by wind strike [leading to] internal expiry and by a vacuity of visceral *qi*.

Licorice Decoction
甘草湯 *gān cǎo tāng*

甘草 芍藥（各五兩） 通草（三兩，《產寶》用當歸） 羊肉（三斤）。

甘草	gān cǎo	Root of Glycyrrhiza uralensis	五兩 5 liǎng	15g
芍藥	sháo yào	Root of Paeonia albiflora	五兩 5 liǎng	15g
通草*	tōng cǎo	Pith in the stalk of Tetrapanax papyriferus	三兩 3 liǎng	9g
羊肉	yáng ròu	Meat of Capra hircus	三斤 3 jīn	144g

上四味，㕮咀，以水一斗六升煮肉，取一斗，去肉內藥，煮取六升，去滓。分五服，日三夜二。

Pound the above four ingredients. Cook the meat in one *dǒu* and six *shēng* of water to obtain one *dǒu*. Remove the meat, add the drugs, and decoct them to obtain six *shēng*. Discard the dregs. Divide into five doses and take it three times during the day and twice at night.

* *Sòng* editors' note: "The *Chǎn Bǎo* uses *dāng guī* (當歸 Root of Angelica polimorpha)."

LINE 3.18

羊肉湯治產後中風，久絕不產，月水不利，乍赤乍白，及男子虛勞冷盛方。

Sheep or Goat's Meat Decoction treats postpartum wind strike with chronic infertility and failure to bear children, inhibited menstruation, and abruptly alternating red and white [vaginal discharge], as well as vacuity taxation and exuberant cold in men.

Sheep or Goat's Meat Decoction
羊肉湯 yáng ròu tāng

羊肉（二斤）成擇大蒜（去皮，切，三升）香豉（三升）。

羊肉	yáng ròu	Meat of Capra hircus or Ovis aries	二斤 2 jīn	96g
大蒜, 去皮 , 切	dà suàn, qù pí, qiē	Bulb of Allium sativum, leafed-out, peeled and chopped	三升 3 shēng	72g
香豉	xiāng chǐ	Preparation of Fermented Glycine max	三升 3 shēng	72g

上三味，以水一斗三升煮取五升，去滓，內酥一升，更煮取三升，分溫三服。

Decoct the above three ingredients in one *dǒu* and three *shēng* of water to obtain five *shēng*. Discard the dregs, add one *shēng* of butter, and decoct it again to obtain three *shēng*. Divide it into three doses and take it heated.

LINE 3.19

葛根湯治產後中風，口噤痙痹，氣息迫急，眩冒困頓，並產後諸疾方。

Pueraria Decoction treats postpartum wind strike, clenched mouth, tetany, and impediment, distressed and rapid breathing, veiling dizziness and drowsiness, as well as the various [other] postpartum diseases.

Pueraria Decoction
葛根湯 gé gēn tāng

葛根 生薑（各六兩） 獨活（四兩） 當歸（三兩） 甘草 桂心 茯苓 石膏 人參 白朮 芎藭 防風（各二兩）。

葛根	gé gēn	Root of Pueraria lobata	六兩 6 liǎng	18g
生薑	shēng jiāng	Fresh root of Zingiber officinale	六兩 6 liǎng	18g
獨活	dú huó	Root and rhizome of Angelica pubescens	四兩 4 liǎng	12g
當歸	dāng guī	Root of Angelica polimorpha	三兩 3 liǎng	9g
甘草	gān cǎo	Root of Glycyrrhiza uralensis	二兩 2 liǎng	6g

桂心	guì xīn	Shaved inner bark of Cinnamomum cassia	二兩 2 liǎng	6g
茯苓	fú líng	Dried fungus of Poria cocos	二兩 2 liǎng	6g
石膏	shí gāo	Gypsum	二兩 2 liǎng	6g
人參	rén shēn	Root of Panax ginseng	二兩 2 liǎng	6g
白朮	bái zhú	Rhizome of Atractylodes macrocephala	二兩 2 liǎng	6g
川芎	chuān xiōng	Root of Ligusticum wallichii	二兩 2 liǎng	6g
防風	fáng fēng	Root of Ledebouriella divaricata	二兩 2 liǎng	6g

上十二味，㕮咀，以水一斗二升煮取三升，去滓。分三服，日三。

Pound the above twelve ingredients and decoct in one *dǒu* and two *shēng* of water to obtain three *shēng*. Discard the dregs. Divide into three doses and take three times a day.

LINE 3.20

治產後中風，防風酒方。

Saposhnikovia Wine treats postpartum wind strike.

Saposhnikovia Wine
防風酒 *fáng fēng jiǔ*

防風 獨活（各一升） 女萎 桂心（各二兩） 茵芋（一兩） 石斛（五兩）。

防風	fáng fēng	Root of Ledebouriella divaricata	一升 1 shēng	24g
獨活	dú huó	Root and rhizome of Angelica pubescens	一升 1 shēng	24g
女萎	nǔ wěi	Stalk of Clematis apiifolia	二兩 2 liǎng	6g
桂心	guì xīn	Shaved inner bark of Cinnamomum cassia	二兩 2 liǎng	6g
茵芋	yīn yù	Foliage and stalk of Skimmia reevesiana	一兩 1 liǎng	3g
石斛	shí hú	Whole plant of Dendrobium nobile	五兩 5 liǎng	15g

上六味，㕮咀，以酒二斗漬三宿。初服一合，稍加至三四合，日三。

Pound the above six ingredients and soak for three nights in two *dǒu* of liquor. At first, take one *gě* per dose, then increase it gradually to a maximum of three or four *gě*, taken three times a day.

LINE 3.21

治產後中風，木防已膏方。

Woody Fangji Paste treats postpartum wind strike.

Woody Fangji Paste
木防己膏 *mù fáng jǐ gāo*

木防己（半升）茵芋（五兩）。

木防己	mù fáng jǐ	Root of Cocculus trilobus	半升	0.5 shēng	12g
茵芋	yīn yù	Foliage and stalk of Skimmia reevesiana	五兩	5 liǎng	15g

上二味，哎咀，以苦酒九升漬一宿，豬膏四升煎，三上三下，膏成，炙手摩千遍，瘥。

Pound the above two ingredients and soak for one night in nine *shēng* of bitter liquor. Heat it in four *shēng* of pork lard, letting it rise and settle three times, until the salve is done. Massage it in with warm hands, rubbing [the patient] a thousand times, and she will recover.

LINE 3.22

治產後中柔風，舉體疼痛，自汗出者，及餘百疾方。

This prescription treats mild cases of postpartum wind strike with pain all over the body and spontaneous sweating, as well as the other myriad diseases.

Formula

獨活（八兩）當歸（四兩）。

獨活	dú huó	Root and rhizome of Angelica pubescens	八兩	8 liǎng	24g
當歸	dāng guī	Root of Angelica polimorpha	四兩	4 liǎng	12g

上二味，哎咀，以酒八升煮取四升，去滓。分四服，日三夜一，取微汗。若上氣者，加桂心二兩，不瘥更作。

Pound the above two ingredients and decoct in eight *shēng* of liquor to obtain four *shēng*. Discard the dregs. Divide into four doses and take three times during the day and once at night. Induce light sweating.

In cases of *qì* ascent, add two *liǎng* of *guì xīn* (桂心Shaved inner bark of Cinnamomum cassia). If she fails to recover, make another batch.*

---

*   *Sòng* editors' note: "Master Gě uses only *dú huó* 獨活 as a single agent. The *Xiǎo Pǐn Fāng* adds *dāng guī* 當歸."

LINE 3.23

治產後中風流腫，浴湯方。

This bath decoction treats postpartum wind strike with drifting swelling.[1]

Formula

鹽（五升，熬令赤）雞毛（一把，燒作灰）。

鹽，熬令赤	yán, āo lìng chì	salt, toasted until glowing red	五升 5 shēng	120g
雞毛，燒作灰	jī máo, shāo zuò huī	Feathers of Gallus gallus domesticus, charred into ashes	一把 1 bǎ	1 handful

上二味，以水一石煮鹽作湯，內雞毛灰著湯中。適冷暖以浴，大良。又浴婦人陰冷腫痛。凡風腫，面欲裂破者，以紫湯一服瘥，神效。紫湯是炒黑豆作者。

Of the two ingredients above, boil the salt in one *dàn* of water to make a decoction, then add the chicken feather ashes to the hot liquid. Bathe in this at whatever temperature she likes. It is very good. Also, bathe a woman's genitals if they are cold, swollen, or painful. In all cases of wind swelling with [the skin of] the face about to crack, give her one dose of *Purple Decoction* and she will recover. Divine efficacy. *Purple Decoction* is made from fried *hēi dòu* (黑豆 Seed of Glycine soja).[2]

---

1.   流腫 *liú zhǒng*: an accumulation of water, pus, or blood that moves around in the body. I interpret 流 as "drifting" (rather than as a type of swelling that is "streaming" in the sense of leaking fluids) based on similar expressions such as 流痧 *liú shā* (drifting sand syndrome, a condition of toxic heat *qì* moving around in the body, erupting as skin papules or swellings at various times and places (see Wiseman and Féng, *Practical Dictionary*, p. 512, and 《中華醫學大辭典》 p. 1064) or 流火 *liú huǒ* (drifting fire, a condition of wind impediment that is called as such because the pain moves around (see 《中華醫學大辭典》 p. 1062). See also 張登本, 主編《內經辭典》 p. 304.

2.   紫湯 *zǐ tāng*: Due to its location within this prescription, this could mean to make the infusion by mixing the charred chicken feathers into a base of *hēi dòu* 黑豆 decoction rather than salt water. Or it could mean to orally take *Purple Decoction* in conjuction with the bath treatment. For instructions on making soybean decoction, see the first prescrip-

tion in this section, "*Soybean Purple Decoction*," in Line 3.2 (pp. 268 - 270) above.

LINE 3.24

治產後中風，頭面手臂通滿方。

This prescription treats postpartum wind strike with fullness throughout the head, face, hands, and shoulders.

大豆三升，以水六升煮取一升半，去豆澄清，更煎取一升，內白朮八兩，附子三兩，獨活三兩，生薑八兩，添水一斗，煎取五升，內好酒五升，合煎，取五升，去滓，分五服，日三夜二。間粥頻服三劑。

Cook three *shēng* of *dà dòu* (大豆 Seed of Glycine max) in six *shēng* of water to obtain one and a half *shēng*. Remove the beans and clarify it by letting the impurities settle to the bottom. Simmer it again to obtain one *shēng*. Add eight *liǎng* of *bái zhú* (白朮 Rhizome of Atractylodes macrocephala), three *liǎng* of *fù zǐ* (附子 Lateral root of Aconitum carmichaeli), three *liǎng* of *dú huó* (獨活 Root and rhizome of Angelica pubescens), and eight *liǎng* of *shēng jiāng* (生薑 Fresh root of Zingiber officinale). Increase the water by adding one *dǒu*, and simmer it to obtain five *shēng*. Add five *shēng* of good liquor and simmer it all together to obtain five *shēng*. Discard the dregs. Divide into five doses and take three times a day and twice at night. Take three preparations [of the medicine] in small doses, separated by gruel.*

---

*   間粥 *jiàn zhōu*: This means to eat some gruel in between taking the medicine.

LINE 3.25

茯神湯治產後忽苦心中衝悸，或志意不定，恍恍惚惚，言語錯謬，心虛所致方。

Root Poria Decoction treats sudden discomfort from surging palpitations* in the center of the heart after childbirth, possibly with instability of the will, severe abstraction, and deranged and absurd speech, all of which are caused by heart vacuity.

Root Poria Decoction

茯神湯 *fú shén tāng*

茯神（四兩）人參 茯苓（各三兩）芍藥 甘草 當歸 桂心（各一兩）生薑（八兩）大棗（三十枚）。

茯神	fú shén	Sclerotium (i.e., white, hardened core in the center) of Poria cocos	四兩 4 liǎng	12g
人參	rén shēn	Root of Panax ginseng	三兩 3 liǎng	9g
茯苓	fú líng	Dried fungus of Poria cocos	三兩 3 liǎng	9g
芍藥	sháo yào	Root of Paeonia albiflora	一兩 1 liǎng	3g
甘草	gān cǎo	Root of Glycyrrhiza uralensis	一兩 1 liǎng	3g
當歸	dāng guī	Root of Angelica polimorpha	一兩 1 liǎng	3g
桂心	guì xīn	Shaved inner bark of Cinnamomum cassia	一兩 1 liǎng	3g
生薑	shēng jiāng	Fresh root of Zingiber officinale	八兩 8 liǎng	24g
大棗	dà zǎo	Mature fruit of Ziziphus jujuba	三十枚 30 méi	30 pcs

上九味，㕮咀，以水一斗煮取三升，去滓。分三服，日三，甚良。

Pound the above nine ingredients and decoct in one *dǒu* of water to obtain three *shēng*. Discard the dregs. Divide into three doses and take three times a day. Excellent.

*   衝悸 *chōng jì*: The *Sūn Zhēn Rén* edition has 惊悸 *jīng jì* (fright palpitations) instead.

LINE 3.26

遠志湯治產後忽苦心中衝悸不定，志意不安，言語錯誤，惚惚憒憒，情不自覺方。

Polygala Decoction treats sudden discomfort from surging palpitations and instability in the center of the heart, a disquieted will, deranged and false speech, severe confusion and muddleheadedness, and lack of awareness of one's own affects.

Polygala Decoction
遠志湯 *yuǎn zhì tāng*

遠志 人參 甘草 當歸 桂心 麥門冬（各二兩） 芍藥（一兩） 茯苓（五兩） 生薑（六兩） 大棗（二十枚）。

遠志	yuǎn zhì	Root of Polygala tenuifolia	二兩 2 liǎng	6g
人參	rén shēn	Root of Panax ginseng	二兩 2 liǎng	6g
甘草	gān cǎo	Root of Glycyrrhiza uralensis	二兩 2 liǎng	6g
當歸	dāng guī	Root of Angelica polimorpha	二兩 2 liǎng	6g

桂心	guì xīn	Shaved inner bark of Cinnamomum cassia	二兩 2 liǎng	6g
麥門冬	mài mén dōng	Tuber of Ophiopogon japonicus	二兩 2 liǎng	6g
芍藥	sháo yào	Root of Paeonia albiflora	一兩 1 liǎng	3g
茯苓	fú líng	Dried fungus of Poria cocos	一兩 1 liǎng	3g
生薑	shēng jiāng	Fresh root of Zingiber officinale	六兩 6 liǎng	18g
大棗	dà zǎo	Mature fruit of Ziziphus jujuba	二十枚 20 méi	20 pcs

上十味，㕮咀，以水一斗煮取三升，去滓。分三服，日三，羸者分四服。產後得此，正是心虛所致。無當歸，用芎藭。若其人心胸中逆氣，加半夏三兩。

Pound the above ten ingredients and decoct in one *dǒu* of water to obtain three *shēng*. Discard the dregs. Divide into three doses and take three times a day. For markedly emaciated patients, divide into four doses. If she has contracted this after childbirth, it is directly caused by heart vacuity. If you do not have *dāng guī* 當歸, use *chuān xiōng* (川芎 Root of Ligusticum wallichii). In cases of counterflow *qì* in the center of the person's heart and chest, add three *liǎng* of *bàn xià* (半夏 Rhizome of Pinellia ternata).

LINE 3.27

茯苓湯治產後暴苦心悸不定，言語謬錯，恍恍惚惚，心中憒憒，此皆心虛所致方。

Poria Decoction treats fulminant discomfort from heart palpitations after childbirth with absurd and deranged speech, severe abstraction, and muddle-headedness in the center of the heart; all of which are caused by heart vacuity.

Poria Decoction
茯苓湯 *fú líng tāng*

茯苓（五兩）甘草 芍藥 桂心（各二兩）生薑（六兩）當歸（二兩）麥門冬（一升）大棗（三十枚）。

茯苓	fú líng	Dried fungus of Poria cocos	五兩 5 liǎng	15g
甘草	gān cǎo	Root of Glycyrrhiza uralensis	二兩 2 liǎng	6g
芍藥	sháo yào	Root of Paeonia albiflora	二兩 2 liǎng	6g
桂心	guì xīn	Shaved inner bark of Cinnamomum cassia	二兩 2 liǎng	6g
生薑	shēng jiāng	Fresh root of Zingiber officinale	六兩 6 liǎng	18g

當歸	dāng guī	Root of Angelica polimorpha	二兩 2 liǎng	6g
麥門冬	mài mén dōng	Tuber of Ophiopogon japonicus	一升 1 shēng	24g
大棗	dà zǎo	Mature fruit of Ziziphus jujuba	三十枚 30 méi	30 pcs

上八味，㕮咀，以水一斗煮取三升，去滓。分三服，日三。無當歸，可用
芎藭。若苦心志不定，加人參二兩，亦可內遠志二兩；若苦煩悶短氣，加生
竹葉一升，先以水一斗三升煮竹葉，取一斗，內藥；若有微風，加獨活三
兩，麻黃二兩，桂心二兩，用水一斗五升；若䯍項苦急，背膊強者，加獨
活，葛根各三兩，麻黃，桂心各二兩，生薑八兩，用水一斗半。

Pound the above eight ingredients and decoct in one *dǒu* of water to obtain three *shēng*. Discard the dregs. Divide into three doses and take three times a day. If you don't have *dāng guī* 當歸, you can substitute *chuān xiōng* (川芎 Root of Ligusticum wallichii). For discomfort from instability in the heart and will, add two *liǎng* of *rén shēn* (人參 Root of Panax ginseng). You can also add two *liang* of *yuǎn zhì* (遠志 Root of Polygala tenuifolia). For discomfort from vexation, oppression, and shortness of breath, add one *shēng* of *shēng zhú yè* (生竹葉 Fresh leaves of Phyllostachys). First boil the *zhú yè* 竹葉 in one *dǒu* and three *shēng* of water to obtain one *dǒu*, then add the drugs. In cases of slight wind [conditions], add three *liǎng* of *dú huó* (獨活 Root and rhizome of Angelica pubescens), two *liǎng* of *má huáng* (麻黃 Stalk of Ephedra sinica), and two *liǎng* of *guì xīn* (桂心 Shaved inner bark of Cinnamomum cassia), and use one *dǒu* and five *shēng* of water. For rigidity, discomfort, and tension in the neck, and rigidity in the back and upper arms, add three *liǎng* each of *dú huó* 獨活 and *gé gēn* (葛根 Root of Pueraria lobata), two *liǎng* each of *má huáng* 麻黃 and *guì xīn* 桂心, and eight *liǎng* of *shēng jiāng* (生薑 Fresh root of Zingiber officinale), and use one and a half *dǒu* of water.

LINE 3.28

安心湯治產後心衝悸不定，恍恍惚惚，不自知覺，言語錯誤，虛煩短氣，志
意不定，此是心虛所致方。

Heart-Quieting Decoction treats postpartum surges, palpitations, and instability in the heart, severe abstraction, lack of self-awareness, deranged and false speech, vacuity vexation and shortness of breath, and instability of the will, all of which are caused by heart vacuity.

Heart-Quieting Decoction
安心湯 *ān xīn tāng*

遠志 甘草（各二兩）人參 茯神 當歸 芍藥（各三兩）麥門冬（一升）大棗
（三十枚）。

遠志	yuǎn zhì	Root of Polygala tenuifolia	二兩 2 liǎng	6g
甘草	gān cǎo	Root of Glycyrrhiza uralensis	二兩 2 liǎng	6g
人參	rén shēn	Root of Panax ginseng	三兩 3 liǎng	9g
茯神	fú shén	Sclerotium (i.e., white, hardened core in the center) of Poria cocos	三兩 3 liǎng	9g
當歸	dāng guī	Root of Angelica polimorpha	三兩 3 liǎng	9g
芍藥	sháo yào	Root of Paeonia albiflora	三兩 3 liǎng	9g
麥門冬	mài mén dōng	Tuber of Ophiopogon japonicus	一升 1 shēng	24g
大棗	dà zǎo	Mature fruit of Ziziphus jujuba	三十枚 30 méi	30 pcs

上八味，㕮咀，以水一斗煮取三升，去滓。分三服，日三。若苦虛煩短氣者，加淡竹葉二升，水一斗二升煮竹葉，取一斗，內藥。若胸中少氣者，益甘草為三兩，善。

Pound the above eight ingredients and decoct in one *dǒu* of water to obtain three *shēng*. Discard the dregs. Divide into three doses and take three times a day. For discomfort from vacuity vexation and shortness of breath, add two *shēng* of *dàn zhú yè* (淡竹葉 Leaves of Lopatherum gracile). Decoct the *zhú yè* 竹葉 in one *dǒu* and two *shēng* of water to obtain one *dǒu* and [then] add the [other] drugs. In cases of shortage of *qì* in the center of the chest, it is good to increase the *gān cǎo* 甘草 to three *liǎng*.

LINE 3.29

甘草丸治產後心虛不足，虛悸，心神不安，吸吸乏氣，或若恍恍惚惚，不自覺知者方。

Licorice Pills treat postpartum vacuity and insufficiency in the heart, vacuity palpitations, disquieted heart spirit, lack of *qì* in spite of heavy inhalations, and possibly severe abstraction and lack of self-awareness.

Licorice Pills
甘草丸 *gān cǎo wán*

甘草（三兩）人參（二兩）遠志（三兩）麥門冬（二兩）昌蒲（三兩）澤瀉（一兩）桂心（一兩）乾薑（二兩）茯苓（二兩）大棗（五十枚）。

甘草	gān cǎo	Root of Glycyrrhiza uralensis	三兩 3 liǎng	9g
人參	rén shēn	Root of Panax ginseng	二兩 2 liǎng	6g
遠志	yuǎn zhì	Root of Polygala tenuifolia	三兩 3 liǎng	9g

麥門冬	mài mén dōng	Tuber of Ophiopogon japonicus	二兩 2 liǎng	6g
菖蒲	chāng pú	Rhizome of Acorus gramineus	三兩 3 liǎng	9g
澤瀉	zé xiè	Rhizome of Alisma plantago-aquatica	一兩 1 liǎng	3g
桂心	guì xīn	Shaved inner bark of Cinnamomum cassia	一兩 1 liǎng	3g
乾薑	gān jiāng	Dried root of Zingiber officinale	二兩 2 liǎng	6g
茯苓	fú líng	Dried fungus of Poria cocos	二兩 2 liǎng	6g
大棗	dà zǎo	Mature fruit of Ziziphus jujuba	五十枚 50 méi	50 pcs

上十味，末之，蜜丸如大豆。酒服二十丸，日四五服，夜再服，不知稍加。若無澤瀉，以白朮代之；若胸中冷，增乾薑。

Pulverize the above ten ingredients and [mix with] honey to make pills the size of soybeans. Take twenty pills in liquor, four or five doses a day and two at night. If no effect is noticed, gradually increase [the dosage]. If you do not have *zé xiè* 澤瀉, substitute *bái zhú* (白朮 Rhizome of Atractylodes macrocephala) for it. In cases of cold in the center of the chest, increase the [amount of] *gān jiāng* 乾薑.

LINE 3.30

人參丸治產後大虛心悸，志意不安，不自覺，恍惚恐畏，夜不得眠，虛煩少氣方。

Ginseng Pills treat serious postpartum vacuity heart palpitations, disquietude of the mind, lack of self-awareness, abstraction and panic, inability to sleep at night, and vacuity vexation and shortage of *qì*.

Ginseng Pills
人參丸 *rén shēn wán*

人參 甘草 茯苓（各三兩） 麥門冬 昌蒲 澤瀉 署預 乾薑（各二兩） 桂心（一兩） 大棗（五十枚）。

人參	rén shēn	Root of Panax ginseng	三兩 3 liǎng	9g
甘草	gān cǎo	Root of Glycyrrhiza uralensis	三兩 3 liǎng	9g
茯苓	fú líng	Dried fungus of Poria cocos	三兩 3 liǎng	9g
麥門冬	mài mén dōng	Tuber of Ophiopogon japonicus	二兩 2 liǎng	6g
菖蒲	chāng pú	Rhizome of Acorus gramineus	二兩 2 liǎng	6g

澤瀉	zé xiè	Rhizome of Alisma plantago-aquatica	二兩 2 liǎng	6g
薯蕷	shǔ yù	Root of Dioscorea opposita	二兩 2 liǎng	6g
乾薑	gān jiāng	Dried root of Zingiber officinale	二兩 2 liǎng	6g
桂心	guì xīn	Shaved inner bark of Cinnamomum cassia	一兩 1 liǎng	3g
大棗	dà zǎo	Mature fruit of Ziziphus jujuba	五十枚 50 méi	50 pcs

上十味，末之，以蜜棗膏和丸如梧子。未食酒服二十丸，日三夜一，不知稍增。若有遠志，內二兩為善。若風氣，內當歸，獨活三兩。亦治男子虛損心悸。

Pulverize the above ten ingredients and mix with honey and jujube paste to make pills the size of firmiana seeds. Take twenty pills in liquor before meals, three times during the day and once at night. If no effect is noticed, gradually increase [the dosage]. If you have *yuǎn zhì* (遠志 Root of Polygala tenuifolia), adding two *liǎng* is excellent. In cases of wind *qì*, add three *liǎng* [each] of *dāng guī* (當歸 Root of Angelica polimorpha) and *dú huó* (獨活 Root and rhizome of Angelica pubescens). It also treats vacuity detriment heart palpitations in men.

LINE 3.31

大遠志丸治產後心虛不足，心下虛悸，志意不安，恍恍惚惚，腹中拘急痛，夜臥不安，胸中吸吸少氣，內補傷損，益氣，安定心神，亦治虛損方。

Major Polygala Pills treat postpartum vacuity and insufficiency in the heart, vacuity palpitations below the heart, disquietude of the mind, severe abstraction, hypertonicity and pain in the center of the abdomen, disquieted sleep at night, and shortage of *qì* in the center of the chest in spite of heavy inhalations. This prescription internally supplements injuries, boosts *qì*, and settles the heart spirit. It also treats vacuity detriment.

Major Polygala Pills
大遠志丸 *dà yuǎn zhì wán*

遠志 甘草 茯苓 麥門冬 人參 當歸 白朮 澤瀉 獨活 昌蒲 (各三兩) 署預 阿膠 (各二兩) 乾薑 (四兩) 乾地黃 (五兩) 桂心 (三兩) 。

遠志	yuǎn zhì	Root of Polygala tenuifolia	三兩 3 liǎng	9g
甘草	gān cǎo	Root of Glycyrrhiza uralensis	三兩 3 liǎng	9g
茯苓	fú líng	Dried fungus of Poria cocos	三兩 3 liǎng	9g
麥門冬	mài mén dōng	Tuber of Ophiopogon japonicus	三兩 3 liǎng	9g

人參	rén shēn	Root of Panax ginseng	三兩 3 liǎng	9g
當歸	dāng guī	Root of Angelica polimorpha	三兩 3 liǎng	9g
白朮	bái zhú	Rhizome of Atractylodes macrocephala	三兩 3 liǎng	9g
澤瀉	zé xiè	Rhizome of Alisma plantago-aquatica	三兩 3 liǎng	9g
獨活	dú huó	Root and rhizome of Angelica pubescens	三兩 3 liǎng	9g
菖蒲	chāng pú	Rhizome of Acorus gramineus	三兩 3 liǎng	9g
薯蕷	shǔ yù	Root of Dioscorea opposita	二兩 2 liǎng	6g
阿膠	ē jiāo	Gelatinous glue produced from Equus asinus	二兩 2 liǎng	6g
乾薑	gān jiāng	Dried root of Zingiber officinale	四兩 4 liǎng	12g
乾地黃	gān dì huáng	Dried root of Rehmannia glutinosa	五兩 5 liǎng	15g
桂心	guì xīn	Shaved inner bark of Cinnamomum cassia	三兩 3 liǎng	9g

上十五味，末之，蜜和如大豆，未食溫酒服二十丸，日三，不知稍增至五十丸。若太虛，身體冷，少津液，加鍾乳三兩為善。

Pulverize the above fifteen ingredients and mix with honey [into pills the size] of soybeans. Take twenty pills in heated liquor before meals three times a day. If no effect is noticed, gradually increase [the dose] to a maximum of fifty pills. In cases of extreme vacuity, with a cold body and shortage of fluids, it is excellent to add three *liǎng* of *zhōng rǔ* (鍾乳 Stalactite).

4. Heart and Abdominal Pain 心腹痛

LINE 4.1

蜀椒湯治產後心痛，此大寒冷所為方。

Sì-Chuān Zanthoxylum Decoction treats postpartum heart pain, which is a condition caused by severe cold.

Sì-Chuān Zanthoxylum Decoction
蜀椒湯 *shǔ jiāo tāng*

蜀椒（二合） 芍藥（一兩） 當歸 半夏 甘草 桂心 人參 茯苓（各二兩） 蜜
（一升） 生薑汁（五合）。

蜀椒	shǔ jiāo	Seed capsules of Zanthoxylum bungeanum	二合 2 gě	14ml
芍藥	sháo yào	Root of Paeonia albiflora	一兩 1 liǎng	3g
當歸	dāng guī	Root of Angelica polimorpha	二兩 2 liǎng	6g
半夏	bàn xià	Rhizome of Pinellia ternata	二兩 2 liǎng	6g
甘草	gān cǎo	Root of Glycyrrhiza uralensis	二兩 2 liǎng	6g
桂心	guì xīn	Shaved inner bark of Cinnamomum cassia	二兩 2 liǎng	6g
人參	rén shēn	Root of Panax ginseng	二兩 2 liǎng	6g
茯苓	fú líng	Dried fungus of Poria cocos	二兩 2 liǎng	6g
米	mǐ	Seed of Oryza sativa	一升 1 shēng	24g
生薑汁	shēng jiāng zhī	Fresh root of Zingiber officinale juice	五合 5 gě	35ml

上十味，哎咀，以水九升煮椒令沸，然後內諸藥，煮取二升半，去滓，內
薑汁及蜜，煎取三升。一服五合，漸加至六合。禁勿冷食。

Pound the above ten ingredients. Decoct the *shǔ jiāo* 蜀椒 in nine *shēng* of water, bringing them to a rolling boil; then add all the [other] drugs. Decoct it to obtain two and a half *shēng*, remove the dregs, add the *shēng jiāng zhī* 生薑汁 and honey, and simmer to obtain three *shēng*. Take five *gě* per dose, gradually increasing it to six *gě*. Prohibition: do not consume cool [substances]!

LINE 4.2

大巖蜜湯治產後心痛方。

Major Rock Honey Decoction treats postpartum heart pain.

Major Rock Honey Decoction
大巖蜜湯 *dà yán mì tāng*[1]

乾地黃 當歸 獨活 甘草 芍藥 桂心 細辛 小草（各二兩） 吳茱萸（一升） 乾薑（三兩）。

乾地黃	gān dì huáng	Dried root of Rehmannia glutinosa	二兩 2 liǎng	6g
當歸	dāng guī	Root of Angelica polimorpha	二兩 2 liǎng	6g
獨活	dú huó	Root and rhizome of Angelica pubescens	二兩 2 liǎng	6g
甘草	gān cǎo	Root of Glycyrrhiza uralensis	二兩 2 liǎng	6g
芍藥	sháo yào	Root of Paeonia albiflora	二兩 2 liǎng	6g
桂心	guì xīn	Shaved inner bark of Cinnamomum cassia	二兩 2 liǎng	6g
細辛	xì xīn	Complete plant including root of Asarum heteropoides	二兩 2 liǎng	6g
小草	xiǎo cǎo	Stalk and foliage of Polygala tenuifolia	二兩 2 liǎng	6g
吳茱萸	wú zhū yú	Unripe fruit of Evodia rutaecarpa	一升 1 shēng	24g
乾薑	gān jiāng	Dried root of Zingiber officinale	三兩 3 liǎng	9g

上十味，㕮咀，以水九升煮取三升，內蜜五合重煮，分三服，日三。

Pound the above ten ingredients and decoct in nine *shēng* of water to obtain three *shēng*. Add five *gě* of *mǐ* (米 Seed of Oryza sativa) and decoct it again. Divide into three doses and take three times a day.[2]

1.　巖蜜 *yán mì*: is a synonym for 石蜜 *shí mì*. This is honey of a pure color, collected from mountain precipices (《中華醫學大辭典》 pp. 838 and 344). Another prescription with the identical name is found in the *Qiān Jīn Fāng* in the volume on wind conditions in the section on "bandit wind" (賊風 *zéi fēng*). It is indicated for "bandit wind with gripping pain in the abdomen, as well as flying corpse run-away outpouring with irregular eruptions, prodding the heart, intestinal fullness, and stabbing below the ribs as if with an awl, as well as being the governing prescription for lesser *yīn* cold damage (《千金方》 8:3)." Its ingredients overlap somewhat with the prescription above, indicating the close connection between the various postpartum conditions and a wind-related etiology.

2.   *Sòng* editors' note: "*Hú Qià* does not use *dú huó* 獨活, *guì xīn* 桂心, or *xiǎo cǎo* 小草. *Qiān Jīn Yì Fāng* does not use *mǐ* 米."

LINE 4.3

乾地黃湯治產後兩脅滿痛，兼除百病方。

Dried Rehmannia Decoction treats postpartum fullness and pain in both ribsides, while simultaneously eliminating the myriad diseases.

Dried Rehmannia Decoction
干地黃湯 *gān dì huáng tāng*

乾地黃 芍藥（各三兩） 當歸 蒲黃（各二兩） 生薑（五兩） 桂心（六兩） 甘草（一兩） 大棗（二十枚）。

乾地黃	gān dì huáng	Dried root of Rehmannia glutinosa	三兩 3 liǎng	9g
芍藥	sháo yào	Root of Paeonia albiflora	三兩 3 liǎng	9g
當歸	dāng guī	Root of Angelica polimorpha	二兩 2 liǎng	6g
蒲黃	pú huáng	Pollen of Typha angustata	二兩 2 liǎng	6g
生薑	shēng jiāng	Fresh root of Zingiber officinale	五兩 5 liǎng	15g
桂心	guì xīn	Shaved inner bark of Cinnamomum cassia	六兩 6 liǎng	18g
甘草	gān cǎo	Root of Glycyrrhiza uralensis	一兩 1 liǎng	3g
大棗	dà zǎo	Mature fruit of Ziziphus jujuba	二十枚 20 méi	20 pcs

上八味，咬咀，以水一斗煮取二升半，去滓。分服，日三。

Pound the above eight ingredients and decoct in one *dǒu* of water to obtain two and a half *shēng*. Discard the dregs. Divide into [three]* doses and take three times a day.

*   分服 *fēn fú*: I have filled in the number according to the *Sūn Zhēn Rén* edition, which has 分三服 *fēn sān fú* (divide into three doses).

LINE 4.4

治產後苦少腹痛，芍藥湯方。

Peony Decoction treats postpartum discomfort from pain in the lesser abdomen.

Peony Decoction
芍藥湯 *sháo yào tāng*

芍藥（六兩）桂心（三兩）甘草（二兩）膠飴（八兩）生薑（三兩）大棗（十二枚）。

芍藥	sháo yào	Root of Paeonia albiflora	六兩 6 liǎng	18g
桂心	guì xīn	Shaved inner bark of Cinnamomum cassia	三兩 3 liǎng	9g
甘草	gān cǎo	Root of Glycyrrhiza uralensis	二兩 2 liǎng	6g
膠飴	jiāo yí	Malt candy	八兩 8 liǎng	24g
生薑	shēng jiāng	Fresh root of Zingiber officinale	三兩 3 liǎng	9g
大棗	dà zǎo	Mature fruit of Ziziphus jujuba	十二枚 12 méi	12 pcs

上六味，咬咀，以水七升煮取四升，去滓，內膠飴令烊。分三服，日三。

Pound the above six ingredients and decoct in seven *shēng* of water to obtain four *shēng*. Discard the dregs, add the malt candy, and let it dissolve. Divide into three doses and take three times a day.

LINE 4.5

當歸湯治婦人寒疝，虛勞不足，若產後腹中絞痛方。

Chinese Angelica Decoction treats women's cold mounting, vacuity taxation and insufficiency, and gripping pain in the center of the abdomen after childbirth.

Chinese Angelica Decoction
當歸湯 *dāng guī tāng*

當歸（二兩）生薑（五兩）芍藥（二兩）羊肉（一斤）。

當歸	dāng guī	Root of Angelica polimorpha	二兩 2 liǎng	6g
生薑	shēng jiāng	Fresh root of Zingiber officinale	五兩 5 liǎng	15g
芍藥[1]	sháo yào	Root of Paeonia albiflora	二兩 2 liǎng	6g
羊肉	yáng ròu	Meat of Capra hircus	一斤 1 jīn	48g

上四味，㕮咀，以水八升煮羊肉熟，取汁煎藥，得三升。適寒溫服七合，日三。

Pound the above four ingredients. Cook the sheep or goat's meat in eight *shēng* of water until well-done and take the liquid to simmer the drugs to obtain three *shēng*. Take seven *gě* at whatever temperature she likes three times a day.[2]

1. *Sòng* editors' note: "The *Zǐ Mǔ Mì Lù* uses *gān cǎo* (甘草 Root of Glycyrrhiza uralensis)."

2. Sòng editors' note: "The *Jīn Guì Yào Luè* and *Hú Qià* do not use *sháo yào* 芍藥 and call it *Minor Sheep or Goat's Meat Decoction*."

LINE 4.6

治產後腹中疾痛，桃仁芍藥湯方。

Peach Kernel and Peony Decoction treats postpartum pain in the center of the abdomen.*

Peach Kernel and Peony Decoction
桃仁芍藥湯 *táo rén sháo yào tāng*

桃仁（半升）芍藥 芎藭 當歸 乾漆 桂心 甘草（各二兩）。

桃仁	táo rén	Seed of Prunus persica	半升 0.5 shēng	12g
芍藥	sháo yào	Root of Paeonia albiflora	二兩 2 liǎng	6g
川芎	chuān xiōng	Root of Ligusticum wallichii	二兩 2 liǎng	6g
當歸	dāng guī	Root of Angelica polimorpha	二兩 2 liǎng	6g
乾漆	gān qī	Dried sap of Rhus verniciflua	二兩 2 liǎng	6g
桂心	guì xīn	Shaved inner bark of Cinnamomum cassia	二兩 2 liǎng	6g
甘草	gān cǎo	Root of Glycyrrhiza uralensis	二兩 2 liǎng	6g

上七味，㕮咀，以水八升煮取三升，分三服。

Pound the above seven ingredients and decoct in eight *shēng* of water to obtain three *shēng*. Divide into three doses.

*   This prescription is missing in the *Sūn Zhēn Rén* edition.

LINE 4.7

羊肉湯治產後及傷身，大虛，上氣，腹痛，兼微風方。

Sheep or Goat's Meat Decoction treats great vacuity, *qì* ascent, abdominal pain, and simultaneous slight wind that occur after child birth or as a result of physical damage.[1]

Sheep or Goat's Meat Decoction
羊肉湯 *yáng ròu táng*

肥羊肉（二斤，如無，用獐，鹿肉） 茯苓 黃芪 乾薑（各三兩） 甘草 獨活 桂心 人參（各二兩） 麥門冬（七合） 生地黃（五兩） 大棗（十二枚）。

肥羊肉，如無，用獐，鹿肉	féi yáng ròu, rú wú, yòng zhāng, lù ròu	Unrendered fat of Capra hircus or Ovis aries. If unavailable, then use *zhāng* or *lù* meat.	二斤 2 jīn	96g
茯苓	fú líng	Dried fungus of Poria cocos	三兩 3 liǎng	9g
黃芪	huáng qí	Root of Astragalus membranaceus	三兩 3 liǎng	9g
乾薑[2]	gān jiāng	Dried root of Zingiber officinale	三兩 3 liǎng	9g
甘草	gān cǎo	Root of Glycyrrhiza uralensis	二兩 2 liǎng	6g
獨活	dú huó	Root and rhizome of Angelica pubescens	二兩 2 liǎng	6g
桂心	guì xīn	Shaved inner bark of Cinnamomum cassia	二兩 2 liǎng	6g
人參	rén shēn	Root of Panax ginseng	二兩 2 liǎng	6g
麥門冬	mài mén dōng	Tuber of Ophiopogon japonicus	七合 7 gě	49ml
生地黃	shēng dì huáng	Fresh root of Rehmannia glutinosa	五兩 5 liǎng	15g
大棗	dà zǎo	Mature fruit of Ziziphus jujuba	十二枚 12 méi	12 pcs

上十一味，㕮咀，以水二斗煮肉取一斗，去肉內藥，煮取三升半，去滓。分四服，日三夜一。

Pound the above eleven ingredients. Cook the meat in *two* dǒu of water to obtain one dǒu, remove the meat, and add the drugs. Decoct to obtain three and a half *shēng*, discard the dregs, and divide into four doses. Take three times a day and once at night.

1.   傷身 *shāng shēn*: The *Sūn Zhēn Rén* edition has 傷寒 *shāng hán* instead, which makes perhaps more sense. The sentence would then read as follows: "*Sheep or Goat's Meat*

Decoction treats …after childbirth or related to cold damage."

2.   *Sòng* editors' note: "The Qiān *Jīn Yì Fāng* does not include *gān jiāng* 乾薑."

LINE 4.8

羊肉當歸湯治產後腹中心下切痛，不能食，往來寒熱，若中風乏氣力方。

Sheep or Goat's Meat and Chinese Angelica Decoction treats postpartum cutting pain in the center of the abdomen and below the heart with inability to eat, alternating [aversion to] cold and heat [effusion], and lack of *qì* and strength as in wind strike.[1]

Sheep or Goat's Meat and Chinese Angelica Decoction
羊肉當歸湯 *yáng ròu dāng guī tāng*

羊肉（三斤）當歸 黃芩（《肘後》用黃芪）芎藭 甘草 防風（各二兩，《肘後》用人參）芍藥（三兩）生薑（四兩）。

羊肉	yáng ròu	Meat of Capra hircus or Ovis aries	三斤 3 jīn	144g
當歸	dāng guī	Root of Angelica polimorpha	二兩 2 liǎng	6g
黃芩[2]	huáng qín	Root of Scutellaria baicalensis	二兩 2 liǎng	6g
川芎	chuān xiōng	Root of Ligusticum wallichii	二兩 2 liǎng	6g
甘草	gān cǎo	Root of Glycyrrhiza uralensis	二兩 2 liǎng	6g
防風[3]	fáng fēng	Root of Ledebouriella divaricata	二兩 2 liǎng	6g
芍藥	sháo yào	Root of Paeonia albiflora	三兩 3 liǎng	9g
生薑	shēng jiāng	Fresh root of Zingiber officinale	四兩 4 liǎng	12g

上八味，㕮咀，以水一斗二升先煮肉熟，減半，內餘藥，煎取三升，去滓，分三服，日三。

Pound the above eight ingredients. First cook the meat in one *dǒu* and two *shēng* of water until it is well-done and [the liquid is] reduced to half, then add the remaining drugs and decoct them to obtain three *shēng*. Discard the dregs, divide into three doses, and take three times a day.[4]

1.   This prescription is found in the *Wài Tái Mì Yào*, where it is called "*Sheep or Goat's Meat Decoction.*" It is missing in the *Sūn Zhēn Rén* edition.
2.   *Sòng* editors' note: "The *Zhǒu Hòu Fāng* uses *huáng qí* (黃芪 Root of Astragalus membranaceus)."
3.   *Sòng* editors' note: "The *Zhǒu Hòu Fāng* also uses *rén shēn* (人參 Root of Panax ginseng)."
4.   The *Hú Qià* substitutes *huáng qí* 黃芪 for *huáng qín* 黃芩 and *bái zhú* (白朮 Rhizome of

Atractylodes macrocephala) for *sháo yào* 芍藥. *Zǐ Mǔ Mì Lù* substitutes *guì xīn* (桂心 Shaved inner bark of Cinnamomum cassia) for *fáng fēng* 防風 and adds seventeen pieces of *dà zǎo* (大棗 Mature fruit of Ziziphus jujuba).

LINE 4.8

羊肉杜仲湯治產後腰痛，欬嗽方。

Sheep or Goat's Meat and Eucommia Decoction treats postpartum lumbar pain and cough.

Sheep or Goat's Meat and Eucommia Decoction
羊肉杜仲湯 *yáng ròu dù zhòng tāng*

羊肉（四斤）杜仲 紫菀（各三兩）五味子 細辛 款冬花 人參 厚朴 芎藭 附子 萆薢 甘草 黃芪（各二兩）當歸 桂心 白朮（各三兩）生薑（八兩）大棗（三十枚）。

羊肉	yáng ròu	Meat of Capra hircus or Ovis aries	四斤 4 jīn	192g
杜仲	dù zhòng	Bark of Eucommia ulmoidis	三兩 3 liǎng	9g
紫菀	zǐ wǎn	Root and rhizome of Aster tataricus	三兩 3 liǎng	9g
五味子	wǔ wèi zǐ	Fruit of Schisandra chinensis	二兩 2 liǎng	6g
細辛	xì xīn	Complete plant including root of Asarum heteropoides	二兩 2 liǎng	6g
款冬花	kuǎn dōng huā	Flower of Tussilago farfara	二兩 2 liǎng	6g
人參	rén shēn	Root of Panax ginseng	二兩 2 liǎng	6g
厚朴	hòu pò	Bark of Magnolia officinalis	二兩 2 liǎng	6g
川芎	chuān xiōng	Root of Ligusticum wallichii	二兩 2 liǎng	6g
附子	fù zǐ	Lateral root of Aconitum carmichaeli	二兩 2 liǎng	6g
萆薢	bì xiè	Rhizome of Dioscorea hypoglauca	二兩 2 liǎng	6g
甘草	gān cǎo	Root of Glycyrrhiza uralensis	二兩 2 liǎng	6g
黃芪	huáng qí	Root of Astragalus membranaceus	二兩 2 liǎng	6g
當歸	dāng guī	Root of Angelica polimorpha	三兩 3 liǎng	9g
桂心	guì xīn	Shaved inner bark of Cinnamomum cassia	三兩 3 liǎng	9g
白朮	bái zhú	Rhizome of Atractylodes macrocephala	三兩 3 liǎng	9g
生薑	shēng jiāng	Fresh root of Zingiber officinale	八兩 8 liǎng	24g

| 大棗 | dà zǎo | Mature fruit of Ziziphus jujuba | 三十枚 30 méi | 30 pcs |

上十八味，哎咀，以水二斗半煮肉，取汁一斗五升，去肉內藥，煎取三升半，去滓，分五服，日三夜二。

Pound the above eighteen ingredients. Cook the meat in two and a half *dǒu* of water to obtain one *dǒu* and five *shēng* of liquid. Remove the meat, add the drugs, and simmer to obtain three and a half *shēng*. Discard the dregs and divide into five doses. Take three times during the day and twice at night.

LINE 4.9

羊肉生地黃湯治產後三日腹痛，補中益藏，強氣力，消血方。

Sheep or Goat's Meat and Fresh Rehmannia Decoction treats postpartum abdominal pain [that lasts] for three days, by supplementing the center and boosting the viscera, strengthening *qì*, and dispersing blood.

Sheep or Goat's Meat and Fresh Rehmannia Decoction
羊肉生地黃湯 *yáng ròu shēng dì huáng tāng*

羊肉（三斤）生地黃（切，二升）桂心 當歸 甘草 芎藭 人參（各二兩）芍藥（三兩）。

羊肉	yáng ròu	Meat of Capra hircus or Ovis aries	三斤 3 jīn	144g
生地黃, 切	shēng dì huáng, qiē	Fresh root of Rehmannia glutinosa, chopped	二兩 2 liǎng	6g
桂心	guì xīn	Shaved inner bark of Cinnamomum cassia	二兩 2 liǎng	6g
當歸	dāng guī	Root of Angelica polimorpha	二兩 2 liǎng	6g
甘草	gān cǎo	Root of Glycyrrhiza uralensis	二兩 2 liǎng	6g
川芎	chuān xiōng	Root of Ligusticum wallichii	二兩 2 liǎng	6g
人參	rén shēn	Root of Panax ginseng	二兩 2 liǎng	6g
芍藥	sháo yào	Root of Paeonia albiflora	三兩 3 liǎng	9g

上八味，哎咀，以水二斗煮肉，取一斗，去肉內藥，煎取三升，分四服，日三夜一。

Pound the above eight ingredients. Cook the meat in two *dǒu* of water to obtain one *dǒu*. Remove the meat, add the drugs, and simmer to obtain three *shēng*. Divide into four doses and take three times during the day and once at night.

LINE 4.10

內補當歸建中湯治產後虛羸不足，腹中疞痛[1]不止，吸吸少氣，或苦小腹拘急，痛引腰背，不能飲食，產後一月日得服四五劑為善，令人丁壯方。

Internally Supplementing Chinese Angelica Center-Fortifying Decoction[2] treats postpartum vacuity emaciation and insufficiency with incessant gripping pain in the center of the abdomen, shortage of *qì* in spite of heavy inhalations, possibly with hypertonicity and pain in the lower abdomen that stretches to the lumbus and back, and inability to eat or drink. If she can take four or five preparations during the first month postpartum,[3] this is good and will make her strong and healthy.

Internally Supplementing Chinese Angelica Center-Fortifying Decoction
內補當歸建中湯 *nèi bǔ dāng guī jiàn zhōng tāng*

當歸（四兩）芍藥（六兩）甘草（二兩）生薑（六兩）桂心（三兩）大棗（十枚）。

當歸	dāng guī	Root of Angelica polimorpha	四兩 4 liǎng		12g
芍藥	sháo yào	Root of Paeonia albiflora	六兩 6 liǎng		18g
甘草	gān cǎo	Root of Glycyrrhiza uralensis	二兩 2 liǎng		6g
生薑	shēng jiāng	Fresh root of Zingiber officinale	六兩 6 liǎng		18g
桂心	guì xīn	Shaved inner bark of Cinnamomum cassia	三兩 3 liǎng		9g
大棗	dà zǎo	Mature fruit of Ziziphus jujuba	十枚 10 méi		10 pcs

上六味，㕮咀，以水一斗煮取三升，去滓。分三服，一日令盡。若大虛，內飴糖六兩，湯成內之於火上，飴消。若無生薑，則以乾薑三兩代之；若其人去血過多，崩傷內竭不止，加地黃六兩，阿膠二兩，合八種，湯成去滓，內阿膠；若無當歸，以芎藭代之。

Pound the above six ingredients and decoct in one *dǒu* of water to obtain three *shēng*. Remove the dregs. Divide into three doses and use it up within one day. In cases of severe vacuity, add six *liǎng* of *yí táng* (飴糖 Malt sugar), adding it to the finished decoction and returning this to the flame until the sugar is melted. If you do not have *shēng jiāng* 生薑, substitute three *liǎng* of *gān jiāng* (乾薑 Dried root of Zingiber officinale) for it. If the patient is suffering from excessive bleeding and flooding damage with incessant internal exhaustion, add six *liǎng* of *dì huáng* (地黃 Root of Rehmannia glutinosa) and two *liǎng* of *ē jiāo* (阿膠 Gelatinous glue produced from Equus asinus), making a total of eight ingredients; add the *ē jiāo* 阿膠 to the finished decoction after removing the dregs. If you don't have *dāng guī* 當歸, substitute *chuān xiōng* (川芎 Root of Ligusticum wallichii) for it.[4]

1. 疞痛 *jiǎo tòng*: Obscure character, defined in the *Shuō Wén Jiě Zì* as 腹中急 *fù zhōng jí* (tension in the abomen), and paraphrased in the *Rén Mín* edition as 绞痛 *jiǎo tòng* (gripping pain).

2. 內補當歸建中湯 *nèi bǔ dāng guī jiàn zhōng tāng*: The *Sūn Zhēn Rén* edition instead has 內補當歸湯達中 *nèi bǔ dāng guī tāng dá zhōng*: *Internally Supplementing Chinese Angelica Decoction*: It reaches the center and…

3. 產後一月日得服四五劑 *chǎn hòu yī yuè rì dé fú sì wǔ jì*: The *Huá Xià* edition and *Rén Mín* edition punctuate between 月 *yuè* and 日 *rì*, suggesting the following interpretation: "During the first month postpartum, if she can take four or five batches daily..." However, this clearly contradicts the instructions below to "use [one preparation] up in one day." Moreover, it is common in gynecological literature to count the critical postpartum period in days, most frequently in the first hundred days postpartum (產後百日 *chǎn hòu bǎi rì*). It is likely that the expression "the days of the first month postpartum" is identical to the standard expression, 產後滿月 *chǎn hòu mǎn yuè* (fulfilling one month postpartum), which the *Ishimpô* explains this way: "The reason that fulfilling the month does not mean counting a full thirty days is because it means to skip over one month. If the birth was in the first month, skipping one month means to skip over the second month and enter the third month" (《醫心方》 23:19).

4. The *Sūn Zhēn Rén* edition adds here a prescription for "*Internally Supplementing Rehmannia Decoction*," indicated for "women's postpartum vacuity with *qì* and blood exhaustion and expiry, abstraction of the essence spirit, occasional pain in the center of the abdomen, and inability to get food down." This prescription is not found in other editions of the *Qiān Jīn Fāng*.

LINE 4.11

內補芎藭湯治婦人產後虛羸，及崩傷過多，虛竭，腹中絞痛方。

Internally Supplementing Chuānxiōng Decoction treats women's postpartum vacuity emaciation as well as excessive flooding damage, with vacuity exhaustion and gripping pain in the center of the abdomen.

Internally Supplementing Chuānxiōng Decoction
內補芎藭湯 *nèi bǔ xiōng qióng tāng*

芎藭 乾地黃（各四兩） 芍藥（五兩） 桂心（二兩） 甘草 乾薑（各三兩）
大棗（四十枚）。

川芎	chuān xiōng	Root of Ligusticum wallichii	四兩 4 liǎng	12g
乾地黃	gān dì huáng	Dried root of Rehmannia glutinosa	四兩 4 liǎng	12g

芍藥	sháo yào	Root of Paeonia albiflora	五兩 5 liǎng	15g
桂心	guì xīn	Shaved inner bark of Cinnamomum cassia	二兩 2 liǎng	6g
甘草	gān cǎo	Root of Glycyrrhiza uralensis	三兩 3 liǎng	9g
乾薑	gān jiāng	Dried root of Zingiber officinale	三兩 3 liǎng	9g
大棗	dà zǎo	Mature fruit of Ziziphus jujuba	四十枚 40 méi	40 pcs

上七味，㕮咀，以水一斗二升煮取三升，去滓，分三服，日三，不瘥復作，至三劑。若有寒，苦微下*，加附子三兩。治婦人虛羸，少氣傷絕，腹中拘急痛，崩傷虛竭，面目無色，及唾吐血，甚良。

Pound the above seven ingredients and decoct in one *dǒu* and two *shēng* of water to obtain three *shēng*. Discard the dregs, divide into three doses, and take three times a day. If she fails to recover, make it repeatedly, up to a total of three preparations. In cases of cold and a slight discharge, add three *liǎng* of *fù zǐ* (附子 Lateral root of Aconitum carmichaeli). [This prescription] is excellent for treating women's vacuity emaciation with shortage of *qì* [to the point of] damage or expiry, hypertonicity and pain in the center of the abdomen, flooding damage vacuity exhaustion, lack of color in the face and eyes, as well as spitting and vomiting blood.

* 　　微下 *wēi xià*: This refers to a slight vaginal discharge, a common symptom of cold-related conditions.

LINE 4.12

大補中當歸湯治產後虛損不足，腹中拘急，或溺血，少腹苦痛，或從高墮下犯內，及金瘡血多內傷，男子亦宜服之方。

Major Center-supplementing Chinese Angelica Decoction treats postpartum vacuity detriment and insufficiency, tension in the center of the abdomen, possibly with bloody urine, bitter pain in the lower abdomen, internal assault [due to] falling from a high place, as well as excessive bleeding and internal damage from incised wounds. It is also suitable for men to take.

Major Center-Supplementing Chinese Angelica Decoction
大補中當歸湯 *dà bǔ zhōng dāng guī tāng*

當歸 續斷 桂心 芎藭 乾薑 麥門冬（各三兩） 芍藥（四兩） 吳茱萸（一升） 乾地黃（六兩） 甘草 白芷（各二兩） 大棗（四十枚）。

當歸	dāng guī	Root of Angelica polimorpha	三兩 3 liǎng	9g
續斷	xù duàn	Root of Dipsacus asper	三兩 3 liǎng	9g
桂心	guì xīn	Shaved inner bark of Cinnamomum cassia	三兩 3 liǎng	9g
川芎	chuān xiōng	Root of Ligusticum wallichii	三兩 3 liǎng	9g
乾薑	gān jiāng	Dried root of Zingiber officinale	三兩 3 liǎng	9g
麥門冬	mài mén dōng	Tuber of Ophiopogon japonicus	三兩 3 liǎng	9g
芍藥	sháo yào	Root of Paeonia albiflora	四兩 4 liǎng	12g
吳茱萸	wú zhū yú	Unripe fruit of Evodia rutaecarpa	一升 1 shēng	24g
乾地黃	gān dì huáng	Dried root of Rehmannia glutinosa	六兩 6 liǎng	18g
甘草	gān cǎo	Root of Glycyrrhiza uralensis	二兩 2 liǎng	6g
白芷	bái zhǐ	Root of Angelica dahurica	二兩 2 liǎng	6g
大棗	dà zǎo	Mature fruit of Ziziphus jujuba	四十枚 40 méi	40 pcs

上十二味，㕮咀，以酒一斗漬藥一宿，明旦以水一斗合煮取五升，去滓。分五服，日三夜二。有黃芪，入二兩益佳。

Pound the above twelve ingredients and soak the drugs in one *dǒu* of liquor over one night. At dawn on the next day, decoct them with one *dǒu* of water to obtain five *shēng* and discard the dregs. Divide into five doses and take three times during the day and twice at night.[1] If you have *huáng qí* (黃芪 Root of Astragalus membranaceus), adding two *liǎng* increases the benefits [of this prescription] even further.[2]

1.　*Sòng* editors' note: "The *Sūn Zhēn Rén* edition adds: 'If it is not enough, you can increase the water by one *shēng*.'"
2.　*Sòng* editors' note: "Following this, the same edition adds a prescription for '*Evodia Wine*,' for the treatment of 'soreness and pain in the center of the abdomen.'"

LINE 4.13

桂心酒治產後疹痛，及卒心腹痛方。

Cinnamon Bark Wine treats postpartum chronic ailments˙ and pain, as well as sudden heart and abdominal pain.

Cinnamon Bark Wine
桂心酒 *guì xīn jiǔ*

桂心三兩，以酒三升煮取二升，去滓，分三服，日三。

Decoct three *liǎng* of *guì xīn* (桂心 Shaved inner bark of Cinnamomum cassia) in three *shēng* of liquor to obtain two *shēng*. Discard the dregs, divide into three doses, and take three times a day.

*　　疹 *chèn*: In modern TCM, this character is pronounced *zhěn* and refers to "papules" or specifically to "measles" (syn. 疢 *chèn*, 胎毒 *tāi dú*, or 麻疹 *má zhěn*). Sūn Sī-Miǎo uses it here in an alternative meaning that is explained by Zhāng Zhòng-Jǐng as follows: 疹 為久病也 *chèn wéi jiǔ bìng yě* ("*Chèn* means a long-term illness." quoted in 張登本, 主編《內經辭典》 p. 356). It is highly unlikely that this section on postpartum abdominal pain would include a prescription for heat-related skin rashes. Moreover, the single ingredient, *guì xīn* 桂心, is a warming drug that is contraindicated in heat conditions. The *Sūn Zhēn Rén* edition has 疼 *téng* (aches) instead.

LINE 4.14

生牛膝酒治產後腹中苦痛方。

Fresh Achyranthes Wine treats bitter postpartum pain in the center of the abdomen.

Fresh Achyranthes Wine
生牛膝酒 *shēng niú xī jiǔ*

生牛膝五兩，以酒五升煮取二升，去滓，分二服。若用乾牛膝根，以酒漬之一宿，然後可煮。

Decoct five *liǎng* of *shēng niú xī* (生牛膝 Fresh root of Achyranthes bidentata) in five *shēng* of liquor to obtain two *shēng*. Discard the dregs and divide into two doses. If using *gān niú xī gēn* (乾牛膝根 Dried root of Achyranthes bidentata), soak it in the liquor over one night. After that, you can decoct it.

LINE 4.15

治產後腹中如弦，當堅痛，無聊賴方。

The [following] prescription treats postpartum [tension] like a bowstring in the center of the abdomen with persistent hardness and pain that is not bound to a specific location.˙

當歸末二方寸匕，內蜜一升煎之，適寒溫頓服之。

[Take] two square-inch spoons of pulverized *dāng guī* (當歸 Root of Angelica polimorpha) and simmer it in one *shēng* of honey. Quaff in a single dose at whatever temperature she likes.

* 　　無聊賴 *wú liáo lài*: The interpretation of this phrase is questionable. Alternatively, the *Sūn Zhēn Rén* edition has 無情賴 *wú qíng lài* (lacking affect and shame), a version that is entirely possible, given the context of postpartum abdominal tension and hardness. (《孫真人千金方》3:8).

LINE 4.16

吳茱萸湯治婦人先有寒冷，胸滿痛，或心腹刺痛，或嘔吐食少，或腫，或寒，或下痢，氣息綿惙欲絕，產後益劇，皆主之方。

Evodia Decoction treats women who prior [to childbirth suffered from] presence of cold, fullness and pain in the chest, possibly stabbing pain in the heart and abdomen, or retching and vomiting and reduced eating, swelling, coldness, or diarrhea, and faint and labored breathing verging on expiry, and whose symptoms have increased dramatically after childbirth. [This prescription] governs them all:

Evodia Decoction
吳茱萸湯 *wú zhū yú tāng*

吳茱萸（二兩）防風 桔梗 乾薑 甘草 細辛 當歸（各十二銖）乾地黃（十八銖）。

吳茱萸	wú zhū yú	Unripe fruit of Evodia rutaecarpa	二兩 2 liǎng	6g
防風	fǎng fēng	Root of Ledebouriella divaricata	十二銖 12 zhū	1.5g
桔梗	jié gěng	Root of Platycodon grandiflorum	十二銖 12 zhū	1.5g
乾薑	gān jiāng	Dried root of Zingiber officinale	十二銖 12 zhū	1.5g
甘草	gān cǎo	Root of Glycyrrhiza uralensis	十二銖 12 zhū	1.5g
細辛	xì xīn	Complete plant including root of Asarum heteropoides	十二銖 12 zhū	1.5g
當歸	dāng guī	Root of Angelica polimorpha	十二銖 12 zhū	1.5g
乾地黃	gān dì huáng	Dried root of Rehmannia glutinosa	十八銖 18 zhū	2.25g

上八味，㕮咀，以水四升煮取一升半，去滓，分再服。

Pound the above eight ingredients and decoct in four *shēng* of water to obtain one and a half *shēng*. Discard the dregs and divide into two doses.

LINE 4.17

蒲黃湯治產後餘疾，胸中少氣，腹痛，頭疼，餘血未盡，除腹中脹滿欲死方。

Typha Pollen Decoction treats residual disease after childbirth [such as] shortage of *qì* in the center of the chest, abdominal pain, headaches, and incomplete elimination of residual blood, by eliminating life-threatening distention and fullness in the center of the abdomen.

Typha Pollen Decoction
蒲黃湯 *pú huáng tāng*

蒲黃（五兩）桂心 芎藭（各一兩）桃仁（二十枚）芒消（一兩）生薑 生地黃（各五兩）大棗（十五枚）。

蒲黃	pú huáng	Pollen of Typha angustata	五兩 5 liǎng	15g
桂心	guì xīn	Shaved inner bark of Cinnamomum cassia	一兩 1 liǎng	3g
川芎	chuān xiōng	Root of Ligusticum wallichii	一兩 1 liǎng	3g
桃仁	táo rén	Seed of Prunus persica	二十枚 20 méi	20 pcs
硭硝	máng xiāo	Hydrated sodium sulfate	一兩 1 liǎng	3g
生薑	shēng jiāng	Fresh root of Zingiber officinale	五兩 5 liǎng	15g
生地黃	shēng dì huáng	Fresh root of Rehmannia glutinosa	五兩 5 liǎng	15g
大棗	dà zǎo	Mature fruit of Ziziphus jujuba	十五枚15 méi	15 pcs

上八味，咬咀，以水九升煮取二升半，去滓，內芒消。分三服，日三。良驗。

Pound the above eight ingredients and decoct in nine *shēng* of water to obtain two and a half *shēng*. Discard the dregs and add the *máng xiāo* 硭硝. Divide into three doses and take three times a day. Good results.

LINE 4.18

敗醬湯治產後疹痛引腰腹中，如錐刀所刺方。

Patrinia Decoction treats chronic postpartum pain stretching to the lumbus and center of the abdomen, as if being stabbed with an awl or knife.

Patrinia Decoction
敗醬湯 bài jiàng tāng

敗醬（三兩） 桂心 芎藭（各一兩半） 當歸（一兩）。

敗醬	bài jiàng	Whole plant with root of Patrinia villosa	三兩 3 liǎng	9g
桂心	guì xīn	Shaved inner bark of Cinnamomum cassia	一兩半 1.5 liǎng	4.5g
川芎	chuān xiōng	Root of Ligusticum wallichii	一兩半 1.5 liǎng	4.5g
當歸	dāng guī	Root of Angelica polimorpha	一兩 1 liǎng	3g

上四味，㕮咀，以清酒二升四斗微火煮取二升，去滓。適寒溫服七合，日三服，食前服之。

Pound the above four ingredients and decoct in two *shēng* of clear liquor and four *shēng* of water over a small flame to obtain two *shēng*. Discard the dregs, and take seven *gě* [as a dose] at whatever temperature she likes. Take three doses before meals.[1]

*   *Sòng* editors' note: "The *Qiān Jīn Yì Fāng* uses only *bài jiàng* 敗醬 as a single ingredient."

LINE 4.19

芎藭湯治產後腹痛方。

Chuānxiōng Decoction treats postpartum abdominal pain.

Chuānxiōng Decoction
芎藭湯 xiōng qióng tāng

芎藭 甘草（各二兩） 蒲黃 女萎（各一兩半） 芍藥 大黃（各三十銖） 當歸（十八銖） 桂心 桃仁 黃芪（《千金翼》作黃芩） 前胡（各一兩） 生地黃（一升）。

川芎	chuān xiōng	Root of Ligusticum wallichii	二兩 2 liǎng	6g
甘草	gān cǎo	Root of Glycyrrhiza uralensis	二兩 2 liǎng	6g
蒲黃	pú huáng	Pollen of Typha angustata	一兩半 1.5 liǎng	4.5g
女萎	nǚ wěi	Stalk of Clematis apiifolia	一兩半 1.5 liǎng	4.5g
芍藥	sháo yào	Root of Paeonia albiflora	三十銖 30 zhū	3.75g

大黃	dà huáng	Root of Rheum palmatum	三十銖 30 zhū	3.75g
當歸	dāng guī	Root of Angelica polimorpha	十八銖 18 zhū	2.25g
桂心	guì xīn	Shaved inner bark of Cinnamomum cassia	一兩 1 liǎng	3g
桃仁	táo rén	Seed of Prunus persica	一兩 1 liǎng	3g
黃芪*	huáng qí	Root of Astragalus membranaceus	一兩 1 liǎng	3g
前胡	qián hú	Root of Peucedanum praeruptorum	一兩 1 liǎng	3g
生地黃	shēng dì huáng	Fresh root of Rehmannia glutinosa	一升 1 shēng	24g

上十二味，㕮咀，以水一斗，酒三升合煮取二升，去滓。分四服，日三夜一。

Pound the above twelve ingredients and simmer in a blend of one *dǒu* of water and three *shēng* of liquor to obtain two *shēng*. Discard the dregs, divide into four doses, and take three times a day and once at night.

*   *Sòng* editors' note: "The *Qiān Jīn Yì Fāng* uses *huáng qín* (黃芩 Root of Scutellaria baicalensis)."

LINE 4.20

獨活湯治產後腹痛，引腰背拘急痛方。

Pubescent Angelica Decoction treats postpartum abdominal pain with hypertonicity and pain stretching to the lumbus and back.

Pubescent Angelica Decoction
獨活湯 *dú huó tāng*

獨活 當歸 桂心 芍藥 生薑（各三兩）甘草（二兩）大棗（二十枚）。

獨活	dú huó	Root and rhizome of Angelica pubescens	三兩 3 liǎng	9g
當歸	dāng guī	Root of Angelica polimorpha	三兩 3 liǎng	9g
桂心	guì xīn	Shaved inner bark of Cinnamomum cassia	三兩 3 liǎng	9g
芍藥	sháo yào	Root of Paeonia albiflora	三兩 3 liǎng	9g
生薑	shēng jiāng	Fresh root of Zingiber officinale	三兩 3 liǎng	9g

| 甘草 | gān cǎo | Root of Glycyrrhiza uralensis | 二兩 2 liǎng | 6g |
| 大棗 | dà zǎo | Mature fruit of Ziziphus jujuba | 二十枚 20 méi | 20 pcs |

上七味，㕮咀，以水八升煮取三升，去滓。分三服，服相去如人行十里久進之。

Pound the above seven ingredients and decoct in eight *shēng* of water to obtain three *shēng*. Discard the dregs. Divide into three doses and take them separated by the length of time it takes a person to walk ten *lǐ*.

LINE 4.21

芍藥黃芪湯治產後心腹痛方。

Peony and Astragalus Decoction treats postpartum heart and abdominal pain.[1]

Peony and Astragalus Decoction
芍藥黃芪湯 *sháo yào huáng qí tāng*

芍藥（四兩）黃芪 白芷 桂心 生薑 人參 芎藭 當歸 乾地黃 甘草（各二兩）
茯苓（三兩）大棗（十枚）。

芍藥	sháo yào	Root of Paeonia albiflora	四兩 4 liǎng	12g
黃芪	huáng qí	Root of Astragalus membranaceus	二兩 2 liǎng	6g
白芷	bái zhǐ	Root of Angelica dahurica	二兩 2 liǎng	6g
桂心	guì xīn	Shaved inner bark of Cinnamomum cassia	二兩 2 liǎng	6g
生薑	shēng jiāng	Fresh root of Zingiber officinale	二兩 2 liǎng	6g
人參	rén shēn	Root of Panax ginseng	二兩 2 liǎng	6g
川芎	chuān xiōng	Root of Ligusticum wallichii	二兩 2 liǎng	6g
當歸	dāng guī	Root of Angelica polimorpha	二兩 2 liǎng	6g
乾地黃	gān dì huáng	Dried root of Rehmannia glutinosa	二兩 2 liǎng	6g
甘草	gān cǎo	Root of Glycyrrhiza uralensis	二兩 2 liǎng	6g
茯苓	fú líng	Dried fungus of Poria cocos	三兩 3 liǎng	9g
大棗	dà zǎo	Mature fruit of Ziziphus jujuba	十枚 10 méi	10 pcs

上十二味，㕮咀，以酒，水各五升合煮，取三升，去滓。先食服一升，日三。

Pound the above twelve ingredients and decoct in a mix of five *shēng* each of liquor and water to obtain three *shēng*. Discard the dregs. Take one *shēng* before meals three times a day.[2]

1.   The *Sūn Zhēn Rén* edition instead has: 治產後止痛方 *zhì chǎn hòu zhǐ tòng fāng* (a post-partum treatment for stopping pain).

2.   *Sòng* editors' note: "The *Qiān Jīn Yì Fāng* lacks *rén shēn* 人參, *dāng guī* 當歸, *chuān xiōng* 川芎, *dà huáng* 大黃, and *fú líng* 茯苓, using a total of seven ingredients."

LINE 4.22

治產後腹脹痛，不可忍者方。

[The following] prescription treats unbearable postpartum pain in the abdomen and intestines:

煮黍黏根為飲，一服即愈。

Simmer *shǔ nián gēn* (黍粘根 Root of Arctium lappa) to make a drink. A single dose promptly causes recovery.

LINE 4.23

治婦人心痛方。

[The following] prescription treats women's heart pain.[*]

布裹鹽如彈丸，燒作灰，酒服之愈。

Wrap a pellet-sized amount of salt in cloth, char into ashes, and take in liquor for recovery.

*   *Sòng* editors' note: "In the *Sūn Zhēn Rén* edition, this and the following two prescriptions are found in chapter 8 of this volume on "Miscellaneous Treatments.""

LINE 4.24

又方

Another prescription:

燒秤鎚投酒中服，亦佳。

It is also good to heat a steelyard weight, immerse it in liquor, and then drink [the liquor].

LINE 4.25

又方

Another prescription:

炒大豆投酒中服，佳。

It is good to fry soybeans, put them in liquor, and then drink it.

5. Malign Dew 惡露

Translator's note: Malign dew is a standard technical term referring to lochia, the discharge from the vagina or uterus following childbirth. The most common problem in this category is "incomplete elimination of malign dew" (惡露不盡 *è lù bù jìn*), a condition overlapping partly with the biomedical condition of lochiorrhea. I have chosen to translate it literally in order to stress the difference to the biomedical understanding of this process. Similar to ideas regarding menstruation, Sūn Sī-Miǎo regards the elimination of malign substances (惡物 *è wù*) as essential for women's recovery from childbirth. While a continued or excessive flow of postpartum blood is also seen as debilitating in the *Qiān Jīn Fāng*, much greater emphasis is placed on the dangers caused by the continuing presence of stale or rotting blood (敗血 *bài xuè*) in the woman's abdomen after childbirth. This is reflected in the choice of medicinals in the following prescriptions: they mostly encourage the flow and elimination of blood and the break-up of bound and hardened blood.

LINE 5.1

乾地黃湯治產後惡露不盡 , 除諸疾 , 補不足方 。

Dried Rehmannia Decoction treats incomplete elimination of malign dew after childbirth, by eliminating the various sicknesses and supplementing insufficiencies.

Dried Rehmannia Decoction
干地黃湯 *gān dì huáng tāng*

乾地黃 (三兩) 芎藭 桂心 黃芪 當歸 (各二兩) 人參 防風 茯苓 細辛 芍藥 甘草 (各一兩) 。

乾地黃	gān dì huáng	Dried root of Rehmannia glutinosa	三兩 3 liǎng	9g
川芎	chuān xiōng	Root of Ligusticum wallichii	二兩 2 liǎng	6g
桂心	guì xīn	Shaved inner bark of Cinnamomum cassia	二兩 2 liǎng	6g
黃芪	huáng qí	Root of Astragalus membranaceus	二兩 2 liǎng	6g
當歸	dāng guī	Root of Angelica polimorpha	二兩 2 liǎng	6g
人參	rén shēn	Root of Panax ginseng	一兩 1 liǎng	3g

防風	fáng fēng	Root of Ledebouriella divaricata	一兩 1 liǎng	3g
茯苓	fú líng	Dried fungus of Poria cocos	一兩 1 liǎng	3g
細辛	xì xīn	Complete plant including root of Asarum heteropoides	一兩 1 liǎng	3g
芍藥	sháo yào	Root of Paeonia albiflora	一兩 1 liǎng	3g
甘草	gān cǎo	Root of Glycyrrhiza uralensis	一兩 1 liǎng	3g

上十一味，㕮咀，以水一斗煮取三升，去滓。分三服，日再夜一。

Pound the above eleven ingredients and decoct in one *dǒu* of water to obtain three *shēng*. Discard the dregs. Divide into three doses and take twice a day and once at night.

LINE 5.2

桃仁湯治產後往來寒熱，惡露不盡方。

Peach Kernel Decoction treats alternating [aversion to] cold and heat [effusion] and incomplete elimination of malign dew after childbirth.

Peach Kernel Decoction
桃仁湯 *táo rén tāng*

桃仁（五兩）吳茱萸（二升）黃芪 當歸 芍藥（各三兩）生薑 醍醐（百鍊酥）柴胡（各八兩）。

桃仁	táo rén	Seed of Prunus persica	五兩 5 liǎng	15g
吳茱萸	wú zhū yú	Unripe fruit of Evodia rutaecarpa	二升 2 shēng	48g
黃芪	huáng qí	Root of Astragalus membranaceus	三兩 3 liǎng	9g
當歸	dāng guī	Root of Angelica polimorpha	三兩 3 liǎng	9g
芍藥	sháo yào	Root of Paeonia albiflora	三兩 3 liǎng	9g
生薑	shēng jiāng	Fresh root of Zingiber officinale	八兩 8 liǎng	24g
醍醐, 百鍊酥	tí hú , bǎi liàn sū	Ghee from butter melted one hundred times	八兩 8 liǎng	24g
柴胡	chái hú	Root of Bupleurum chinense	八兩 8 liǎng	24g

上八味，㕮咀，以酒一斗，水二升合煮，取三升，去滓。適寒溫，先食服一升，日三。

Pound the above eight ingredients and decoct in a mix of one *dǒu* of liquor and two *shēng* of water, to obtain three *shēng*. Discard the dregs. Take one *shēng* before meals at whatever temperature she likes three times a day.

LINE 5.3

澤蘭湯治產後惡露不盡，腹痛不除，小腹急痛，痛引腰背，少氣力方。

Lycopus Decoction treats incomplete elimination of malign dew after childbirth, with abdominal pain that cannot be relieved, tension and pain in the lower abdomen, pain stretching to the lumbus and back, and shortage of *qì* and strength.

Lycopus Decoction
澤蘭湯 *zé lán tāng*

澤蘭 當歸 生地黃（各二兩） 甘草（一兩半） 生薑（三兩） 芍藥（一兩） 大棗（十枚）。

澤蘭	zé lán	Foliage and stalk of Lycopus lucidus	二兩 2 liǎng	6g
當歸	dāng guī	Root of Angelica polimorpha	二兩 2 liǎng	6g
生地黃	shēng dì huáng	Fresh root of Rehmannia glutinosa	二兩 2 liǎng	6g
甘草	gān cǎo	Root of Glycyrrhiza uralensis	一兩半 1.5 liǎng	4.5g
生薑	shēng jiāng	Fresh root of Zingiber officinale	三兩 3 liǎng	9g
芍藥	sháo yào	Root of Paeonia albiflora	一兩 1 liǎng	3g
大棗	dà zǎo	Mature fruit of Ziziphus jujuba	十枚 10 méi	10 pcs

上七味，㕮咀，以水九升煮取三升，去滓。分三服，日三。墮身欲死，服亦瘥。

Pound the above seven ingredients and decoct in nine *shēng* of water to obtain three *shēng*. Discard the dregs. Divide into three doses and take three times a day. It also causes recovery in cases of miscarriage* [when the patient is] on the verge of death.

---

* 墮身 *duò shēn*: Lit. "fall of the body." This could also mean "in cases of falling," but given the context here of gynecological prescriptions, I read it as a synonym for the more common 墮胎 *duò tāi* (lit. "fall of the fetus," in modern TCM usually referring to abortion).

LINE 5.4

甘草湯治產乳餘血不盡，逆搶心胸，手足逆冷，脣乾，腹脹，短氣方。

Licorice Decoction treats incomplete elimination of the residual blood after childbirth and nursing, [to the point where it] counterflows and prods the heart and chest, with counterflow cold in hands and feet, dried lips, abdominal distention, and shortness of breath.

Licorice Decoction
甘草湯 *gān cǎo tāng*

甘草 芍藥 桂心 阿膠（各三兩） 大黃（四兩）。

甘草	gān cǎo	Root of Glycyrrhiza uralensis	三兩 3 liǎng	9g
芍藥	sháo yào	Root of Paeonia albiflora	三兩 3 liǎng	9g
桂心	guì xīn	Shaved inner bark of Cinnamomum cassia	三兩 3 liǎng	9g
阿膠	ē jiāo	Gelatinous glue produced from Equus asinus	三兩 3 liǎng	9g
大黃	dà huáng	Root of Rheum palmatum	四兩 4 liǎng	12g

上五味，哎咀，以東流水一斗煮取三升，去滓，內阿膠令烊。分三服。一服入腹中，面即有顏色。一日一夜盡此三升，即下腹中惡血一二升，立瘥。當養之如新產者。

Pound the above five ingredients and decoct in one *dǒu* of east-flowing water to obtain three *shēng*. Discard the dregs, add the *ē jiāo* 阿膠, and let it melt. Divide into three doses. When the first dose has entered the abdomen, her face will promptly regain its color. After using up the full three *shēng* in one day and night, she will then discharge one to two *shēng* of malign blood from inside the abdomen. This will establish her recovery. You should nurture her like a new mother.

LINE 5.5

大黃湯治產後惡露不盡方。

Rhubarb Decoction treats incomplete elimination of malign dew after childbirth.

Rhubarb Decoction
大黃湯 *dà huáng tāng*

大黃 當歸 甘草 生薑 牡丹 芍藥（各三兩） 吳茱萸（一升）。

大黃	dà huáng	Root of Rheum palmatum	三兩 3 liǎng	9g
當歸	dāng guī	Root of Angelica polimorpha	三兩 3 liǎng	9g
甘草	gān cǎo	Root of Glycyrrhiza uralensis	三兩 3 liǎng	9g
生薑	shēng jiāng	Fresh root of Zingiber officinale	三兩 3 liǎng	9g
牡丹	mǔ dān	Bark of the root of Paeonia suffruticosa	三兩 3 liǎng	9g
芍藥	sháo yào	Root of Paeonia albiflora	三兩 3 liǎng	9g
吳茱萸	wú zhū yú	Unripe fruit of Evodia rutaecarpa	一升 1 shēng	24g

上七味，㕮咀，以水一斗煮取四升，去滓。分四服，一日令盡。加人參二兩，名人參大黃湯。

Pound the above seven ingredients and decoct in one *dǒu* of water to obtain four *shēng*. Discard the dregs. Divide into four doses and finish [the entire batch] in one day. If you add two *liǎng* of *rén shēn* (人參 Root of Panax ginseng), it is called *Ginseng and Rhubarb Decoction*.

LINE 5.6

治產後往來寒熱，惡露不盡，柴胡湯方。

Bupleurum Decoction treats alternating [aversion to] cold and heat [effusion] and incomplete elimination of malign dew after childbirth.

Bupleurum Decoction
柴胡湯 *chái hú tāng*

柴胡（八兩）桃仁（五十枚）當歸 黃芪 芍藥（各三兩）生薑（八兩）吳茱萸（二升）。

柴胡	chái hú	Root of Bupleurum chinense	八兩 8 liǎng	24g
桃仁	táo rén	Seed of Prunus persica	五十枚 50 méi	50 pcs
當歸	dāng guī	Root of Angelica polimorpha	三兩 3 liǎng	9g
黃芪	huáng qí	Root of Astragalus membranaceus	三兩 3 liǎng	9g
芍藥	sháo yào	Root of Paeonia albiflora	三兩 3 liǎng	9g
生薑	shēng jiāng	Fresh root of Zingiber officinale	八兩 8 liǎng	24g
吳茱萸	wú zhū yú	Unripe fruit of Evodia rutaecarpa	二升 2 shēng	48g

上七味，㕮咀，以水一斗三升煮取三升，去滓。先食服一升，日三。

Pound the above seven ingredients and decoct in one *dǒu* and three *shēng* of water to obtain three *shēng*. Discard the dregs. Take one *shēng* before meals three times a day.*

*   *Sòng* editors' notes: "The *Qiān Jīn Yì Fāng* uses one *dǒu* of clear liquor to decoct the drugs."

LINE 5.7

蒲黃湯治產後餘疾，有積血不去，腹大短氣，不得飲食，上衝胸脅，時時煩憒逆滿，手足惕疼，胃中結熱方。

Typha Pollen Decoction treats residual sickness after childbirth,[1] [such as] the presence of accumulated blood that fails to be removed, enlarged abdomen and shortness of breath, inability to eat and drink, upward surges [of *qi*] into the chest and ribsides; recurrent vexation, muddleheadedness, and counterflow fullness, soreness in the hands and feet, and heat bind in the center of the stomach.

Typha Pollen Decoction
蒲黃湯 *pú huáng tāng*

蒲黃（半兩）大黃 芒消 甘草 黃芩（各一兩）大棗（三十枚）。

蒲黃	pú huáng	Pollen of Typha angustata	半兩 0.5 liǎng	1.5g
大黃	dà huáng	Root of Rheum palmatum	一兩 1 liǎng	3g
硭硝	máng xiāo	Hydrated sodium sulfate	一兩 1 liǎng	3g
甘草	gān cǎo	Root of Glycyrrhiza uralensis	一兩 1 liǎng	3g
黃芩	huáng qín	Root of Scutellaria baicalensis	一兩 1 liǎng	3g
大棗	dà zǎo	Mature fruit of Ziziphus jujuba	三十枚 30 méi	30 pcs

上六味，㕮咀，以水五升煮取一升，清朝服，至日中下。若不止，進冷粥半盞即止。若不下，與少熱飲，自下。人羸者，半之。

Pound the above six ingredients and decoct in five *shēng* of water to obtain one *shēng*. Take at daybreak, and she will discharge [the blood] by midday.[2] If [the discharge] does not stop, eating half a small cup of cool rice gruel will make it stop. If there is no discharge, give her something hot to drink and she will spontaneously discharge. If the patient suffers from marked emaciation, half [the prescription].[3]

1.   餘疾 *yú jí*: I interpret this literally as referring to conditions that were caused by and are left over from the taxation and exhaustion of childbirth. But it is also possible to read it

as "conditions caused by residual blood after childbirth," since 余血 *yú xuè* is a standard term for the old blood remaining in the uterus after childbirth that is elsewhere called "malign dew." In any case, from the list of symptoms it is quite clear that this prescription addresses the problem of residual blood accumulating in the abdomen after childbirth.

2. 清朝服至日中下 *qīng cháo fú zhì rì zhōng xià*: The Chinese critical editions punctuate between 日中 and 下, suggesting the following interpretation: "Take it from daybreak until the middle of the day. There will be discharge..." I prefer to punctuate between 服 and 日中, based on a similar but slightly longer version of this prescription in the *Qiān Jīn Yì Fāng*: 清朝服至日中當利 若下不止... "Take it at daybreak. Arriving at midday, [her discharge] should be disinhibited. If the discharge does not stop..." (《千金翼方》6:4), in the prescription for *Rhubarb Decoction* (大黃湯 *dà huáng tāng*).

3. *Sòng* editors' notes: "The *Qiān Jīn Yì Fāng* calls it *Rhubarb Decoction* and does not use *máng xiāo* 硭硝."

LINE 5.8

治產後餘疾，惡露不除，積聚作病，血氣結搏，心腹疼痛，銅鏡鼻湯方。

Bronze Mirror Knob Decoction treats residual sickness after childbirth, failure to eliminate malign dew, accumulations and gatherings that are causing disease, blood and *qì* binding and contending with each other, and pain in the heart and abdomen.

Bronze Mirror Knob Decoction
銅鏡鼻湯 *tóng jìng bí tāng*

銅鏡鼻（十八銖，燒末）大黃（二兩半）乾地黃 芍藥 芎藭 乾漆 芒消（各二兩）亂髮（如雞子大，燒）大棗（三十枚）。

銅鏡鼻，燒末	tóng jìng bí, shāo mò	Bronze mirror knob, burnt and pulverized	十八銖 18 zhū	2.25g
大黃	dà huáng	Root of Rheum palmatum	二兩半 2.5 liǎng	7.5g
乾地黃	gān dì huáng	Dried root of Rehmannia glutinosa	二兩 2 liǎng	6g
芍藥	sháo yào	Root of Paeonia albiflora	二兩 2 liǎng	6g
川芎	chuān xiōng	Root of Ligusticum wallichii	二兩 2 liǎng	6g
乾漆	gān qī	Dried sap of Rhus verniciflua	二兩 2 liǎng	6g
硭硝	máng xiāo	Hydrated sodium sulfate	二兩 2 liǎng	6g
亂髮，燒	luàn fà, shāo	Matted hair, burnt	如雞子大 rú jī zǐ dà	an amount the size of a chicken egg

大棗	dà zǎo	Mature fruit of Ziziphus jujuba	三十枚 30 méi	30 pcs

上九味，㕮咀，以水七升煮取二升二合，去滓，內髮灰鏡鼻末，分三服。

Of the nine ingredients above, pound and decoct [the drugs] in seven *shēng* of water to obtain two *shēng* and two *gě*. Discard the dregs, add the ashed hair and pulverized mirror knob, and divide into three doses.

LINE 5.9

小銅鏡鼻湯治如前狀方。

Minor Bronze Mirror Knob Decoction treats the same conditions as above.

Minor Bronze Mirror Knob Decoction
小銅鏡鼻湯 *xiǎo tóng jìng bí tāng*

銅鏡鼻（十銖，燒末）大黃 甘草 黃芩 芒消 乾地黃（各二兩）桃仁（五十枚）。

銅鏡鼻, 燒末	tóng jìng bí, shāo mò	Bronze mirror knob, burnt and pulverized	十銖 10 zhū	1.25g
大黃	dà huáng	Root of Rheum palmatum	二兩 2 liǎng	6g
甘草	gān cǎo	Root of Glycyrrhiza uralensis	二兩 2 liǎng	6g
黃芩	huáng qín	Root of Scutellaria baicalensis	二兩 2 liǎng	6g
硭硝	máng xiāo	Hydrated sodium sulfate	二兩 2 liǎng	6g
乾地黃	gān dì huáng	Dried root of Rehmannia glutinosa	二兩 2 liǎng	6g
桃仁	táo rén	Seed of Prunus persica	五十枚 50 méi	50 pcs

上七味，㕮咀，以酒六升煮取三升，去滓，內鏡鼻末，分三服。亦治遁尸心腹痛，及三十六尸疾。

Pound the above seven ingredients and decoct in six *shēng* of liquor to obtain three *shēng*. Discard the dregs, add the pulverized mirror knob, and divide into three doses. It also treats heart and abdominal pain from vanishing corpse [syndrome], as well as the thirty-six corpse diseases.*

---

*   *Sòng* editors' notes: "三十六尸疾 *sān shí liù shī jí*: This is not a standard technical term but most likely refers to all the varieties of corpse disease, 尸病 *shī bìng*. The *Bìng Yuán Lùn* discusses the varieties of corpse disease in twelve entries and explains in the introduction to this section: "The human body is inhabited by the three corpses and the various worms, which are all born with the person. These worms shun blood. Their malignancy can connect with ghosts. Often they link with and draw in external evil, causing trouble and injury for the person. When [the evil] erupts, it appears like this: Sometimes it is deep down and secret and one doesn't know where the discomfort lies, but there is no place that is not malign. Sometimes the abdomen is painful and the intestines are tense.... Sometimes the mind is confused. It alters its appearance very frequently. The condition is generally the same but there are small differences. Nevertheless, since one prescription treats them all, they are all called corpse disease." (《病源論》 23:2:1-12). Vanishing corpse (遁尸 *dùn shī*) is one variety of corpse disease which "lodges and conceals itself between the muscles and the blood channels. It arises and becomes active if there has been an offense against prohibitions, causing distention, fullness, and stabbing pain in the heart and abdomen, tense and panting *qì* that attacks both rib-sides and surges upward against the heart and chest. It subsides and then recurs and flares up again. It lodges, then vanishes without dispersing and is therefore called vanishing corpse (《病源論》 23:2:3)."

LINE 5.10

治產後兒生處空，流血不盡，小腹絞痛，梔子湯方。

Gardenia Decoction treats postpartum emptiness in the place where the fetus was engendered with inexhaustible bleeding and gripping pain in the lower abdomen.

Gardenia Decoction
梔子湯 *zhī zǐ tāng*

梔子三十枚，以水一斗煮取六升，內當歸，芍藥各二兩，蜜五合，生薑五兩，羊脂一兩於梔子汁中，煎取二升。分三服，日三。

Decoct thirty pieces of *zhī zǐ* (梔子 Fruit of Gardenia jasminoides) in one *dǒu* of water to obtain six *shēng*. Add two *liǎng* each of *dāng guī* (當歸 Root of Angelica polimorpha) and *sháo yào* (芍藥 Root of Paeonia albiflora), five *gě* of *mǐ* (米 Seed of Oryza sativa), five *liǎng* of *shēng jiāng* (生薑 Fresh root of Zingiber officinale), and one *liǎng* of *yáng zhī* (羊脂 Unrendered fat of Capra hircus) to the gardenia juice and simmer to obtain two *shēng*. Divide into three doses and take three times a day.

LINE 5.11

治產後三日至七日，腹中餘血未盡，絞痛強滿，氣息不通，生地黃湯方。

Fresh Rehmannia Decoction treats incomplete elimination of the residual blood in the abdomen with gripping pain, rigidity and fullness, and stopped breathing, during the third to seventh days postpartum.

Fresh Rehmannia Decoction
生地黃湯 shēng dì huáng tāng

生地黃（五兩）生薑（三兩）大黃 芍藥 茯苓 細辛 桂心 當歸甘草 黃芩（各一兩半）大棗（二十枚）。

生地黃	shēng dì huáng	Fresh root of Rehmannia glutinosa	五兩 5 liǎng	15g
生薑	shēng jiāng	Fresh root of Zingiber officinale	二兩 2 liǎng	6g
大黃	dà huáng	Root of Rheum palmatum	一兩半 1.5 liǎng	4.5g
芍藥	sháo yào	Root of Paeonia albiflora	一兩半 1.5 liǎng	4.5g
茯苓	fú líng	Dried fungus of Poria cocos	一兩半 1.5 liǎng	4.5g
細辛	xì xīn	Complete plant including root of Asarum heteropoides	一兩半 1.5 liǎng	4.5g
桂心	guì xīn	Shaved inner bark of Cinnamomum cassia	一兩半 1.5 liǎng	4.5g
當歸	dāng guī	Root of Angelica polimorpha	一兩半 1.5 liǎng	4.5g
甘草	gān cǎo	Root of Glycyrrhiza uralensis	一兩半 1.5 liǎng	4.5g
黃芩	huáng qín	Root of Scutellaria baicalensis	一兩半 1.5 liǎng	4.5g
大棗	dà zǎo	Mature fruit of Ziziphus jujuba	二十枚 20 méi	20 pcs

上十一味，㕮咀，以水八升煮取二升半，去滓。分三服，日三。

Pound the above eleven ingredients and decoct in eight *shēng* of water to obtain two and a half *shēng*. Discard the dregs. Divide into three doses and take three times a day.

LINE 5.12

治新產後有血，腹中切痛，大黃乾漆湯方。

Rhubarb and Lacquer Decoction treats [continuing] presence of blood [in the uterus] right after childbirth* with cutting pain in the center of the abdomen.

Rhubarb and Lacquer Decoction
大黃干漆湯 dà huáng gān qī tāng

大黃 乾漆 乾地黃 桂心 乾薑（各二兩）。

大黃	dà huáng	Root of Rheum palmatum	二兩 2 liǎng	6g
乾漆	gān qī	Dried sap of Rhus verniciflua	二兩 2 liǎng	6g
乾地黃	gān dì huáng	Dried root of Rehmannia glutinosa	二兩 2 liǎng	6g
桂心	guì xīn	Shaved inner bark of Cinnamomum cassia	二兩 2 liǎng	6g
乾薑	gān jiāng	Dried root of Zingiber officinale	二兩 2 liǎng	6g

上五味，㕮咀，以水三升，清酒五升煮取三升，去滓。溫服一升，血當下；若不瘥，明旦服一升；滿三服，病無不瘥。

Pound the above five ingredients and decoct in three *shēng* of water and five *shēng* of clear liquor to obtain three *shēng*. Discard the dregs. Taking one *shēng* warm should precipitate the blood. If she fails to recover, take another *shēng* at the next daybreak. When she has used up all three doses, the disease is bound to have been cured.

* 新產後有血 *xīn chǎn hòu yǒu xuè*: In this context, this phrase does not mean that the prescription treats postpartum bleeding, as a modern reader trained in biomedicine might suspect, but, to the contrary, that it treats blood remaining in the uterus after childbirth, or in other words, the incomplete elimination of malign dew. This becomes clear in the latter half of this prescription where Sūn Sī-Miǎo states directly that it should induce the precipitation of blood (血當下 *xuè dāng xià*).

LINE 5.13

治產後血不去，麻子酒方。

Cannabis Fruit Wine treats failure to eliminate blood after childbirth.

Cannabis Fruit Wine
麻子酒 *má zǐ jiǔ*

麻子五升，擣，以酒一斗漬一宿，明旦去滓。溫服一升，先食服；不瘥，夜服一升，不吐下。忌房事一月。將養如初產法。

Pound five *shēng* of *má zǐ* (麻子 Seed of Cannabis sativa) and soak in one *dǒu* of liquor over one night. At the next dawn, discard the dregs. Take one *shēng* warm before meals. If she fails to recover, take another *shēng* at night. [The medicine] will not make her vomit, but [only] discharge [the blood].˙ Prohibit sexual activity for the first month and nurture her according to the methods for newly delivered [mothers].

* 不吐下 *bù tú xià*: My interpretation of this phrase is based on a similar statement in the next prescription, which specifies that *Cimicifuga Decoction* is supposed to make her vomit in order to discharge the blood. Vomiting is a common side-effect which was often associated with the efficacy of the medicine. Especially in the context of expelling something from the abdomen, whether a dead fetus, a living child in a stalled labor, a retained placenta, or lochia, many prescriptions are intended to cause vomiting in order to induce the abdominal muscles to contract, thereby stimulating the discharge.

LINE 5.14

治產後惡物不盡，或經一月，半歲，一歲，升麻湯方。

Cimicifuga Decoction treats incomplete elimination of malign substances after childbirth, whether a month, half a year, or one year have passed.

Cimicifuga Decoction
升麻湯 *shēng má tāng*

升麻三兩，以清酒五升煮取二升，去滓。分再服，當吐下惡物，勿怪，良。

Decoct three *liǎng* of *shēng má* (升麻 Rhizome of Cimifuga foetida) in five *shēng* of clear liquor to obtain two *shēng* and discard the dregs. Divide into two doses. [The medicine] is supposed to induce vomiting and [thereby] discharge the malign substance. Do not consider this strange; it is good.

LINE 5.15

治產後惡血不盡，腹中絞刺痛不可忍方。

[The following] prescription treats incomplete elimination of malign blood after childbirth with unbearable gripping and stabbing pain in the center of the abdomen.

Formula

大黃 黃芩 桃仁（各三兩）桂心 甘草 當歸（各二兩）芍藥（四兩）生地黃（六兩）。

大黃	dà huáng	Root of Rheum palmatum	三兩 3 liǎng	9g
黃芩	huáng qín	Root of Scutellaria baicalensis	三兩 3 liǎng	9g
桃仁	táo rén	Seed of Prunus persica	三兩 3 liǎng	9g

桂心	guì xīn	Shaved inner bark of Cinnamomum cassia	二兩 2 liǎng	6g
甘草	gān cǎo	Root of Glycyrrhiza uralensis	二兩 2 liǎng	6g
當歸	dāng guī	Root of Angelica polimorpha	二兩 2 liǎng	6g
芍藥	sháo yào	Root of Paeonia albiflora	四兩 4 liǎng	12g
生地黃	shēng dì huáng	Fresh root of Rehmannia glutinosa	六兩 6 liǎng	18g

上八味，㕮咀，以水九升煮取二升半，去滓，食前分三服。

Pound the above eight ingredients and decoct in nine *shēng* of water to obtain two and a half *shēng*. Discard the dregs. Take before meals, divided into three doses.

LINE 5.16

治產後漏血不止方。

[The following] prescription treats incessant spotting of blood after childbirth.

露蜂房 敗船茹。

| 露蜂房 | lù fēng fáng | Nest of Polistes mandarinus |
| 敗船茹 | bài chuán rú | Shavings of entangled Phyllostachys bambusoides roots |

上二味，等分作灰，取酪若漿服方寸匕，日三。

[Char] equal amounts of the above two ingredients into ashes. Take koumiss or fermented millet drink and take a square-inch spoon [of the medicine] in it three times a day.

LINE 5.17

又方

Another prescription:

Formula

大黃（三兩）芒消（一兩）桃仁（三十枚）水蛭（三十枚）虻蟲（三十枚）甘草 當歸（各二兩）蟅蟲（四十枚）。

大黃	dà huáng	Root of Rheum palmatum	三兩 3 liǎng	9g
硭硝	máng xiāo	Hydrated sodium sulfate	一兩 1 liǎng	3g
桃仁	táo rén	Seed of Prunus persica	三十枚 30 méi	30 pcs
水蛭	shuǐ zhì	Dried body of Whitmania pigra	三十枚 30 méi	30 pcs
虻蟲	méng chóng	Dried body of the female of Tabanus bivittatus	三十枚 30 méi	30 pcs
甘草	gān cǎo	Root of Glycyrrhiza uralensis	二兩 2 liǎng	6g
當歸	dāng guī	Root of Angelica polimorpha	二兩 2 liǎng	6g
蟅蟲	zhè chóng	Entire dried body of the female of Eupolyphaga sinensis	四十枚 40 méi	40 pcs

上八味，哎咀，以水三升，酒二升合煮，取三升，去滓。分三服，當下血。

Pound the above eight ingredients and decoct in a mix of three *shēng* of water and two *shēng* of liquor, to obtain three *shēng*. Discard the dregs and divide into three doses. It should precipitate the blood.

LINE 5.18

又方

Another prescription:

Formula

桂心 蠐螬 (各二兩) 栝樓根 牡丹 (各三兩) 豉 (一升) 。

桂心	guì xīn	Shaved inner bark of Cinnamomum cassia	二兩 2 liǎng	6g
蠐螬	qí cáo	Dried larva of Holotrichia diomphalia	二兩 2 liǎng	6g
栝蔞根	guā lóu gēn	Root of Trichosanthes kirilowii	三兩 3 liǎng	9g
牡丹	mǔ dān	Bark of the root of Paeonia suffruticosa	三兩 3 liǎng	9g
[豆]豉	[dòu] chǐ	Preparation of Glycine max	一升 1 shēng	24g

上五味，哎咀，以水八升煮取三升，去滓，分三服。

Pound the above five ingredients, decoct in eight *shēng* of water to obtain three *shēng*, and discard the dregs. Divide into three doses.[*]

*   *Sòng* editors' notes: "At this point, the *Sūn Zhēn Rén* edition inserts two prescriptions, one for postpartum wind strike with drifting swelling (identical with the bath infusion from chapter three of volume three, on Line 3.23 above p. 286), and one for unbearable abdominal and intestinal pain.

LINE 5.19

治產後血不可止者方。

[The following] prescription treats incessant postpartum bleeding.

乾昌蒲三兩，以清酒五升漬，煮取三升，分再服，即止。

Soak three *liǎng* of dried *chāng pú* (菖蒲 Rhizome of Acorus gramineus) in five shēng of clear liquor and decoct it to obtain three *shēng*. Take it divided into two doses, and [the bleeding] will promptly stop.

LINE 5.20

治產後惡血不除，四體並惡方。

[The following] prescription treats failure to eliminate malign blood after childbirth, with simultaneous malignancy in the four limbs.

續骨木二十兩，破如筹子大，以水一斗煮取三升。分三服，相去如人行十里久，間食粥。或小便數，或惡血下，即瘥。此木得三遍煮。

Break twenty *liǎng* of *xù gǔ mù* (續骨木 Stems of Sambucus williamsii) into pieces the size of counting tallies and decoct in one *dǒu* of water to obtain three *shēng*. Divide into three doses [and take] them separated from each other by the length of time it takes a person to walk ten *lǐ*. In between, eat rice gruel. [The medicine] might [cause her to] urinate frequently or discharge malign blood, either of which indicates recovery. This wood may be decocted three times.*

*   This means that you can use the same wood to make three batches of this medicine.

LINE 5.21

治產後下血不盡，煩悶，腹痛方。

[The following] prescription treats incomplete descent of blood after childbirth, with vexation, oppression, and abdominal pain.

Formula

羚羊角（燒成炭，刮取三兩）芍藥（二兩，熬令黃）枳實（一兩，細切，熬令黃）。

羚羊角,燒成炭,刮取	líng yáng jiǎo, shāo chéng tàn, guā qǔ	Horn of the male Saiga tatarica, charred into ashes and shaved	三兩 3 liǎng	9g
芍藥,熬令黃	sháo yào, āo lìng huáng	Root of Paeonia albiflora, roasted until yellow	二兩 2 liǎng	6g
枳實,細切,熬令黃	zhǐ shí, xì qiē āo lìng huáng	Unripe fruit of Poncirus trifoliata, finely chopped and roasted until yellow	一兩 1 liǎng	3g

上三味，治下篩，煮水作湯。服方寸匕，日再夜一，稍加至二匕。

Finely pestle and sift the above three ingredients. Boil water to make a hot liquid. Take a square-inch spoon [of the medicine in the hot water], twice during the day and once at night, gradually increasing [the dosage] to two spoons.

LINE 5.22

又方

Another prescription:

鹿角燒成炭，擣篩。煮豉汁，服方寸匕，日三夜再，稍加至二七。不能用豉清，煮水作湯用方。

Char *lù jiǎo* (鹿角 Ossified antler or antler base of Cervus nippon) into ashes and pound and sift it. Boil leaven juice and take a square-inch spoon in this three times during the day and twice at night, gradually increasing [the dosage] to two spoons. If you cannot use leaven juice, make a decoction with boiled water and use that instead.

LINE 5.23

又方

Another prescription:

擣生藕取汁，飲二升，甚驗。

Pound fresh lotus to make juice and drink two *shēng*. Best results.

LINE 5.24

又方

Another prescription:

生地黃汁一升，酒三合和，溫頓服之。

Mix one *shēng* of *shēng dì huáng zhī* (生地黃汁 Juice from the fresh root of Rehmannia glutinosa) with three *gě* of liquor and quaff heated in a single dose.

LINE 5.25

又方

Another prescription:

赤小豆，擣散，取東流水和服方寸匕，不瘥便服。

Grind *chì xiǎo dòu* (赤小豆 Fruit of Phaseolus calcaratus) into a powder and take a square-inch spoon mixed into east-flowing water. If she fails to recover, take another dose.

LINE 5.26

治產後血瘕痛方。

The following prescription treats painful blood conglomerations after childbirth.

古鐵一斤，秤鐵斧頭鐵杵亦得，炭火燒令赤，內酒五升中，稍熱服之，神妙。

Heat one *jīn* of old iron — steelyard weights, ax heads, or iron pestles can all be used — over a charcoal fire until glowing red. Immerse it in five *shēng* of liquor and drink [the liquor when it is still] slightly hot. [This prescription has] wondrous [results].

LINE 5.27

治婦人血瘕，心腹積聚，乳餘疾，絕生，小腹堅滿，貫臍中熱，腰背痛，小便不利，大便難，不下食，有伏虫，臚脹，癰疽腫，久寒留熱，胃管有邪氣方。

[The following] prescription treats women's blood conglomerations, accumulations and gatherings in the heart and abdomen, residual sickness from childbearing, and interrupted fertility,* with [the symptoms of] hardness and fullness in the lower abdomen, heat running through the center of the navel, pain in the lumbus and back, inhibited urination, difficult defecation, inability to get food down, presence of latent worms, distention in the front part of the abdomen, welling- and flat-abscesses and swelling, chronic cold and retained heat, and presence of evil *qì* in the stomach duct.

Formula

半夏（一兩六銖） 石膏 藜蘆 牡蒙 蓯蓉（各十八銖） 桂心 乾薑（各一兩）烏喙（半兩） 巴豆（六十銖，研如膏）。

半夏	bàn xià	Rhizome of Pinellia ternata	一兩 1 liǎng 六銖 6 zhū	3.75g
石膏	shí gāo	Gypsum	十八銖 18 zhū	2.25g
藜蘆	lí lú	Root and rhizome of Veratrum nigrum	十八銖 18 zhū	2.25g
牡蒙	mǔ méng	Root of Paris quadrifolia	十八銖 18 zhū	2.25g
蓯蓉	cōng róng	Stalk of Cistanche salsa	十八銖 18 zhū	2.25g
桂心	guì xīn	Shaved inner bark of Cinnamomum cassia	一兩 1 liǎng	3g
乾薑	gān jiāng	Dried root of Zingiber officinale	一兩 1 liǎng	3g
烏喙	wū huì	Main tuber of Aconitum carmichaeli	半兩 0.5 liǎng	1.5g
巴豆,研如膏	bā dòu, yán rú gāo	Seed of Croton tiglium, ground into a paste	六十銖 60 zhū	7.5g

上九味，末之，蜜丸如小豆。服二丸，日三。及治男子疝病。

Pulverize the above nine ingredients and mix with honey into pills the size of azuki beans. Take two pills [per dose] three times a day. [This prescription] also treats mounting disease in men.

---

*　　　　絕生 *jué shēng*: I interpret this as a synonym for the more common technical term 絕產 *jué chǎn* (lit. "interruption of [the woman's ability to] give birth").

LINE 5.28

治婦人血瘕痛方。

[The following] prescription treats women's blood conglomerations and pain.

Formula

乾薑（一兩）烏賊骨（一兩）。

乾薑	gān jiāng	Dried root of Zingiber officinale	一兩 1 liǎng	3g
烏賊骨	wū zéi gǔ	Calcified shell of Sepiella main-droni	一兩 1 liǎng	3g

上二味，治下篩，酒服方寸匕，日三。

Finely pestle and sift the above two ingredients and take a square-inch spoon in liquor three times a day.

LINE 5.29

又方

Another prescription:

末桂溫酒服方寸匕，日三。

Take a square-inch spoon of pulverized cinnamon in liquor three times a day.

6. Diarrhea 下痢

LINE 6.1

膠蠟湯治產後三日內，下諸雜五色痢方。

Ass Hide Glue and Bee's Wax Decoction treats five-color diarrhea[1] in the first three days postpartum, with the discharge of various [substances] all mixed together.

Ass Hide Glue and Bee's Wax Decoction
膠蠟湯 *jiāo là tāng*

阿膠（一兩） 蠟（如簿棋三枚） 當歸（一兩半） 黃連（二兩） 黃蘗（一兩） 陳廩米（一升）。

阿膠	ē jiāo	Gelatinous glue produced from Equus asinus	一兩 1 liǎng	3g
蠟	là	Secretion of Apis cerana	如簿棋三枚 rú bo qí sān méi	an amount the size of three chess pieces
當歸	dāng guī	Root of Angelica polimorpha	一兩半 1.5 liǎng	4.5g
黃連	huáng lián	Rhizome of Coptis chinensis	二兩 2 liǎng	6g
黃蘗	huáng bò	Bark of Phellodendron amurense	一兩 1 liǎng	3g
陳廩米	chén lǐn mǐ	Seed of Oryza sativa	一升 1 shēng	24g

上六味，㕮咀，以水八升煮米蟹目沸，去米內藥，煮取二升，去滓，內膠蠟令烊。分四服，一日令盡。

Pound the above six ingredients and cook the rice in eight *shēng* of water to a crab-eye boil.[2] Remove the rice, add the drugs, and decoct it to obtain two *shēng*. Discard the dregs, add the *ē jiāo* 阿膠 and *là* 蠟, and let them melt. Divide into four doses and finish [the whole preparation] in one day.

1. 五色痢 *wǔ sè lì*: This refers to a subcategory of *lì* that is a combination of the other types of diarrhea, namely red diarrhea (赤痢 *chì lì*, feces containing blood), white diarrhea (白痢 *bái lì*, diarrhea with pus in the feces), yellow diarrhea (黃痢 *huáng lì*) green-blue diarrhea (青痢 *qīng lì*), or water and grain diarrhea (水穀痢 *shuǐ gǔ lì*). See (《病源 論》17:16).

2. 蟹目沸 *xiè mù fèi*: 蟹目 ("crab eyes") is a standard expression for describing the appearance of the tiny air bubbles that rise to the surface when water first starts boiling. Thus, the entire phrase here does not mean to boil the rice until it has the appearance of crab eyes, but to cook it by simmering it gently.

LINE 6.2

治產後餘寒下痢，便膿血赤白，日數十行，腹痛，時時下血，桂蜜湯方。

Cinnamon and Honey Decoction treats postpartum residual cold and red or white diarrhea with pus and blood in the stool, dozens of bowel movements a day, abdominal pain, and recurring descent of blood.

Cinnamon and Honey Decoction
桂蜜湯 *guì mì tāng*

桂心（二兩） 蜜（一升） 附子（一兩） 乾薑 甘草（各二兩） 當歸（二 兩） 赤石脂（十兩）。

桂心	guì xīn	Shaved inner bark of Cinnamomum cassia	二兩 2 liǎng	6g
米	mǐ	Seed of Oryza sativa	一升 1 shēng	24g
附子	fù zǐ	Lateral root of Aconitum carmichaeli	一兩 1 liǎng	3g
乾薑	gān jiāng	Dried root of Zingiber officinale	二兩 2 liǎng	6g
甘草	gān cǎo	Root of Glycyrrhiza uralensis	二兩 2 liǎng	6g
當歸	dāng guī	Root of Angelica polimorpha	二兩 2 liǎng	6g
赤石脂	chì shí zhī	Halloysite	十兩 10 liǎng	30g

上七味，㕮咀，以水六升煮取三升，去滓內蜜，煎一兩沸。分三服，日 三。

Pound the above seven ingredients and decoct in six *shēng* of water to obtain three *shēng*. Discard the dregs, add the honey and simmer it, bringing it to a rolling boil once or twice. Divide into three doses and take three times a day.

LINE 6.3

治產後下赤白，腹中絞痛，湯方。

[The following] decoction treats postpartum red and white discharge* with gripping pain in the center of the abdomen.

Formula

芍藥 乾地黃（各四兩） 甘草 阿膠 艾葉 當歸（各八兩）。

芍藥	sháo yào	Root of Paeonia albiflora	四兩 4 liǎng	12g
乾地黃	gān dì huáng	Dried root of Rehmannia glutinosa	四兩 4 liǎng	12g
甘草	gān cǎo	Root of Glycyrrhiza uralensis	八兩 8 liǎng	24g
阿膠	ē jiāo	Gelatinous glue produced from Equus asinus	八兩 8 liǎng	24g
艾葉	ài yè	Dry-roasted foliage of Artemisia argyi	八兩 8 liǎng	24g
當歸	dāng guī	Root of Angelica polimorpha	八兩 8 liǎng	24g

上六味，㕮咀，以水七升煮取二升半，去滓，內膠令烊，分三服。

Pound the above six ingredients and decoct in seven *shēng* of water to obtain two and a half *shēng*. Discard the dregs, add the *ē jiāo* 阿膠 and let it melt. Divide into three doses.

---

*   下赤白 *xià chì bái*: This refers to a discharge containing blood and pus. I read this in this context as a synonym for 赤白痢 *chì bái lì* (red and white diarrhea), not as referring to vaginal discharge.

LINE 6.4

治產後赤白下久不斷，身面悉腫方。

[The following] prescription treats chronic and incessant red and white discharge after childbirth, with pervasive swelling of the body and face.

Formula

大豆（一升，微熬） 小麥（一升） 吳茱萸（半升） 蒲黃（一升）。

大豆, 微熬	dà dòu, wēi āo	Seed of Glycine max, slightly toasted	一升 1 shēng	24g
小麥	xiǎo mài	Seed or flour of Triticum aestivum	一升 1 shēng	24g
吳茱萸	wú zhū yú	Unripe fruit of Evodia rutaecarpa	半升 0.5 shēng	12g
蒲黃	pú huáng	Pollen of Typha angustata	一升 1 shēng	24g

上四味，以水九升煮取三升，去滓，分三服。此方神驗。亦可以水五升，酒一斗煎取四升，分四服。

Decoct the above four ingredients in nine *shēng* of water to obtain three *shēng*. Discard the dregs and divide into three doses. This prescription has divine results. One can also simmer [the ingredients] in five *shēng* of water and one *dǒu* of liquor to obtain four *shēng* and then divide it into four doses.

LINE 6.5

治產後痢赤白，心腹刺痛方。

[The following] prescription treats red and white diarrhea after childbirth with stabbing pain in the heart and abdomen.

Formula

薤白（一兩）當歸（二兩）酸石榴皮（三兩）地榆（四兩）粳米（五合）。

薤白	xiè bái	Stalk of Allium macrostemon	一兩 1 liǎng	3g
當歸	dāng guī	Root of Angelica polimorpha	二兩 2 liǎng	6g
酸石榴皮	suān shí liú pí	Sour rind of the fruit of Punica granatum	三兩 3 liǎng	9g
地榆	dì yú	Root of Sanguisorba officinalis	四兩 4 liǎng	12g
粳米	jīng mǐ	Seed of the non-glutinous variety of Oryza sativa	五合 5 gě	35ml

上五味，㕮咀，以水六升煮取二升半，去滓，分三服。

Pound the above five ingredients and decoct in six *shēng* of water to obtain two and a half *shēng*. Discard the dregs and divide into three doses.˙

*   *Sòng* editors' note: "The *Bì Xiào Fāng* adds one *liǎng* of *hòu pò* (厚朴 Bark of Magnolia officinalis) and 1.5 *liǎng* each of *ē jiāo* (阿膠 Gelatinous glue produced from Equus asinus), *rén shēn* (人參 Root of Panax ginseng), *gān cǎo* (甘草 Root of Glycyrrhiza uralensis), and *huáng lián* (黃連 Rhizome of Coptis chinensis)."

LINE 6.6

治產後下痢赤白，腹痛，當歸湯方。

Chinese Angelica Decoction treats red and white diarrhea after childbirth with abdominal pain.

Chinese Angelica Decoction
當歸湯 *dāng guī tāng*

當歸 (三兩) 乾薑 白朮 (各二兩) 芎藭 (二兩半) 甘草 白艾 (熟者) 附子 (各一兩) 龍骨 (三兩)。

當歸	dāng guī	Root of Angelica polimorpha	三兩 3 liǎng	9g
乾薑	gān jiāng	Dried root of Zingiber officinale	二兩 2 liǎng	6g
白朮	bái zhú	Rhizome of Atractylodes macrocephala	二兩 2 liǎng	6g
川芎	chuān xiōng	Root of Ligusticum wallichii	二兩半 2.5 liǎng	7.5g
甘草	gān cǎo	Root of Glycyrrhiza uralensis	一兩 1 liǎng	3g
白艾,熟者	bái ài, shú zhě	Foliage of Crossostephium chinense, cooked	一兩 1 liǎng	3g
附子	fù zǐ	Lateral root of Aconitum carmichaeli	一兩 1 liǎng	3g
龍骨	lóng gǔ	Os draconis	三兩 3 liǎng	9g

上八味，咬咀，以水六升煮取二升，去滓。分三服，一日令盡。

Pound the above eight ingredients and decoct in six *shēng* of water to obtain two *shēng*. Discard the dregs and divide into three doses. Use [the medicine] up in one day.

LINE 6.7

治產後下痢兼虛極，白頭翁湯方。

Pulsatilla Decoction treats postpartum diarrhea concurrent with vacuity extreme.

Pulsatilla Decoction
白頭翁湯 *bái tóu wēng tāng*

白頭翁（二兩） 阿膠 秦皮 黃連 甘草（各二兩） 黃蘗（三兩）。

白頭翁	bái tóu wēng	Root of Pulsatilla chinensis	二兩 2 liǎng	6g
阿膠	ē jiāo	Gelatinous glue produced from Equus asinus	二兩 2 liǎng	6g
秦皮	qín pí	Bark of the trunk of Fraxinus rhunchophylla	二兩 2 liǎng	6g
黃連	huáng lián	Rhizome of Coptis chinensis	二兩 2 liǎng	6g
甘草	gān cǎo	Root of Glycyrrhiza uralensis	二兩 2 liǎng	6g
黃蘗	huáng bò	Bark of Phellodendron amurense	三兩 3 liǎng	9g

上六味，㕮咀，以水七升煮取二升半，去滓，內膠令烊。分三服，日三。

Pound the above six ingredients and decoct in seven *shēng* of water to obtain two and a half *shēng*. Discard the dregs, add the *ē jiāo* 阿膠 and let it melt. Divide into three doses and take three times a day.

LINE 6.8

治產後早起中風冷，泄痢及帶下，鱉甲湯方。

Turtle Shell Decoction treats wind and cold strike caused by rising too early after childbirth, with diarrhea and vaginal discharge.

Turtle Shell Decoction
鱉甲湯 *biē jiǎ tāng*

鱉甲（如手大） 當歸 黃連 乾薑（各二兩） 黃蘗（長一尺,廣三寸）。

鱉甲	biē jiǎ	Dorsal shell of Amyda sinensis	如手大 rú shǒu dà	an amount the size of a hand
當歸	dāng guī	Root of Angelica polimorpha	二兩 2 liǎng	6g
黃連	huáng lián	Rhizome of Coptis chinensis	二兩 2 liǎng	6g
乾薑	gān jiāng	Dried root of Zingiber officinale	二兩 2 liǎng	6g
黃蘗	huáng bò	Bark of Phellodendron amurense	長一尺,廣三寸 cháng 1 chǐ, guǎng sān cùn	30cm long, 3 cm wide

上五味，哎咀，以水七升煮取三升，去滓。分三服，日三。

Pound the above five ingredients and decoct in seven *shēng* of water to obtain three *shēng*. Discard the dregs. Divide into three doses and take three times a day.*

*   *Sòng* editors' note: "The *Qiān Jīn Yì Fāng* adds one *liǎng* of *bái tóu wēng* (白頭翁 Root of Pulsatilla chinensis)."

LINE 6.9

龍骨丸治產後虛冷，下血及穀下晝夜無數，兼治產後惡露不斷方。

Dragon Bone Pills treat postpartum vacuity cold with bloody and grain diarrhea[1] that occurs innumerable times during the day and at night, as well as incessant [flow of] malign dew after childbirth.

Dragon Bone Pills
龍骨丸 *lóng gǔ wán*

龍骨（四兩）乾薑 甘草 桂心（各二兩）。

龍骨	lóng gǔ	Os draconis	四兩	4 liǎng	12g
乾薑	gān jiāng	Dried root of Zingiber officinale	二兩	2 liǎng	6g
甘草	gān cǎo	Root of Glycyrrhiza uralensis	二兩	2 liǎng	6g
桂心	guì xīn	Shaved inner bark of Cinnamomum cassia	二兩	2 liǎng	6g

上四味，末之，蜜和，暖酒服二十丸如梧子，日三。

Pulverize the above four ingredients and mix with honey [to make pills]. Take twenty pills the size of firmiana seeds in warm liquor three times a day. [2]

1.   下血及穀下 *xià xuè jí gǔ xià*: Lit. "descent of blood as well as grain discharge." I interpret 穀下 as describing the symptoms of a type of diarrhea that is usually referred to by the technical term 水穀痢 *shuǐ gǔ lì* (grain and water diarrhea). This condition is caused by a vacuity of spleen and stomach *qì*, resulting in their failure to digest solids and fluids, so that they are discharged as diarrhea without being digested properly. See (《病源論》 17:1) for a lengthy explanation of the pathology and etiology of this condition.
2.   *Sòng* editors' note: "Another [version of this] prescription adds two *liǎng* each of *rén shēn* (人參 Root of Panax ginseng) and *dà huáng* (大黃 Root of Rheum palmatum)."

LINE 6.10

阿膠丸治產後虛冷洞下，心腹絞痛，兼泄瀉不止方。

Ass Hide Glue Pills treat postpartum throughflux diarrhea* from vacuity cold, with gripping pain in the heart and abdomen and concurrent incessant diarrhea.

Ass Hide Glue Pills
阿膠丸 *ē jiāo wán*

阿膠（四兩） 人參 甘草 龍骨 桂心 乾地黃 白朮 黃連 當歸 附子（各二兩）
。

阿膠	ē jiāo	Gelatinous glue produced from Equus asinus	四兩 4 liǎng	12g
人參	rén shēn	Root of Panax ginseng	二兩 2 liǎng	6g
甘草	gān cǎo	Root of Glycyrrhiza uralensis	二兩 2 liǎng	6g
龍骨	lóng gǔ	Os draconis	二兩 2 liǎng	6g
桂心	guì xīn	Shaved inner bark of Cinnamomum cassia	二兩 2 liǎng	6g
乾地黃	gān dì huáng	Dried root of Rehmannia glutinosa	二兩 2 liǎng	6g
白朮	bái zhú	Rhizome of Atractylodes macrocephala	二兩 2 liǎng	6g
黃連	huáng lián	Rhizome of Coptis chinensis	二兩 2 liǎng	6g
當歸	dāng guī	Root of Angelica polimorpha	二兩 2 liǎng	6g
附子	fù zǐ	Lateral root of Aconitum carmichaeli	二兩 2 liǎng	6g

上十味，末之，蜜丸如梧子。溫酒服二十丸，日三。

Pulverize the above ten ingredients and mix with honey into pills the size of firmiana seeds. Take twenty pills in warm liquor three times a day.

---

*　　　洞下 *dòng xià*: extreme diarrhea, potentially with retching and vomiting, caused by a failure of the digestive functions. It is most commonly found in the compound 洞泄 *dòng xiè*, which in modern TCM, is defined as "most severe diarrhea until [the contents of the stomach] are emptied out and nothing is left" (《中華醫學大辭典》 p. 906).

LINE 6.11

澤蘭湯治產後餘疾，寒下*凍膿，裏急，胸脅滿痛，欬嗽嘔血，寒熱，小便赤黃，大便不利方。

Lycopus Decoction treats residual sickness after childbirth with cold discharge that is icy and contains pus, abdominal urgency, fullness and pain in the chest and rib-sides, coughing and vomiting of blood, [aversion to] cold and heat [effusion], red and yellow urine, and inhibited defecation.

Lycopus Decoction
澤蘭湯 *zé lán tāng*

澤蘭（二十四銖）石膏（二十四銖）當歸（十八銖）遠志（三十銖）甘草 厚朴（各十八銖）藁本 芎藭（各十五銖）乾薑 人參 桔梗 乾地黃（各十二銖）白朮 蜀椒 白芷 柏子仁 防風 山茱萸 細辛（各九銖）桑白皮 麻子仁（各半升）。

澤蘭	zé lán	Foliage and stalk of Lycopus lucidus	十四銖	24 zhū	3g
石膏	shí gāo	Gypsum	十四銖	24 zhū	3g
當歸	dāng guī	Root of Angelica polimorpha	十八銖	18 zhū	2.25g
遠志	yuǎn zhì	Root of Polygala tenuifolia	三十銖	30 zhū	3.75g
甘草	gān cǎo	Root of Glycyrrhiza uralensis	十八銖	18 zhū	2.25g
厚朴	hòu pò	Bark of Magnolia officinalis	十八銖	18 zhū	2.25g
藁本	gǎo běn	Rhizome and root of Ligusticum sinense	十五銖	15 zhū	1.875g
川芎	chuān xiōng	Root of Ligusticum wallichii	十五銖	15 zhū	1.875g
乾薑	gān jiāng	Dried root of Zingiber officinale	十二銖	12 zhū	1.5g
人參	rén shēn	Root of Panax ginseng	十二銖	12 zhū	1.5g
桔梗	jié gěng	Root of Platycodon grandiflorum	十二銖	12 zhū	1.5g
乾地黃	gān dì huáng	Dried root of Rehmannia glutinosa	十二銖	12 zhū	1.5g
白朮	bái zhú	Rhizome of Atractylodes macrocephala	九銖	9 zhū	1.125g
蜀椒	shǔ jiāo	Seed capsules of Zanthoxylum bungeanum	九銖	9 zhū	1.125g
白芷	bái zhǐ	Root of Angelica dahurica	九銖	9 zhū	1.125g
柏子仁	bǎi zǐ rén	Seed of Platycladus orientalis	九銖	9 zhū	1.125g
防風	fáng fēng	Root of Ledebouriella divaricata	九銖	9 zhū	1.125g
山茱萸	shān zhū yú	Fruit of Cornus officinalis	九銖	9 zhū	1.125g
細辛	xì xīn	Complete plant including root of Asarum heteropoides	九銖	9 zhū	1.125g
桑白皮	sāng bái pí	Bark of the root of Morus alba	半升	0.5 shēng	12g
麻子仁	má zǐ rén	Seed of Cannabis sativa	半升	0.5 shēng	12g

上二十一味，㕮咀，以水一斗五升先內桑白皮，煮取七升半，去之，內諸藥，煮取三升五合，去滓，分三服。

Pound the above twenty-one ingredients. First, decoct the *sāng bái pí* 桑白皮 in one *dǒu* and five *shēng* of water to obtain seven and a half *shēng*. Remove it, add all the [remaining] drugs and decoct to obtain three *shēng* and five *gě*. Discard the dregs and divide into three doses.

*   寒下 *hán xià*: This refers to discharge caused by contracting cold after birth. See the description of "cold diarrhea" (冷痢 *lěng lì*) in the *Bìng Yuán Lùn*: "Caused by wind strike, it is characterized by the discharge of green, white, or black matter (《病源論》 17:11).

LINE 6.12

治產後下痢，乾地黃湯方

Dried Rehmannia Decoction treats postpartum diarrhea.

Dried Rehmannia Decoction
干地黃湯 *gān dì huáng tāng*

乾地黃（三兩）白頭翁 黃連（各一兩）蜜蠟（一方寸）阿膠（如手掌大一枚）。

乾地黃	gān dì huáng	Dried root of Rehmannia glutinosa	三兩 3 liǎng	9g
白頭翁	bái tóu wēng	Root of Pulsatilla chinensis	一兩 1 liǎng	3g
黃連	huáng lián	Rhizome of Coptis chinensis	一兩 1 liǎng	3g
蜜蠟	mì là	Wax of Apis cerana	一方寸 1 fāng cùn	7.5g
阿膠	ē jiāo	Gelatinous glue produced from Equus asinus	如手掌大一枚 rú shǒu zhǎng dà 1 méi	1 pc the size of the palm of a hand

上五味，㕮咀，以水五升煮取二升半，去滓，內膠蠟令烊。分三服，日三。

Pound the above five ingredients and decoct in five *shēng* of water to obtain two and a half *shēng*. Discard the dregs, add the *ē jiāo* 阿膠 and wax, and let them melt. Divide into three doses and take three times a day.˙

---

* *Sòng* editors' note: "The *Qiān Jīn Yì Fāng* adds one *liǎng* of *gān jiāng* (乾薑 Dried root of Zingiber officinale)."

LINE 6.13

治產後忽著寒熱，下痢，生地黃湯方。

Fresh Rehmannia Decoction treats suddenly occurring [aversion to] cold and heat [effusion] with diarrhea after childbirth.

Fresh Rehmannia Decoction
生地黃湯 *shēng dì huáng tāng*

生地黃（五兩）甘草 黃連 桂心（各一兩）大棗（二十枚）淡竹葉（二升，一作竹皮）赤石脂（二兩）。

生地黃	shēng dì huáng	Fresh root of Rehmannia glutinosa	五兩 5 liǎng	15g
甘草	gān cǎo	Root of Glycyrrhiza uralensis	一兩 1 liǎng	3g
黃連	huáng lián	Rhizome of Coptis chinensis	一兩 1 liǎng	3g
桂心	guì xīn	Shaved inner bark of Cinnamomum cassia	一兩 1 liǎng	3g
大棗	dà zǎo	Mature fruit of Ziziphus jujuba	二十枚 20 méi	20 pcs
淡竹葉	dàn zhú yè	Leaves of Lopatherum gracile	二升 2 shēng	48g
赤石脂	chì shí zhī	Halloysite	二兩 2 liǎng	6g

上七味，㕮咀，以水一斗煮竹葉，取七升，去滓內藥，煮取二升半。分三服，日三。

Pound the above seven ingredients. Decoct the bamboo leaves in one *dǒu* of water to obtain seven *shēng*. Discard the dregs and add the [remaining] drugs. Decoct to obtain two and a half *shēng*. Divide into three doses and take three times a day.*

---

* *Sòng* editors' note: "Another [version of this] prescription uses *zhú pí* (竹皮 Shavings of the stripped core Phyllostachys stalks) instead of *dàn zhú yè* 淡竹葉."

LINE 6.14

治產後下痢，藍青丸方。

Indigo Residue Pills treat postpartum diarrhea.

Indigo Residue Pills
藍青丸 *lán qīng wán*

藍青（熬）附子 鬼臼 蜀椒（各一兩半）厚朴 阿膠 甘草（各二兩 艾葉 龍骨 黃連 當歸（各三兩）黃蘗 茯苓 人參（各一兩）。

藍青, 熬	lán qīng, āo	Dye produced from the foliage of Isatis tinctoria, cooked	一兩半 1.5 liǎng	4.5g
附子	fù zǐ	Lateral root of Aconitum carmichaeli	一兩半 1.5 liǎng	4.5g
鬼臼	guǐ jiù	Root of Dysosma versipellis	一兩半 1.5 liǎng	4.5g
蜀椒	shǔ jiāo	Seed capsules of Zanthoxylum bungeanum	一兩半 1.5 liǎng	4.5g
厚朴	hòu pò	Bark of Magnolia officinalis	二兩 2 liǎng	6g
阿膠	ē jiāo	Gelatinous glue produced from Equus asinus	二兩 2 liǎng	6g
甘草	gān cǎo	Root of Glycyrrhiza uralensis	二兩 2 liǎng	6g
艾葉	ài yè	Dry-roasted foliage of Artemisia argyi	三兩 3 liǎng	9g
龍骨	lóng gǔ	Os draconis	三兩 3 liǎng	9g
黃連	huáng lián	Rhizome of Coptis chinensis	三兩 3 liǎng	9g
當歸	dāng guī	Root of Angelica polimorpha	三兩 3 liǎng	9g
黃蘗	huáng bò	Bark of Phellodendron amurense	一兩 1 liǎng	3g
茯苓	fú líng	Dried fungus of Poria cocos	一兩 1 liǎng	3g
人參	rén shēn	Root of Panax ginseng	一兩 1 liǎng	3g

上十四味，末之，蜜和丸如梧子。空腹，每服以飲下二十丸。

Pulverize the above fourteen ingredients and mix with honey into pills the size of firmiana seeds. On an empty stomach, take twenty pills at a time by drinking them with liquid.[*]

* *Sòng* editors' note: "Another [version of this] prescription adds four *liǎng* of *chì shí zhī* (赤石脂 Halloysite)."

LINE 6.15

治產後虛冷下痢，赤石脂丸方。

Halloysite Pills treat diarrhea from postpartum vacuity cold.

Halloysite Pills
赤石脂丸 *chì shí zhī wán*

赤石脂（三兩） 當歸 白朮 黃連 乾薑 秦皮 甘草（各二兩） 蜀椒 附子（各一兩）。

赤石脂	chì shí zhī	Halloysite	三兩 3 liǎng	9g
當歸	dāng guī	Root of Angelica polimorpha	二兩 2 liǎng	6g
白朮	bái zhú	Rhizome of Atractylodes macrocephala	二兩 2 liǎng	6g
黃連	huáng lián	Rhizome of Coptis chinensis	二兩 2 liǎng	6g
乾薑	gān jiāng	Dried root of Zingiber officinale	二兩 2 liǎng	6g
秦皮	qín pí	Bark of the trunk of Fraxinus rhunchophylla	二兩 2 liǎng	6g
甘草	gān cǎo	Root of Glycyrrhiza uralensis	二兩 2 liǎng	6g
蜀椒	shǔ jiāo	Seed capsules of Zanthoxylum bungeanum	一兩 1 liǎng	3g
附子	fù zǐ	Lateral root of Aconitum carmichaeli	一兩 1 liǎng	3g

上九味，末之，蜜丸如梧子。酒服二十丸，日三。

Pulverize the above nine ingredients and mix with honey into pills the size of firmiana seeds. Take twenty pills in liquor[1] three times a day.[2]

1. 酒服 *jiǔ fú*: The *Sūn Zhēn Rén* edition instead has: 煮米飲服... *zhǔ mǐ yǐn fú* "cook rice and take [the medicine] ... in its liquid."
2. *Sòng* editors' note: "The *Qiān Jīn Yì Fāng* processes [the ingredients] into a powder, to take a square-inch spoon in liquid on an empty stomach."

LINE 6.16

治產後下痢，赤散方。

Red Powder treats postpartum diarrhea.

Red Powder
赤散 *chì sǎn*

赤石脂（三兩） 桂心（一兩） 代赭（三兩）。

赤石脂	chì shí zhī	Halloysite	三兩 3 liǎng	9g
桂心	guì xīn	Shaved inner bark of Cinnamomum cassia	一兩 1 liǎng	3g
代赭	dài zhě	Hematite	三兩 3 liǎng	9g

上三味，治下篩。酒服方寸匕，日三，十日愈。

Finely pestle and sift the above three ingredients. Take a square-inch spoon in liquor three times a day. After ten days, she will recover.

LINE 6.17

治產後下痢，黑散方。

Black Powder treats postpartum diarrhea.

Black Powder
黑散 *hēi sǎn*

麻黃 貫眾 桂心（各一兩） 甘草（三兩） 乾漆（三兩） 細辛（二兩）。

麻黃	má huáng	Stalk of Ephedra sinica	一兩 1 liǎng	3g
貫眾	guàn zhòng	Rhizome of Aspidium crassirhizoma	一兩 1 liǎng	3g
桂心	guì xīn	Shaved inner bark of Cinnamomum cassia	一兩 1 liǎng	3g
甘草	gān cǎo	Root of Glycyrrhiza uralensis	三兩 3 liǎng	9g
乾漆	gān qī	Dried sap of Rhus verniciflua	三兩 3 liǎng	9g
細辛	xì xīn	Complete plant including root of Asarum heteropoides	二兩 2 liǎng	6g

上六味，治下篩。酒服五撮，日再，五日愈。

Finely pestle and sift the above six ingredients. Take a five-fingered pinch in liquor twice a day, and she will recover after five days. *

---

*   *Sòng* editors' note: "Taking it with wheat gruel is particularly excellent."
Although this sentence is not marked as commentary in the modern critical editions, it is missing in the *Sūn Zhēn Rén* edition and is therefore most likely a later addition.

LINE 6.18

治產後下痢，黃散方。

Yellow Powder treats postpartum diarrhea.

Yellow Powder
黃散 *huáng sǎn*

黃連（二兩）黃芩 蟅蟲 乾地黃（各一兩）。

黃連	huáng lián	Rhizome of Coptis chinensis	二兩 2 liǎng	6g
黃芩	huáng qín	Root of Scutellaria baicalensis	一兩 1 liǎng	3g
蟅蟲	zhè chóng	Entire dried body of the female of Eupolyphaga sinensis	一兩 1 liǎng	3g
乾地黃	gān dì huáng	Dried root of Rehmannia glutinosa	一兩 1 liǎng	3g

上四味，治下篩。酒服方寸匕，日三，十日愈。

Finely pestle and sift the above four ingredients. Take a square-inch spoon in liquor three times a day, and she will recover after ten days.

LINE 6.19

治產後痢，龍骨散方。

Dragon Bone Powder treats postpartum diarrhea.

Dragon Bone Powder
龍骨散 *lóng gǔ sǎn*

五色龍骨 黃蘗根皮（蜜炙令焦）代赭 赤石脂 艾（各一兩半）黃連（二兩）。

五色龍骨	wǔ sè lóng gǔ	Five color Os draconis	一兩半 1.5 liǎng	4.5g
黃蘗根皮，蜜炙令焦	huáng bò gēn pí, mì zhì lìng jiāo	Bark of Phellodendron amurense, mix fried in honey until burnt	一兩半 1.5 liǎng	4.5g
代赭	dài zhě	Hematite	一兩半 1.5 liǎng	4.5g
赤石脂	chì shí zhī	Halloysite	一兩半 1.5 liǎng	4.5g

| 艾[葉] | ài [yè] | [Dry-roasted foliage of] Artemisia argyi | 一兩半 1.5 liǎng | 4.5g |
| 黃連 | huáng lián | Rhizome of Coptis chinensis | 二兩 2 liǎng | 6g |

上六味，治下篩，飲服方寸匕，日三。

Finely pestle and sift the above six ingredients. Take a square-inch spoon in liquid three times a day.

7. Strangury and Thirst 淋渴

Translator's note: In modern Chinese, 渴 is identical with the English "thirst," but its original meaning, which is preserved in the more restricted medical use of this term, is defined in the *Shuō Wén Jiě Zì*: "The meaning of 渴 is water that is dried up and evaporated. Later, the character 竭 is used [to convey this nuanced meaning]." (渴義為水乾涸後作竭 *kě yì wéi shuǐ gān hé hòu zuò jié*; 《說文解字》 11a). In medical literature, it refers to the pathological drying up of fluids inside the body, identical to the English "dehydration." This section is entitled "prescriptions for treating postpartum frequent urination" (治產後小便數方 *zhì chǎn hòu xiǎo biàn shù fāng*) in the *Sūn Zhēn Rén* edition.

LINE 7.1

治產後小便數兼渴，栝樓湯方。

Trichosanthes Decoction treats postpartum urinary frequency concurrent with thirst.

Trichosanthes Decoction
栝樓湯 *guā lóu tāng*

栝樓根 黃連（各二兩） 人參（三兩） 大棗（十五枚） 甘草（二兩） 麥門冬（二兩） 桑螵蛸（二十枚） 生薑（三兩）。

栝蔞根	guā lóu gēn	Root of Trichosanthes kirilowii	二兩 2 liǎng	6g
黃連	huáng lián	Rhizome of Coptis chinensis	二兩 2 liǎng	6g
人參	rén shēn	Root of Panax ginseng	三兩 3 liǎng	9g
大棗	dà zǎo	Mature fruit of Ziziphus jujuba	十五枚 15 méi	15 pcs
甘草	gān cǎo	Root of Glycyrrhiza uralensis	二兩 2 liǎng	6g
麥門冬	mài mén dōng	Tuber of Ophiopogon japonicus	二兩 2 liǎng	6g
桑螵蛸	sāng piāo xiāo	Cocoon-like egg capsules of Paratenodera sinensis	二十枚 20 méi	20 pcs
生薑	shēng jiāng	Fresh root of Zingiber officinale	三兩 3 liǎng	9g

上八味，哎咀，以水七升煮取二升半，分三服。

Pound the above eight ingredients and decoct in seven *shēng* of water to obtain two and a half *shēng*. Divide into three doses.

LINE 7.2

治產後小便數，雞膍胵湯方。

Chicken Gizzard Lining[1] Decoction treats postpartum urinary frequency.

Chicken Gizzard Lining Decoction
雞膍胵湯 *jī pí zhì tāng*

雞膍胵（二十具[2]）雞腸（三具，洗）乾地黃 當歸 甘草（各二兩）麻黃（四兩）厚朴 人參（各三兩）生薑（五兩）大棗（二十枚）。

雞膍胵	jī pí zhì	Dried skin from the inside the gizzard of Gallus gallus domesticus	二三具 2 or 3 jù	2 or 3 sets
雞腸, 洗	jī cháng, xǐ	Intestine of Gallus gallus domesticus, washed	三具 3 jù[3]	3 sets
乾地黃	gān dì huáng	Dried root of Rehmannia glutinosa	二兩 2 liǎng	6g
當歸	dāng guī	Root of Angelica polimorpha	二兩 2 liǎng	6g
甘草	gān cǎo	Root of Glycyrrhiza uralensis	二兩 2 liǎng	6g
麻黃	má huáng	Stalk of Ephedra sinica	四兩 4 liǎng	12g
厚朴	hòu pò	Bark of Magnolia officinalis	三兩 3 liǎng	9g
人參	rén shēn	Root of Panax ginseng	三兩 3 liǎng	9g
生薑	shēng jiāng	Fresh root of Zingiber officinale	五兩 5 liǎng	15g
大棗	dà zǎo	Mature fruit of Ziziphus jujuba	二十枚 20 méi	20 pcs

上十味，㕮咀，以水一斗煮膍胵及腸大棗，取七升，去滓，內諸藥，煎取三升半，分三服。

Pound the above ten ingredients. Cook the gizzard linings, intestines, and *dà zǎo* 大棗 in one *dǒu* of water to obtain seven *shēng*, and discard the dregs. Add all the [remaining] drugs, simmer to obtain three and a half *shēng* and divide into three doses.

1. 雞膍胵 *jī pí zhì*: In contemporary TCM, this drug is more commonly called 雞內金 *jī nèi jīn*.
2. 二十具 *èr shí jù*: In spite of the fact that this textual version is found in most modern Chinese editions, as well as the *Sūn Zhēn Rén* edition, I interpret this as a textual corrup-

tion and read it instead as 二三具 *èr sān jù*, which is the version of this text found in the *Sì Kù Quán Shū* edition. My reasoning is based on the fact that the normal amount of this ingredient in similar prescriptions is one or two sets (see, for example, the many prescriptions quoted for this drug in (《本草綱目》48, 1721). The equivalent prescription in the *Qiān Jīn Yì Fāng* does, however, also call for twenty sets (《千金翼方》7:7).

3. The *Sūn Zhēn Rén* edition calls for only one set.

LINE 7.3

治婦人結氣成淋，小便引痛，上至小腹，或時溺血，或如豆汁，或如膠飴，
每發欲死，食不生肌，面目萎黃，師所不能治方。

[The following] prescription treats women's strangury caused by *qì* bind, pain during urination that stretches all the way up to the lower abdomen, possibly occasional bloody urine or urine that resembles bean juice or malt candy, bringing her close to death every time it flares up, eating without engendering flesh, and a withered yellow complexion in the face and eyes. [It cures cases that even] a master is unable to treat.

Formula

貝齒（四枚，燒作末）葵子（一升）石膏（五兩，碎）滑石（二兩，末）
。

貝齒, 燒作末	bèi chǐ, shāo zuò mò	The shell of Monetaria moneta, charred and pulverized	四枚 4 méi	4 pcs
葵子	kuí zǐ	Seed of Malva verticillata	一升 1 shēng	24g
石膏, 碎	shí gāo, suì	Gypsum, crushed into pieces	五兩 5 liǎng	15g
滑石, 末	huá shí, mò	Talcum, pulverized	二兩 2 liǎng	6g

上四味，以水七升煮二物，取二升，去滓，內二末及豬脂一合，更煎三沸。
分三服，日三，不瘥再合服。

Of the four ingredients above, decoct the two [coarse] substances in seven *shēng* of water to obtain two *shēng*. Discard the dregs and add the two powders together with one *gě* of pork lard and simmer it again, bringing it to a rolling boil three times.* Divide into three doses and take three times a day. If she fails to recover, compound a second [batch] and take it.

---

*   This means that the *kuí zǐ* 葵子 and *shí gāo* 石膏 should be decocted first and then strained out before the pulversized *bèi chǐ* 貝齒 and *huá shí* 滑石 are added together with the pork fat.

LINE 7.4

治產後卒淋，氣淋，血淋，石淋，石韋湯方。

Pyrrosia Decoction treats sudden strangury after childbirth,[1] *qì* strangury, blood strangury, and stone strangury.[2]

Pyrrosia Decoction
石韋湯 *shí wéi tāng*

石韋（二兩）　榆皮（五兩）　黃芩（二兩）　大棗（三十枚）　通草（二兩）
甘草（二兩）　葵子（二升）　白朮（《產寶》用芍藥）　生薑（各三兩）。

石韋	shí wéi	Foliage of Pyrrosia lingua	二兩 2 liǎng	6g
榆[白]皮	yú [bái] pí	The fibrous inner bark of the root or trunk of Ulmus pumila	五兩 5 liǎng	15g
黃芩	huáng qín	Root of Scutellaria baicalensis	二兩 2 liǎng	6g
大棗	dà zǎo	Mature fruit of Ziziphus jujuba	三十枚 30 méi	30 pcs
通草	tōng cǎo	Pith in the stalk of Tetrapanax papyriferus	二兩 2 liǎng	6g
甘草	gān cǎo	Root of Glycyrrhiza uralensis	二兩 2 liǎng	6g
葵子	kuí zǐ	Seed of Malva verticillata	二升 2 shēng	48g
白朮[3]	bái zhú	Rhizome of Atractylodes macrocephala	三兩 3 liǎng	9g
生薑	shēng jiāng	Fresh root of Zingiber officinale	三兩 3 liǎng	9g

上九味，㕮咀，以水八升煮取二升半，分三服。

Pound the above nine ingredients and decoct in eight *shēng* of water to obtain two and a half *shēng*. Divide into three doses.[4]

1. It is not clear from the Chinese whether this prescription treats sudden strangury after childbirth as well as *qì* strangury etc., or whether it treats sudden strangury after childbirth, characterized by the symptoms of *qì* strangury, blood strangury, etc. The latter seems more likely, given both the location of the prescription here, as well as the structure of the introductory sentence in most prescription entries: Usually, a general indication is followed by secondary and more specific signs and symptoms that serve to describe exactly the condition addressed by the prescription.

2. These are all technical terms for different varieties of strangury. As explained in the *Bìng Yuán Lùn*, *qì* strangury (氣淋 *qì lín*) is a type of strangury characterized by a sensation of fullness in the lower abdomen and bladder. It is caused by hot *qì* from the bladder entering the uterus, which then causes *qì* distention in the uterus (《病源論》 14:2:3). Blood

strangury (血淋 *xuè lín*) is described as "extreme cases of heat-related strangury that lead to blood in the urine... In cases of severe exhaustion, [the blood] will scatter and leave its regular channels. It will overflow and percolate into the uterus, creating blood strangury" (《病源論》 14:2:7). Lastly, stone strangury (石淋 *shí lín*) is described as "strangury concurrent with discharge of stones. The kidney governs the fluids. When the fluids are bound, they transform into stones, causing sand-like stones to lodge in the kidney" (《病源論》 14:2:2).

3. *Sòng* editors' note: "The *Chǎn Bǎo* uses *sháo yào* (芍藥 Root of Paeonia albiflora)."

4. *Sòng* editors' note: "The *Jí Yàn Fāng* lacks *gān cǎo* 甘草 and *shēng jiāng* 生薑. Neither Master Cuī, nor the *Chǎn Bǎo*, use *shēng jiāng* 生薑 or *dà zǎo* (大棗 Mature fruit of Ziziphus jujuba)."

LINE 7.5

治產後淋澀，葵根湯方。

Mallow Root Decoction treats postpartum strangury and rough urination.

Mallow Root Decoction
葵根湯 *kuí gēn tāng*

葵根（二兩）車前子（一升）亂髮（燒灰）大黃（各一兩）冬瓜練（七合，一作汁）通草（三兩）桂心 滑石（各一兩）生薑（六兩）。

葵根	kuí gēn	Rhizome of Malva verticillata	二兩 2 liǎng	6g
車前子	chē qián zǐ	Seed of Plantago asiatica	一升 1 shēng	24g
亂髮, 燒灰	luàn fà, shāo huī	Matted hair, burnt into ashes	一兩 1 liǎng	3g
大黃	dà huáng	Root of Rheum palmatum	一兩 1 liǎng	3g
冬瓜練˙	dōng guā liàn	Pulp of Benincasa hispida	七合 7 gě	49ml
通草	tōng cǎo	Pith in the stalk of Tetrapanax papyriferus	三兩 3 liǎng	9g
桂心	guì xīn	Shaved inner bark of Cinnamomum cassia	一兩 1 liǎng	3g
滑石	huá shí	Talcum	一兩 1 liǎng	3g
生薑	shēng jiāng	Fresh root of Zingiber officinale	六兩 6 liǎng	18g

上九味，㕮咀，以水七升煮取二升半，分三服。

Pound the above nine ingredients and decoct in sven *shēng* of water to obtain two and a half *shēng*. Divide into three doses.

* *Sòng* editors' note: "The *Qiān Jīn Yì Fāng* does not use *dōng guā liàn* 冬瓜練. Another [version] uses *dōng guā zhī* (冬瓜汁 Juice of Benincasa hispida)."

LINE 7.6

治產後淋，茅根湯方。

Imperata Decoction treats postpartum strangury.

Imperata Decoction
茅根湯 *máo gén tāng*

白茅根（一斤）瞿麥（四兩）地脉（二兩）桃膠 甘草（各一兩）鯉魚齒
（一百枚）人參（二兩）茯苓（四兩）生薑（三兩）。

白茅根	bái máo gēn	Imperata cylindrica	一斤 1 jīn	48g
瞿麥	qú mài	Entire plant, including flowers, of Dianthus superbus	四兩 4 liǎng	12g
地麥	dì mài*	Fruit of Kochia scoparia	二兩 2 liǎng	6g
桃膠	táo jiāo	Sap emerging from the bark of the trunk of Prunus persica	一兩 1 liǎng	3g
甘草	gān cǎo	Root of Glycyrrhiza uralensis	一兩 1 liǎng	3g
鯉魚齒	lǐ yú chǐ	Teeth of Cyprinus carpio	一百枚 100 méi	100 pcs
人參	rén shēn	Root of Panax ginseng	二兩 2 liǎng	6g
茯苓	fú líng	Dried fungus of Poria cocos	四兩 4 liǎng	12g
生薑	shēng jiāng	Fresh root of Zingiber officinale	三兩 3 liǎng	9g

上九味，㕮咀，以水一斗煮取二升半，分三服。

Pound the above nine ingredients and decoct in one *dǒu* of water to obtain two and a half *shēng*. Divide into three doses.

* 地脉 *dì mài*: This compound is not found elsewhere in the materia medica literature. In a similar version of this prescription in the *Qiān Jīn Yì Fāng*, however, Sūn Sī-Miǎo uses 地麥 *dì mài* instead, which is a common synonym for 地膚子 *dì fū zǐ*, kochia fruit (《千金翼方》 7:7). I therefore assume that 脉 *mài* here is a scribal error for 麥, especially since the main pharmaceutical function of kochia is to disinhibit urination (《中藥大辭典》 #1403), which exactly fits the purpose of this prescription.

LINE 7.7

治產後淋，滑石散方。

Talcum Powder treats postpartum strangury.

Talcum Powder
滑石散 *huá shí sǎn*

滑石（五兩）通草 車前子 葵子（各四兩）。

滑石	huá shí	Talcum	五兩	5 liǎng	15g
通草	tōng cǎo	Pith in the stalk of Tetrapanax papyriferus	四兩	4 liǎng	12g
車前子	chē qián zǐ	Seed of Plantago asiatica	四兩	4 liǎng	12g
葵子	kuí zǐ	Seed of Malva verticillata	四兩	4 liǎng	12g

上四味，治下篩。酢漿水服方寸匕，稍加至二匕。

Finely pestle and sift the above four ingredients. Take a square-inch spoon [per dose] in fermented millet drink, gradually increasing [the dosage] to two spoons.

LINE 7.8

治產後虛渴，少氣力，竹葉湯方。

Bamboo Leaf Decoction treats postpartum vacuity thirst with lack of *qì* and strength.

Bamboo Leaf Decoction
竹葉湯 *zhú yè tāng*

竹葉（三升）甘草 茯苓 人參（各一兩）小麥（五合）生薑（三兩）大棗（十四枚）半夏（三兩）麥門冬（五兩）。

竹葉	zhú yè	Leaves of Phyllostachys	三兩	3 liǎng	9g
甘草	gān cǎo	Root of Glycyrrhiza uralensis	一兩	1 liǎng	3g
茯苓	fú líng	Dried fungus of Poria cocos	一兩	1 liǎng	3g
人參	rén shēn	Root of Panax ginseng	一兩	1 liǎng	3g

小麥	xiǎo mài	Seed or flour of Triticum aestivum	五合 5 gě	35ml
生薑	shēng jiāng	Fresh root of Zingiber officinale	三兩 3 liǎng	9g
大棗	dà zǎo	Mature fruit of Ziziphus jujuba	十四枚 14 méi	14 pcs
麥門冬	mài mén dōng	Tuber of Ophiopogon japonicus	三兩 3 liǎng	9g
半夏	bàn xià	Rhizome of Pinellia ternata	五兩 5 liǎng	15g

上九味，㕮咀，以水九升煮竹葉，小麥，取七升，去滓內諸藥，更煎取二升半，一服五合，日三夜一。

Pound the above nine ingredients. Boil the *zhú yè* 竹葉 and *xiǎo mài* 小麥 in nine *shēng* of water to obtain seven *shēng*. Discard the dregs and add all the [remaining] drugs. Simmer it again to obtain two and a half *shēng*. Take five *gě* per dose, three times a day and once at night.

LINE 7.9

治產後渴不止，栝樓湯方。

Trichosanthes Decoction treats incessant strangury after childbirth.

Trichosanthes Decoction
栝樓湯 *guā lóu tāng*

栝樓根（四兩） 人參（三兩） 甘草（二兩，崔氏不用） 麥門冬（三兩）
大棗（二十枚） 土瓜根（五兩，崔氏用蘆根） 乾地黃（二兩）。

栝蔞根	guā lóu gēn	Root of Trichosanthes kirilowii	四兩 4 liǎng	12g
人參	rén shēn	Root of Panax ginseng	三兩 3 liǎng	9g
甘草[1]	gān cǎo	Root of Glycyrrhiza uralensis	二兩 2 liǎng	6g
麥門冬	mài mén dōng	Tuber of Ophiopogon japonicus	三兩 3 liǎng	9g
大棗	dà zǎo	Mature fruit of Ziziphus jujuba	二十枚 20 méi	20 pcs
土瓜根[2]	tǔ guā gēn	Root of Trichosanthes cucumerina	五兩 5 liǎng	15g
乾地黃	gān dì huáng	Dried root of Rehmannia glutinosa	二兩 2 liǎng	6g

上七味，㕮咀，以水一斗二升煮取六升，分六服。

Pound the above seven ingredients and decoct in one *dǒu* and two *shēng* of water to obtain six *shēng*. Divide into six doses.

1. *Sòng* editors' note: "Master Cuī does not use *gān cǎo* 甘草."
2. *Sòng* editors' note: "Master Cuī uses *lú gēn* (蘆根 Rhizome of Phragmites communis)."

363

8. Miscellaneous Treatments 雜治

Translator's note: This is perhaps one of the most interesting gynecological categories since it consists of any treatments regarded as specific to women that do not fall into the categories of childbirth-related conditions (volume two and the previous sections in volume three) or conditions related to menstruation and vaginal discharge (volume four). The conditions in this section thus constitute truly gendered illnesses and offer a wealth of information regarding the medical interpretation of the female body and its gender-specific strengths and weaknesses. While placed in the volume on postpartum conditions, they are not directly related to childbearing, except for the fact that the taxation from childbearing reinforces or exacerbates many insuffiencies and weaknesses that were considered typical of the female body.

LINE 8.1

治婦人勞氣，食氣，胃滿吐逆，其病頭重結痛，小便赤黃，大下氣方。

Major Qì-Precipitating Formula treats women's taxation *qì* and food *qì*,[1] fullness in the stomach and counterflow vomiting, and the [related] symptoms of heaviness and binding pain in the head and reddish or yellow urine.[2]

Major Qì-Precipitating Formula
大下氣方 *dà xià qì fāng*

烏頭 黃芩 巴豆（各半兩） 半夏（三兩） 大黃（八兩） 戎鹽（一兩半） 蟅蟲 桂心 苦參（各十八銖） 人參 消石（各一兩）。

烏頭	wū tóu	Main tuber of Aconitum carmichaeli	半兩 0.5 liǎng	1.5g
黃芩	huáng qín	Root of Scutellaria baicalensis	半兩 0.5 liǎng	1.5g
巴豆	bā dòu	Seed of Croton tiglium	半兩 0.5 liǎng	1.5g
半夏	bàn xià	Rhizome of Pinellia ternata	三兩 3 liǎng	9g
大黃	dà huáng	Root of Rheum palmatum	八兩 8 liǎng	24g
戎鹽	róng yán	Halite	一兩半 1.5 liǎng	4.5g

蟅蟲	zhè chóng	Entire dried body of the female of Eupolyphaga sinensis	十八銖 18 zhū	2.25g
桂心	guì xīn	Shaved inner bark of Cinnamomum cassia	十八銖 18 zhū	2.25g
苦參	kǔ shēn	Root of Sophora flavescens	十八銖 18 zhū	2.25g
人參	rén shēn	Root of Panax ginseng	一兩 1 liǎng	3g
消石	xiāo shí	Niter	一兩 1 liǎng	3g

上十一味，末之，以蜜，青牛膽拌和，擣三萬杵，丸如梧子。宿不食，酒服五丸，安臥須臾當下。下黃者，小腹積也；青者，疝也；白者，內風也；如水者，留飲也；青如粥汁，膈上邪氣也；血如腐肉者，傷也；赤如血者，乳餘疾也；如蟲刺者，蠱也；下已必渴，渴飲粥，飢食酥糜，三日後當溫食，食必肥濃，三十日平復。亦名破積烏頭丸，主心腹積聚，氣悶脹，疝瘕，內傷瘀血，產乳餘疾，及諸不足。

Pulverize the above eleven ingredients and blend them well with honey and green cow bile. Pound [the mixture] with a pestle thirty-thousand times and [shape into] pills the size of firmiana seeds. After fasting overnight, take five pills in liquor, lie down and rest. After a moment, [the medicine] should cause a vaginal discharge. If the discharge is yellow, it indicates an accumulation in the lower abdomen; If it is green, it indicates mounting. If it is white, it indicates internal wind. If it is like water, it indicates retained fluids. If it is green and of a rice gruel- or juice-like consistency, it indicates evil *qì* above the diaphragm. If it is bloody and like rotten flesh, it is an injury. If it is red and blood-like, it is a residual sickness [caused by] childbearing. If it feels like an irritation from worms, it is *gǔ* toxin. After the discharge stops, she will invariably be thirsty. For the thirst, drink rice gruel; for hunger, eat butter porridge. After three days, she should [start] eat[ing] warm solid foods, which must be rich and concentrated. She will recover after thirty days. [This prescription] is also called *Accumulation-Breaking Aconite Pills*. It is the governing prescription for accumulations and gatherings in the heart and abdomen, *qì* oppression and distention, mounting-conglomerations and blood stasis from internal damage, residual sicknesses from childbearing, as well as the various insufficiencies.

1. 勞氣食氣 *láo qì shí qì*: These terms are not attested elsewhere (as, for example, in such likely places as the discussion of *qì* disorders in the *Bìng Yuán Lùn*, 《病源論》 13:1-25). The phrase could be interpreted as "*qì* conditions due to taxation and *qì* conditions due to food." For possible hints on what this might mean, compare with Sūn Sī-Miǎo's explanation of the etiology for the conditions to be treated by this prescription at the end of the prescription. The *Bìng Yuán Lùn* does have an entry on "*qì* symptoms" (氣候 *qì hòu*) in the gynecological section. It explains that "*qì* disorder is caused by vacuity in the lungs... Worrying, pondering, fear, or anger, or an inappropriate dwelling or diet can all damage and stir lung *qì*, engendering illness" (《病源論》 37:14). Cháo Yuán-Fāng distinguishes between the pathologies of vacuity *qì* and repletion *qì*, and cold *qì* and hot *qì*, but nowhere mentions the terms *láo qì* or *shí qì*. Given the context, it is likely that Sūn Sī-Miǎo is referring to vacuity *qì*, especially since its main symptom, according to the *Bìng Yuán Lùn*, is "descent of *qì*," which Sūn Sī-Miǎo also mentions among the symptoms treated by this prescription.

2.   This prescription is missing in the *Sūn Zhēn Rén* edition, which instead quotes two pre-
        scriptions for bloody urine (one of them recommending to drink the husband's charred
        and pulverized fingernails in liquor).

LINE 8.2

治婦人汗血，吐血，尿血，下血，竹箹湯方。

Bamboo Shavings Decoction treats women's sweating of blood, vomiting blood, bloody
urine, and descent of blood.

Bamboo Shavings Decoction
竹茹湯 *zhú rú tāng*

竹箹（二升） 乾地黃（四兩） 人參 芍藥 桔梗 芎藭 當歸 甘草 桂心（各一
兩）。

竹茹	zhú rú	Shavings of the stripped core Phyllos-tachys stalks	二升 2 shēng	48g
乾地黃	gān dì huáng	Dried root of Rehmannia glutinosa	四兩 4 liǎng	12g
人參	rén shēn	Root of Panax ginseng	一兩 1 liǎng	3g
芍藥	sháo yào	Root of Paeonia albiflora	一兩 1 liǎng	3g
桔梗	jié gěng	Root of Platycodon grandiflorum	一兩 1 liǎng	3g
川芎	chuān xiōng	Root of Ligusticum wallichii	一兩 1 liǎng	3g
當歸	dāng guī	Root of Angelica polimorpha	一兩 1 liǎng	3g
甘草	gān cǎo	Root of Glycyrrhiza uralensis	一兩 1 liǎng	3g
桂心	guì xīn	Shaved inner bark of Cinnamomum cas-sia	一兩 1 liǎng	3g

上九味，㕮咀，以水一斗煮取三升，分三服。

Pound the above nine ingredients and decoct in one *dǒu* of water to obtain three *shēng*.
Divide into three doses.

LINE 8.3

治婦人自少患風，頭眩眼疼方。

[The following] prescription treats women's wind problems that have troubled her her
since childhood, dizziness of the head, and eye pain.

Formula

石南（一方用石韋）　細辛　天雄　茵芋（各二兩）　山茱萸　乾薑（各三兩）　署預　防風　貫眾　獨活　蘼蕪（各四兩）。

石楠*	shí nán	Dry-roasted foliage of Photinia serrulata	二兩 2 liǎng	6g
細辛	xì xīn	Complete plant including root of Asarum heteropoides	二兩 2 liǎng	6g
天雄	tiān xióng	Mature root of Aconitum carmichaeli	二兩 2 liǎng	6g
茵芋	yīn yù	Foliage and stalk of Skimmia reevesiana	二兩 2 liǎng	6g
山茱萸	shān zhū yú	Fruit of Cornus officinalis	三兩 3 liǎng	9g
乾薑	gān jiāng	Dried root of Zingiber officinale	三兩 3 liǎng	9g
薯蕷	shǔ yù	Root of Dioscorea opposita	四兩 4 liǎng	12g
防風	fáng fēng	Root of Ledebouriella divaricata	四兩 4 liǎng	12g
貫眾	guàn zhòng	Rhizome of Aspidium crassirhizoma	四兩 4 liǎng	12g
獨活	dú huó	Root and rhizome of Angelica pubescens	四兩 4 liǎng	12g
蘼蕪	mí wú	Foliage and sprout of Ligusticum wallichii	四兩 4 liǎng	12g

上十一味，㕮咀，以酒三斗漬五日。初飲二合，日三，稍稍加之。

Pound the above eleven ingredients and soak in three *dǒu* of liquor for five days. At first drink two *gě* [per dose] three times a day, then increase the amount very gradually.

* *Sòng* editors' note: "Another [version of this] prescription uses *shí wéi* (石韋 Foliage of Pyrrosia lingua)."

LINE 8.4

治婦人經服硫黃丸，忽患頭痛項冷，冷歇又心胸煩熱，眉骨眼眥瘭痛，有時生瘡，喉中乾燥，四體痛癢方。

[The following] prescription treats women's sudden sickness due to the regular consumption of *Sulphur Pills*,* headaches and coldness in the neck, and when the cold stops, vexing heat in the heart and chest, itching and pain in the eyebrow bones and corners of the eyes, occasional formation of sores, dryness in the throat, and pain and itching in the four limbs.

Formula

栝樓根 麥門冬 龍膽（各三兩） 大黃（二兩） 土瓜根（八兩） 杏仁（二升）。

栝蔞根	guā lóu gēn	Root of Trichosanthes kirilowii	三兩 3 liǎng	9g
麥門冬	mài mén dōng	Tuber of Ophiopogon japonicus	三兩 3 liǎng	9g
龍膽	lóng dǎn	Root and rhizome of Gentiana scabra	三兩 3 liǎng	9g
大黃	dà huáng	Root of Rheum palmatum	二兩 2 liǎng	6g
土瓜根	tǔ guā gēn	Root of Trichosanthes cucumerina	八兩 8 liǎng	24g
杏仁	xìng rén	Dried seed of Prunus armeniaca	二升 2 shēng	48g

上六味，末之，蜜丸。飲服如梧子十枚，日三服，漸加之。

Pulverize the above six ingredients and mix with honey into pills. Take ten pills the size of firmiana seeds in liquid, three doses a day, and gradually increase [the dosage].

* 硫磺丸 *liú huáng wán*: Sulphur is classified as toxic and very hot, and should therefore not be taken over a long period. See, for example, (《中華醫學大辭典》 p. 1392), and (《神農本草經》 3:216).

LINE 8.5

治婦人患癖，按時如有三五個而作水聲，殊不得寢食，常心悶方。

[The following] prescription treats women's problems with aggregations that, when pressed, feel as if there were three to five [lumps] and make a water-like sound, extraordinary inability to sleep or eat, and constant oppression in the heart.

牽牛子三升，治下篩。飲服方寸匕，日一服。三十服後可服好硫黃一兩。

Finely pestle and sift three *shēng* of *qiān niú zǐ* (牽牛子 Seed of Pharbitis nil). Take a square-inch spoon in liquid, one dose a day. After thirty doses, she may take one *liǎng* of high-quality sulphur.

LINE 8.6

治婦人忽與鬼交通方。

[The following] prescription treats women's sudden intercourse with ghosts.[1]

Formula

松脂（二兩）雄黃（一兩，末）。

| 松脂 | sōng zhī | Rosin of Pinus massoniana | 二兩 2 liǎng | 6g |
| 雄黃, 末 | xióng huáng, mò | Realgar, pulverized | 一兩 1 liǎng | 3g |

上二味，先烊松脂，乃內雄黃末，以虎爪攪令相得，藥成，取如雞子中黃，夜臥以著燻籠中燒，令病人取鼻向其上，以被自覆，惟出頭，勿令過熱及令氣得泄也。

Of the two ingredients above, first melt the *sōng zhī* 松脂 and then add the *xióng huáng* 雄黃. Stir it with a tiger claw until it is well-blended and the medicine is done. Take an amount the size of the yolk in a chicken egg and, at bedtime, burn it inside an incense burner. Make the patient inhale it up her nose,[2] and cover her with a quilt, allowing only the head to stick out. Do not let her get overheated, but allow the *qì* to drain out.[3]

1. 與鬼交通 *yǔ guǐ jiāo tōng*: This gynecological disease is described in detail in the *Bìng Yuán Lùn*: Explained in terms very similar to wind evil, it is caused by vacuity in the internal organs, which has weakened the hold of the spirit, allowing ghosts to invade. Its symptoms are inability to recognize others, speaking and laughing as if interacting with an invisible presence, and occasional crying and grief (《病源論》 40:4). It appears that "intercourse" in this context refers not necessarily to sexual intercourse, but to any sort of interaction. Contrary to cases of spirit possession, the ghost does not possess the person but remains an external presence who engages the mind of the afflicted. In a prescription for this condition in the *Ishimpô*, however, the interaction clearly has sexual overtones. This is evidenced both by the etiology of the illness, namely "lack of intercourse between *yīn* and *yáng* (陰陽不交 *yīn yáng bù jiāo*, i.e., lack of sex), causing deep and intense desires and wants," as well as the treatment: "Make the woman have intercourse with a man without spilling essence, day and night without stopping. If she is encumbered, do not exceed seven days. She will invariably recover" (《醫心方》 21:30).
2. 令病人取鼻向其上 *lìng bìng rén qǔ bí xiàng qí shàng*: This means that you should make her lean over the incense burner and inhale the burning medicine through her nose. This is the textual version found in the *Sūn Zhēn Rén* edition and *Rén Mín* edition. The *Huá Xià* edition and the version of this prescription in the *Ishimpô* instruct instead to "make the patient take [the incense burner?] herself and hoist herself on top of it" (令病人取自升其上 *lìng bìng rén qǔ zì shēng qí shàng*).
3. 勿令過熱及令氣得泄也 *wù lìng guò rè jí lìng qì dé xiè*: *qì* could refer here either to the fumes of the medicine, meaning that the patient should allow the fumes to escape after inhaling them; or it could refer to the pathogenic substance called ghost *qì* (鬼氣 *guǐ qì*), which needs to be drained away for the woman to recover from this condition. As a third alternative, one could read the sentence in this way: "Do not allow her to get overheated or allow her *qì* to drain."

LINE 8.7

厚朴湯治婦人下焦勞冷，膀胱腎氣損弱，白汁與小便俱出者方。

Officinal Magnolia Bark Decoction treats women's taxation cold in the lower burner, detriment and weakness of bladder and kidney *qì*, and discharge of a white liquid with urination.

Officinal Magnolia Bark Decoction
厚朴湯 *hòu pò tāng*

厚朴如手大，長四寸，以酒五升煮兩沸，去滓，取桂一尺末之，內汁中調和，一宿勿食，且頓服之。

Decoct a piece of *hòu pò* (厚朴 Bark of Magnolia officinalis) the size of a hand, four *cùn* long, in five *shēng* of liquor, bringing it to a rolling boil twice, and discard the dregs. Take one *chǐ* of cinnamon and pulverize it. Add it to the liquid and mix it in. After fasting overnight, quaff it in the morning in a single dose.

LINE 8.8

溫經湯主婦人小腹痛方。

Menses-Warming Decoction is the governing prescription for women's pain in the lower abdomen.

Menses-Warming Decoction
溫經湯 *wēn jīng tāng*

茯苓（六兩） 芍藥（三兩） 薏苡仁（半升） 土瓜根（三兩）。

茯苓	fú líng	Dried fungus of Poria cocos	六兩 6 liǎng	18g
芍藥	sháo yào	Root of Paeonia albiflora	三兩 3 liǎng	9g
薏苡仁	yì yǐ rén	Seed kernel of Coix lachryma-jobi	半升 0.5 shēng	12g
土瓜根	tǔ guā gēn	Root of Trichosanthes cucumerina	三兩 3 liǎng	9g

上四味，㕮咀，以酒三升漬一宿，且加水七升煎取二升，分再服。

Pound the above four ingredients and soak overnight in three *shēng* of liquor. In the morning, add seven *shēng* of water and simmer to obtain two *shēng*. Divide into two doses.

LINE 8.9

治婦人胸滿心下堅，咽中帖帖，如有炙肉臠，吐之不出，咽之不下，半夏厚朴湯方。

Pinellia and Officinal Magnolia Bark Decoction treats women's fullness in the chest and hardness below the heart, and stickiness in the throat as if there were pieces of roasted meat [lodged there] that she can neither vomit up nor swallow down.

Pinellia and Officinal Magnolia Bark Decoction

半夏厚朴湯 *bàn xià hòu pò tāng*

半夏（一升）厚朴（三兩）茯苓（四兩）生薑（五兩）蘇葉（二兩）。

半夏	bàn xià	Rhizome of Pinellia ternata	一升 1 shēng	24g
厚朴	hòu pò	Bark of Magnolia officinalis	三兩 3 liǎng	9g
茯苓	fú líng	Dried fungus of Poria cocos	四兩 4 liǎng	12g
生薑	shēng jiāng	Fresh root of Zingiber officinale	五兩 5 liǎng	15g
蘇葉	sū yè	Foliage of Perilla frutescens	二兩 2 liǎng	6g

上五味，哎咀，以水七升煮取四升。分四服，日三夜一，不瘥頻服。一方無蘇葉，生薑。

Pound the above five ingredients and decoct in seven *shēng* of water to obtain four *shēng*. Divide into four doses and take three times a day and once at night. If she fails to recover, take it continuously. Another [version of this] prescription does not include *sū yè* 蘇葉 and *shēng jiāng* 生薑.*

*   This last comment is also found in the *Sūn Zhēn Rén* edition and is therefore likely to have been a part of the original text.

LINE 8.10

治婦人氣方。

[The following] prescription treats women's *qì* [pathologies].

平旦服烏牛尿，日一，止。

Right before daybreak, drink the urine of a black cow, once a day, then [the condition] will stop.*

* *Sòng* editors' note: "At this point, the *Sūn Zhēn Rén* edition adds three prescriptions for heart pain that are in the other editions found at the very end of chapter four of volume one, on 'heart and abdominal pain.'" See above, in chapter four of volume three, in Lines 4.23-25 (pp. 315 - 316).

LINE 8.11

治婦人胸中伏氣，昆布丸方。

Kelp Pills treat women's latent *qì* in the center of the chest.[1]

Kelp Pills
昆布丸 *kūn bù wán*

昆布 海澡 芍藥 桂心 人參 白石英 款冬花 桑白皮（各二兩） 茯苓 鍾乳 柏子仁（各二兩半） 紫菀 甘草（各一兩） 乾薑（一兩六銖） 吳茱萸 五味子 細辛（各一兩半） 杏仁（百枚） 橘皮 蘇子（各五合）。

昆布	kūn bù	Leaf-shaped body of Laminaria japonica	二兩半 2.5 liǎng	7.5g
海藻	hǎi zǎo	Whole plant of Sargassum fusiforme	二兩半 2.5 liǎng	7.5g
芍藥	sháo yào	Root of Paeonia albiflora	二兩半 2.5 liǎng	7.5g
桂心	guì xīn	Shaved inner bark of Cinnamomum cassia	二兩半 2.5 liǎng	7.5g
人參	rén shēn	Root of Panax ginseng	二兩半 2.5 liǎng	7.5g
白石英	bái shí yīng	White quartz	二兩半 2.5 liǎng	7.5g
款冬花	kuǎn dōng huā	Flower of Tussilago farfara	二兩半 2.5 liǎng	7.5g
桑白皮	sāng bái pí	Bark of the root of Morus alba	二兩半 2.5 liǎng	7.5g
茯苓	fú líng	Dried fungus of Poria cocos	二兩半 2.5 liǎng	7.5g
鐘乳	zhōng rǔ	Stalactite	二兩半 2.5 liǎng	7.5g
柏子仁	bǎi zǐ rén	Seed of Platycladus orientalis	二兩半 2.5 liǎng	7.5g
紫菀	zǐ wǎn	Root and rhizome of Aster tataricus	一兩 1 liǎng	3g
甘草	gān cǎo	Root of Glycyrrhiza uralensis	一兩 1 liǎng	3g
乾薑	gān jiāng	Dried root of Zingiber officinale	一兩六銖 1 liǎng 6 zhū	3.75g
吳茱萸	wú zhū yú	Unripe fruit of Evodia rutaecarpa	一兩半 1.5 liǎng	4.5g
烏頭	wū tóu	Main tuber of Aconitum carmichaeli	一兩半 1.5 liǎng	4.5g

五味子	wǔ wèi zǐ	Fruit of Schisandra chinensis	一兩半 1.5 liǎng	4.5g
細辛	xì xīn	Complete plant including root of Asarum heteropoides	一兩半 1.5 liǎng	4.5g
杏仁	xìng rén	Dried seed of Prunus armeniaca	百枚 100 méi	100 pcs
橘皮	jú pí	Peel of Citrus reticulata	五合 5 gě	35ml
蘇子	sū zǐ	Seed of Perilla frutescens	五合 5 gě	35ml

上二十味，末之，蜜和。酒服二十丸如梧子，日再，加至四十丸。

Pulverize the above twenty ingredients and mix with honey. Take twenty pills the size of firmiana seeds in liquor twice a day, increasing [the dosage] to a maximum of forty pills.

*   伏氣 *fú qì*: This term could refer to a condition caused by dampness and heat lying latent in the channels. Suffering from abnormal aches and pains and red and swollen feet, the patient herself feels very hot, but is cold when touched by others (See 《中華醫學大辭典》 p. 536), which unfortunately does not give the source of this information). Although the *Bìng Yuán Lùn* dedicates an entire volume to *qì* disorders (《病源論》 13, which includes such entries as "bound *qì*," "roaming *qì*," or "*qì* ascent"), it does not discuss "latent *qì*." *Fú qì* could also quite literally refer to "deep-lying [i.e., shallow] breathing."

LINE 8.12

治婦人無故憂恚，胸中迫塞，氣不下方。

[The following] prescription treats women's anxiety and rage without cause, distress and blockage in the center of the chest, and failure to precipitate *qì*.

Formula

芍藥 滑石 黃連 石膏 前胡 山茱萸（各一兩六銖） 大黃 細辛 麥門冬（各一兩） 半夏（十八銖） 桂心（半兩） 生薑（一兩）。

芍藥	sháo yào	Root of Paeonia albiflora	一兩六銖 1 liǎng 6 zhū	3.75g
滑石	huá shí	Talcum	一兩六銖 1 liǎng 6 zhū	3.75g
黃連	huáng lián	Rhizome of Coptis chinensis	一兩六銖 1 liǎng 6 zhū	3.75g
石膏	shí gāo	Gypsum	一兩六銖 1 liǎng 6 zhū	3.75g
前胡	qián hú	Root of Peucedanum praeruptorum	一兩六銖 1 liǎng 6 zhū	3.75g
山茱萸	shān zhū yú	Fruit of Cornus officinalis	一兩六銖 1 liǎng 6 zhū	3.75g

大黃	dà huáng	Root of Rheum palmatum	一兩 1 liǎng	3g
細辛	xì xīn	Complete plant including root of Asarum heteropoides	一兩 1 liǎng	3g
麥門冬	mài mén dōng	Tuber of Ophiopogon japonicus	一兩 1 liǎng	3g
半夏	bàn xià	Rhizome of Pinellia ternata	十八銖 18 zhū	2.25g
桂心	guì xīn	Shaved inner bark of Cinnamomum cassia	半兩 0.5 liǎng	1.5g
生薑	shēng jiāng	Fresh root of Zingiber officinale	一兩 1 liǎng	3g

上十二味，末之，蜜丸如梧子。酒服二十丸，加至三十丸，日三服。

Pulverize the above twelve ingredients and [make] honey pills the size of firmiana seeds. Take twenty pills [per dose] in liquor, increasing it to a maximum of thirty pills, three doses a day.

LINE 8.13

婦人斷產方。

[The following] prescription interrupts childbearing.[1]

蠶子故紙方一尺，燒為末，酒服之，終身不產。

Burn and pulverize a one-*chǐ* square of old silkworm paper[2] and take it in liquor. She will not bear children for the rest of her life.

---

1. 斷產 *duàn chǎn*: This means that it is intended to induce sterility for birth control, which in this case is permanent as the concluding sentence states.
2. 蠶子故紙 *cán zǐ gù zhǐ*: 蠶紙 *cán zhǐ* (silkworm paper) is a synonym for 蠶連 *cán lián*, the paper used in silkworm production for collecting the eggs laid by the silkworm moths in order to raise further silkworms. This ingredient clearly has symbolic and magical powers, given the strong association of sericulture with women's work. See Francesca Bray, *Technology and Gender*, pp. 183-191, for the gendered significance of textile production. The *Qiān Jīn Yì Fāng*, records an almost identical prescription, but using "old silkworm cloth" (故蠶子布 *gù cán zǐ bù*) instead (《千金翼方》 5:4).

LINE 8.14

又方

Another prescription:

油煎水銀一日勿息。空肚服棗大一枚，永斷，不損人。

Simmer mercury in oil for an entire day without stopping. On an empty stomach, take a jujube-sized piece. [Her reproductive capacity] will be interrupted forever, but it will not harm her.

LINE 8.15

治勞損，產後無子，陰中冷溢出，子門閉，積年不瘥，身體寒冷方。

[The following] prescription treats taxation detriment and infertility after childbirth, cold spilling out from the vagina, closure of the infant's gate[1] that has lasted for several consecutive years without recovery, and coldness of the body.

Formula

防風（一兩半） 桔梗（三十銖） 人參（一兩） 昌蒲 半夏 丹參 厚朴 乾薑 紫菀 杜衡（各十八銖） 秦艽 白薟 牛膝 沙參（各半兩）。

防風	fáng fēng	Root of Ledebouriella divaricata	一兩半 1.5 liǎng	4.5g
桔梗	jié gěng	Root of Platycodon grandiflorum	三十銖 30 zhū	3.75g
人參	rén shēn	Root of Panax ginseng	一兩 1 liǎng	3g
菖蒲	chāng pú	Rhizome of Acorus gramineus	十八銖 18 zhū	2.25g
半夏	bàn xià	Rhizome of Pinellia ternata	十八銖 18 zhū	2.25g
丹參	dān shēn	Root of Salvia miltiorrhiza	十八銖 18 zhū	2.25g
厚朴	hòu pò	Bark of Magnolia officinalis	十八銖 18 zhū	2.25g
乾薑	gān jiāng	Dried root of Zingiber officinale	十八銖 18 zhū	2.25g
紫菀	zǐ wǎn	Root and rhizome of Aster tataricus	十八銖 18 zhū	2.25g
杜蘅	dù héng	Rhizome and root, or whole plant of Asarum forbesii	十八銖 18 zhū	2.25g
秦艽	qín jiāo	Root of Gentiana macrophylla	半兩 0.5 liǎng	1.5g
白薟	bái liǎn	Root of Ampelopsis japonica	半兩 0.5 liǎng	1.5g
牛膝	niú xī	Root of Achyranthes bidentata	半兩 0.5 liǎng	1.5g
沙參	shā shēn	Root of Adenophora tetraphylla	半兩 0.5 liǎng	1.5g

上十四味，末之，白蜜和丸如小豆。食後服十五丸，日三服。不知，增至二十丸，有身止。夫不在，勿服之。服藥後七日方合陰陽。

Pulverize the above fourteen ingredients and mix with white honey into pills the size of azuki beans. Take fifteen pills after meals three times a day. If no effect is noticed, increase [the dosage] to a maximum of twenty pills. Stop when she is with child. Do not take them when the husband is not present.[2] Exactly seven days after taking the medicine, unite *yīn* and *yáng* [in sexual intercourse].

1. 子門閉 *zǐ mén bì*: *Zǐ mén* refers to a woman's genitals in the context of her ability to receive the man's essence. As an anatomical location, it refers to the vagina in general, but possibly in the restricted sense of the cervix. "Infant's gate blockage" is a common explanation for infertility. Contrast with "jade gate," which refers to the anterior part of the vagina, often in the restricted context of that of virgins (see next prescription).
2. This warning probably indicates the aphrodisiac effect of the medicine. Otherwise, it might suggest iatrogenic side-effects so that the medicine should only be taken when there is a good chance of achieving the intended effect of a pregnancy.

LINE 8.16

治產後癖瘦，玉門冷，五加酒方。

Acanthopanax Liquor treats postpartum aggregations, emaciation, and cold in the jade gate.[1]

Acanthopanax Liquor
五加酒 *wǔ jiā jiǔ*

五加皮（二升）枸杞子（二升）乾地黃 丹參（各二兩）杜仲（一斤）乾薑（三兩）天門冬（四兩）蛇床子（一升）乳床（半斤）。

五加皮	wǔ jiā pí	Root bark of Acanthopanax gracilistylus	二升 2 shēng	48g
枸杞子	gǒu qǐ zǐ	Fruit of Lycium chinensis	二升 2 shēng	48g
乾地黃	gān dì huáng	Dried root of Rehmannia glutinosa	二兩 2 liǎng	6g
丹參	dān shēn	Root of Salvia miltiorrhiza	二兩 2 liǎng	6g
杜仲	dù zhòng	Bark of Eucommia ulmoidis	一斤 1 jīn	48g
乾薑	gān jiāng	Dried root of Zingiber officinale	三兩 3 liǎng	9g
天門冬	tiān mén dōng	Tuber of Asparagus cochinchinensis	四兩 4 liǎng	12g
蛇床子	shé chuáng zǐ	Fruit of Cnidium monnieri	一升 1 shēng	24g
乳床	rǔ chuáng[2]	rǔchuáng	半斤 0.5 jīn	24g

上九味，㕮咀，以絹袋子盛，酒三斗漬三宿。一服五合，日再，稍加至十合，佳。

Pound the above nine ingredients and pack them into a silk bag. Soak it for three nights in three *dǒu* of liquor. Take five *gě* [of the liquor] per dose twice a day, gradually increasing it to a maximum of ten *gě*. It is good.

1. 玉門 *yù mén*: a technical term referring to the vagina in general and mostly used in the context of sexual intercourse. In contrast to the "infant's gate" mentioned above, it might refer specifically to the entrance of the vagina. Sometimes it is used in a restricted sense as that of virgins (see 《病源論》 37:24, and above).
2. 乳床: An identifiable drug name that might be a scribal error for *rǔ xiāng* (乳香 Frankincense).

LINE 8.17

治子門閉 , 血聚腹中生肉癥 , 藏寒所致方。

[The following] prescription treats closure of the infant's gate and blood accumulating in the center of the abdomen that is generating concretions in the flesh, a condition that is caused by cold in the viscera.

Formula

生地黃汁 (三升) 生牛膝汁 (一斤) 乾漆 (半斤) 。

生地黃汁	shēng dì huáng zhī	Fresh root of Rehmannia glutinosa juice	三升 3 shēng	72g
生牛膝汁	shēng niú xī zhī	Fresh root of Achyranthes bidentata juice	一斤 1 jīn	48g
乾漆	gān qī	Dried sap of Rhus verniciflua	半斤 0.5 jīn	24g

上三味 , 先擣漆為散 , 內汁中攪 , 微火煎為丸。酒服如梧子三丸 , 日再。若覺腹中痛 , 食後服之。

Of the three ingredients above, first grind the *gān qī* 乾漆 into powder, then add the juices and stir it. Heat it over a small flame and make pills. Take three pills the size of firmiana seeds in liquor twice a day. If she experiences pain in the center of the abdomen [as a consequence of taking the pills], take them after meals.

LINE 8.18

治產勞 , 玉門開而不閉方。

[The following] prescription treats childbirth taxation, [causing] the jade gate to stay open and not close.˙

Formula

硫黃（四兩）　吳茱萸（一兩半）　菟絲子（一兩六銖）　蛇床子（一兩）。

硫磺	liú huáng	Sulphur	四兩 4 liǎng	12g
吳茱萸	wú zhū yú	Unripe fruit of Evodia rutaecarpa	一兩半 1.5 liǎng	4.5g
菟絲子	tù sī zǐ	Seed of Cuscuta chinensis	一兩六銖 1 liǎng 6 zhū	3.75g
蛇床子	shé chuáng zǐ	Fruit of Cnidium monnieri	一兩 1 liǎng	3g

上四味，為散，以水一升煎二方寸匕，洗玉門，日再。

Make a powder with the above four ingredients. Heat two square-inch spoons [of this] in one *shēng* of water and wash the jade gate with it twice a day.

---

* Compare this with the prescriptions above, Line 8.15 and 8.16. It is worth noticing how the terms "infant's gate" and "jade gate" are understood differently here: While it is pathological for the infant's gate to be closed (as in the expression 子門閉 *zǐ mén bì*, "closure of the infant's gate"), it is equally pathological for the jade gate to remain open after childbirth (玉門開 *yù mén kāi*).

LINE 8.19

治產後陰道開不閉方。

[The following] prescription treats postpartum openness and failure of the *yīn* path˙ to close.

石灰一斗，熬令燒草，以水二斗投之，適寒溫，入汁中坐漬之，須臾復易，坐如常法。已效，千金不傳。

Toast one *dǒu* of limestone to the point where it can set grass on fire, and put it into two *dǒu* of water. Adjust the temperature and immerse [the patient] in the liquid, sitting down to soak [the genitals]. After a short while, repeat [the treatment] with a changed [liquid]. Sit as usual. Of proven efficacy, do not transmit it [even] for a thousand pieces of gold.

---

* 陰道 *yīn dào*: the vagina.

LINE 8.20

治婦人陰脱¹，黃芩散方。

Scutellaria Powder treats women's vaginal prolapse.

Scutellaria Powder
黃芩散 *huáng qín sǎn*

黃芩 蝟皮 當歸（各半兩）芍藥（一兩）牡蠣 竹皮（各二兩半）狐莖（一具，《千金翼》用松皮）。

黃芩	huáng qín	Root of Scutellaria baicalensis	半兩 0.5 liǎng	1.5g
蝟皮	wèi pí	Skin of Erinaceus europaeus	半兩 0.5 liǎng	1.5g
當歸	dāng guī	Root of Angelica polimorpha	半兩 0.5 liǎng	1.5g
芍藥	sháo yào	Root of Paeonia albiflora	一兩 1 liǎng	3g
牡蠣	mǔ lì	Shell of Ostrea rivularis	二兩半 2.5 liǎng	7.5g
竹皮	zhú pí	Shavings of the stripped core Phyllostachys stalks	二兩半 2.5 liǎng	7.5g
狐莖²	hú jīng	Penis of Vulpes vulpes	一具 1 jù	1 set

上七味，治下篩。飲服方寸匕，日三。禁舉重房勞，勿冷食。

Finely pestle and sift the above seven ingredients. Take a square-inch spoon in fluid three times a day. Restrict lifting of heavy weights and bedchamber taxation, as well as the consumption of cold foods.

---

1. 陰脱 *yīn tuō*. A common gynecological category, explained by Cháo Yuán-Fāng in this way: "The uterine network vessels are damaged and injured and the uterus is depleted. Cold *qì* surges down, causing the uterus to protrude outwards (挺出 *tǐng chū*). This condition is called "downward prolapse" (下脱 *xià tuō*). It can also be caused by childbirth-related expenditure of strength and suppression of *qì*..." (《病源論》 40:117). In modern literature, *yīn tuō* is often translated as "uterine prolapse," but it covers a much wider range and at the same time more specific connotations than that biomedical term in modern TCM. In one sense, *tuō* refers to the pathological loss of flesh, as in the definition of *tuō* in the oldest Chinese dictionary as "perishing flesh and emaciation" (脱消肉臞也 *tuō xiāo ròu qū yě* (《說文解字》 p. 364). Wiseman and Féng's translation as "desertion" (*Practical Dictionary*, p. 124), paraphrased as "critical loss," reflects this literal meaning nicely, as in such compounds as "*qì* desertion" (氣脱 *qì tuō*). In its widest sense, 陰脱 can therefore refer to a critical loss of *yīn*, in opposition to patterns of 陽脱, *yáng* desertion. In this case, it is synonymous with the term 亡陰 *wáng yīn* (*yīn* collapse), defined by Wiseman and Féng as a "critical pattern of wearing of *yīn*-blood" (ibid., p. 709). In

the context of early Chinese gynecology, however, 陰脫 has the more restricted meaning of vaginal prolapse, due to a failure of the vagina to close after childbirth. This is based on the more restricted meaning of 陰 as genitals, and of 脫 as "slipping out, dislocating" (i.e., from the inside of the abdomen). To my knowledge, Sūn Sī-Miǎo uses the term exclusively in this restricted sense, and the translation as "*yīn* desertion" reflects a later usage.

2. *Sòng* editors' note: "The *Qiān Jīn Yì Fāng* uses sōng pí (松皮 Bark of Pinus massoniana)."

LINE 8.21

治婦人陰脫，硫黃散方。

Sulphur Powder treats women's vaginal prolapse.

Sulphur Powder
硫磺散 *liú huáng sǎn*

硫黃 烏賊骨（各半兩） 五味子（三銖）。

硫磺	liú huáng	Sulphur	半兩 0.5 liǎng	1.5g
烏賊骨	wū zéi gǔ	Calcified shell of Sepiella maindroni	半兩 0.5 liǎng	1.5g
五味子	wǔ wèi zǐ	Fruit of Schisandra chinensis	三銖 3 zhū	0.375g

上三味，治下篩，以粉其上良，日再三粉之。

Finely pestle and sift the above three ingredients. It is best applied as a powder to [the protruding genitals]. Powder [the genitals] two or three times a day.

LINE 8.22

治婦人陰脫，當歸散方。

Chinese Angelica Powder treats women's vaginal prolapse.

Chinese Angelica Powder
當歸散 *dāng guī sǎn*

當歸 黃芩（各二兩） 芍藥（一兩六銖） 蝟皮（半兩） 牡蠣（二兩半）。

當歸	dāng guī	Root of Angelica polimorpha	二兩 2 liǎng	6g
黃芩	huáng qín	Root of Scutellaria baicalensis	二兩 2 liǎng	6g
芍藥	sháo yào	Root of Paeonia albiflora	一兩六銖 1 liǎng 6 zhū	3.75g
蝟皮	wèi pí	Skin of Erinaceus europaeus	半兩 0.5 liǎng	1.5g
牡蠣	mǔ lì	Shell of Ostrea rivularis	二兩半 2.5 liǎng	7.5g

上五味，治下篩。酒服方寸匕，日三。禁舉重，良。

Finely pestle and sift the above five ingredients. Take a square-inch spoon in liquor three times a day. Restrict lifting of heavy weights. [This prescription] is good.

LINE 8.23

治產後陰下脫方。

[The following] prescription treats postpartum prolapse of the genitals.

蛇床子一升布裹，炙熨之。亦治產後陰中痛。

Wrap one *shēng* of *shé chuáng zǐ* (蛇床子 Fruit of Cnidium monnieri) in a cloth, heat it and apply it as a hot compress. It also treats postpartum pain in the genitals.

LINE 8.24

治婦人陰下脫，若脫肛方。

[The following] prescription treats women's prolapse of the genitals as well as prolapse of the anus.[*]

羊脂煎訖，適冷暖以塗上。以鐵精傳脂上，多少令調，以火炙布令暖，以熨肛上，漸推內之。

Fry sheep or goat fat thoroughly. [Let it cool down to a] comfortable temperature and spread it on [the genitals]. Take iron ash and apply it on top of the fat, adjusting the amount as you go along. Heat a cloth over the fire until warm and apply it as a hot compress over the anus. Gently push it back in.

---

[*]   脫肛 *tuō gāng*. Since the anus is related to the large intestine, vacuity cold there will cause its *qì* to surge downward and push the anus out. The condition can also be caused

by excessive use of force during childbirth (see 《病源論》 40:113).

LINE 8.25

[又方]

[Another prescription:]

末磁石，酒服方寸匕，日三。

Pulverize magnetite and take a square-inch spoon in liquor three times a day.

LINE 8.26

治產後陰下脫方。

[The following] prescription treats postpartum vaginal prolapse.

燒人屎為末，酒服方寸匕，日三。

Char human feces and pulverize them. Take a square-inch spoon in liquor three times a day.

LINE 8.27

又方

Another prescription:

燒弊帚頭為灰，酒服方寸匕。

Char an old broom top into ashes and take a square-inch spoon in liquor.

LINE 8.28

又方

Another prescription:

Formula

皂莢（半兩）半夏 大黃 細辛（各十八銖）蛇床子（三十銖）。

皂莢	zào jiá	Fruit of Gleditsia sinensis	半兩 0.5 liǎng	1.5g
半夏	bàn xià	Rhizome of Pinellia ternata	十八銖 18 zhū	2.25g
大黃	dà huáng	Root of Rheum palmatum	十八銖 18 zhū	2.25g
細辛	xì xīn	Complete plant including root of Asarum heteropoides	十八銖 18 zhū	2.25g
蛇床子	shé chuáng zǐ	Fruit of Cnidium monnieri	三十銖 30 zhū	3.75g

上五味，治下篩，以薄絹囊盛，大如指，內陰中，日二易，即瘥。

Finely pestle and sift the above five ingredients. Pack them into a fine silken bag, the size of a finger. Insert it into the vagina, change it twice a day, and she will recover promptly.

LINE 8.29

又方

Another prescription:

鱉頭五枚，燒末，以井花水服方寸匕，日三。

Char and pulverize five turtle heads. Take a square-inch spoon in well-flower water three times a day.

LINE 8.29

又方

Another prescription:

Formula

蜀椒 吳茱萸（各一升）戎鹽（如雞子大）。

蜀椒	shǔ jiāo	Seed capsules of Zanthoxylum bungeanum	一升 1 shēng	24g
吳茱萸	wú zhū yú	Unripe fruit of Evodia rutaecarpa	一升 1 shēng	24g

戎鹽	róng yán	Halite	如雞子大 rú jī zǐ dà	an amount the size of a chicken egg

上三味，皆熬令變色，治末，以綿裹如半雞子大，內陰中，日一易，二十日瘥。

Slowly heat the above three ingredients together until they change color, then finely pestle them into a powder. Wrap an amount the size of half a chicken egg in thin silk cloth, and insert into the vagina. Change it once a day, and in twenty days she will recover.

LINE 8.30

治陰下挺出方。

[The following] prescription treats vaginal protrusion.

Formula

蜀椒 烏頭 白及（各半兩）。

蜀椒*	shǔ jiāo	Seed capsules of Zanthoxylum bungeanum	半兩 0.5 liǎng	1.5g
烏頭	wū tóu	Main tuber of Aconitum carmichaeli	半兩 0.5 liǎng	1.5g
白芨	bái jí	Rhizome of Bletilla striata	半兩 0.5 liǎng	1.5g

上三味，治末，以方寸匕綿裹，內陰中入三寸，腹中熱易之，日一度，明旦乃復著，七日愈。

Finely pestle the above three ingredients into a powder. Wrap a square-inch spoon [of the powder] in thin silk cloth and insert it into the vagina, three *cùn* deep. When [she feels] heat in the abdomen, change it, once a day. Then reapply it the next morning, and after seven days she will recover.

*   *Sòng* editors' note: "The *Guǎng Jì Fāng* does not use *shǔ jiāo* 蜀椒."

LINE 8.31

治產後藏中風，陰腫痛，當歸洗湯方。

Chinese Angelica Wash Decoction treats postpartum wind strike in the viscera and vaginal swelling and pain.

Chinese Angelica Wash Decoction
當歸洗湯 *dāng guī xǐ tāng*

當歸 獨活 白芷 地榆（各三兩） 敗醬（《千金翼》不用） 礬石（各二兩）
。

當歸	dāng guī	Root of Angelica polimorpha	三兩	3 liǎng	9g
獨活	dú huó	Root and rhizome of Angelica pubescens	三兩	3 liǎng	9g
白芷	bái zhǐ	Root of Angelica dahurica	三兩	3 liǎng	9g
地榆	dì yú	Root of Sanguisorba officinalis	三兩	3 liǎng	9g
敗醬*	bài jiàng	Whole plant with root of Patrinia villosa	二兩	2 liǎng	6g
礬石	fán shí	Alum	二兩	2 liǎng	6g

上六味，㕮咀，以水一斗半煮取五升。適冷煖，稍稍洗陰，日三。

Pound the above six ingredients and decoct in one and a half *dǒu* of water to obtain five *shēng*. Adjust the temperature and rinse the genitals with this gently three times a day.

*   *Sòng* editors' note: "The *Qiān Jīn Yì Fāng* does not use *bài jiàng* 敗醬."

LINE 8.32

治產後陰腫痛方。

[The following] prescription treats postpartum vaginal swelling and pain.

熟擣桃仁傅之，良，日三度。

It is good to apply thoroughly pounded *táo rén* (桃仁 Seed of Prunus persica) three times a day.

LINE 8.33

治男女陰瘡膏方。

[The following] salve treats men's and and women's genital sores.

Formula

米粉（一酒杯）芍藥 黃芩 牡蠣 附子 白芷（各十八銖）。

米粉	mǐ fěn	Flour of Oryza sativa	一酒杯 1 jiǔ bēi	1 wine-cup full
芍藥	sháo yào	Root of Paeonia albiflora	十八銖 18 zhū	2.25g
黃芩	huáng qín	Root of Scutellaria baicalensis	十八銖 18 zhū	2.25g
牡蠣	mǔ lì	Shell of Ostrea rivularis	十八銖 18 zhū	2.25g
附子	fù zǐ	Lateral root of Aconitum carmi-chaeli	十八銖 18 zhū	2.25g
白芷	bái zhǐ	Root of Angelica dahurica	十八銖 18 zhū	2.25g

上六味，哎咀，以不中水豬膏一斤煎之於微火上，三下三上，候白芷黃，膏成，絞去滓，內白粉，和令相得，傅瘡上。並治口瘡。

Pound the above six ingredients. Simmer [the ingredients] over a small flame in one *jīn* of pork lard that does not contain any water, bringing it to a boil and then letting it settle three times. When the *bái zhǐ* 白芷 has turned yellow, the salve is done. Wring out and discard the dregs, add the white flour and mix until well-blended. Apply it on the sore. It also treats mouth sores.

LINE 8.34

治陰中痛，生瘡方。

[The following] prescription treats pain in the vagina and formation of sores.

Formula

羊脂（一斤）杏仁（一升）當歸 白芷 芎藭（各一兩）。

羊脂	yáng zhī	Unrendered fat of Capra hircus	一斤 1 jīn	48g
杏仁	xìng rén	Dried seed of Prunus armeniaca	一升 1 shēng	24g
當歸	dāng guī	Root of Angelica polimorpha	一兩 1 liǎng	3g
白芷	bái zhǐ	Root of Angelica dahurica	一兩 1 liǎng	3g
川芎	chuān xiōng	Root of Ligusticum wallichii	一兩 1 liǎng	3g

上五味，末之，以羊脂和諸藥，內缽中，置甑內蒸之三升米頃，藥成。取如大豆，綿裹內陰中，日一易。

Pulverize the above five ingredients. Combine all the drugs with the sheep or goat fat and put it in a bowl. Set this inside a rice steamer and steam it for the duration of time it would take to cook three shēng of rice. Then the medicine is done. Take an amount the size of a soybean, wrap it in thin silk cloth, and insert it into the vagina, changing it once a day.

LINE 8.35

治陰中癢，如蟲行狀方。

[The following] prescription treats itching in the vagina, resembling the movement of worms.

Formula

礬石（十八銖） 芎藭（一兩） 丹砂（少許）。

礬石	fán shí	Alum	十八銖 18 zhū	2.25g
川芎	chuān xiōng	Root of Ligusticum wallichii	一兩 1 liǎng	3g
丹砂	dān shā	Mercuric sulfide	少許 shǎo xǔ	a small amount

上三味，治下篩，以綿裹藥，著陰中，蟲自死。

Finely pestle and sift the above three ingredients. Wrap the drugs in thin silk cloth and apply it to the inside of the vagina. The worms will die on their own.

LINE 8.36

治男女陰蝕略盡方。

[The following] prescription treats men's and women's genital erosion* to the point of almost total destruction.

Formula

蝦蟆 兔屎。

| 蝦蟆 | há má | Whole body of Rana limnocharis |
| 兔屎 | tù shǐ | Feces of Oryctolagus domesticus |

上二味，等分為末，以傅瘡上。

Pulverize equal portions of the above two ingredients and apply on top of the sores.

* 陰蝕 *yīn shí*: I follow Wiseman and Féng's terminology (*Practical Dictionary*, p. 241) because it reflects the literal meaning of the term well. This term refers to a type of genital sore, generally in women, that is caused by evil fire from the seven affects and leads to ulceration of the external genitals, unbearable itching, [sensation of] worms and pain in the genitals, and, in chronic cases, to rotting flesh in the vagina, foul-smelling vaginal discharge, sharp pain, emaciation and gradual erosion of the internal organs, to the point of death (《中華醫學大辭典》, p. 598). In the most literal sense, 蝕 originally refers to the gradual erosion and destruction that is caused by worms eating flesh. For a more common example of the use of 蝕, the compound 骨蝕 *gǔ shí* (bone erosion) is explained in the *Líng Shū* as internal damage to the bones, caused by heat overcoming cold and rotting the flesh and muscles (《靈樞》 75).

LINE 8.37

又方

Another prescription:[1]

當歸 芍藥 甘草 蛇床子 (各一兩) 地榆 (三兩) 。

當歸	dāng guī	Root of Angelica polimorpha	一兩 1 liǎng	3g
芍藥	sháo yào	Root of Paeonia albiflora	一兩 1 liǎng	3g
甘草	gān cǎo	Root of Glycyrrhiza uralensis	一兩 1 liǎng	3g
蛇床子[2]	shé chuáng zǐ	Fruit of Cnidium monnieri	一兩 1 liǎng	3g
地榆	dì yú	Root of Sanguisorba officinalis	三兩 3 liǎng	9g

上五味，㕮咀，以水五升煮取二升，洗之，日三夜二。

Pound the above five ingredients and decoct in five *shēng* of water to obtain two *shēng*. Wash [the sores] with this three times a day and twice at night.

1. This and the following two prescriptions are found later in this section in the *Sūn Zhēn Rén* edition. In their place, we find two prescriptions, one for postpartum abdominal pain and one for incessant vaginal bleeding after the first sexual intercourse of virgins. For the rest of this section, the *Sūn Zhēn Rén* edition contains almost the same prescriptions as

the *Sòng* revisions, but in no apparent order of arrangement. In contrast, the *Sòng* revision arranges the prescriptions in the following order: first treatments for vaginal protrusion, then for vaginal sores, and then for vaginal bleeding due to sexual intercourse (whether in virgins or due to injury from a man). It concludes the volume with a collection of moxibustion prescriptions for inhibited menstruation and infertility.

2. *Sòng* editors' note: "Another [version of this] prescription uses *chuān xiōng* (川芎 Root of Ligusticum wallichii)."

LINE 8.38

又方

Another prescription:

Formula

蒲黃（一升）水銀（一兩）。

| 蒲黃 | pú huáng | Pollen of Typha angustata | 一升 1 shēng | 24g |
| 水銀 | shuǐ yín | Mercury | 一兩 1 liǎng | 3g |

上二味，研之，以粉上。

Grind the above two ingredients and apply as a powder on [the sores].

LINE 8.39

又方

Another prescription:

肥豬肉（十斤），以水煮取熟，去肉，盆中浸之，冷易，不過三兩度。亦治陰中癢，有蟲。

Cook ten *jīn* of fatty pork in water until well-done. Take out the meat, place [the liquid] in a bowl and soak [the sores].]When the liquid] has cooled off, change it. Do not exceed two or three [treatments]. It also treats itching and presence of worms in the vagina.

LINE 8.40

治男女陰中瘡，濕癢方。

[The following] prescription treats men's and women's genital sores and damp itching.

Formula

黃連 梔子 甘草 黃蘗（各一兩） 蛇床子（二兩）。

黃連	huáng lián	Rhizome of Coptis chinensis	一兩 1 liǎng	3g
梔子	zhī zǐ	Fruit of Gardenia jasminoides	一兩 1 liǎng	3g
甘草	gān cǎo	Root of Glycyrrhiza uralensis	一兩 1 liǎng	3g
黃蘗	huáng bò	Bark of Phellodendron amurense	一兩 1 liǎng	3g
蛇床子	shé chuáng zǐ	Fruit of Cnidium monnieri	二兩 2 liǎng	6g

上五味，治下篩，以粉瘡上，無汁，以豬脂和塗之。深者，用綿裏內瘡中，日二。

Finely pestle and sift the above five ingredients. Powder the sores with this. If there is no fluid [leaking from the sores], mix it with pork lard and spread it on. If they are deep [inside the vagina], wrap [the powder] in thin silk cloth and insert it to where the sores are, twice a day.

LINE 8.41

治陰中癢入骨困方。

[The following] prescription treats vaginal itching that is entering the bones, causing encumbrance.

Formula

大黃 黃芩 黃芪（各一兩） 芍藥（半兩） 玄參 丹參（各十八銖） 吳茱萸（三十銖）。

大黃	dà huáng	Root of Rheum palmatum	一兩 1 liǎng	3g
黃芩	huáng qín	Root of Scutellaria baicalensis	一兩 1 liǎng	3g
黃芪	huáng qí	Root of Astragalus membranaceus	一兩 1 liǎng	3g
芍藥	sháo yào	Root of Paeonia albiflora	半兩 0.5 liǎng	1.5g
玄參	xuán shēn	Root of Scrophularia ningpoensis	十八銖 18 zhū	2.25g
丹參	dān shēn	Root of Salvia miltiorrhiza	十八銖 18 zhū	2.25g

| 吳茱萸 | wú zhū yú | Unripe fruit of Evodia rutaecarpa | 三十銖 30 zhū | 3.75g |

上七味，治下篩，酒服方寸匕，日三。

Finely pestle and sift the above seven ingredients. Take a square-inch spoon in liquor three times a day.

LINE 8.42

又方

Another prescription:

狼牙兩把，以水五升煮取一升，洗之，日五六度。

Decoct two handfuls of *láng yá* (狼牙 Root of Potentilla cryptotaenia) in five *shēng* of water to obtain one *shēng*. Rinse [the vagina] with this, five or six times a day.

LINE 8.43

治陰瘡方。

[The following] prescription treats vaginal sores.

Formula

蕪荑 芎藭 黃芩 甘草 礬石 雄黃 附子 白芷 黃連。

蕪荑	wú yí	Processed fruit of Ulmus macrocarpa	六銖 6 zhū	0.75g
川芎	chuān xiōng	Root of Ligusticum wallichii	六銖 6 zhū	0.75g
黃芩	huáng qín	Root of Scutellaria baicalensis	六銖 6 zhū	0.75g
甘草	gān cǎo	Root of Glycyrrhiza uralensis	六銖 6 zhū	0.75g
礬石	fán shí	Alum	六銖 6 zhū	0.75g
雄黃	xióng huáng	Realgar	六銖 6 zhū	0.75g
附子	fù zǐ	Lateral root of Aconitum carmichaeli	六銖 6 zhū	0.75g
白芷	bái zhǐ	Root of Angelica dahurica	六銖 6 zhū	0.75g
黃連	huáng lián	Rhizome of Coptis chinensis	六銖 6 zhū	0.75g

上九味，各六銖，㕮咀，以豬膏四兩合煎，傅之。

Pound six *zhū* of each of the above nine ingredients and simmer them with four *liǎng* of pork fat. Apply [to the sores].

LINE 8.44

治女人交接輒血出方。

[The following] prescription treats women's [vaginal] bleeding that occurs as soon as they engage in sexual intercourse.

Formula

桂心 伏龍肝（各二兩）。

桂心	guì xīn	Shaved inner bark of Cinnamomum cassia	二兩 2 liǎng	6g
伏龍肝	fú lóng gān	Stove earth	二兩 2 liǎng	6g

上二味，為末，酒服方寸匕，立止。

Pulverize the above two ingredients and take a square-inch spoon in liquor. It will stop [the bleeding] immediately.

LINE 8.45

治童女交接，陽道違理，及為佗物所傷，血出流離不止方。

[The following] prescription treats unstoppable [vaginal] bleeding in virgins after [their first] sexual intercourse, if the male organ has violated the regular order of things, or if [the vagina] has been damaged by other objects.

取釜低墨少許，研胡麻以傅之。

Take a small amount of soot from the bottom of a pan and grind it with *hú má* (胡麻 Black seed of Sesamum indicum). Apply it [to the vagina].

LINE 8.46

又方

Another prescription:

燒青布並髮灰傳之，立愈。

Char green-blue cloth together with hair into ashes and apply it [to the vagina]. She will promptly recover.

LINE 8.47

又方

Another prescription:

燒繭絮灰傳之。

Char silkworm cocoons into ashes and apply [to the vagina].

LINE 8.48

治合陰陽輒痛不可忍方。

[The following] prescription treats unbearable pain at the moment of uniting *yīn* and *yáng*.

Formula

黃連（一兩半） 牛膝 甘草（各一兩）。

黃連	huáng lián	Rhizome of Coptis chinensis	一兩半 1.5 liǎng	4.5g
牛膝	niú xī	Root of Achyranthes bidentata	一兩 1 liǎng	3g
甘草	gān cǎo	Root of Glycyrrhiza uralensis	一兩 1 liǎng	3g

上三味，㕮咀，以水四升煮取二升，洗之，日四度。

Pound the above three ingredients and decoct in four *shēng* of water to obtain two *shēng*. Wash [the genitals] with this four times a day.

LINE 8.49

治女人傷於丈夫，四體沈重，噓吸，頭痛方。

[The following] prescription treats women's [idsorders resulting from] damage by their husband,[1] heaviness of the four limbs, huffing and gasping, and headache.

Formula

生地黃（八兩）芍藥（五兩）香豉（一升）蔥白（一升）生薑（四兩）甘草（二兩）。

生地黃	shēng dì huáng	Fresh root of Rehmannia glutinosa	八兩 8 liǎng	24g
芍藥	sháo yào	Root of Paeonia albiflora	五兩 5 liǎng	15g
香豉	xiāng chǐ	Preparation of Fermented Glycine max	一升 1 shēng	24g
蔥白	cōng bái	Stalk of Allium fistulosum	一升 1 shēng	24g
生薑	shēng jiāng	Fresh root of Zingiber officinale	四兩 4 liǎng	12g
甘草	gān cǎo	Root of Glycyrrhiza uralensis	二兩 2 liǎng	6g

上六味，㕮咀，以水七升煮取二升半。分三服，不瘥重作。慎房事。（《集驗方》無生薑甘草。）

Pound the above six ingredients and decoct in seven *shēng* of water to obtain two and a half *shēng*. Divide into three doses, and, if she fails to recover, make it again. Beware of sexual activity.[2]

---

1. Based on context, it is clear that Sūn Sī-Miǎo refers here specifically to vaginal injuries sustained during sexual intercourse, as described in the prescriptions above.
2. *Sòng* editors' note: "The *Jí Yàn Fāng* does not use *shēng jiāng* 生薑 and *gān cǎo* 甘草."

LINE 8.50

治婦人陰陽過度，玉門疼痛，小便不通，白玉湯方。

White Jade Decoction treats women's [conditions resulting from] excessive sexual activity,* pain in the jade gate, and blocked urination.

White Jade Decoction
白玉湯 *bái yù tāng*

白玉（一兩半）白术（五兩）澤瀉　蓯蓉（各二兩）當歸（五兩）。

白玉	bái yù	Fine slivers of white jade	一兩半 1.5 liǎng	4.5g
白朮	bái zhú	Rhizome of Atractylodes macrocephala	五兩 5 liǎng	15g
澤瀉	zé xiè	Rhizome of Alisma plantago-aquatica	二兩 2 liǎng	6g
蓯蓉	cōng róng	Stalk of Cistanche salsa	二兩 2 liǎng	6g
當歸	dāng guī	Root of Angelica polimorpha	五兩 5 liǎng	15g

上五味，哎咀，先以水一斗煎玉五十沸，去玉內藥，煎取二升。分再服，相去一炊頃。

Pound the above five ingredients. First, simmer the jade in one *dǒu* of water, bringing it to a rolling boil fifty times. Then remove the jade, add the drugs, and simmer to obtain two *shēng*. Divide into two doses and [take them] separated from each other by the amount of time it takes to cook a meal.

* 治婦人陰陽過度 *zhì fù rén yīn yáng guò dù*: The *Sūn Zhēn Rén* edition has an alternate version with a slightly different, but significant emphasis: 治因其夫陰陽過度 *zhì yīn qí fū yīn yáng guò dù* (treats [conditions] caused by the husband's excessive sexual activity). In this wording, the husband is explicitly blamed for his wife's sickness, expressing Sūn Sī-Miǎo's paternalistic concern for his female patients and the apparently not too rare possibility of women being physically injured by their husbands' sexual excess and unlimited access to their wives' bodies.

LINE 8.51

治動胎見血，腰痛，小腹疼，月水不通，陰中腫痛方。

[The following] prescription treats bleeding [during pregnancy] after the fetus has been stirred,[1] pain in the lumbus and lower abdomen, blocked menstruation,[2] and swelling and pain in the vagina.

Formula

蒲黃（二兩）蔥白（一斤，切）當歸（二兩，切）吳茱萸 阿膠（各一兩）。

蒲黃	pú huáng	Pollen of Typha angustata	二兩 2 liǎng	6g
蔥白, 切	cōng bái, qiē	Stalk of Allium fistulosum, chopped	一斤 1 jīn	48g
當歸, 切	dāng guī, qiē	Root of Angelica polimorpha, chopped	二兩 2 liǎng	6g
吳茱萸	wú zhū yú	Unripe fruit of Evodia rutaecarpa	一兩 1 liǎng	3g

| 阿膠 | ē jiāo | Gelatinous glue produced from Equus asinus | 一兩 1 liǎng | 3g |

上五味，以水九升煮取二升半，去滓，內膠令烊，分三服。

Decoct the above five ingredients in nine *shēng* of water to obtain two and a half *shēng*. Discard the dregs and add the *ē jiāo* 阿膠, letting it melt. Divide into three doses.

1. 動胎 *dòng tāi*: Before this phrase, the *Sūn Zhēn Rén* edition inserts the three characters 傷丈夫 *shāng zhàng fū* (damaged by the husband). Given the fact that this prescription appears here in the context of treatments for miscellaneous problems caused by sexual intercourse (see the preceding and following prescriptions) rather than in the section on pregnancy (volume 2, chapter 4, section g on bleeding in pregnancy), it is most likely that this prescription refers specifically to cases where the fetus has been harmed by the husband's sexual activity, which is then also causing the following symptoms. To distinguish it, the condition of fetal unrest is always called 胎動 *tāi dòng*.

2. It is not clear if this refers to the long-term effects of a damaged fetus (and presumably subsequent miscarriage) in the pregnancy, or if this is a separate condition addressed by this prescription. I interpret it here as yet another symptom caused by injury from sexual intercourse during pregnancy for two reasons: First, the prescriptions in this section appear to have been consciously placed together in related etiological groups. The prescriptions preceding and following this one all concern pathologies caused by injuries sustained during sexual intercourse. In addition, Sūn Sī-Miǎo's prescriptions all follow a fairly strict pattern: First, the etiology is named, and then the secondary symptoms are listed. In general, when a prescription treats several unrelated conditions, these are linked by 及 *jí* (as well as), to clearly mark the dual application of a prescription (see, for example, chapter two of volume three, Line 2.10 (pp. 264 - 265) or chapter three of volume three, on Line 3.2 (pp. 268 - 270) above).

LINE 8.52

治妊娠為夫所動欲死，單行竹瀝汁方。

Single Agent Bamboo Sap Juice treats patients on the verge of death from being stirred by their husband[1] during pregnancy.

Single Agent Bamboo Sap Juice
單行竹瀝汁 *dān xíng zhú lì zhī*

取淡竹斷兩頭節，火燒中央，器盛兩頭得汁，飲之，立效。

Take bland bamboo and break off a section with two ends.[2] Roast the middle of it over a fire and catch the juice from both ends in a container. Drinking it has immediate efficacy.

1. 為夫所動欲死 *wéi fū suǒ dòng yù sǐ*: While this phrase, at first sight and out of its medical context, could also be understood in a more psychological sense as "having been aroused/disturbed by their husbands and wanting to die," the context of this prescription, as well as the consistent usage of *yù sǐ* throughout this text as "on the verge of death," make it quite clear that this prescription is a treatment for cases of life-threatening physical abuse [in the context of sexual intercourse] in pregnancy.

2. 兩頭節 *liǎng tóu jié*: This means that the piece is still sealed at either end.

LINE 8.53

治傷丈夫，苦頭痛，欲嘔，心悶，桑根白皮湯方。

Mulberry Bark Decoction treats damage by the husband, headache, tendency to retch, and heart oppression.

Mulberry Bark Decoction
桑根白皮湯 *sāng gēn bái pí tāng*

桑根白皮（半兩）乾薑（二兩）桂心（五寸）大棗（二十枚）。

桑根白皮	sāng gēn bái pí	Bark of the root of Morus alba	半兩 0.5 liǎng	1.5g
乾薑	gān jiāng	Dried root of Zingiber officinale	二兩 2 liǎng	6g
桂心	guì xīn	Shaved inner bark of Cinnamomum cassia	五寸 5 cùn	3g
大棗	dà zǎo	Mature fruit of Ziziphus jujuba	二十枚 20 méi	20 pcs

上四味，㕮咀，以酒一斗煮取三升，去滓，分三服，適衣，無令汗出。

Pound the above four ingredients and decoct in one *dǒu* of liquor to obtain three *shēng*. Discard the dregs and divide into three doses. Adjust her clothing to prevent her from sweating [as a result of taking the medicine].

LINE 8.54

治嫁痛單行方。

[The following] is a single agent prescription for treating wedding pain.˙

大黃十八銖，以好酒一升煮三沸，頻服之，良。

Decoct eighteen *zhū* of *dà huáng* (大黃 Root of Rheum palmatum) in one *shēng* of good liquor, bringing it to a boil three times. Quaff it in a single dose. Good.

---

*   嫁痛 *jià tòng*: Explained in the *Zhōng Huá Yī Xué Dà Cí Diǎn* as "the pain experienced by newly-wed girls resulting from injury to their vagina on their wedding night (《中華醫學大辭典》 p. 1501).

LINE 8.55

治小戶嫁痛連日方。

[The following] prescription treats wedding pain [resulting from] a small entrance [to the vagina], which has continued for several days.

Formula

甘草（三兩）芍藥（半兩）生薑（十八銖）桂心（六銖）。

甘草	gān cǎo	Root of Glycyrrhiza uralensis	三兩 3 liǎng	9g
芍藥	sháo yào	Root of Paeonia albiflora	半兩 0.5 liǎng	1.5g
生薑	shēng jiāng	Fresh root of Zingiber officinale	十八銖 18 zhū	2.25g
桂心	guì xīn	Shaved inner bark of Cinnamomum cassia	六銖 6 zhū	0.75g

上四味，㕮咀，以酒二升煮三沸，去滓。盡服，神效。

Pound the above four ingredients and decoct in two *shēng* of liquor, bringing it to a boil three times. Discard the dregs. Take it all. Divinely effective.

LINE 8.56

又方

Another prescription:

牛膝五兩，以酒三升煮取半，去滓，分三服。

Decoct five *liǎng* of *niú xī* (牛膝 Root of Achyranthes bidentata) in three *shēng* of liquor until reduced to half. Discard the dregs and divide into three doses.

LINE 8.57

治小戶嫁痛方。

[The following] prescription treats wedding pain [resulting from] a small entrance.

烏賊骨，燒為屑，酒服方寸匕，日三。

Char *wū zéi gǔ* (烏賊骨 Calcified shell of Sepiella maindroni) and break it into pieces. Take a square-inch spoon in liquor three times a day.

LINE 8.58

治陰寬大，令窄小方。

[The following] prescription treats a wide and large vagina, making it narrow and small.

Formula

兔屎 乾漆（各半兩）鼠頭骨（二枚）雌雞肝（二個，陰乾百日）。

兔屎	tù shǐ	Feces of Oryctolagus domesticus	半兩 0.5 liǎng	1.5g
乾漆	gān qī	Dried sap of Rhus verniciflua	半兩 0.5 liǎng	1.5g
鼠頭骨	shǔ tóu gǔ	Head of Rattus norvegicus	二枚 2 méi	2 pcs
雌雞肝，陰乾百日	cī jī gān, yīn gān bǎi rì	Liver of Gallus gallus domesticus, dried in the shade for 100 days	二個 2 gè	2 pcs

上四味，末之，蜜丸如小豆，月初七日*合時，著一丸陰頭，令徐徐內之。三日知，十日小，五十日如十五歲童女。

Make a powder with the above four ingredients and mix with honey into pills the size of azuki beans. Have intercourse on the seventh day from the beginning of the month[1] and, at that time, place one pill on the top of the penis and insert it little by little. After three days, you will notice [an effect]; after ten days, [the vagina] will have shrunk; and after fifty days, it will be like that of a fifteen-year-old virgin.

---

*   月初七日 *yuè chū qī rì*: The *Sūn Zhēn Rén* edition has 七月七日 *qī yuè qī rì* (on the seventh day of the seventh month) instead.

LINE 8.59
治陰冷令熱方。

[The following] prescription treats a cold vagina by making it hot.

內食茱萸於牛膽中令滿，陰乾百日。每取二七枚綿裹之，齒嚼令碎，內陰中，良久，熱如火。

Fill a cow's gallbladder with *shí zhū yú* (食茱萸 Fruit of Zanthoxylum ailanthoides) to the top and dry it in the shade for one hundred days. Take two times seven pieces [out of it] per dose, wrap them in thin silk cloth, chew them with your teeth to crush them, and insert into the vagina. [Leave the suppository in] for a good long time [until] it is hot like fire.

LINE 8.60

Moxibustion Treatments

(一) 月水不利，賁豚上下，並無子：灸四滿三十壯，穴在丹田兩邊相去各一寸半，丹田在臍下二寸是也。(二) 婦人胞落頹：灸臍中三百壯。(三) 又：灸身交五十壯，三報，在臍下橫文中。(四) 又：灸背脊當臍五十壯。(五) 又：灸玉泉五十壯，三報。(六) 又：灸龍門二十壯，三報，在玉泉下，女人入陰內外之際。此穴卑令廢不針灸。(七) 婦人胞下垂，注陰下脫：灸俠玉泉三寸，隨年壯，三報。(八) 婦人陰冷腫痛：灸歸來三十壯，三報，俠玉泉五寸是其穴。(九) 婦人欲斷產：灸右踝上一寸三壯，即斷。

(1) For inhibited urination and running piglet [causing her *qì* to surge] up and down, as well as for infertility: Burn 30 moxa cones on Fourfold Fullness.[1] The points are located on both sides of the cinnabar field, each one and a half *cùn* to the side. The cinnabar field is located two *cùn* below the navel.

(2) For [the treatment of] women's drooping uterus: Burn 300 moxa cones on the center of the navel. [Burn] 300 cones.

(3) Again: Burn 50 cones on Bodily Intersection. Repeat three times. It is located in the middle of the horizontal line below the navel.

(4) Again: Burn 50 cones on the point where the spinal chord is opposite the navel.

(5) Again: Burn 50 cones on Jade Spring.[2] Repeat three times.

(6) Again: Burn 20 cones on Dragon Gate.[3] Repeat three times. It is located below Jade Spring, at the border of the internal and external parts of a woman's genitals.[4] This point

is inferior and therefore discontinued nowadays and not needled or cauterized [any more].

(7) For [the treatment of] women [suffering from] a low-hanging uterus that is pouring into the vagina and has prolapsed down: Burn moxa cones on the point three *cùn* to both sides of Jade Spring, the number of cones corresponding to her age. Repeat three times.

(8) For [the treatment of] women [suffering from] vaginal coldness, swelling, and pain: Burn 30 cones on Return.[5] Repeat three times. This point is located five *cùn* to both sides of Jade Spring.

(9) For [the treatment of] women desiring to interrupt their childbearing: Burn three cones of moxa on a point that is located] one *cùn* above the right ankle, and they will promptly stop [bearing children].

1. 四滿 *sì mǎn*: KI-14, a pair of points used in modern TCM for lesser abdominal pain, diarrhea, menstrual irregularities, vaginal discharge, infertility, hernia, seminal emission, and urinary dribbling (李經緯, 主編. 《中醫大辭典》 p. 468). Sūn Sī-Miǎo elsewhere uses them for treating inhibited menstruation, upward and downward surging blood, as well as infertility (《千金翼方》 26:2). According to the *Sūn Zhēn Rén* edition, the points are located only one *cùn* to each side of the cinnabar field, which is located 3 *cùn* below the navel.

2. 身交 *shēn jiāo*: Not a standard acupuncture point. According to modern acupuncture texts, located either 0.3 or 3 *cùn* below the navel and indicated for such conditions as constipation, urinary problems, and vaginal discharge (李經緯, 主編.《中醫大辭典》 p. 881).

3. 玉泉 *yù quán*: Not a standard acupuncture point name, but the *Qiān Jīn Yì Fāng* also recommends to cauterize this point for treating repeated miscarriages by increasing her ability to carry a pregnancy to terms (《千金翼方》 26:2). It states there that it is identical with 中極 *zhōng jī* (Central Pole, CV-3), which is confirmed by the *Zhēn Jiǔ Jiǎ Yǐ Jīng*. This is used in modern TCM to supplement the kidneys and *yáng*, regulate menstruation, stop leucorrhea, warm essence, and regulate the bladder (see 李經緯, 主編.《中醫大辭典》 p. 266).

4. 龍門 *lóng mén* (Dragon Gate): Not a standard acupuncture point. In the *Bìng Yuán Lùn*, this term is used as the name for the entrance to the vagina in women who are married but have never given birth (《病源論》 137:24). The *Qiān Jīn Yì Fāng* describes its location in slightly different terms as located "above the outer edge of the genitals."

5. 歸來 *guī lái*: ST-29.

Bèi Jí Qiān Jīn Yào Fāng

備急千金要方

Volume 4

卷第四

1. Supplementing and Boosting 補益

Translator's note: Contrary to Sūn Sī-Miǎo's usual practice of loosely adopting the categorization of women's conditions found in the *Bìng Yuán Lùn*, this section has no equivalent in that text. Instead, the *Bìng Yuán Lùn* dedicates two full volumes to the various symptoms of "vacuity taxation" (虛勞 *xū lǎo*), which are, however, not addressed specifically to women. This divergence is probably based on the fact that the subject of supplementing and boosting became increasingly important in the clinical practice of gynecology, but was of minor significance from an etiological perspective.

LINE 1.1

論曰凡婦人欲求美色，肥白罕比，年至七十與少不殊者，勿服紫石英，令人色黑，當服鍾乳澤蘭丸也。

Essay: In all cases when a woman wishes for a beautiful complexion, so glistening white that few can compare, and looking youthful even as she approaches seventy years of age, do not let her take *zǐ shí yīng* (紫石英 Fluorite). It will darken her complexion. She should take *Stalactite and Lycopus Pills*.*

---

*   This introductory essay and warning is located later in the *Sūn Zhēn Rén* edition (after line 1.8 below), which could indicate that it constitutes a later insertion. Perhaps the darkening effect of *zǐ shí yīng* 紫石英 on a woman's complexion was a more recent medical discovery that contradicted earlier practices. The *Shén Nóng Běn Cǎo Jīng*, for example, still categorizes *zǐ shí yīng* 紫石英 as non-toxic (無毒 *wú dú*). It recommends taking it for "supplementing insufficiencies, and for [treating] women's wind-cold in the uterus, infertility, and lack of off-spring for ten years. If taken long-term, it warms the center, lightens the body, and extends one's years" (《神農本草經》 2:103). It would therefore be the ideal ingredient for addressing the symptoms in this section and is indeed included in a majority of the prescriptions, contrary to the warning in the introductory essay. The prescription for *Stalactite and Lycopus Pills* is found below, Line 1.9 (pp. 414 - 415).

LINE 1.2

柏子仁丸治婦人五勞七傷，羸冷瘦削，面無顏色，飲食減少，貌失光澤，及產後斷緒無子，能久服，令人肥白補益方。

Arborvitae Seed Pills treat women's five taxations and seven damages, thinness, coldness, marked emaciation, and whittling, lack of color in the face, deficient [intake of] food and drink, a lusterless appearance, as well as postpartum lack of descendants and infertility. This prescription can be taken for a long period of time and will make the person fat and white by supplementing and boosting.[1]

Arborvitae Seed Pills
柏子仁丸 *bǎi zǐ rén wán*

柏子仁 黃芪 乾薑 紫石英（各二兩） 蜀椒（一兩半） 杜仲 當歸 甘草 芎藭（各四十二銖） 厚朴 桂心 桔梗 赤石脂 蓯蓉 五味子 白朮 細辛 獨活 人參 石斛 白芷 芍藥（各一兩） 澤蘭（二兩六銖） 藁本 蕪荑（各十八銖） 乾地黃 烏頭（一方作牛膝） 防風（各三十銖）鍾乳 白石英（各二兩）。

柏子仁	bǎi zǐ rén	Seed of Platycladus orientalis	二兩 2 liǎng	6g
黃芪	huáng qí	Root of Astragalus membranaceus	二兩 2 liǎng	6g
乾薑	gān jiāng	Dried root of Zingiber officinale	二兩 2 liǎng	6g
紫石英	zǐ shí yīng	Fluorite	二兩 2 liǎng	6g
蜀椒	shǔ jiāo	Seed capsules of Zanthoxylum bungeanum	一兩半 1.5 liǎng	4.5g
杜仲	dù zhòng	Bark of Eucommia ulmoidis	四十二銖 42 zhū	5.25g
當歸	dāng guī	Root of Angelica polimorpha	四十二銖 42 zhū	5.25g
甘草	gān cǎo	Root of Glycyrrhiza uralensis	四十二銖 42 zhū	5.25g
川芎	chuān xiōng	Root of Ligusticum wallichii	四十二銖 42 zhū	5.25g
厚朴	hòu pò	Bark of Magnolia officinalis	一兩 1 liǎng	3g
桂心	guì xīn	Shaved inner bark of Cinnamomum cassia	一兩 1 liǎng	3g
桔梗	jié gěng	Root of Platycodon grandiflorum	一兩 1 liǎng	3g
赤石脂	chì shí zhī	Halloysite	一兩 1 liǎng	3g
蓯蓉	cōng róng	Stalk of Cistanche salsa	一兩 1 liǎng	3g
五味子	wǔ wèi zǐ	Fruit of Schisandra chinensis	一兩 1 liǎng	3g
白朮	bái zhú	Rhizome of Atractylodes macrocephala	一兩 1 liǎng	3g
細辛	xì xīn	Complete plant including root of Asarum heteropoides	一兩 1 liǎng	3g
獨活	dú huó	Root and rhizome of Angelica pubescens	一兩 1 liǎng	3g
人參	rén shēn	Root of Panax ginseng	一兩 1 liǎng	3g
石斛	shí hú	Whole plant of Dendrobium nobile	一兩 1 liǎng	3g

白芷	bái zhǐ	Root of Angelica dahurica	一兩 1 liǎng	3g
芍藥	sháo yào	Root of Paeonia albiflora	一兩 1 liǎng	3g
澤蘭	zé lán	Foliage and stalk of Lycopus lucidus	二兩 六銖 2 liǎng 6 zhū	6.75g
藁本	gǎo běn	Rhizome and root of Ligusticum sinense	十八銖 18 zhū	2.25g
蕪荑	wú yí	Processed fruit of Ulmus macrocarpa	十八銖 18 zhū	2.25g
乾地黃	gān dì huáng	Dried root of Rehmannia glutinosa	三十銖 30 zhū	3.75g
烏頭[2]	wū tóu	Main tuber of Aconitum carmichaeli	三十銖 30 zhū	3.75g
防風	fáng fēng	Root of Ledebouriella divaricata	三十銖 30 zhū	3.75g
鐘乳	zhōng rǔ	Stalactite	二兩 2 liǎng	6g
白石英	bái shí yīng	White quartz	二兩 2 liǎng	6g

上三十味，為末，蜜和。酒服二十丸如梧子，不知加至三十丸。

Pulverize the above thirty ingredients and mix with honey. Take twenty pills the size of firmiana seeds in liquor. If you notice no effect, increase [the dosage] to a maximum of thirty pills.[3]

1. For this and the following formula, information about the specific quantities of each ingredient vary somewhat from one edition to the next. I follow the *Huá Xià* edition, as it seems in general to be the most carefully edited in regards to such details. No footnotes in the Chinese critical editions explain these textual variations.

2. *Sòng* editors' note: "Another [version of this] prescription uses *niú xī* (牛膝 Root of Achyranthes bidentata)."

3. *Sòng* editors' note: "The *Qiān Jīn Yì Fāng* does not use *wū tóu* 烏頭, but includes half a *liǎng* each of *lóng gǔ* (龍骨 Os draconis), *fáng kuí* (防葵 unknown), *fú líng* (茯苓 Dried fungus of Poria cocos), and *qín jiāo* (秦艽 Root of Gentiana macrophylla), using a total of 33 ingredients. [It states that this prescription] treats hemilateral withering after childbirth."

LINE 1.3

大五石澤蘭丸治婦人風虛寒中，腹內雷鳴，緩急，風頭痛寒熱，月經不調，繞臍惻惻痛，或心腹痞堅，逆害飲食，手足常冷，多夢紛紜，身體痹痛，榮衛不和，虛弱不能動搖，及產後虛損，并宜服此方。

Major Five Stones and Lycopus Pills treat women's[1] wind vacuity and cold strike, thunderous rumbling in the abdomen, [alternating] slackening and tensing, wind headache, [aversion to] cold and heat [effusion], irregular menstruation, anguishing pain around the navel, possibly with glomus and hardness in the heart or abdomen, counterflow harming the ability to eat and drink, constant cold in the hands and feet, profuse confused dreams, impediment pain in the whole body, imbalance between defense and construction, vacuity and weakness [to the point of] being unable to move and stir, as well as postpartum vacuity detriment. This prescription is appropriate to take for all these [conditions].

Major Five Stones and Lycopus Pills
大五石澤蘭丸 *dà wǔ shí zé lán wán*

鍾乳 禹餘糧 紫石英 甘草 黃芪（各二兩半） 石膏 白石英 蜀椒 乾薑（各二兩） 澤蘭（二兩六銖） 當歸 桂心 芎藭 厚朴 柏子仁 乾地黃 細辛 茯苓 五味子 龍骨（各一兩半） 石斛 遠志 人參 續斷 白朮 防風 烏頭（各三十銖） 山茱萸 紫菀（各一兩） 白芷 藁本 蕪荑（各十八銖）。

鐘乳	zhōng rǔ	Stalactite	二兩半 2.5 liǎng	7.5g
禹餘糧	yǔ yú liáng	Limonite	二兩半 2.5 liǎng	7.5g
紫石英	zǐ shí yīng	Fluorite	二兩半 2.5 liǎng	7.5g
甘草	gān cǎo	Root of Glycyrrhiza uralensis	二兩半 2.5 liǎng	7.5g
黃芪	huáng qí	Root of Astragalus membranaceus	二兩半 2.5 liǎng	7.5g
石膏	shí gāo	Gypsum	二兩 2 liǎng	6g
白石英	bái shí yīng	White quartz	二兩 2 liǎng	6g
蜀椒	shǔ jiāo	Seed capsules of Zanthoxylum bungeanum	二兩 2 liǎng	6g
乾薑	gān jiāng	Dried root of Zingiber officinale	二兩 2 liǎng	6g
澤蘭	zé lán	Foliage and stalk of Lycopus lucidus	二兩 六銖 2 liǎng 6 zhū	6.75g
當歸	dāng guī	Root of Angelica polimorpha	一兩半 1.5 liǎng	4.5g
桂心	guì xīn	Shaved inner bark of Cinnamomum cassia	一兩半 1.5 liǎng	4.5g
川芎	chuān xiōng	Root of Ligusticum wallichii	一兩半 1.5 liǎng	4.5g
厚朴	hòu pò	Bark of Magnolia officinalis	一兩半 1.5 liǎng	4.5g
柏子仁	bǎi zǐ rén	Seed of Platycladus orientalis	一兩半 1.5 liǎng	4.5g
乾地黃	gān dì huáng	Dried root of Rehmannia glutinosa	一兩半 1.5 liǎng	4.5g
細辛	xì xīn	Complete plant including root of Asarum heteropoides	一兩半 1.5 liǎng	4.5g
茯苓	fú líng	Dried fungus of Poria cocos	一兩半 1.5 liǎng	4.5g
五味子	wǔ wèi zǐ	Fruit of Schisandra chinensis	一兩半 1.5 liǎng	4.5g
龍骨	lóng gǔ	Os draconis	一兩半 1.5 liǎng	4.5g
石斛	shí hú	Whole plant of Dendrobium nobile	三十銖 30 zhū	3.75g
遠志	yuǎn zhì	Root of Polygala tenuifolia	三十銖 30 zhū	3.75g
人參	rén shēn	Root of Panax ginseng	三十銖 30 zhū	3.75g

續斷	xù duàn	Root of Dipsacus asper	三十銖 30 zhū	3.75g
白朮	bái zhú	Rhizome of Atractylodes macro-cephala	三十銖 30 zhū	3.75g
防風	fáng fēng	Root of Ledebouriella divaricata	三十銖 30 zhū	3.75g
烏頭	wū tóu	Main tuber of Aconitum carmichaeli	三十銖 30 zhū	3.75g
山茱萸	shān zhū yú	Fruit of Cornus officinalis	一兩 1 liǎng	3g
紫菀	zǐ wǎn	Root and rhizome of Aster tataricus	一兩 1 liǎng	3g
白芷	bái zhǐ	Root of Angelica dahurica	十八銖 18 zhū	2.25g
藁本	gǎo běn	Rhizome and root of Ligusticum sinense	十八銖 18 zhū	2.25g
蕪荑	wú yí	Processed fruit of Ulmus macrocarpa	三十銖 30 zhū	3.75g

上三十二味，為末，蜜和丸如梧子大。酒服二十丸，加至三十丸。

Pulverize the above thirty-two ingredients and mix with honey into pills the size of firmiana seeds. Take twenty pills [per dose] in liquor, increasing [the dosage] to a maximum of thirty pills.[2]

1. The *Sūn Zhēn Rén* edition has 產後 *chǎn hòu* (postpartum) instead of 婦人 *fù rén* (women).

2. *Sòng* editors' note: "The *Qiān Jīn Yì Fāng* includes 2 *liǎng* of *yáng qǐ shí* (陽起石 Actinolite)."

LINE 1.4

小五石澤蘭丸治婦人勞冷虛損，飲食減少，面無光色，腹中冷痛，經候不調，吸吸少氣無力，補益溫中方。

Minor Five Stones and Lycopus Pills treat women's taxation cold and vacuity detriment, reduced [intake of] food and drink, lack of luster and color in the face, coldness and pain in the center of the abdomen, menstrual irregularities, and shortage of *qì* and lack of strength in spite of frequent inhalations, by supplementing and boosting and warming the center.

Minor Five Stones and Lycopus Pills
小五石澤蘭丸 *xiǎo wǔ shí zé lán wán*

鍾乳 紫石英 礬石（各一兩半） 白石英 赤石脂 當歸 甘草（各四十二銖） 石膏 陽起石 乾薑（各二兩） 澤蘭（二兩六銖） 蓯蓉 龍骨 桂心（各二兩半） 白朮 芍藥 厚朴 人參 蜀椒 山茱萸（各三十銖） 柏子仁 藁本（各一兩） 蕪

莄（十八銖）。

鐘乳	zhōng rǔ	Stalactite	一兩半 1.5 liǎng	4.5g
紫石英	zǐ shí yīng	Fluorite	一兩半 1.5 liǎng	4.5g
礬石	fán shí	Alum	一兩半 1.5 liǎng	4.5g
白石英	bái shí yīng	White quartz	四十二銖 42 zhū	5.25g
赤石脂	chì shí zhī	Halloysite	四十二銖 42 zhū	5.25g
當歸	dāng guī	Root of Angelica polimorpha	四十二銖 42 zhū	5.25g
甘草	gān cǎo	Root of Glycyrrhiza uralensis	四十二銖 42 zhū	5.25g
石膏	shí gāo	Gypsum	二兩 2 liǎng	6g
陽起石	yáng qǐ shí	Actinolite	二兩 2 liǎng	6g
乾薑	gān jiāng	Dried root of Zingiber officinale	二兩 2 liǎng	6g
澤蘭	zé lán	Foliage and stalk of Lycopus lucidus	二兩 六銖 2 liǎng 6 zhū	6.75g
蓯蓉	cōng róng	Stalk of Cistanche salsa	二兩半 2.5 liǎng	7.5g
龍骨	lóng gǔ	Os draconis	二兩半 2.5 liǎng	7.5g
桂心	guì xīn	Shaved inner bark of Cinnamomum cassia	二兩半 2.5 liǎng	7.5g
白朮	bái zhú	Rhizome of Atractylodes macro-cephala	三十銖 30 zhū	3.75g
芍藥	sháo yào	Root of Paeonia albiflora	三十銖 30 zhū	3.75g
厚朴	hòu pò	Bark of Magnolia officinalis	三十銖 30 zhū	3.75g
人參	rén shēn	Root of Panax ginseng	三十銖 30 zhū	3.75g
蜀椒	shǔ jiāo	Seed capsules of Zanthoxylum bungeanum	三十銖 30 zhū	3.75g
山茱萸	shān zhū yú	Fruit of Cornus officinalis	三十銖 30 zhū	3.75g
柏子仁	bǎi zǐ rén	Seed of Platycladus orientalis	一兩 1 liǎng	3g
藁本	gǎo běn	Rhizome and root of Ligusticum sinense	一兩 1 liǎng	3g
蕪荑	wú yí	Processed fruit of Ulmus macrocarpa	十八銖 18 zhū	2.25g

上二十三味，為末，蜜和丸如梧子大。酒服二十丸，加至三十丸，日三。

Pulverize the above twenty-three ingredients and mix with honey into pills the size of firm-iana seeds. Take twenty pills [per dose] in liquor, increasing [the dosage] to a maximum of thirty pills, three times a day.

LINE 1.5

增損澤蘭丸治產後百病，理血氣，補虛勞方。

Modified Lycopus Pills treat the myriad postpartum diseases by regulating blood and *qi* and supplementing vacuity taxation.*

Modified Lycopus Pills
增損澤蘭丸 *zēng sǔn zé lán wán*

澤蘭 甘草 當歸 芎藭（各四十二銖）附子 乾薑 白朮 白芷 桂心細辛（各一兩）防風 人參 牛膝（各三十銖） 柏子仁 乾地黃 石斛（各三十六銖） 厚朴 藁本 蕪荑（各半兩） 麥門冬（二兩）。

澤蘭	zé lán	Foliage and stalk of Lycopus lucidus	四十二銖 42 zhū	5.25g
甘草	gān cǎo	Root of Glycyrrhiza uralensis	四十二銖 42 zhū	5.25g
當歸	dāng guī	Root of Angelica polimorpha	四十二銖 42 zhū	5.25g
川芎	chuān xiōng	Root of Ligusticum wallichii	四十二銖 42 zhū	5.25g
附子	fù zǐ	Lateral root of Aconitum carmichaeli	一兩 1 liǎng	3g
乾薑	gān jiāng	Dried root of Zingiber officinale	一兩 1 liǎng	3g
白朮	bái zhú	Rhizome of Atractylodes macro-cephala	一兩 1 liǎng	3g
白芷	bái zhǐ	Root of Angelica dahurica	一兩 1 liǎng	3g
桂心	guì xīn	Shaved inner bark of Cinnamomum cassia	一兩 1 liǎng	3g
細辛	xì xīn	Complete plant including root of Asarum heteropoides	一兩 1 liǎng	3g
防風	fáng fēng	Root of Ledebouriella divaricata	三十銖 30 zhū	3.75g
人參	rén shēn	Root of Panax ginseng	三十銖 30 zhū	3.75g
牛膝	niú xī	Root of Achyranthes bidentata	三十銖 30 zhū	3.75g
柏子仁	bǎi zǐ rén	Seed of Platycladus orientalis	三十六銖 36 zhū	4.5g
乾地黃	gān dì huáng	Dried root of Rehmannia glutinosa	三十六銖 36 zhū	4.5g
石斛	shí hú	Whole plant of Dendrobium nobile	三十六銖 36 zhū	4.5g
厚朴	hòu pò	Bark of Magnolia officinalis	半兩 0.5 liǎng	1.5g
藁本	gǎo běn	Rhizome and root of Ligusticum sinense	半兩 0.5 liǎng	1.5g
蕪荑	wú yí	Processed fruit of Ulmus macrocarpa	半兩 0.5 liǎng	1.5g
麥門冬	mài mén dōng	Tuber of Ophiopogon japonicus	二兩 2 liǎng	6g

上二十味，為末，蜜和丸如梧子。空腹酒下十五丸，至二十丸。

Pulverize the above twenty ingredients and mix with honey into pills the size of firmiana seeds. On an empty stomach, down fifteen pills [per dose] in liquor. Increase [the dosage] to a maximum of 20 pills.

*   This prescription is missing in the *Sūn Zhēn Rén* edition.

LINE 1.6

大補益當歸丸治產後虛羸不足，胸中少氣，腹中拘急疼痛，或引腰背痛，或所下過多，血不止，虛竭乏氣，晝夜不得眠，及崩中，面目脫色，唇乾口燥，亦治男子傷絕，或從高墮下，內有所傷，藏虛吐血，及金瘡傷犯皮肉方。

*Major Supplementing and Boosting Chinese Angelica Pills** treat postpartum vacuity emaciation and insufficiency, shortage of *qì* in the chest, hypertonicity and pain in the abdomen, possibly with pain stretching to the lumbus and back, or with excessive vaginal discharge, incessant bleeding, vacuity drain of *qì*, inability to sleep by day or night, as well as center flooding, loss of color in the face and eyes, and dry lips and mouth. It also treats men's injury[-related] expiry, whether due to a fall from a high place, the presence of internal injury, vacuity of the viscera and blood ejection, or a flesh injury from an incised wound.

Major Supplementing and Boosting Chinese Angelica Pills
大補益當歸丸 *dà bǔ yì dāng guī wán*

當歸 芎藭 續斷 乾薑 阿膠 甘草（各四兩） 白朮 吳茱萸 附子 白芷（各三兩） 桂心 芍藥（各二兩） 乾地黃（十兩）。

當歸	dāng guī	Root of Angelica polimorpha	四兩 4 liǎng	12g
川芎	chuān xiōng	Root of Ligusticum wallichii	四兩 4 liǎng	12g
續斷	xù duàn	Root of Dipsacus asper	四兩 4 liǎng	12g
乾薑	gān jiāng	Dried root of Zingiber officinale	四兩 4 liǎng	12g
阿膠	ē jiāo	Gelatinous glue produced from Equus asinus	四兩 4 liǎng	12g
甘草	gān cǎo	Root of Glycyrrhiza uralensis	四兩 4 liǎng	12g
白朮	bái zhú	Rhizome of Atractylodes macro-cephala	三兩 3 liǎng	9g
吳茱萸	wú zhū yú	Unripe fruit of Evodia rutaecarpa	三兩 3 liǎng	9g

附子	fù zǐ	Lateral root of Aconitum carmichaeli	三兩 3 liǎng	9g
白芷	bái zhǐ	Root of Angelica dahurica	三兩 3 liǎng	9g
桂心	guì xīn	Shaved inner bark of Cinnamomum cassia	二兩 2 liǎng	6g
芍藥	sháo yào	Root of Paeonia albiflora	二兩 2 liǎng	6g
乾地黃	gān dì huáng	Dried root of Rehmannia glutinosa	十兩 10 liǎng	30g

上十三味，為末，蜜和丸如梧子大。酒服二十丸，日三夜一，不知加至五十丸。若有真蒲黃，加一升，絕妙。

Pulverize the above thirteen ingredients and mix with honey into pills the size of firmiana seeds. Take twenty pills in liquor three times during the day and once at night. If you notice no effect, increase [the dosage] to a maximum of fifty pills. If true *pú huáng* (蒲黃 Pollen of Typha angustata) is available, adding one *shēng* is of the utmost excellence.

*   *Sòng* editors' note: "In the *Sūn Zhēn Rén* edition, this prescription is called *Internally Supplementing Major Chinese Angelica Pills* (內補大當歸丸 *nèi bǔ dà dāng guī wán*), but the actual prescription is identical."

LINE 1.7

白芷丸治產後所下過多，及崩中傷損，虛竭少氣，面目脫色，腹中痛方。

Dahurian Angelica Pills treat the postpartum [conditions of] excessive vaginal discharge and center flooding [from] injuries, exhaustion and shortage of *qì*, loss of color in the face and eyes, and pain in the center of the abdomen.

Dahurian Angelica Pills
白芷丸 *bái zhǐ wán*

白芷（五兩）乾地黃（四兩）續斷 乾薑 當歸 阿膠（各三兩）附子（一兩）。

白芷	bái zhǐ	Root of Angelica dahurica	五兩 5 liǎng	15g
乾地黃	gān dì huáng	Dried root of Rehmannia glutinosa	四兩 4 liǎng	12g
續斷	xù duàn	Root of Dipsacus asper	三兩 3 liǎng	9g
乾薑	gān jiāng	Dried root of Zingiber officinale	三兩 3 liǎng	9g
當歸	dāng guī	Root of Angelica polimorpha	三兩 3 liǎng	9g
阿膠	ē jiāo	Gelatinous glue produced from Equus asinus	三兩 3 liǎng	9g

附子	fù zǐ	Lateral root of Aconitum carmichaeli	一兩 1 liǎng	3g

上七味，為末，蜜和丸如梧子大。酒服二十丸，日四五服。無當歸，芎藭代；入蒲黃一兩，妙；無續斷，大薊根代。

Pulverize the above seven ingredients and mix with honey into pills the size of firmiana seeds. Take twenty pills in liquor four or five times a day. If you don't have *dāng guī* 當歸, substitute *chuān xiōng* (川芎 Root of Ligusticum wallichii). Adding one *liǎng* of *pú huáng* (蒲黃 Pollen of Typha angustata) is excellent. If you don't have *xù duàn* 續斷, substitute *dà jì gēn* (大薊根 Root of Cirsium japonicum).

LINE 1.8

紫石英柏子仁丸治女子遇冬天時行溫風，至春夏病熱，頭痛，熱毒風虛，百脈沈重，下赤白，不思飲食，而頭眩心悸，酸忄斯凘恍惚，不能起居方。

Fluorite and Arborvitae Seed Pills treat women suffering from heat disease in the spring and summer after being exposed to unseasonably warm wind in the winter, headache, heat toxin wind vacuity, heaviness in the hundred channels, red and white vaginal discharge, no thought of food or drink, dizziness in the head and heart palpitations, distress, anxiety, and abstraction, and inability to [go on with their] daily life.

Fluorite and Arborvitae Seed Pills
紫石英柏子仁丸 *zǐ shí yīng bǎi zǐ rén wán*

紫石英 柏子仁（各三兩） 烏頭 桂心 當歸 山茱萸 澤瀉 芎藭 石斛 遠志 寄生 蓯蓉 乾薑 甘草（各二兩） 蜀椒 杜蘅 辛夷（各一兩） 細辛（一兩半）。

紫石英	zǐ shí yīng	Fluorite	三兩 3 liǎng	9g
柏子仁	bǎi zǐ rén	Seed of Platycladus orientalis	三兩 3 liǎng	9g
烏頭	wū tóu	Main tuber of Aconitum carmichaeli	二兩 2 liǎng	6g
桂心	guì xīn	Shaved inner bark of Cinnamomum cassia	二兩 2 liǎng	6g
當歸	dāng guī	Root of Angelica polimorpha	二兩 2 liǎng	6g
山茱萸	shān zhū yú	Fruit of Cornus officinalis	二兩 2 liǎng	6g
澤瀉	zé xiè	Rhizome of Alisma plantago-aquatica	二兩 2 liǎng	6g
川芎	chuān xiōng	Root of Ligusticum wallichii	二兩 2 liǎng	6g
石斛	shí hú	Whole plant of Dendrobium nobile	二兩 2 liǎng	6g
遠志	yuǎn zhì	Root of Polygala tenuifolia	二兩 2 liǎng	6g

寄生	jì shēng	Branches and foliage of Viscum coloratum	二兩 2 liǎng	6g
蓯蓉	cōng róng	Stalk of Cistanche salsa	二兩 2 liǎng	6g
乾薑	gān jiāng	Dried root of Zingiber officinale	二兩 2 liǎng	6g
甘草	gān cǎo	Root of Glycyrrhiza uralensis	二兩 2 liǎng	6g
蜀椒	shǔ jiāo	Seed capsules of Zanthoxylum bungeanum	一兩 1 liǎng	3g
杜蘅[1]	dù héng	Rhizome and root, or whole plant of Asarum forbesii	一兩 1 liǎng	3g
蕪荑	wú yí	Processed fruit of Ulmus macrocarpa	一兩 1 liǎng	3g
細辛	xì xīn	Complete plant including root of Asarum heteropoides	一兩半 1.5 liǎng	4.5g

上十八味，為末，蜜和丸如梧子。酒服二十丸，漸加至三十丸，日三服。

Pulverize the above eighteen ingredients and mix with honey into pills the size of firmiana seeds. Take twenty pills in liquor, gradually increasing [the dosage] to a maximum of thirty pills, three times a day.[2]

1. *Sòng* editors' note: "Another [version of this] prescription has *dù zhòng* (杜仲 Bark of Eucommia ulmoidis)."
2. *Sòng* editors' note: "Another [version of this] prescription adds 1 *liǎng* of *mǔ lì* (牡蠣 Shell of Ostrea rivularis)."
   Following this prescription, the *Sūn Zhēn Rén* edition inserts the short essay that is placed at the beginning of this chapter in the other editions.

LINE 1.9

鍾乳澤蘭丸治婦人久虛羸瘦，四肢百體煩疼，臍下結冷，不能食，面目瘀黑，憂恚不樂，百病方。

Stalactite and Lycopus Pills treat women's myriad diseases of chronic vacuity emaciation, vexation and pain in the four limbs and all over the body, binding cold below the navel, inability to eat, bruises and black spots in the face and eyes, and anxiety, rage, and unhappiness.

Stalactite and Lycopus Pills
鍾乳澤蘭丸 *zhōng rǔ zé lán wán*

鍾乳（三兩）澤蘭（三兩六銖）防風（四十二銖）人參 柏子仁 麥門冬 乾

地黃 石膏 石斛（各一兩半）芎藭 甘草 白芷 牛膝 山茱萸 署預 當歸 藁本（各三十銖）細辛 桂心（各一兩）蕪荑（半兩）艾葉（十八銖）。

鐘乳	zhōng rǔ	Stalactite	三兩 3 liǎng	9g
澤蘭	zé lán	Foliage and stalk of Lycopus lucidus	三兩六銖 3 liǎng 6 zhū	9.75g
防風	fáng fēng	Root of Ledebouriella divaricata	四十二銖 42 zhū	5.25g
人參	rén shēn	Root of Panax ginseng	一兩半 1.5 liǎng	4.5g
柏子仁	bǎi zǐ rén	Seed of Platycladus orientalis	一兩半 1.5 liǎng	4.5g
麥門冬	mài mén dōng	Tuber of Ophiopogon japonicus	一兩半 1.5 liǎng	4.5g
乾地黃	gān dì huáng	Dried root of Rehmannia glutinosa	一兩半 1.5 liǎng	4.5g
石膏	shí gāo	Gypsum	一兩半 1.5 liǎng	4.5g
石斛	shí hú	Whole plant of Dendrobium nobile	一兩半 1.5 liǎng	4.5g
川芎	chuān xiōng	Root of Ligusticum wallichii	三十銖 30 zhū	3.75g
甘草	gān cǎo	Root of Glycyrrhiza uralensis	三十銖 30 zhū	3.75g
白芷	bái zhǐ	Root of Angelica dahurica	三十銖 30 zhū	3.75g
牛膝	niú xī	Root of Achyranthes bidentata	三十銖 30 zhū	3.75g
山茱萸	shān zhū yú	Fruit of Cornus officinalis	三十銖 30 zhū	3.75g
當歸	dāng guī	Root of Angelica polimorpha	三十銖 30 zhū	3.75g
藁本	gǎo běn	Rhizome and root of Ligusticum sinense	三十銖 30 zhū	3.75g
細辛	xì xīn	Complete plant including root of Asarum heteropoides	一兩 1 liǎng	3g
桂心	guì xīn	Shaved inner bark of Cinnamomum cassia	一兩 1 liǎng	3g
蕪荑	wú yí	Processed fruit of Ulmus macrocarpa	半兩 0.5 liǎng	1.5g
艾葉	ài yè	Dry-roasted foliage of Artemisia argyi	十八銖 18 zhū	2.25g

上二十一味，為末，蜜和丸如梧子。酒服二十丸，加至四十丸，日二服。

Pulverize the above twenty-one ingredients and mix with honey into pills the size of firmiana seeds. Take twenty pills in liquor, increasing [the dosage] to a maximum of forty pills, two times a day.

LINE 1.10

大澤蘭丸治婦人虛損，及中風餘病，疝瘕，陰中冷痛；或頭風入腦，寒痹，筋攣緩急，血閉無子，面上遊風去來，目淚出，多涕唾，忽忽如醉；或胃中冷逆胸中，嘔不止，及泄痢淋瀝；或五藏六腑寒熱不調，心下痞急，邪氣咳逆；或漏下赤白，陰中腫痛，胸脅支滿；或身體皮膚中澀如麻豆，苦癢，痰癖結氣；或四肢拘攣，風行周身，骨節疼痛，目眩無所見；或上氣惡寒，泗淅如瘧；或喉痹，鼻齆，風癇癲疾；或月水不通，魂魄不定，飲食無味，並產後內衄，無所不治，服之令人有子。

Major Lycopus Pills treat women's vacuity detriment as well as residual wind strike diseases, mounting-conglomerations, and coldness and pain in the vagina; or wind in the head entering the brain, cold impediment, slackening and tensing of the sinews, blood blockage[1] and infertility, intermittent roaming wind on the face, tearing of the eyes, increased sniveling and salivating, and confusion as if she was intoxicated; or coldness in the stomach counterflowing into the chest, incessant retching, diarrhea, and dribbling urination; or an imbalance of hot and cold in the five viscera and six bowels, glomus and tension below the heart, and evil *qì* cough counterflow; or white and red vaginal spotting, swelling and pain in the vagina, and propping fullness[2] in the chest and rib-sides; or roughness of the skin all over the body resembling measles, uncomfortable itching, phlegm aggregations, and *qì* bind; or hypertonicity in the four limbs, wind circulating in the body, pain in the bones and joints, and blinding dizziness in the eyes; or *qì* ascent and aversion to cold, and shivering from cold as if in malaria; or throat impediment, nose congestion,[3] and wind convulsions and topsy-turviness; or menstrual stoppage, instability of the *hún* and *pò* souls, and lack of appetite for food or drink; as well as treating postpartum internal spontaneous bleeding. There is no [condition] that these [pills] cannot treat. Taking these [pills] will allow the patient to be with child.

Major Lycopus Pills
大澤蘭丸 *dà zé lán wán*

澤蘭（二兩六銖）藁本 當歸 甘草（各一兩十八銖）紫石英（三兩）芎藭乾地黃 柏子仁 五味子（各一兩半）桂心 石斛 白朮（一兩六銖）白芷 蓯蓉厚朴 防風 署預 茯苓 乾薑 禹餘糧 細辛 卷柏（各一兩）蜀椒 人參 杜仲 牛膝 蛇床子 續斷 艾葉 蕪荑（各十八銖）赤石脂 石膏（各二兩）。

澤蘭	zé lán	Foliage and stalk of Lycopus lucidus	二兩六銖 2 liǎng 6 zhū	6.75g
藁本	gǎo běn	Rhizome and root of Ligusticum sinense	一兩十八銖 1 liǎng 18 zhū	5.25g
當歸	dāng guī	Root of Angelica polimorpha	一兩十八銖 1 liǎng 18 zhū	5.25g
甘草	gān cǎo	Root of Glycyrrhiza uralensis	一兩十八銖 1 liǎng 18 zhū	5.25g
紫石英	zǐ shí yīng	Fluorite	三兩 3 liǎng	9g
川芎	chuān xiōng	Root of Ligusticum wallichii	一兩半 1.5 liǎng	4.5g
乾地黃	gān dì huáng	Dried root of Rehmannia glutinosa	一兩半 1.5 liǎng	4.5g
柏子仁	bǎi zǐ rén	Seed of Platycladus orientalis	一兩半 1.5 liǎng	4.5g

五味子	wǔ wèi zǐ	Fruit of Schisandra chinensis	一兩半 1.5 liǎng	4.5g
桂心	guì xīn	Shaved inner bark of Cinnamomum cassia	一兩六銖 1 liǎng 6 zhū	3.75g
石斛	shí hú	Whole plant of Dendrobium nobile	一兩六銖 1 liǎng 6 zhū	3.75g
白朮	bái zhú	Rhizome of Atractylodes macro-cephala	一兩六銖 1 liǎng 6 zhū	3.75g
白芷	bái zhǐ	Root of Angelica dahurica	一兩 1 liǎng	3g
蓯蓉	cōng róng	Stalk of Cistanche salsa	一兩 1 liǎng	3g
厚朴	hòu pò	Bark of Magnolia officinalis	一兩 1 liǎng	3g
防風	fáng fēng	Root of Ledebouriella divaricata	一兩 1 liǎng	3g
薯蕷	shǔ yù	Root of Dioscorea opposita	一兩 1 liǎng	3g
茯苓	fú líng	Dried fungus of Poria cocos	一兩 1 liǎng	3g
乾薑	gān jiāng	Dried root of Zingiber officinale	一兩 1 liǎng	3g
禹餘糧	yǔ yú liáng	Limonite	一兩 1 liǎng	3g
細辛	xì xīn	Complete plant including root of Asarum heteropoides	一兩 1 liǎng	3g
卷柏	juǎn bǎi	Entire plant of Selaginella tama-riscina	一兩 1 liǎng	3g
蜀椒	shǔ jiāo	Seed capsules of Zanthoxylum bungeanum	十八銖 18 zhū	2.25g
人參	rén shēn	Root of Panax ginseng	十八銖 18 zhū	2.25g
杜仲	dù zhòng	Bark of Eucommia ulmoidis	十八銖 18 zhū	2.25g
牛膝	niú xī	Root of Achyranthes bidentata	十八銖 18 zhū	2.25g
蛇床子	shé chuáng zǐ	Fruit of Cnidium monnieri	十八銖 18 zhū	2.25g
續斷	xù duàn	Root of Dipsacus asper	十八銖 18 zhū	2.25g
艾葉	ài yè	Dry-roasted foliage of Artemisia argyi	十八銖 18 zhū	2.25g
蕪荑	wú yí	Processed fruit of Ulmus macrocarpa	十八銖 18 zhū	2.25g
楮實子	chǔ shí zǐ	Fruit of Broussonetia papyrifera	二兩 2 liǎng	6g
石膏	shí gāo	Gypsum	二兩 2 liǎng	6g

上三十二味，為末，蜜和丸如梧子大。酒服二十丸，至四十丸。久赤白痢，去乾地黃，石膏，麥門冬，柏子仁，加大麥蘖，陳麴，龍骨，阿膠，黃連各一兩半；有鍾乳，加三兩，良。

Pulverize the above thirty-two ingredients and mix with honey into pills the size of firmiana seeds. Take twenty pills [per dose] in liquor, increasing [the dosage] to a maximum of forty pills. For chronic red or white diarrhea, leave out the *gān dì huáng* 乾地黃, *shí gāo* 石膏, *mài mén dōng* 麥門冬, and *bǎi zǐ rén* 柏子仁, but add one and a half *liǎng* each of *dà mài niè* (大麥蘗 Shoots of Hordeum vulgare), *chén qū* (陳麵 Medicated leaven), *lóng gǔ* (龍骨 Os draconis), *ē jiāo* (阿膠 Gelatinous glue produced from Equus asinus), and *huáng lián* (黃連 Rhizome of Coptis chinensis). If you have *zhōng rǔ* (鐘乳 Stalactite), adding three *liǎng* is good.[4]

1. 血閉 *xuè bì*: While not a common expression, it is most probably a synonym for menstrual blockage (經閉 *jīng bì*, i.e., amenorrhea) in this context.

2. 支滿 *zhī mǎn*: A technical term referring to a sensation of fullness under the arch of the ribs. In the *Sù Wèn*, it is used with slight variation in meaning: It refers to a condition of fullness in the abdomen: "As for stomach malaria, it causes people to also suffer from additional diseases. They tend to be hungry and yet are unable to eat, and if they do eat, they [suffer from] propping fullness and an enlarged abdomen" (《素文》36). Alternatively, it can refer specifically to the sensation of fullness in the upper part of the body: "As for heart diseases, there is pain in the center of the chest and propping fullness in the rib-sides" (《素文》 22). I follow the terminology suggested by Nigel Wiseman who explains his use of "propping" in the sense that the pain of the condition is making the patient sit erect as if propped up. In modern TCM, the term has come to be used exclusively in this latter sense to refer to fullness in the chest or rib-sides (Wiseman and Féng, *Practical Dictionary*, p. 468). This is also the sense of the term in the prescription above.

3. 鼻齆 *bí wèng*: A pathology of nose blockage, manifesting as inhibition in the nose, nasal speech, and inability to smell. To paraphrase the explanation in the *Bìng Yuán Lùn*, a vacuity of lung *qì* allows the evil *qì* of wind-cold to enter the brain and lodge in the nose, causing nose blockage and inability of *qì* to flow freely and harmoniously (《病源論》48:140).

4. *Sòng* editors' note: "Another [version of this] prescription adds 18 *zhū* of *zhǐ shí* (枳實 Unripe fruit of Poncirus trifoliata) and 1.5 *liǎng mài mén dōng (*麥門冬 Tuber of Ophiopogon japonicus*)."

LINE 1.11

小澤蘭丸治產後虛羸勞冷，身體尪瘦方。

Minor Lycopus Pills treat postpartum vacuity emaciation, taxation cold, and a weak and emaciated body.

Minor Lycopus Pills
小澤蘭丸 *xiǎo zé lán wán*

澤蘭（二兩六銖） 當歸 甘草（各一兩十八銖） 芎藭 柏子仁 防風 茯苓（各一兩） 白芷 蜀椒 藁本 細辛 白术 桂心 蕪荑 人參 食茱萸 厚朴（各十八銖） 石膏（二兩）。

澤蘭	*zé lán*	Foliage and stalk of Lycopus lucidus	二兩六銖 2 liǎng 6 zhū	6.75g

當歸	dāng guī	Root of Angelica polimorpha	一兩十八銖 1 liǎng 18 zhū	5.25g
甘草	gān cǎo	Root of Glycyrrhiza uralensis	一兩十八銖 1 liǎng 18 zhū	5.25g
川芎	chuān xiōng	Root of Ligusticum wallichii	一兩 1 liǎng	3g
柏子仁	bǎi zǐ rén	Seed of Platycladus orientalis	一兩 1 liǎng	3g
防風	fáng fēng	Root of Ledebouriella divaricata	一兩 1 liǎng	3g
茯苓	fú líng	Dried fungus of Poria cocos	一兩 1 liǎng	3g
白芷	bái zhǐ	Root of Angelica dahurica	十八銖 18 zhū	2.25g
蜀椒	shǔ jiāo	Seed capsules of Zanthoxylum bungeanum	十八銖 18 zhū	2.25g
藁本	gǎo běn	Rhizome and root of Ligusticum sinense	十八銖 18 zhū	2.25g
細辛	xì xīn	Complete plant including root of Asarum heteropoides	十八銖 18 zhū	2.25g
白朮	bái zhú	Rhizome of Atractylodes macro-cephala	十八銖 18 zhū	2.25g
桂心	guì xīn	Shaved inner bark of Cinnamomum cassia	十八銖 18 zhū	2.25g
蕪荑	wú yí	Processed fruit of Ulmus macrocarpa	十八銖 18 zhū	2.25g
人參	rén shēn	Root of Panax ginseng	十八銖 18 zhū	2.25g
食茱萸	shí zhū yú	Fruit of Zanthoxylum ailanthoides	十八銖 18 zhū	2.25g
厚朴	hòu pò	Bark of Magnolia officinalis	十八銖 18 zhū	2.25g
石膏	shí gāo	Gypsum	二兩 2 liǎng	6g

上十八味，為末，蜜和丸如梧子大。酒服二十丸，日三服，稍加至四十丸。無疾者，依此方春秋二時常服一劑，甚良。有病虛羸黃瘦者，服如前。一方無茯苓，石膏，有芍藥，乾薑。

Pulverize the above eighteen ingredients and mix with honey into pills the size of firmiana seeds. Take twenty pills [per dose] in liquor three times a day, gradually increasing [the dosage] to a maximum of forty pills. For [women] who are free from disease, it is excellent to follow this prescription and always take one batch each in the two seasons of spring and fall. For patients suffering from vacuity emaciation with a yellow complexion, take it as [recommended] above.*

*   *Sòng* editors' note: "Another [version of this] prescription does not use *fú líng* 茯苓 or *shí gāo* 石膏, but includes *sháo yào* (芍藥 Root of Paeonia albiflora) and *gān jiāng* (乾薑 Dried root of Zingiber officinale).
Hú Qià lists fifteen ingredients, leaving out *bǎi zǐ rén* 柏子仁, *rén shēn* 人參, and *shí zhū yú* 食茱萸. He instructs to heat all ingredients until they change color, except for the *xì xīn* 細辛 and *guì xīn* 桂心, which are used raw, and then to make a powder, mix it with honey into pellet-sized pills, and to take them in heated liquor. The *Qiān Jīn Yì Fāng* does not use *fú líng* 茯苓 or *shí zhū yú* 食茱萸, but includes one *liǎng* of *gān jiāng* 乾薑."

LINE 1.12

紫石英天門冬丸主風冷在子宮，有子常墮落，或始為婦便患心痛，仍成心疾
[1]，月水都未曾來，服之肥充，令人有子。

Fluorite and Asparagus Pills are the governing prescription for wind-cold in the infant's
palace[2] [causing] habitual miscarriage [in women who do] become pregnant, or for
discomfort from heart pain in recently married women, which can subsequently turn into
heart racing; or for a complete absence of menstruation from childhood on. Taking these
[pills] will make her fat and plump and cause her to be with child.

Fluorite and Asparagus Pills
紫石英天門冬丸 *zǐ shí yīng tiān mén dōng wán*

紫石英 天門冬 禹餘糧（各三兩） 蕪荑 烏頭 蓯蓉 桂心 甘草 五味子 柏子仁
石斛 人參 澤瀉（一作澤蘭） 遠志 杜仲（各二兩） 蜀椒 卷柏 寄生 石南 雲
母 當歸（一作辛夷） 烏賊骨（各一兩）。

紫石英	zǐ shí yīng	Fluorite	三兩 3 liǎng	9g
天門冬	tiān mén dōng	Tuber of Asparagus cochinchinensis	三兩 3 liǎng	9g
禹餘糧	yǔ yú liáng	Limonite	三兩 3 liǎng	9g
蕪荑	wú yí	Processed fruit of Ulmus macrocarpa	二兩 2 liǎng	6g
烏頭	wū tóu	Main tuber of Aconitum carmichaeli	二兩 2 liǎng	6g
蓯蓉	cōng róng	Stalk of Cistanche salsa	二兩 2 liǎng	6g
桂心	guì xīn	Shaved inner bark of Cinnamomum cassia	二兩 2 liǎng	6g
甘草	gān cǎo	Root of Glycyrrhiza uralensis	二兩 2 liǎng	6g
五味子	wǔ wèi zǐ	Fruit of Schisandra chinensis	二兩 2 liǎng	6g
柏子仁	bǎi zǐ rén	Seed of Platycladus orientalis	二兩 2 liǎng	6g
石斛	shí hú	Whole plant of Dendrobium nobile	二兩 2 liǎng	6g
人參	rén shēn	Root of Panax ginseng	二兩 2 liǎng	6g
澤瀉[3]	zé xiè	Rhizome of Alisma plantago-aquatica	二兩 2 liǎng	6g
遠志	yuǎn zhì	Root of Polygala tenuifolia	二兩 2 liǎng	6g
杜仲	dù zhòng	Bark of Eucommia ulmoidis	二兩 2 liǎng	6g
蜀椒	shǔ jiāo	Seed capsules of Zanthoxylum bungeanum	一兩 1 liǎng	3g

卷柏	juǎn bǎi	Entire plant of Selaginella tamariscina	一兩 1 liǎng	3g
寄生	jì shēng	Branches and foliage of Viscum coloratum	一兩 1 liǎng	3g
石楠	shí nán	Dry-roasted foliage of Photinia serrulata	一兩 1 liǎng	3g
雲母	yún mǔ	Muscovite	一兩 1 liǎng	3g
當歸⁴	dāng guī	Root of Angelica polimorpha	一兩 1 liǎng	3g
烏賊骨	wū zéi gǔ	Calcified shell of Sepiella maindroni	一兩 1 liǎng	3g

上二十二味，為末，蜜和為丸，梧子大。酒服二十丸，日二服，加至四十丸。

Pulverize the above twenty-two ingredients and mix with honey into pills the size of firmiana seeds. Take twenty pills [per dose] in liquor, two doses a day, increasing [the dosage] to a maximum of forty pills.

1. 心疾 *xīn jí*: Throughout the *Qiān Jīn Fāng*, the term *jí* is mostly used in the sense of "disease." It seems possible, if not likely, though that it carries here the more specific connotation of "racing," as it does in contemporary TCM, where it is used mostly in the context of pulse diagnosis.
2. Coldness in the uterus is one of the primary causes of infertility. "Infant's palace" (子宮 *zǐ gōng*) is a term for the uterus that emphasizes its gestational function of housing the fetus.
3. *Sòng* editors' note: "Another [version of this] prescription has *zé lán* (澤蘭 Foliage and stalk of Lycopus lucidus)."
4. *Sòng* editors' note: "Another [version of this] prescription has *xīn yí* (辛夷 Flower of Magnolia liliflora)."

LINE 1.13

三石澤蘭丸治風虛不足，通血脈，補寒冷方。

Three Stones and Lycopus Pills treat wind vacuity and insufficiency by freeing the flow of blood in the channels and by supplementing [in] cold [conditions].

Three Stones and Lycopus Pills
三石澤蘭丸 *sān shí zé lán wán*

鍾乳 白石英（各四兩） 紫石英 防風 藁本 茯神（各一兩六銖） 澤蘭（二兩六銖） 黃芪 石斛 石膏（各二兩） 甘草 當歸 芎藭（各一兩十八銖） 白术 桂心 人參 乾薑 獨活 乾地黃（各一兩半） 白芷 桔梗 細辛 柏子仁 五味子 蜀

椒 黃芩 蓯蓉 芍藥 秦艽 防葵（各一兩） 厚朴 蕪菁（各十八銖）。

鐘乳	zhōng rǔ	Stalactite	四兩 4 liǎng	12g
白石英	bái shí yīng	White quartz	四兩 4 liǎng	12g
紫石英	zǐ shí yīng	Fluorite	一兩六銖 1 liǎng 6 zhū	3.75g
防風	fáng fēng	Root of Ledebouriella divaricata	一兩六銖 1 liǎng 6 zhū	3.75g
藁本	gǎo běn	Rhizome and root of Ligusticum sinense	一兩六銖 1 liǎng 6 zhū	3.75g
茯神	fú shén	Sclerotium (i.e., white, hardened core in the center) of Poria cocos	一兩六銖 1 liǎng 6 zhū	3.75g
澤蘭	zé lán	Foliage and stalk of Lycopus lucidus	二兩六銖 2 liǎng 6 zhū	6.75g
黃芪	huáng qí	Root of Astragalus membranaceus	二兩 2 liǎng	6g
石斛	shí hú	Whole plant of Dendrobium nobile	二兩 2 liǎng	6g
石膏	shí gāo	Gypsum	二兩 2 liǎng	6g
甘草	gān cǎo	Root of Glycyrrhiza uralensis	一兩十八銖 1 liǎng 18 zhū	5.25g
當歸	dāng guī	Root of Angelica polimorpha	一兩十八銖 1 liǎng 18 zhū	5.25g
川芎	chuān xiōng	Root of Ligusticum wallichii	一兩十八銖 1 liǎng 18 zhū	5.25g
白朮	bái zhú	Rhizome of Atractylodes macro-cephala	一兩半 1.5 liǎng	4.5g
桂心	guì xīn	Shaved inner bark of Cinnamomum cassia	一兩半 1.5 liǎng	4.5g
人參	rén shēn	Root of Panax ginseng	一兩半 1.5 liǎng	4.5g
乾薑	gān jiāng	Dried root of Zingiber officinale	一兩半 1.5 liǎng	4.5g
獨活	dú huó	Root and rhizome of Angelica pube-scens	一兩半 1.5 liǎng	4.5g
乾地黃	gān dì huáng	Dried root of Rehmannia glutinosa	一兩半 1.5 liǎng	4.5g
白芷	bái zhǐ	Root of Angelica dahurica	一兩 1 liǎng	3g
桔梗	jié gěng	Root of Platycodon grandiflorum	一兩 1 liǎng	3g
細辛	xì xīn	Complete plant including root of Asarum heteropoides	一兩 1 liǎng	3g
柏子仁	bǎi zǐ rén	Seed of Platycladus orientalis	一兩 1 liǎng	3g
五味子	wǔ wèi zǐ	Fruit of Schisandra chinensis	一兩 1 liǎng	3g
蜀椒	shǔ jiāo	Seed capsules of Zanthoxylum bungeanum	一兩 1 liǎng	3g
黃芩	huáng qín	Root of Scutellaria baicalensis	一兩 1 liǎng	3g

蓯蓉	cōng róng	Stalk of Cistanche salsa	一兩 1 liǎng	3g
芍藥	sháo yào	Root of Paeonia albiflora	一兩 1 liǎng	3g
秦艽	qín jiāo	Root of Gentiana macrophylla	一兩 1 liǎng	3g
防葵	fáng kuí	unknown	一兩 1 liǎng	3g
厚朴	hòu pò	Bark of Magnolia officinalis	十八銖 18 zhū	2.25g
蕪荑	wú yí	Processed fruit of Ulmus macrocarpa	十八銖 18 zhū	2.25g

上三十二味，為末，蜜和丸如梧子大。酒服二十丸，加至三十丸，日二三服。

Pulverize the above thirty-two ingredients and mix with honey into pills the size of firmiana seeds. Take twenty pills in liquor two or three times a day, increasing [the dosage] to a maximum of thirty pills.

*   *Sòng* editors' note: "They are also called *Dendrobium and Lycopus Pills.*"

LINE 1.14

大平胃澤蘭丸治男子女人五勞七傷諸不足，定志意，除煩滿，手足虛冷羸瘦，及月水往來不調，體不能動等病方。

Major Stomach-Calming Lycopus Pills treat the five taxations and seven damages and the various insufficiencies in men and women, by stabilizing the will and eliminating vexing fullness [and by treating] vacuity cold in the hands and feet with marked emaciation, irregular onset and ending of the menses, and inability to move the body.

Major Stomach-Calming Lycopus Pills
大平胃澤蘭丸 *dà píng wèi zé lán wán*

澤蘭 細辛 黃芪 鍾乳（各三兩）柏子仁 乾地黃（各二兩半）大黃 前胡 遠志 紫石英（各二兩）芎藭 白朮 蜀椒（各一兩半）白芷 丹參 梔子 芍藥 桔梗 秦艽 沙參 桂心 厚朴 石斛 苦參 人參 麥門冬 乾薑（各一兩）附子（六兩）吳茱萸 麥糵（各五合）陳麴（一升）棗（五十枚，作膏）。

澤蘭	zé lán	Foliage and stalk of Lycopus lucidus	三兩 3 liǎng	9g
細辛	xì xīn	Complete plant including root of Asarum heteropoides	三兩 3 liǎng	9g
黃芪	huáng qí	Root of Astragalus membranaceus	三兩 3 liǎng	9g
鐘乳	zhōng rǔ	Stalactite	三兩 3 liǎng	9g

柏子仁	bǎi zǐ rén	Seed of Platycladus orientalis	二兩半 2.5 liǎng	7.5g
乾地黃	gān dì huáng	Dried root of Rehmannia glutinosa	二兩半 2.5 liǎng	7.5g
大黃	dà huáng	Root of Rheum palmatum	二兩 2 liǎng	6g
前胡	qián hú	Root of Peucedanum praeruptorum	二兩 2 liǎng	6g
遠志	yuǎn zhì	Root of Polygala tenuifolia	二兩 2 liǎng	6g
紫石英	zǐ shí yīng	Fluorite	二兩 2 liǎng	6g
川芎	chuān xiōng	Root of Ligusticum wallichii	一兩半 1.5 liǎng	4.5g
白朮	bái zhú	Rhizome of Atractylodes macro-cephala	一兩半 1.5 liǎng	4.5g
蜀椒	shǔ jiāo	Seed capsules of Zanthoxylum bungeanum	一兩半 1.5 liǎng	4.5g
白芷	bái zhǐ	Root of Angelica dahurica	一兩 1 liǎng	3g
丹參	dān shēn	Root of Salvia miltiorrhiza	一兩 1 liǎng	3g
栀子[1]	zhī zǐ	Fruit of Gardenia jasminoides	一兩 1 liǎng	3g
芍藥	sháo yào	Root of Paeonia albiflora	一兩 1 liǎng	3g
桔梗	jié gěng	Root of Platycodon grandiflorum	一兩 1 liǎng	3g
秦艽	qín jiāo	Root of Gentiana macrophylla	一兩 1 liǎng	3g
沙參	shā shēn	Root of Adenophora tetraphylla	一兩 1 liǎng	3g
桂心	guì xīn	Shaved inner bark of Cinnamomum cassia	一兩 1 liǎng	3g
厚朴	hòu pò	Bark of Magnolia officinalis	一兩 1 liǎng	3g
石斛	shí hú	Whole plant of Dendrobium nobile	一兩 1 liǎng	3g
苦參	kǔ shēn	Root of Sophora flavescens	一兩 1 liǎng	3g
人參	rén shēn	Root of Panax ginseng	一兩 1 liǎng	3g
麥門冬	mài mén dōng	Tuber of Ophiopogon japonicus	一兩 1 liǎng	3g
乾薑	gān jiāng	Dried root of Zingiber officinale	一兩 1 liǎng	3g
附子	fù zǐ	Lateral root of Aconitum carmichaeli	六兩 6 liǎng	18g
吳茱萸	wú zhū yú	Unripe fruit of Evodia rutaecarpa	五合 5 gě	35ml
麥蘖	mài niè	Shoots of Hordeum vulgare	五合 5 gě	35ml
陳麴	chén qū	Medicated leaven	一升 1 shēng	24g
[大]棗, 作膏	[dà] zǎo, zuò gāo	Mature fruit of Ziziphus jujuba, processed into a paste	五十枚 50 méi	50 pcs

上三十二味，為末，蜜和丸如梧子大。酒服二十丸，加至三十丸，令人肥健。

Pulverize the above thirty-two ingredients and mix with honey into pills the size of firmiana seeds. Take twenty pills in liquor, increasing [the dosage] to a maximum of thirty pills. It makes the person fat and healthy.[2]

1. *Sòng* editors' note: "Another [version of this] prescription has *zhǐ shí* (枳實 Unripe fruit of Poncirus trifoliata)."
2. *Sòng* editors' note: "Another version [of this prescription] does not use *gān jiāng* 乾薑, but includes three *liǎng* of *dāng guī* (當歸 Root of Angelica polimorpha)."

LINE 1.15

澤蘭散治產後風虛方。

Lycopus Powder treats postpartum wind vacuity.

Lycopus Powder
澤蘭散 *zé lán sǎn*

澤蘭（九分）禹餘糧 防風（各十分）石膏 白芷 乾地黃 赤石脂 肉蓯蓉 鹿茸 芎藭（各八分）藁本 蜀椒 白朮 柏子仁（各五分）桂心 甘草 當歸 乾薑（各七分）蕪荑 細辛 厚朴（各四分）人參（三分）。

澤蘭	zé lán	Foliage and stalk of Lycopus lucidus	九分 9 fēn	6.75g
禹餘糧	yǔ yú liáng	Limonite	十分 10 fēn	7.5g
防風	fáng fēng	Root of Ledebouriella divaricata	十分 10 fēn	7.5g
石膏	shí gāo	Gypsum	八分 8 fēn	6g
白芷	bái zhǐ	Root of Angelica dahurica	八分 8 fēn	6g
乾地黃	gān dì huáng	Dried root of Rehmannia glutinosa	八分 8 fēn	6g
赤石脂	chì shí zhī	Halloysite	八分 8 fēn	6g
肉蓯蓉	ròu cōng róng	Fleshy stalk of Cistanche salsa	八分 8 fēn	6g
鹿茸	lù róng	Pilose antler of Cervus nippon	八分 8 fēn	6g
川芎	chuān xiōng	Root of Ligusticum wallichii	八分 8 fēn	6g
藁本	gǎo běn	Rhizome and root of Ligusticum sinense	五分 5 fēn	3.75g
蜀椒	shǔ jiāo	Seed capsules of Zanthoxylum bungeanum	五分 5 fēn	3.75g
白朮	bái zhú	Rhizome of Atractylodes macrocephala	五分 5 fēn	3.75g
柏子仁	bǎi zǐ rén	Seed of Platycladus orientalis	五分 5 fēn	3.75g
桂心	guì xīn	Shaved inner bark of Cinnamomum cassia	七分 7 fēn	5.25g
甘草	gān cǎo	Root of Glycyrrhiza uralensis	七分 7 fēn	5.25g

當歸	dāng guī	Root of Angelica polimorpha	七分 7 fēn	5.25g
乾薑	gān jiāng	Dried root of Zingiber officinale	七分 7 fēn	5.25g
蕪荑	wú yí	Processed fruit of Ulmus macrocarpa	四分 4 fēn	3g
細辛	xì xīn	Complete plant including root of Asarum heteropoides	四分 4 fēn	3g
厚朴	hòu pò	Bark of Magnolia officinalis	四分 4 fēn	3g
人參	rén shēn	Root of Panax ginseng	三分 3 fēn	2.25g

上二十二味，治下篩。酒服方寸匕，日三，以意增之。

Finely pound and sift the above twenty-two ingredients. Take a square-inch spoon in liquor three times a day, increasing it at will.

427

2. Menstrual Stoppage 月水不通

Translator's note: The terminology Sūn Sī-Miǎo employs in this chapter to refer to different degrees of menstrual flow is quite specific: It ranges from "inhibition" (不利 *bù lì*), through "stasis" (瘀 *yū*), to "blockage" (月閉 *yuè bì*), and to the most severe case of "stoppage" (不通 *bù tōng*), which describes the total obstruction and absence of menstrual flow.

LINE 2.1

桃仁湯治婦人月水不通方。

Peach Kernel Decoction treats women's menstrual stoppage.

Peach Kernel Decoction
桃仁湯 *táo rén tāng*

桃仁 朴消 牡丹皮 射干 土瓜根 黃芩（各三兩） 芍藥 大黃 柴胡（各四兩）
牛膝 桂心（各二兩） 水蛭 虻蟲（各七十枚）。

桃仁	táo rén	Seed of Prunus persica	三兩 3 liǎng	9g
朴消	pò xiāo	Impure mirabilite	三兩 3 liǎng	9g
牡丹皮	mǔ dān pí	Bark of the root of Paeonia suffruticosa	三兩 3 liǎng	9g
射干	shè gān	Rhizome of Belamcanda chinensis	三兩 3 liǎng	9g
土瓜根	tǔ guā gēn	Root of Trichosanthes cucumerina	三兩 3 liǎng	9g
黃芩	huáng qín	Root of Scutellaria baicalensis	三兩 3 liǎng	9g
芍藥	sháo yào	Root of Paeonia albiflora	四兩 4 liǎng	12g
大黃	dà huáng	Root of Rheum palmatum	四兩 4 liǎng	12g
柴胡	chái hú	Root of Bupleurum chinense	四兩 4 liǎng	12g
牛膝	niú xī	Root of Achyranthes bidentata	二兩 2 liǎng	6g
桂心	guì xīn	Shaved inner bark of Cinnamomum cassia	二兩 2 liǎng	6g

| 水蛭 | shuǐ zhì | Dried body of Whitmania pigra | 七十枚 70 méi | 70 pcs |
| 虻蟲 | méng chóng | Dried body of the female of Tabanus bivittatus | 七十枚 70 méi | 70 pcs |

上十三味，㕮咀，以水九升煮取二升半，去滓，分三服。

Pound the above thirteen ingredients and decoct in nine *shēng* of water to obtain two and a half *shēng*. Discard the dregs and divide into three doses.

LINE 2.2

乾薑丸治婦人寒熱，羸瘦，酸消怠惰，胸中支滿，肩背脊重痛，腹裡堅滿積聚，或痛不可忍，引腰小腹痛，四肢煩疼，手足厥逆，寒至肘膝，或煩滿，手足虛熱，意欲投水中，百節盡痛，心下常苦懸痛，時寒時熱，惡心，涎唾喜出，每愛鹹酸甜苦之物，身體或如雞皮，月經不通，大小便苦難，食不生肌。

Dried Ginger Pills treat women's [aversion to] cold and heat [effusion], marked emaciation, soreness, whitttling, and fatigue, propping fullness in the center of the chest, heaviness and pain in the shoulders, back, and spine, hardness, fullness, and accumulations in the abdomen possibly with unbearable pain, pain stretching to the lumbus and the lower abdomen, vexation and aching in the four limbs, reverse flow in the hands and feet, coldness up to the elbows and knees possibly with vexing fullness and vacuity heat in the hands and feet, causing her to want to toss herself into water, extreme pain in the hundred joints, constant discomfort and suspension pain below the heart, alternating [aversion to] cold and heat [effusion], nausea, tendency to drool and salivate, frequent love of salty, sour, sweet, or bitter substances, possibly an [appearance of] the body like chicken skin, menstrual stoppage, discomfort and difficulty during urination and defecation, and eating without engendering flesh.

Dried Ginger Pills
干薑丸 *gān jiāng wán*

乾薑 芎藭 茯苓 消石 杏仁 水蛭 虻蟲 桃仁 蠐螬 蟅蟲（各一兩） 柴胡 芍藥 人參 大黃 蜀椒 當歸（各二兩）。

乾薑	gān jiāng	Dried root of Zingiber officinale	一兩 1 liǎng	3g
川芎	chuān xiōng	Root of Ligusticum wallichii	一兩 1 liǎng	3g
茯苓	fú líng	Dried fungus of Poria cocos	一兩 1 liǎng	3g
消石	xiāo shí	Niter	一兩 1 liǎng	3g
杏仁	xìng rén	Dried seed of Prunus armeniaca	一兩 1 liǎng	3g

水蛭	shuǐ zhì	Dried body of Whitmania pigra	一兩 1 liǎng	3g
虻蟲	méng chóng	Dried body of the female of Tabanus bivittatus	一兩 1 liǎng	3g
桃仁	táo rén	Seed of Prunus persica	一兩 1 liǎng	3g
蠐螬	qí cáo	Dried larva of Holotrichia diomphalia	一兩 1 liǎng	3g
蟅蟲	zhè chóng	Entire dried body of the female of Eupolyphaga sinensis	一兩 1 liǎng	3g
柴胡	chái hú	Root of Bupleurum chinense	二兩 2 liǎng	6g
芍藥	sháo yào	Root of Paeonia albiflora	二兩 2 liǎng	6g
人參	rén shēn	Root of Panax ginseng	二兩 2 liǎng	6g
大黃	dà huáng	Root of Rheum palmatum	二兩 2 liǎng	6g
蜀椒	shǔ jiāo	Seed capsules of Zanthoxylum bungeanum	二兩 2 liǎng	6g
當歸	dāng guī	Root of Angelica polimorpha	二兩 2 liǎng	6g

上十六味，為末，蜜和丸如梧子。空心飲下三丸，不知加至十丸。

Pulverize the above sixteen ingredients and mix with honey into pills the size of firmiana seeds. On an empty stomach, down three pills [per dose] in fluid. If you notice no effect, increase [the dosage] to a maximum of ten pills.*

---

*   *Sòng* editors' note: "The *Qiān Jīn Yì Fāng* [indicates this prescription] for treating women's conglomerations and binds, and conditions below the rib-sides."

LINE 2.3

乾漆湯治月水不通，小腹堅痛不得近方。

Lacquer Decoction treats menstrual stoppage and lower abdominal hardness and pain so severe that she will not let anyone near her.

Lacquer Decoction
干漆湯 *gān qī tāng*

乾漆 葳蕤 芍藥 細辛 甘草 附子（各一兩） 當歸 桂心 芒消 黃芩（各二兩）
大黃（三兩） 吳茱萸（一升）。

乾漆	gān qī	Dried sap of Rhus verniciflua	一兩 1 liǎng	3g
葳蕤	wěi ruí	Rhizome of Polygonatum odoratum	一兩 1 liǎng	3g

芍藥	sháo yào	Root of Paeonia albiflora	一兩 1 liǎng	3g
細辛	xì xīn	Complete plant including root of Asarum heteropoides	一兩 1 liǎng	3g
甘草	gān cǎo	Root of Glycyrrhiza uralensis	一兩 1 liǎng	3g
附子	fù zǐ	Lateral root of Aconitum carmichaeli	一兩 1 liǎng	3g
當歸	dāng guī	Root of Angelica polimorpha	二兩 2 liǎng	6g
桂心	guì xīn	Shaved inner bark of Cinnamomum cassia	二兩 2 liǎng	6g
硭硝	máng xiāo	Hydrated sodium sulfate	二兩 2 liǎng	6g
黃芩	huáng qín	Root of Scutellaria baicalensis	二兩 2 liǎng	6g
大黃	dà huáng	Root of Rheum palmatum	三兩 3 liǎng	9g
吳茱萸	wú zhū yú	Unripe fruit of Evodia rutaecarpa	一升 1 shēng	24g

上十二味，㕮咀，以清酒一斗浸一宿，煮取三升，去滓，內消烊盡，分為三服，相去如一炊頃。

Pound the above twelve ingredients and soak over one night in one *dǒu* of clear liquor. Decoct to obtain three *shēng* and discard the dregs. Add the *máng xiāo* 硭硝 and let it melt completely. Divide into three doses and [take them] separated from each other by the time it takes to cook a meal.

LINE 2.4

芒消湯治月經不通方。

Mirabilite Decoction treats menstrual stoppage.

Mirabilite Decoction
硭硝湯 *máng xiāo tāng*

芒消 丹砂（末） 當歸 芍藥 土瓜根 水蛭（各二兩） 大黃（三兩） 桃仁（一升）。

硭硝	máng xiāo	Hydrated sodium sulfate	二兩 2 liǎng	6g
丹砂, 末	dān shā, mò	Mercuric sulfide, pulverized	二兩 2 liǎng	6g
當歸	dāng guī	Root of Angelica polimorpha	二兩 2 liǎng	6g
芍藥	sháo yào	Root of Paeonia albiflora	二兩 2 liǎng	6g
土瓜根	tǔ guā gēn	Root of Trichosanthes cucumerina	二兩 2 liǎng	6g
水蛭	shuǐ zhì	Dried body of Whitmania pigra	二兩 2 liǎng	6g

大黃	dà huáng	Root of Rheum palmatum	三兩 3 liǎng	9g
桃仁	táo rén	Seed of Prunus persica	一升 1 shēng	24g

上八味，㕮咀，以水九升煮取三升，去滓，內丹砂，芒消，分為三服。

Pound the above eight ingredients and decoct [the last six ingredients] in nine *shēng* of water to obtain three *shēng*. Discard the dregs, add the *dān shā* 丹砂 and *máng xiāo* 硭硝, and divide into three doses.

LINE 2.5

治月經不通，心腹絞痛欲死，通血止痛方。

[The following] prescription treats menstrual stoppage with gripping pain in the heart and abdomen so severe to bring her to the verge of death, by freeing blood and relieving pain.

Formula

當歸 大黃 芍藥（各三兩） 吳茱萸 乾地黃 乾薑 芎藭 虻蟲 水蛭（各二兩） 細辛 甘草 桂心（各一兩） 梔子（十四枚） 桃仁（一升）。

當歸	dāng guī	Root of Angelica polimorpha	三兩 3 liǎng	9g
大黃	dà huáng	Root of Rheum palmatum	三兩 3 liǎng	9g
芍藥	sháo yào	Root of Paeonia albiflora	三兩 3 liǎng	9g
吳茱萸	wú zhū yú	Unripe fruit of Evodia rutaecarpa	二兩 2 liǎng	6g
乾地黃	gān dì huáng	Dried root of Rehmannia glutinosa	二兩 2 liǎng	6g
乾薑	gān jiāng	Dried root of Zingiber officinale	二兩 2 liǎng	6g
川芎	chuān xiōng	Root of Ligusticum wallichii	二兩 2 liǎng	6g
虻蟲	méng chóng	Dried body of the female of Tabanus bivittatus	二兩 2 liǎng	6g
水蛭	shuǐ zhì	Dried body of Whitmania pigra	二兩 2 liǎng	6g
細辛	xì xīn	Complete plant including root of Asarum heteropoides	一兩 1 liǎng	3g
甘草	gān cǎo	Root of Glycyrrhiza uralensis	一兩 1 liǎng	3g
桂心	guì xīn	Shaved inner bark of Cinnamomum cassia	一兩 1 liǎng	3g
梔子仁	zhī zǐ	Fruit of Gardenia jasminoides	十四枚 14 méi	14 pcs
桃仁	táo rén	Seed of Prunus persica	一升 1 shēng	24g

上十四味，㕮咀，以水一斗五升煮取五升，分為五服。

Pound the above fourteen ingredients and decoct in one *dǒu* and five *shēng* of water to obtain five *shēng*. Divide into five doses.*

*   *Sòng* editors' note: "Another edition includes 3 *liǎng* each of *niú xī* (牛膝 Root of Achyranthes bidentata) and *má zǐ rén* (麻子仁 Seed of Cannabis sativa)."

LINE 2.6

桃仁湯治月經不通方。

Peach Kernel Decoction treats menstrual stoppage.[1]

Peach Kernel Decoction
桃仁湯 *táo rén tāng*

桃仁（一升）當歸 土瓜根 大黃 水蛭 虻蟲 芒消（各二兩） 牛膝 麻子仁 桂心（各三兩）。

桃仁	táo rén	Seed of Prunus persica	一升 1 shēng	24g
當歸	dāng guī	Root of Angelica polimorpha	二兩 2 liǎng	6g
土瓜根	tǔ guā gēn	Root of Trichosanthes cucumerina	二兩 2 liǎng	6g
大黃	dà huáng	Root of Rheum palmatum	二兩 2 liǎng	6g
水蛭	shuǐ zhì	Dried body of Whitmania pigra	二兩 2 liǎng	6g
虻蟲	méng chóng	Dried body of the female of Tabanus bivittatus	二兩 2 liǎng	6g
硭硝	máng xiāo	Hydrated sodium sulfate	二兩 2 liǎng	6g
牛膝	niú xī	Root of Achyranthes bidentata	三兩 3 liǎng	9g
麻子仁	má zǐ rén	Seed of Cannabis sativa	三兩 3 liǎng	9g
桂心	guì xīn	Shaved inner bark of Cinnamomum cassia	三兩 3 liǎng	9g

上十味，㕮咀，以水九升煮取三升半，去滓，內消令烊，分為三服。

Pound the above ten ingredients and decoct in nine *shēng* of water to obtain three and a half *shēng*. Discard the dregs, add the *máng xiāo* 硭硝 and let it melt. Divide into three doses.[2]

1. An almost identical prescription with the same name is found at the very beginning of this section (see Line 2.1 above). It has exactly the same purpose of freeing a stopped menstrual flow and uses a very similar combination of ingredients.

2. *Sòng* editors' note: "The *Zhǒu Hòu Fāng* does not use *dāng guī* 當歸 and *má zǐ rén* 麻子仁, but includes three *liǎng* each of *mǔ dān* (牡丹 Bark of the root of Paeonia suffruticosa), *shè gān* (射干 Rhizome of Belamcanda chinensis), *huáng qín* (黃芩 Root of Scutellaria baicalensis), *sháo yào* (芍藥 Root of Paeonia albiflora), and *chái hú* (柴胡 Root of Bupleurum chinense), with a total of thirteen ingredients. The *Qiān Jīn Yì Fāng* does not use *méng chóng* 虻蟲."

LINE 2.7

前胡牡丹湯治婦人盛實，有熱在腹，月經瘀閉不通，及勞熱，熱病後，或因月經來，得熱不通方。

Peucedanum and Moutan Decoction treats women's exuberant repletion, presence of heat in the abdomen, static, blocked, or stopped menstrual flow; as well as menstrual stoppage from taxation heat, after heat diseases, or due to contracting heat at the onset of menstruation.˙

Peucedanum and Moutan Decoction
前胡牡丹湯 *qián hú mǔ dān tāng*

前胡 牡丹 玄參 桃仁 黃芩 射干 旋復花 栝樓根 甘草（各二兩） 芍藥 茯苓 大黃 枳實（各三兩）。

前胡	qián hú	Root of Peucedanum praeruptorum	二兩 2 liǎng	6g
牡丹	mǔ dān	Bark of the root of Paeonia suffruticosa	二兩 2 liǎng	6g
玄參	xuán shēn	Root of Scrophularia ningpoensis	二兩 2 liǎng	6g
桃仁	táo rén	Seed of Prunus persica	二兩 2 liǎng	6g
黃芩	huáng qín	Root of Scutellaria baicalensis	二兩 2 liǎng	6g
射干	shè gān	Rhizome of Belamcanda chinensis	二兩 2 liǎng	6g
旋覆花	xuán fù huā	Flowerhead of Inula britannica	二兩 2 liǎng	6g
栝蔞根	guā lóu gēn	Root of Trichosanthes kirilowii	二兩 2 liǎng	6g
甘草	gān cǎo	Root of Glycyrrhiza uralensis	二兩 2 liǎng	6g
芍藥	sháo yào	Root of Paeonia albiflora	三兩 3 liǎng	9g
茯苓	fú líng	Dried fungus of Poria cocos	三兩 3 liǎng	9g
大黃	dà huáng	Root of Rheum palmatum	三兩 3 liǎng	9g

| 枳實 | zhǐ shí | Unripe fruit of Poncirus trifoliata | 三兩 3 liǎng | 9g |

上十三味，㕮咀，以水一斗煮取三升，分為三服。

Pound the above thirteen ingredients and decoct in one *dǒu* of water to obtain three *shēng*. Divide into three doses.

*　This indication is slightly unusual since a lack of menstrual flow is usually associated with vacuity and the presence of cold. According to the *Bìng Yuán Lùn*, menstrual stoppage is caused by "taxation harming the blood and *qì*, causing vacuity in the body and allowing the contraction of wind-cold. The evil *qì* of wind-cold lodges in the uterus, damages the thoroughfare and controlling vessels and hand greater *yáng* and lesser *yīn* channels, and causes the uterine network vessels to be cut off, so that blood and *qì* stop flowing... Wind-cold damages the blood in the channels. It is the natural characteristic of blood to flow freely when it contracts warmth, and to be inhibited and blocked when it contracts cold. When it is bound and seized by cold, blood binds internally, causing menstrual stoppage (《病源論》 37:23)."

LINE 2.8

乾地黃當歸丸治月水不通，或一月再來，或隔月不至，或多或少，或淋瀝不斷，或來而腰腹刺痛不可忍，四體噓吸不飲食，心腹堅痛，有青黃黑色水下，或如清水，不欲行動，舉體沈重，惟思眠臥，欲食酸物，虛乏黃瘦方。

Dried Rehmannia and Chinese Angelica Pills treat menstrual stoppage or [menstruation] occurring twice in one month or failing to arrive in alternate months, an excessive or scanty menstrual flow, incessant dribbling, or its onset accompanied by unbearable stabbing pain in the lumbus and abdomen, [as well as] in the four limbs, huffing and gasping and failure to eat and drink, hardness and pain in the heart and abdomen, [vaginal] discharge of green, yellow, or black-colored fluid, or discharge like clear water, lack of interest in movement and activity, heaviness when lifting the limbs, only thinking of sleep and rest, desire to eat sour foods, and vacuity, jaundice, and emaciation.[1]

Dried Rehmannia and Chinese Angelica Pills
干地黃當歸丸 *gān dì huáng dāng guī wán*

乾地黃（三兩） 當歸 甘草（各一兩半） 牛膝 芍藥 乾薑 澤蘭 人參 牡丹（各一兩六銖） 丹參 蜀椒 白芷 黃芩 桑耳 桂心（各一兩） 蟅蟲（四十枚） 芎藭（一兩十八銖） 桃仁（二兩） 水蛭 虻蟲（各七十枚） 蒲黃（二合）
。

乾地黃	gān dì huáng	Dried root of Rehmannia glutinosa	三兩 3 liǎng	9g
當歸	dāng guī	Root of Angelica polimorpha	一兩半 1.5 liǎng	4.5g
甘草	gān cǎo	Root of Glycyrrhiza uralensis	一兩半 1.5 liǎng	4.5g
牛膝	niú xī	Root of Achyranthes bidentata	一兩六銖 1 liǎng 6 zhū	3.75g
芍藥	sháo yào	Root of Paeonia albiflora	一兩六銖 1 liǎng 6 zhū	3.75g
乾薑	gān jiāng	Dried root of Zingiber officinale	一兩六銖 1 liǎng 6 zhū	3.75g
澤蘭	zé lán	Foliage and stalk of Lycopus lucidus	一兩六銖 1 liǎng 6 zhū	3.75g
人參	rén shēn	Root of Panax ginseng	一兩六銖 1 liǎng 6 zhū	3.75g
牡丹	mǔ dān	Bark of the root of Paeonia suffruticosa	一兩六銖 1 liǎng 6 zhū	3.75g
丹參	dān shēn	Root of Salvia miltiorrhiza	一兩 1 liǎng	3g
蜀椒	shǔ jiāo	Seed capsules of Zanthoxylum bungeanum	一兩 1 liǎng	3g
白芷	bái zhǐ	Root of Angelica dahurica	一兩 1 liǎng	3g
黃芩	huáng qín	Root of Scutellaria baicalensis	一兩 1 liǎng	3g
桑耳	sāng ěr	Mulberry wood ear	一兩 1 liǎng	3g
桂心	guì xīn	Shaved inner bark of Cinnamomum cassia	一兩 1 liǎng	3g
䗪蟲	zhè chóng	Entire dried body of the female of Eupolyphaga sinensis	四十枚 40 méi	40 pcs
川芎	chuān xiōng	Root of Ligusticum wallichii	一兩十八銖 1 liǎng 18 zhū	5.25g
桃仁	táo rén	Seed of Prunus persica	二兩 2 liǎng	6g
水蛭	shuǐ zhì	Dried body of Whitmania pigra	七十枚 70 méi	70 pcs
虻蟲	méng chóng	Dried body of the female of Tabanus bivittatus	七十枚 70 méi	70 pcs
蒲黃	pú huáng	Pollen of Typha angustata	二合 2 gě	14ml

上二十一味，為末，蜜和丸如梧子大，每日空心酒下十五丸，漸加至三十
丸，以知為度。

Pulverize the above twenty-one ingredients and mix with honey into pills the size of firmiana seeds. Every day, down fifteen pills in liquor on an empty stomach, gradually increasing [the dosage] to a maximum of thirty pills, until an effect is noticed.[2]

1.   This list of symptoms is almost literally identical with the indications for *Chalk Pills* (白堊丸 *bái è wán*), which is found in this place in the *Sūn Zhēn Rén* edition. That prescription is not found anywhere in the other editions.

2.   *Sòng* editors' note: "One edition does not contain [this prescription]."

LINE 2.9

牡丹丸治婦人女子諸病後，月經閉絕不通，及從小來不通，並新產後瘀血不消，服諸湯利血後，餘疢未平，宜服之，取平復方。

Moutan Pills treat menstrual block, interruption, or stoppage in married women and virgins after the various diseases, as well as menstrual stoppage since childhood, and blood stagnation and non-dispersion right after childbirth. After [the woman] has taken the various decoctions to disinhibit blood, when she has not yet recovered from the residual conditions, she should take [these pills] and thereby regain her health.

Moutan Pills
牡丹丸 *mǔ dān wán*

牡丹（三兩）芍藥 玄參 桃仁 當歸 桂心（各二兩）虻蟲 水蛭（各五十枚）蠐螬（二十枚）瞿麥 芎藭 海藻（各一兩）。

牡丹	mǔ dān	Bark of the root of Paeonia suf-fruticosa	三兩 3 liǎng	9g
芍藥	sháo yào	Root of Paeonia albiflora	二兩 2 liǎng	6g
玄參	xuán shēn	Root of Scrophularia ningpoensis	二兩 2 liǎng	6g
桃仁	táo rén	Seed of Prunus persica	二兩 2 liǎng	6g
當歸	dāng guī	Root of Angelica polimorpha	二兩 2 liǎng	6g
桂心	guì xīn	Shaved inner bark of Cinnamomum cassia	二兩 2 liǎng	6g
虻蟲	méng chóng	Dried body of the female of Tabanus bivittatus	五十枚 50 méi	50 pcs
水蛭	shuǐ zhì	Dried body of Whitmania pigra	五十枚 50 méi	50 pcs
蠐螬	qí cáo	Dried larva of Holotrichia di-omphalia	二十枚 20 méi	20 pcs
瞿麥	qú mài	Entire plant, including flowers, of Dianthus superbus	一兩 1 liǎng	3g
川芎	chuān xiōng	Root of Ligusticum wallichii	一兩 1 liǎng	3g

| 海藻 | hǎi zǎo | Whole plant of Sargassum fusiforme | 一兩 1 liǎng | 3g |

上十二味，為末，蜜和丸如梧子大，酒下十五丸，加至二十丸。血盛者，作散，服方寸匕，腹中當轉如沸，血自化成水去；如小便赤少，除桂心用地膚子一兩。

Pulverize the above twelve ingredients and mix with honey into pills the size of firmiana seeds. Down fifteen pills [per dose] in liquor, increasing [the dosage] to a maximum of twenty pills. In cases of blood exuberance, prepare [the drugs into] a powder and take a square-inch spoon. The center of her abdomen should churn as if boiling over. The blood will spontaneously transform into a watery liquid and be expelled. In cases of red or scanty urine, take out the *guì xīn* 桂心 and replace it with one *liǎng* of *dì fū zǐ* (地膚子 Fruit of Kochia scoparia).

LINE 2.10

黃芩牡丹湯治女人從小至大月經未嘗來，顏色萎黃，氣力衰少，飲食無味方。

Scutellaria and Moutan Decoction treats women's complete absence of menstruation from childhood to adulthood, a withered and yellow complexion, weakened *qì* and strength, and inability to taste food and drink.

Scutellaria and Moutan Decoction
黃芩牡丹湯 *huáng qín mǔ dān tāng*

黃芩 牡丹 桃仁 瞿麥 芎藭（各二兩） 芍藥 枳實 射干 海藻 大黃（各三兩）虻蟲（七十牧） 水蛭（五十枚） 蠐螬（十枚）。

黃芩	huáng qín	Root of Scutellaria baicalensis	二兩 2 liǎng	6g
牡丹	mǔ dān	Bark of the root of Paeonia suffruticosa	二兩 2 liǎng	6g
桃仁	táo rén	Seed of Prunus persica	二兩 2 liǎng	6g
瞿麥	qú mài	Entire plant, including flowers, of Dianthus superbus	二兩 2 liǎng	6g
川芎	chuān xiōng	Root of Ligusticum wallichii	二兩 2 liǎng	6g
芍藥	sháo yào	Root of Paeonia albiflora	三兩 3 liǎng	9g
枳實	zhǐ shí	Unripe fruit of Poncirus trifoliata	三兩 3 liǎng	9g
射干	shè gān	Rhizome of Belamcanda chinensis	三兩 3 liǎng	9g
海藻	hǎi zǎo	Whole plant of Sargassum fusiforme	三兩 3 liǎng	9g

大黃	dà huáng	Root of Rheum palmatum	三兩 3 liǎng	9g
虻蟲	méng chóng	Dried body of the female of Tabanus bivittatus	七十枚 70 méi	70 pcs
水蛭	shuǐ zhì	Dried body of Whitmania pigra	五十枚 50 méi	50 pcs
蠐螬	qí cáo	Dried larva of Holotrichia diomphalia	十枚 10 méi	10 pcs

上十三味，㕮咀，以水一斗煮取三升，分三服。服兩劑後，灸乳下一寸黑員際各五十壯。

Pound the above thirteen ingredients and decoct in one *dǒu* of water to obtain three *shēng*. Divide into three doses. After taking two preparations [of this prescription], burn 50 cones of moxa on each side at the point one *cùn* below the nipple, at the edge of the areola of the breast.

LINE 2.11

治月經不通方。

[The following] prescription treats menstrual stoppage.

取葶藶一升為末，蜜丸如彈子大，綿裹，內陰中入三寸。每丸一宿易之，有汁出止。

Take one *shēng* of *tíng lì* (葶藶 Seed of Lepidium apetalum) and pulverize it. [Mix it] with honey [to make] pellet-sized pills, wrap [one] in thin silk cloth, and insert it into the vagina, three *cùn* deep. Leave each pill in over one night and then change it. Stop when there is fluid coming out.

LINE 2.12

乾漆丸治月經不通，百療不瘥方。

Lacquer Pills treat menstrual stoppage and a hundred ailments that fail to improve.

Lacquer Pills
干漆丸 *gān qī wán*

乾漆 土瓜根 射干 芍藥（各一兩半） 牡丹 牛膝 黃芩 桂心 吳茱萸 大黃 柴胡（各一兩六銖） 桃仁 鱉甲（各二兩） 蟅蟲 蠐螬（各四十枚） 水蛭 虻蟲（各七十枚） 大麻仁（四合） 亂髮（雞子大二枚） 菴䕡子（二合）。

乾漆	gān qī	Dried sap of Rhus verniciflua	一兩半 1.5 liǎng	4.5g
土瓜根	tǔ guā gēn	Root of Trichosanthes cucumerina	一兩半 1.5 liǎng	4.5g
射干	shè gān	Rhizome of Belamcanda chinensis	一兩半 1.5 liǎng	4.5g
芍藥	sháo yào	Root of Paeonia albiflora	一兩半 1.5 liǎng	4.5g
牡丹	mǔ dān	Bark of the root of Paeonia suffruticosa	一兩六銖 1 liǎng 6 zhū	3.75g
牛膝	niú xī	Root of Achyranthes bidentata	一兩六銖 1 liǎng 6 zhū	3.75g
黃芩	huáng qín	Root of Scutellaria baicalensis	一兩六銖 1 liǎng 6 zhū	3.75g
桂心	guì xīn	Shaved inner bark of Cinnamomum cassia	一兩六銖 1 liǎng 6 zhū	3.75g
吳茱萸	wú zhū yú	Unripe fruit of Evodia rutaecarpa	一兩六銖 1 liǎng 6 zhū	3.75g
大黃	dà huáng	Root of Rheum palmatum	一兩六銖 1 liǎng 6 zhū	3.75g
柴胡	chái hú	Root of Bupleurum chinense	一兩六銖 1 liǎng 6 zhū	3.75g
桃仁	táo rén	Seed of Prunus persica	二兩 2 liǎng	6g
鱉甲	biē jiǎ	Dorsal shell of Amyda sinensis	二兩 2 liǎng	6g
䗪蟲	zhè chóng	Entire dried body of the female of Eupolyphaga sinensis	四十枚 40 méi	40 pcs
蠐螬	qí cáo	Dried larva of Holotrichia diomphalia	四十枚 40 méi	40 pcs
水蛭	shuǐ zhì	Dried body of Whitmania pigra	七十枚 70 méi	70 pcs
虻蟲	méng chóng	Dried body of the female of Tabanus bivittatus	七十枚 70 méi	70 pcs
大麻仁	dà má rén	Seed of Cannabis sativa	四合 4 gě	28ml
亂髮	luàn fà	Matted hair	雞子大二枚 jī zǐ dà 2 méi	2 pcs the size of chicken eggs
菴䕡子	ān lǘ zǐ	Fruit of Artemisia keiskeana	二合 2 gě	14ml

上二十味，為末，以蜜和為丸。每日酒下十五丸，梧子大，漸加至三十丸，
日三。仍用後浸酒服前丸藥。

Pulverize the above twenty ingredients and mix with honey into pills. Every day, down fifteen pills the size of firmiana seeds in liquor, gradually increasing [the dosage] to a maximum of thirty pills, three times a day. Moreover, use the following steeped wine to take the above pill medicine.

LINE 2.13

浸酒方。

A prescription for steeped wine.

Formula

大麻子（三升）菴䕡子（二升）桃仁（一升）竈屋炱煤（四兩）土瓜根 射干（各六兩）牛膝（八兩）桂心（四兩）。

大麻子	dà má zǐ	Seed of Cannabis sativa	三升 3 shēng	72g
菴䕡子	ān lǘ zǐ	Fruit of Artemisia keiskeana	二升 2 shēng	48g
桃仁	táo rén	Seed of Prunus persica	一升 1 shēng	24g
灶屋炱煤	zào wū tái méi	Kitchen soot	四兩 4 liǎng	12g
土瓜根	tǔ guā gēn	Root of Trichosanthes cucumerina	六兩 6 liǎng	18g
射干	shè gān	Rhizome of Belamcanda chinensis	六兩 6 liǎng	18g
牛膝	niú xī	Root of Achyranthes bidentata	八兩 8 liǎng	24g
桂心	guì xīn	Shaved inner bark of Cinnamomum cassia	四兩 4 liǎng	12g

上八味，咬咀，以清酒三斗，絹袋盛藥浸五宿，以一盞下前丸藥，甚良。 或單服之，亦好。

Pound the above eight ingredients. Pack the drugs into a silk bag and soak them in three *dǒu* of clear liquor for five nights. It is excellent to use one small cup [of this wine] to down the previous pill medicine. Alternatively, taking it alone is also good.

LINE 2.14

當歸丸治女人臍下癥結，刺痛如蟲所嚙，及如錐刀所刺，或赤白帶下，十二 疾，腰背疼痛，月水或在月前或在月後。

Chinese Angelica Pills treat women's aggregations and binds below the navel, stabbing pain as if from biting insects or as if being stabbed with an awl or knife, possibly with red and white vaginal discharge, the twelve [concretion] diseases, pain in the lumbus and back, and early or delayed menstruation.

Chinese Angelica Pills
當歸丸 *dāng guī wán*

當歸 葶藶 附子 吳茱萸 大黃（各二兩） 黃芩 桂心 乾薑 牡丹 芎藭（各一兩半） 細辛 秦椒 柴胡 厚朴（各一兩六銖） 牡蒙（一方無） 甘草（各一兩）虻蟲 水蛭（各五十枚）。

當歸	dāng guī	Root of Angelica polimorpha	二兩 2 liǎng	6g
葶藶	tíng lì	Seed of Lepidium apetalum	二兩 2 liǎng	6g
附子	fù zǐ	Lateral root of Aconitum carmi-chaeli	二兩 2 liǎng	6g
吳茱萸	wú zhū yú	Unripe fruit of Evodia rutaecarpa	二兩 2 liǎng	6g
大黃	dà huáng	Root of Rheum palmatum	二兩 2 liǎng	6g
黃芩	huáng qín	Root of Scutellaria baicalensis	一兩半 1.5 liǎng	4.5g
桂心	guì xīn	Shaved inner bark of Cinnamomum cassia	一兩半 1.5 liǎng	4.5g
乾薑	gān jiāng	Dried root of Zingiber officinale	一兩半 1.5 liǎng	4.5g
牡丹	mǔ dān	Bark of the root of Paeonia suf-fruticosa	一兩半 1.5 liǎng	4.5g
川芎	chuān xiōng	Root of Ligusticum wallichii	一兩半 1.5 liǎng	4.5g
細辛	xì xīn	Complete plant including root of Asarum heteropoides	一兩六銖 1 liǎng 6 zhū	3.75g
秦椒	qín jiāo	Seed capsule of Zanthoxylum bungeanum	一兩六銖 1 liǎng 6 zhū	3.75g
柴胡	chái hú	Root of Bupleurum chinense	一兩六銖 1 liǎng 6 zhū	3.75g
厚朴	hòu pò	Bark of Magnolia officinalis	一兩六銖 1 liǎng 6 zhū	3.75g
牡蒙[1]	mǔ méng	Root of Paris quadrifolia	一兩 1 liǎng	3g
甘草	gān cǎo	Root of Glycyrrhiza uralensis	一兩 1 liǎng	3g
虻蟲	méng chóng	Dried body of the female of Ta-banus bivittatus	五十枚 50 méi	50 pcs
水蛭	shuǐ zhì	Dried body of Whitmania pigra	五十枚 50 méi	50 pcs

上十八味，為末，蜜和丸如梧子大。空心酒下十五丸，日再。有胎，勿服之。

Pulverize the above eighteen ingredients and mix with honey into pills the size of firmiana seeds. On an empty stomach, down fifteen pills in liquor twice a day.[2] Do not take them during pregnancy.[3]

1.   *Sòng* editors' note: "Another [version of this] prescription lacks *mǔ méng* 牡蒙."
2.   The *Sūn Zhēn Rén* edition recommends to "down five pills in liquor on an empty stomach twice a day, increasing [the dosage] to a maximum of ten pills." This is a considerable divergence from the instructions found in the other editions and could reflect contesting medical views regarding the use of strong blood-moving formulas in treating women's menstrual problems.
3.   Since the prescription's intended effect is to break up the bound blood and restore the normal menstrual flow, it would, in the case of a pregnancy, cause an abortion.

LINE 2.15

鱉甲丸治女人小腹中積聚，大如七八寸盤面，上下周流，痛不可忍，手足苦冷，欬噫腥臭，兩脅熱如火炙，玉門冷如風吹，經水不通，或在月前，或在月後，服之三十日便瘥，有孕。此是河內太守魏夫人方。

Turtle Shell Pills treat women's accumulations and gatherings in the center of the lower abdomen that are as big as the surface of a seven or eight *cùn* bowl[1] and move up and down and around, unbearable pain, bitter coldness in the hands and feet, coughing and belching with fishy-smelling breath, heat in both rib-sides as if from a blazing fire, coldness in the jade gate as if the wind was blowing in, and menstrual stoppage or early or late menstruation. After taking these [pills] for thirty days, she will recover and be pregnant. This is a prescription from the wife of Governor Wèi of Hé-Nèi.[2]

Turtle Shell Pills
鱉甲丸 *biē jiǎ wán*

鱉甲 桂心（各一兩半） 蜂房（半兩） 玄參 蜀椒 細辛 人參 苦參 丹參 沙參 吳茱萸（各十八銖） 蟅蟲 水蛭 乾薑 牡丹 附子 皂莢 當歸 芍藥 甘草 防葵（各一兩） 蠐螬（二十枚） 虻蟲 大黃（各一兩六銖）。

鱉甲	biē jiǎ	Dorsal shell of Amyda sinensis	一兩半 1.5 liǎng	4.5g
桂心	guì xīn	Shaved inner bark of Cinnamomum cassia	一兩半 1.5 liǎng	4.5g
防風	fáng fēng	Root of Ledebouriella divaricata	半兩 0.5 liǎng	1.5g

玄參	xuán shēn	Root of Scrophularia ningpoensis	十八銖 18 zhū	2.25g
蜀椒	shǔ jiāo	Seed capsules of Zanthoxylum bungeanum	十八銖 18 zhū	2.25g
細辛	xì xīn	Complete plant including root of Asarum heteropoides	十八銖 18 zhū	2.25g
人參	rén shēn	Root of Panax ginseng	十八銖 18 zhū	2.25g
苦參	kǔ shēn	Root of Sophora flavescens	十八銖 18 zhū	2.25g
丹參	dān shēn	Root of Salvia miltiorrhiza	十八銖 18 zhū	2.25g
沙參	shā shēn	Root of Adenophora tetraphylla	十八銖 18 zhū	2.25g
吳茱萸	wú zhū yú	Unripe fruit of Evodia rutaecarpa	十八銖 18 zhū	2.25g
蟅蟲	zhè chóng	Entire dried body of the female of Eupolyphaga sinensis	一兩 1 liǎng	3g
水蛭	shuǐ zhì	Dried body of Whitmania pigra	一兩 1 liǎng	3g
乾薑	gān jiāng	Dried root of Zingiber officinale	一兩 1 liǎng	3g
牡丹	mǔ dān	Bark of the root of Paeonia suffruticosa	一兩 1 liǎng	3g
附子	fù zǐ	Lateral root of Aconitum carmichaeli	一兩 1 liǎng	3g
皂莢	zào jiá	Fruit of Gleditsia sinensis	一兩 1 liǎng	3g
當歸	dāng guī	Root of Angelica polimorpha	一兩 1 liǎng	3g
芍藥	sháo yào	Root of Paeonia albiflora	一兩 1 liǎng	3g
甘草	gān cǎo	Root of Glycyrrhiza uralensis	一兩 1 liǎng	3g
防葵	fáng kuí	unknown	一兩 1 liǎng	3g
蠐螬	qí cáo	Dried larva of Holotrichia diomphalia	二十枚 20 méi	20 pcs
虻蟲	méng chóng	Dried body of the female of Tabanus bivittatus	一兩六銖 1 liǎng 6 zhū	3.75g
大黃	dà huáng	Root of Rheum palmatum	一兩六銖 1 liǎng 6 zhū	3.75g

上二十四味，為末，蜜和丸如梧子大。酒下七丸，日三，稍加之，以知為度。

Pulverize the above twenty-four ingredients and mix with honey into pills the size of firmiana seeds. Down seven pills in liquor three times a day, gradually increasing [the dosage] until an effect is noticed.

1. The *Sūn Zhēn Rén* edition has instead "大如揲面 *dà rǔ shé miàn*" (the size of a surface for counting yarrow stalks [in divination])."
2. 河內太守魏夫人 *hé nèi tài shǒu wèi fū rén*: During the *Suí* period, Hé-Nèi was the name of a county that corresponds to modern Qìn-Yáng County 沁陽縣 in Hé-Nán 河南. It

is perhaps significant that an elite woman is specifically identified as the source of this highly complex prescription. It proves that women were actively involved not just in the practice of such less esteemed aspects of healthcare as midwifery or simple kitchen recipes, but also in the practice of medical treatment with medicinal decoctions that required a thorough understanding of pharmaceutics, etiology, and therapy. Unfortunately, we still do not know enough about women's role in early Chinese medicine to judge whether Lady Wèi was just a noteworthy exception or a representative of a larger tradition or line of practitioners.

LINE 2.26

又方治婦人因產後虛冷，堅結積在腹內，月經往來不時，苦腹脹滿，繞臍下痛引腰背，手足煩，或冷熱，心悶不欲食。

Another prescription for treating women's vacuity cold due to the after-effects of childbirth, hardness, binding, and accumulations in the abdomen, erratic onset and end of menstruation, discomfort from abdominal distention and fullness, pain around and below the navel stretching to the lumbus and back, vexation in the hands and feet, possibly [aversion to] cold and heat [effusion], and heart oppression and no desire to eat.

Formula

鱉甲（一兩半）乾薑 赤石脂 丹參 禹餘糧 當歸 白芷 乾地黃（各一兩六銖）代赭 甘草 鹿茸 烏賊骨 殭蠶（各十八銖）桂心 細辛 蜀椒 附子（各一兩）。

鱉甲	biē jiǎ	Dorsal shell of Amyda sinensis	一兩半 1.5 liǎng	4.5g
乾薑	gān jiāng	Dried root of Zingiber officinale	一兩六銖 1 liǎng 6 zhū	3.75g
赤石脂	chì shí zhī	Halloysite	一兩六銖 1 liǎng 6 zhū	3.75g
丹參	dān shēn	Root of Salvia miltiorrhiza	一兩六銖 1 liǎng 6 zhū	3.75g
禹餘糧	yǔ yú liáng	Limonite	一兩六銖 1 liǎng 6 zhū	3.75g
當歸	dāng guī	Root of Angelica polimorpha	一兩六銖 1 liǎng 6 zhū	3.75g
白芷[1]	bái zhǐ	Root of Angelica dahurica	一兩六銖 1 liǎng 6 zhū	3.75g
乾地黃	gān dì huáng	Dried root of Rehmannia glutinosa	一兩六銖 1 liǎng 6 zhū	3.75g
代赭	dài zhě	Hematite	十八銖 18 zhū	2.25g

甘草	gān cǎo	Root of Glycyrrhiza uralensis	十八銖 18 zhū	2.25g
鹿茸	lù róng	Pilose antler of Cervus nippon	十八銖 18 zhū	2.25g
烏賊骨	wū zéi gǔ	Calcified shell of Sepiella maindroni	十八銖 18 zhū	2.25g
殭蠶	jiāng cán	Dried 4th or 5th stage larva of the moth of Bombyx mori	十八銖 18 zhū	2.25g
桂心	guì xīn	Shaved inner bark of Cinnamomum cassia	一兩 1 liǎng	3g
細辛	xì xīn	Complete plant including root of Asarum heteropoides	一兩 1 liǎng	3g
蜀椒	shǔ jiāo	Seed capsules of Zanthoxylum bungeanum	一兩 1 liǎng	3g
附子	fù zǐ	Lateral root of Aconitum carmichaeli	一兩 1 liǎng	3g

上十七味，末，蜜和丸如梧子大。空心酒下五丸，加至十丸。

Pulverize the above seventeen ingredients and mix with honey into pills the size of firmiana seeds. On an empty stomach, down five pills [per dose] in liquor, increasing [the dosage] to a maximum of ten pills.[2]

1. *Sòng* editors' note: "Another [version of this] prescription has *bái zhú* (白朮Rhizome of Atractylodes macrocephala)."
2. The *Sūn Zhēn Rén* edition adds the following sentence: "Pork, chicken, dog, or rabbit meat, and raw vegetables and garlic are prohibited."

LINE 2.27

禹餘糧丸治婦人產後積冷堅癖方。

Limonite Pills treat women's postpartum accumulation of cold, hardness, and aggregations.[1]

Limonite pills
禹餘糧丸 *yǔ yú liáng wán*

禹餘糧 烏賊骨 吳茱萸 桂心 蜀椒（各二兩半） 當歸 白朮 細辛 乾地黃 人參 芍藥 芎藭 前胡（各一兩六銖） 乾薑（三兩） 礜石（六銖） 白薇 紫菀 黃芩（各十八銖） 蟅蟲（一兩）。

禹餘糧	yǔ yú liáng	Limonite	二兩半 2.5 liǎng	7.5g
烏賊骨	wū zéi gǔ[2]	Calcified shell of Sepiella main-droni	二兩半 2.5 liǎng	7.5g
吳茱萸	wú zhū yú	Unripe fruit of Evodia rutaecarpa	二兩半 2.5 liǎng	7.5g
桂心	guì xīn	Shaved inner bark of Cinnamomum cassia	二兩半 2.5 liǎng	7.5g
蜀椒	shǔ jiāo	Seed capsules of Zanthoxylum bungeanum	二兩半 2.5 liǎng	7.5g
當歸	dāng guī	Root of Angelica polimorpha	一兩六銖 1 liǎng 6 zhū	3.75g
白朮	bái zhú	Rhizome of Atractylodes macro-cephala	一兩六銖 1 liǎng 6 zhū	3.75g
細辛	xì xīn	Complete plant including root of Asarum heteropoides	一兩六銖 1 liǎng 6 zhū	3.75g
乾地黃	gān dì huáng	Dried root of Rehmannia glutinosa	一兩六銖 1 liǎng 6 zhū	3.75g
人參	rén shēn	Root of Panax ginseng	一兩六銖 1 liǎng 6 zhū	3.75g
芍藥	sháo yào	Root of Paeonia albiflora	一兩六銖 1 liǎng 6 zhū	3.75g
川芎	chuān xiōng	Root of Ligusticum wallichii	一兩六銖 1 liǎng 6 zhū	3.75g
前胡	qián hú	Root of Peucedanum praeruptorum	一兩六銖 1 liǎng 6 zhū	3.75g
乾薑	gān jiāng	Dried root of Zingiber officinale	三兩 3 liǎng	9g
礬石	fán shí	Alum	六銖 6 zhū	0.75g
白薇	bái wēi	Root of Cynanchum atratum	十八銖 18 zhū	2.25g
紫菀	zǐ wǎn	Root and rhizome of Aster tataricus	十八銖 18 zhū	2.25g
黃芩	huáng qín	Root of Scutellaria baicalensis	十八銖 18 zhū	2.25g
蟅蟲	zhè chóng	Entire dried body of the female of Eupolyphaga sinensis	一兩 1 liǎng	3g

上十九味，為末，蜜如丸如梧子。空心酒若飲下二十丸，日二，不知則加之。

Pulverize the above nineteen ingredients and mix with honey into pills the size of firmiana seeds. On an empty stomach, down twenty pills in liquor or [another] beverage twice a day. If no effect is noticed, increase [the dosage].

1.   The *Sūn Zhēn Rén* edition has instead "… treat women's postpartum wasting and cold-ness, hardness, and aggregations."

2.   The *Sūn Zhēn Rén* edition has *wū tóu* (烏頭 Main tuber of Aconitum carmichaeli) instead of *wū zéi gǔ* 烏賊骨.

LINE 2.28

牡蒙丸治婦人產後十二癥病，帶下無子，皆是冷風寒氣，或產後未滿百日，胞胳惡血未盡，便利於懸圊上及久坐，濕寒入裏，結在小腹，牢痛為之積聚，小如雞子，大者如拳，按之跳手隱隱然，或如蟲嚙，或如針刺，氣時搶心，兩脅支滿，不能食，飲食不消化，上下通流，或守胃管，痛連玉門背膊，嘔逆，短氣，汗出，少腹苦寒，胞中創，咳引陰痛，小便自出，子門不正，令人無子，腰胯疼痛，四肢沈重淫躍，一身盡腫，乍來乍去，大便不利，小便淋瀝，或月經不通，或下如腐肉，青黃赤白黑等，如豆汁，夢想不祥方。（亦名紫蓋丸。）

Four-leaved Paris Root Pills treat women's twelve postpartum concretion diseases, vaginal discharge, and infertility, all of which are [related to] the cold *qi* of cool wind. Perhaps the woman, prior to the conclusion of the hundred days postpartum and the complete elimination of malign blood from the uterine network vessels, squatted carelessly over the privy for a long time. [This allowed] dampness and cold to enter inside, to bind in the lower abdomen, to cause firmness and pain, and to form accumulations and gatherings, the smaller ones the size of a chicken egg, the larger ones the size of a fist, slippery and ungraspable when pressed down. [This condition can be accompanied by pain] as if gnawed by worms or stabbed by needles, *qi* intermittently prodding the heart, propping fullness in both rib-sides, inability to eat, failure to disperse and transform food and drink, causing it to flow up and down or to get stuck in the stomach duct, pain all the way from the jade gate to the back and arms, retching counterflow and shortness of breath, sweating, bitter coldness in the lower abdomen, wounds in the uterus,[1] coughing with pain stretching to the genitals, spontaneous urination, a crooked vagina causing infertility, pain in the lumbus and hip, heaviness and random flailing of the four limbs, abruptly occuring extreme swelling all over the entire body, constipation, dribbling urination, a menstrual period that is either stopped or resembles rotten flesh, a blue-green, yellow, red, white, black, or other-colored [substance], or bean juice, and inauspicious dreams and thoughts. ([This prescription] is also called *Purple Canopy Pills*.)[2]

Four-Leaved Paris Root Pills
牡蒙丸 *mǔ méng wán*

牡蒙 厚朴 消石 前胡 乾薑 蟅蟲 牡丹 蜀椒 黃芩 桔梗 茯苓 細辛 葶藶 人參 芎藭 吳茱萸 桂心（各十八銖）大黃（二兩半）附子（一兩六銖）當歸（半兩）。

| 牡蒙 | mǔ méng | Root of Paris quadrifolia | 十八銖 18 zhū | 2.25g |
| 厚朴 | hòu pò | Bark of Magnolia officinalis | 十八銖 18 zhū | 2.25g |

消石	xiāo shí	Niter	十八銖 18 zhū	2.25g
前胡	qián hú	Root of Peucedanum praeruptorum	十八銖 18 zhū	2.25g
乾薑	gān jiāng	Dried root of Zingiber officinale	十八銖 18 zhū	2.25g
䗪蟲	zhè chóng	Entire dried body of the female of Eupolyphaga sinensis	十八銖 18 zhū	2.25g
牡丹	mǔ dān	Bark of the root of Paeonia suf-fruticosa	十八銖 18 zhū	2.25g
蜀椒	shǔ jiāo	Seed capsules of Zanthoxylum bungeanum	十八銖 18 zhū	2.25g
黃芩	huáng qín	Root of Scutellaria baicalensis	十八銖 18 zhū	2.25g
桔梗	jié gěng	Root of Platycodon grandiflorum	十八銖 18 zhū	2.25g
茯苓	fú líng	Dried fungus of Poria cocos	十八銖 18 zhū	2.25g
細辛	xì xīn	Complete plant including root of Asarum heteropoides	十八銖 18 zhū	2.25g
葶藶	tíng lì	Seed of Lepidium apetalum	十八銖 18 zhū	2.25g
人參	rén shēn	Root of Panax ginseng	十八銖 18 zhū	2.25g
川芎	chuān xiōng	Root of Ligusticum wallichii	十八銖 18 zhū	2.25g
吳茱萸	wú zhū yú	Unripe fruit of Evodia rutaecarpa	十八銖 18 zhū	2.25g
桂心	guì xīn	Shaved inner bark of Cinnamomum cassia	十八銖 18 zhū	2.25g
大黃	dà huáng	Root of Rheum palmatum	二兩半 2.5 liǎng	7.5g
附子	fù zǐ	Lateral root of Aconitum carmi-chaeli	一兩六銖 1 liǎng 6 zhū	3.75g
當歸	dāng guī	Root of Angelica polimorpha	半兩 0.5 liǎng	1.5g

上二十味，為末，蜜和，更擣萬杵，丸如梧子大。空心酒服三丸，日三。不知，則加之至五六丸。下赤白青黃物如魚子者，病根出矣。

Pulverize the above twenty ingredients and mix with honey. Then pound [the medicine] again with ten thousand pestle strokes and form pills the size of firmiana seeds. On an empty stomach, take three pills in liquor three times a day. If no effect is noticed, increase [the dosage] to a maximum of five or six pills. When she discharges a red, white, blue-green, or yellow substance of a consistency like fish roe, this is the root of the disease coming out.

1. 胞中創 *bāo zhōng chuàng*: The *Sūn Zhēn Rén* edition has 胞中有瘡 *bāo zhōng yǒu chuāng* instead.
2. 紫蓋丸 *zǐ gài wán*: A purple canopy is one of the emperor's insignia and therefore denotes something of great value.

LINE 2.29

治月經不通，結成癥瘕如石，腹大骨立，宜此破血下癥方。

[The following] prerscription treats menstrual stoppage, [blood] binding and forming rocklike concretions and conglomerations, an enlarged abdomen and protruding bones.[1] [Patients] should take this prescription to break blood and precipitate the concretions.

Formula

大黃 消石（各六兩） 巴豆 蜀椒（各一兩） 代赭 柴胡（熬變色） 水蛭 丹參（熬令紫色） 土瓜根（各三兩） 乾漆 芎藭 乾薑 虻蟲 茯苓（各二兩）。

大黃	dà huáng	Root of Rheum palmatum	六兩 6 liǎng	18g
消石	xiāo shí	Niter	六兩 6 liǎng	18g
巴豆	bā dòu	Seed of Croton tiglium	一兩 1 liǎng	3g
蜀椒	shǔ jiāo	Seed capsules of Zanthoxylum bungeanum	一兩 1 liǎng	3g
代赭	dài zhě	Hematite	三兩 3 liǎng	9g
柴胡, 熬變色	chái hú, āo biàn sè	Root of Bupleurum chinense, slowly roasted until the color changes	三兩 3 liǎng	9g
水蛭	shuǐ zhì	Dried body of Whitmania pigra	三兩 3 liǎng	9g
丹參[2], 熬令紫色	dān shēn, āo lìng zǐ sè	Root of Salvia miltiorrhiza, slowly roasted until it is purple	三兩 3 liǎng	9g
土瓜根	tǔ guā gēn	Root of Trichosanthes cucumerina	三兩 3 liǎng	9g
乾漆	gān qī	Dried sap of Rhus verniciflua	二兩 2 liǎng	6g
川芎	chuān xiōng	Root of Ligusticum wallichii	二兩 2 liǎng	6g
乾薑	gān jiāng	Dried root of Zingiber officinale	二兩 2 liǎng	6g
虻蟲	méng chóng	Dried body of the female of Tabanus bivittatus	二兩 2 liǎng	6g
茯苓	fú líng	Dried fungus of Poria cocos	二兩 2 liǎng	6g

上十四味，為末，巴豆別研，蜜和丸如梧子。空心酒服二丸，未知加至五丸，日再服。

Pulverize the above fourteen ingredients, grinding the croton seed separately. Mix with honey into pills the size of firmiana seeds and take two pills [per dose] in liquor on an empty stomach. If no effect is noticed, increase [the dosage] to a maximum of five pills. Take two doses a day.

1. 骨立 *gǔ lì*: a sign of extreme wasting and emaciation.
2. The *Sūn Zhēn Rén* edition has *dān shā* (丹砂 Mercuric sulfide) instead.
3. *Sòng* editors' note: "The *Qiān Jīn Yì Fāng* does not use *chái hú* 柴胡, *shuǐ zhì* 水蛭, *dān shēn* 丹參, and *tǔ guā gēn* 土瓜根."

LINE 2.30

大虻蟲丸治月經不通六七年，或腫滿氣逆，腹脹瘕痛，宜服此，數有神驗方。

Major Tabanus Pills treat women's menstrual stoppage [that has lasted] for six or seven years, possibly with swelling, fullness, and *qì* counterflow, abdominal distention, conglomerations, and pain. These pills are suitable [for these conditions] and have achieved divine results on numerous occasions.

Major Tabanus Pills
大虻蟲丸 *dà méng chóng wán*

虻蟲（四百枚）蠐螬（一升）乾地黃 牡丹 乾漆 芍藥 牛膝 土瓜根 桂心（各四兩）吳茱萸 桃仁 黃芩 牡蒙（各三兩）茯苓 海藻（各五兩）水蛭（三百枚）芒消（一兩）人參（一兩半）䗪蟲（五合）。

虻蟲	méng chóng	Dried body of the female of Tabanus bivittatus	四百枚 400 méi	400 pcs
蠐螬	qí cáo	Dried larva of Holotrichia diomphalia	一升 1 shēng	24g
乾地黃	gān dì huáng	Dried root of Rehmannia glutinosa	四兩 4 liǎng	12g
牡丹	mǔ dān	Bark of the root of Paeonia suffruticosa	四兩 4 liǎng	12g
乾漆	gān qī	Dried sap of Rhus verniciflua	四兩 4 liǎng	12g
芍藥	sháo yào	Root of Paeonia albiflora	四兩 4 liǎng	12g
土瓜根	tǔ guā gēn	Root of Trichosanthes cucumerina	四兩 4 liǎng	12g
桂心	guì xīn	Shaved inner bark of Cinnamomum cassia	四兩 4 liǎng	12g
吳茱萸	wú zhū yú	Unripe fruit of Evodia rutaecarpa	三兩 3 liǎng	9g
桃仁	táo rén	Seed of Prunus persica	三兩 3 liǎng	9g
黃芩	huáng qín	Root of Scutellaria baicalensis	三兩 3 liǎng	9g
牡蒙	mǔ méng	Root of Paris quadrifolia	三兩 3 liǎng	9g
茯苓	fú líng	Dried fungus of Poria cocos	五兩 5 liǎng	15g

海藻	hǎi zǎo	Whole plant of Sargassum fusiforme	五兩 5 liǎng	15g
水蛭	shuǐ zhì	Dried body of Whitmania pigra	三百枚 300 méi	300 pcs
硭硝	máng xiāo	Hydrated sodium sulfate	一兩 1 liǎng	3g
人參	rén shēn	Root of Panax ginseng	一兩半 1.5 liǎng	4.5g
葶藶	tíng lì	Seed of Lepidium apetalum	五合 5 gě	35ml

上十九味，為末，蜜和丸如梧子大。每日空心酒下七丸，不知加之，日三服。

Pulverize the above nineteen ingredients and mix with honey into pills the size of firmiana seeds. Every day, down seven pills [per dose] in liquor on an empty stomach. If no effect is noticed, increase [the dosage]. Take three doses a day.[1,2]

1. This sentence is missing in the *Sūn Zhēn Rén* edition, which could mean either a textual error or a considerable difference in use, as the prescription would then instruct to take only one dose per day.
2. *Sòng* editors' note: "The *Qiān Jīn Yì Fāng* does not use *máng xiāo* 硭硝 or *rén shēn* 人參."

LINE 2.31

桂心酒治月經不通，結成癥瘕方。

Shaved Cinnamon Bark Wine treats menstrual stoppage and [blood] binding and forming concretions and conglomerations.

Shaved Cinnamon Bark Wine
桂心酒 *guì xīn jiǔ*

桂心 牡丹 芍藥 牛膝 乾漆 土瓜根 牡蒙（各四兩） 吳茱萸（一升） 大黃（三兩） 黃芩 乾薑（各二兩） 虻蟲（二百枚） 蟅蟲 螬蟷 水蛭（各七十枚） 亂髮灰 細辛（各一兩） 殭蠶（五十枚） 大麻仁 竈突墨（三升） 乾地黃（六兩） 虎杖根 鱉甲（各五兩） 菴䕡子（二升）。

桂心	guì xīn	Shaved inner bark of Cinnamomum cassia	四兩 4 liǎng	12g
牡丹	mǔ dān	Bark of the root of Paeonia suffruticosa	四兩 4 liǎng	12g

芍藥	sháo yào	Root of Paeonia albiflora	四兩 4 liǎng	12g
牛膝	niú xī	Root of Achyranthes bidentata	四兩 4 liǎng	12g
乾漆	gān qī	Dried sap of Rhus verniciflua	四兩 4 liǎng	12g
土瓜根	tǔ guā gēn	Root of Trichosanthes cucumerina	四兩 4 liǎng	12g
牡蒙	mǔ méng	Root of Paris quadrifolia	四兩 4 liǎng	12g
吳茱萸	wú zhū yú	Unripe fruit of Evodia rutaecarpa	一升 1 shēng	24g
大黃	dà huáng	Root of Rheum palmatum	三兩 3 liǎng	9g
黃芩	huáng qín	Root of Scutellaria baicalensis	二兩 2 liǎng	6g
乾薑	gān jiāng	Dried root of Zingiber officinale	二兩 2 liǎng	6g
虻蟲	méng chóng	Dried body of the female of Tabanus bivittatus	二百枚 200 méi	200 pcs
蟅蟲	zhè chóng	Entire dried body of the female of Eupolyphaga sinensis	七十枚 70 méi	70 pcs
蠐螬	qí cáo	Dried larva of Holotrichia diomphalia	七十枚 70 méi	70 pcs
水蛭	shuǐ zhì	Dried body of Whitmania pigra	七十枚 70 méi	70 pcs
亂髮灰	luàn fà huī	Matted hair ash	一兩 1 liǎng	3g
細辛	xì xīn	Complete plant including root of Asarum heteropoides	一兩 1 liǎng	3g
殭蠶	jiāng cán	Dried 4th or 5th stage larva of the moth of Bombyx mori	五十枚 50 méi	50 pcs
大麻仁	dà má rén	Seed of Cannabis sativa	三升 3 shēng	72g
灶突墨	zào tú mò	Stove-pipe soot	三升 3 shēng	72g
乾地黃	gān dì huáng	Dried root of Rehmannia glutinosa	六兩 6 liǎng	18g
虎杖根	hǔ zhàng gēn	Root of Polygonum cuspidatum	五兩 5 liǎng	15g
鱉甲	biē jiǎ	Dorsal shell of Amyda sinensis	五兩 5 liǎng	15g
菴䕡子	ān lǘ zǐ	Fruit of Artemisia keiskeana	二升 2 shēng	48g

上二十四味，㕮咀，以酒四斗分兩甕，浸之七日併一甕盛，攪令調，還分作兩甕。初服二合，日二，加至三四合。

Pound the above twenty-four ingredients. [Combine with] four *dǒu* of liquor and divide into two jars. Soak [the drugs] for seven days and then pack all into one jar, stir until they are distibuted evenly, then divide them again into two jars. Initially, take two *gě* twice a day, increasing [the dosage] to a maximum of three or four *gě*.

LINE 2.32

虎杖煎治腹內積聚，虛脹雷鳴，四肢沈重，月經不通，亦治丈夫病方。

Bushy Knotweed Brew treats accumulations and gatherings in the abdomen, vacuity distention and thunderous rumbling, heaviness of the four limbs, and menstrual stoppage. It also treats men's diseases.*

Bushy Knotweed Brew
虎杖煎 *hŭ zhàng jiān*

取高地虎杖根，細剉二斛，以水二石五斗煮取一大斗半，去滓，澄濾令淨，取好淳酒五升和煎，令如餳。每服一合，消息為度，不知則加之。

Pick *hŭ zhàng gēn* (虎杖根 Root of Polygonum cuspidatum) from a high elevation. Break it into fine pieces [and prepare] two *hú*. Decoct it in two *shí* and five *dŏu* of water to obtain one and a half large *dŏu*. Discard the dregs and let the impurities settle to the ground until [the decoction] has cleared. Mix it with five *shēng* of high-quality hard liquor and simmer it down to a syrupy consistency. For each dose, take one *gĕ*. Measure [the effect of the medicine] by whether [the abdominal masses] have disappeared. If no effect is noticed, increase [the dosage].

*   This last sentence is missing in the *Sūn Zhēn Rén* edition.

LINE 2.33

又方治月經閉不通，結瘕，腹大如甕，短氣欲死方。

Another prescription: for treating menstrual block or stoppage, binds and conglomerations, an abdomen enlarged to the size of a jar, and shortage of *qì* to the point of expiry.*

Formula

虎杖根（百斤，去頭去土，暴乾，切）土瓜根 牛膝（各取汁二斗）。

虎杖根, 去頭去土，暴乾，切	hŭ zhàng gēn, qù tóu qù tŭ, bào gān, qiē	Root of Polygonum cuspidatum, with tips and dirt removed, dried in the sun, and chopped	百斤 100 jīn	4,800g
土瓜根, 取汁	tŭ guā gēn, qŭ zhī	Root of Trichosanthes cucumerina juice	二斗 2 dŏu	1400ml
牛膝, 取汁	niú xī, qŭ zhī	Root of Achyranthes bidentata juice	二斗 2 dŏu	1400ml

上三味，㕮咀，以水一斛浸虎杖根一宿，明旦煎取二斗，內土瓜，牛膝

汁，攪令調勻，煎令如餳。每以酒服一合，日再夜一，宿血當下。若病去，
止服。

Pound the above three ingredients. Soak the *hǔ zhàng gēn* 虎杖根 in one *hú* of water overnight, and on the next morning simmer it to obtain two *dǒu*. Add the *tǔ guā gēn* 土瓜根 and *niú xī* 牛膝 juice, stir until evenly blended, and simmer down to a syrupy consistency. Take one *gě* for each [dose] in liquor, twice during the day and once at night. This should precipitate the blood overnight. When the disease has been removed, stop taking it.

*   This and the following four prescriptions are found at the very end of this section in the *Sūn Zhēn Rén* edition.

LINE 2.34

桃仁煎治帶下，經閉不通方。

Peach Kernel Brew treats vaginal discharge and menstrual block or stoppage.

Peach Kernel Brew
桃仁煎 *táo rén jiān*

桃仁 虻蟲（各一升）朴消（五兩）大黃（六兩）。

桃仁	táo rén	Seed of Prunus persica	一升 1 shēng	24g
虻蟲	méng chóng	Dried body of the female of Tabanus bivittatus	一升 1 shēng	24g
朴消	pò xiāo	Impure mirabilite	五兩 5 liǎng	15g
大黃	dà huáng	Root of Rheum palmatum	六兩 6 liǎng	18g

上四味，為末，別治桃仁，以醇苦酒四升內銅鐺中，炭火煎取二升，下大黃，桃仁，虻蟲，等攪勿住手，當欲可丸，下朴消，更攪勿住手，良久出之，可丸乃止。取一丸如雞子黃投酒中，預一宿勿食服之。至晡時，下如大豆汁，或如雞肝，凝血，蝦蟆子，或如膏，此是病下也。

Pulverize the above four ingredients. Finely pestle the *táo rén* 桃仁 separately. Take four *shēng* of concentrated bitter liquor, pour it into a copper pan, and simmer it over a charcoal fire to obtain two *shēng*. Add the *dà huáng* 大黃, *táo rén* 桃仁, *méng chóng* 虻蟲, and stir it evenly* without stopping until it is [thickened to a consistency] where you can form pills. Add the *pò xiāo* 朴消 and stir it again without stopping. After a good long while, remove it [from the fire]. Stop only when [it is thickened sufficiently that] you can form pills. Take a pill the size of an egg yolk and immerse it in liquor. In preparation, fast overnight and then take it. By late afternoon, she will discharge a substance like soybean juice, chicken liver, congealed blood, frog eggs, or lard. This is the disease being discharged.

* 等攪 *děng jiǎo*: Modern critical editions punctuate between 等 and 攪, suggesting an interpretation of 等 in the sense of "and the other ingredients/etc.," as it occurs frequently throughout the text when it follows a list of medicinals. Given the fact that there are no other ingredients in this prescription except for the mirabilite, which is added later, this reading is unlikely. An alternative interpretation of 等 as "in equal proportions" is even less likely because this meaning is found only in the compound 等分 *děng fēn* throughout the rest of the text. It does, moreover, not make sense here since the amount of each medicinal is clearly stated above.

LINE 2.35

治月經不通，臍下堅結，大如杯升，發熱往來，下痢羸瘦，此為氣瘕（一作血瘕）。若生肉癥，不可為也。療之之方。

[The following] prescription treats menstrual stoppage, hard knots below the navel that are the size of a *shēng*-sized cup, intermittent fever, diarrhea, and marked emaciation. This [condition] means *qì* conglomerations (another [edition?] has blood conglomerations).[1] If she has formed flesh concretions,[2] it means that it cannot be treated. This prescription is for curing [the *qì* conglomerations].

Formula

生地黃（三十斤，取汁）乾漆（一斤，為末）。

生地黃, 取汁	shēng dì huáng, qǔ zhī	Fresh root of Rehmannia glutinosa juice	三十斤 30 jīn	1440g
乾漆, 為末	gān qī, wéi mò	Dried sap of Rhus verniciflua, pulverized	一斤 1 jīn	48g

上二味，以漆末內地黃汁中，微火煎令可丸。每服酒下如梧子大三丸，不知加之，常以食後服。

Of the two ingredients above, put the pulverized *gān qī* 乾漆 into the *[shēng] dì huáng zhī* 生地黃汁 juice and simmer over a small flame until [it has thickened enough that] you can make pills. For each dose, down three pills the size of firmiana seeds in liquor. If no effect is noticed, increase [the dosage]. Take it consistently after meals.

1.   The *Sūn Zhēn Rén* edition adds here the words: 可治 *kě zhì* (which is treatable).
2.   肉癥 *ròu zhēng*: This means that the condition has progressed to the point where the masses have a palpable, solid shape.

LINE 2.36

治月經不通，甚極閉塞方。

[The following] prescription treats menstrual stoppage and the most severe type of blockage.

Formula

牛膝（一斤）麻子（三升，蒸）土瓜根（三兩）桃仁（二升）。

牛膝	niú xī	Root of Achyranthes bidentata	一斤 1 jīn	250g
麻子, 蒸	má zǐ, zhēng	Seed of Cannabis sativa, toasted	三升 3 shēng	72g
土瓜根	tǔ guā gēn	Root of Trichosanthes cucumerina	三升 3 shēng	72g
桃仁	táo rén	Seed of Prunus persica	二升 2 shēng	48g

上四味，㕮咀，以好酒一斗五升浸五宿。一服五合，漸加至一升，日三，能多益佳。

Pound the above four ingredients and soak in one *dǒu* and five *shēng* of high-grade liquor for five nights. Take five *gě* per dose, gradually increasing [the dosage] to a maximum of one *shēng*, three times a day. If she is able to drink a lot, the benefits are even better.*

*   This last sentence is not found in the *Sūn Zhēn Rén* edition. It could therefore be an addition by the *Sòng* editors.

LINE 2.37

治產後風冷，留血不去，停結，月水閉塞方。

[The following] prescription treats postpartum wind-cold, failure to remove retained blood, collecting and binding [blood], and menstrual block.

Formula

桃仁 麻子仁（各二升） 菴閭子（一升）。

桃仁	táo rén	Seed of Prunus persica	二升 2 shēng	48g
麻子仁	má zǐ rén	Seed of Cannabis sativa	二升 2 shēng	48g
菴閭子	ān lǘ zǐ	Fruit of Artemisia keiskeana	一升 1 shēng	24g

上三味，㕮咀，以好酒三斗浸五宿。每服五合，日三，稍加至一升。

Pound the above three ingredients and soak in three *dǒu* of high-grade liquor for five nights. Take five *gě* per dose three times a day, gradually increasing [the dosage] to a maximum of one *shēng*.

LINE 2.38

五京丸治婦人腹中積聚，九痛七害，及腰中冷引小腹，害食，得冷便下方。

Five Jīng Pills treat women's accumulations and gatherings in the center of the abdomen, nine pains and seven damages,[1] as well as coldness in the center of the lumbus stretching to the lower abdomen, food damage,[2] and vaginal discharge after contracting cold.[3]

Five Jīng Pills
五京丸 *wǔ jīng wán*

乾薑 蜀椒（各三兩） 附子（一兩） 吳茱萸（一升） 當歸 狼毒 黃芩 牡蠣（各二兩）。

乾薑	gān jiāng	Dried root of Zingiber officinale	三兩 3 liǎng	9g
蜀椒	shǔ jiāo	Seed capsules of Zanthoxylum bungeanum	三兩 3 liǎng	9g
附子	fù zǐ	Lateral root of Aconitum carmichaeli	一兩 1 liǎng	3g
吳茱萸	wú zhū yú	Unripe fruit of Evodia rutaecarpa	一升 1 shēng	24g
當歸	dāng guī	Root of Angelica polimorpha	二兩 2 liǎng	6g
狼毒	láng dú	Root of Stellera chamaejasme	二兩 2 liǎng	6g
黃芩	huáng qín	Root of Scutellaria baicalensis	二兩 2 liǎng	6g
牡蠣	mǔ lì	Shell of Ostrea rivularis	二兩 2 liǎng	6g

上八味，為末，蜜和丸如梧子。初服三丸，日二，加至十丸。此出京氏五

君，故名五京。久患冷困當服之。

Pulverize the above eight ingredients and mix with honey into pills the size of firmiana seeds. Initially take three pills twice a day, then increase [the dosage] to a maximum of ten pills. This prescription has come from the five gentlemen from the Jīng clan[4] and is therefore called "Five Jīng." You should take these for chronic problems with cold encumbrance.

1. 九痛七害 *jiǔ tòng qī hài*: This phrase is part of a standard list of thirty-six types of vaginal discharge that is already found in the *Bìng Yuán Lùn*. It is cited in its entirety below in chapter three of volume four, Line 3.1 (pp. 466 - 468).
2. 害食 *hài shí*: Damage to the body in general, but especially the spleen and stomach, caused by the improper intake or digestion of food. Diet-related conditions are one of the standard "five evils" (五邪 *wǔ xié*) to affect the viscera. The following explanation is found in the *Nàn Jīng*: "Drinking and eating [without restraint], as well as weariness and exhaustion, harm the spleen.... What is meant by 'the five evils'? It is like this. To be hit by wind, to be harmed by heat, to drink and eat [without restraint], as well as weariness and exhaustion, to be harmed by cold, to be hit by humidity, these [conditions] are called the five evils." (《難經》 49, translated in Unschuld, *Nan-ching*, pp. 457-458. See also his translations of several commentaries related to food-damage in the following pages, esp. pp. 464-465).
3. The following prescriptions in this section are missing in the *Sūn Zhēn Rén* edition. The text resumes with the next chapter.
4. 京氏五君 *jīng shì wǔ jūn*: The Jīng clan produced several famous members during the *Hàn* dynasty. The "five gentlemen" therefore apparently refers to five illustrious members of this clan whose exact identity is, however, unclear.

LINE 2.39

雞鳴紫丸治婦人癥瘕積聚方。

Cockcrow Purple Pills treat women's concretions, conglomerations, accumulations, and gatherings.[1]

Cockcrow Purple Pills
雞鳴紫丸 *jī míng zǐ wán*

皂莢（一分）藜蘆 甘草 礬石 烏喙 杏仁 乾薑 桂心 巴豆（各二分）前胡 人參（各四分）代赭（五分）阿膠（六分）大黃（八分）。

皂莢	zào jiá	Fruit of Gleditsia sinensis	一分 1 fēn	.75g
藜蘆	lí lú	Root and rhizome of Veratrum nigrum	二分 2 fēn	1.5g

甘草	gān cǎo	Root of Glycyrrhiza uralensis	二分 2 fēn	1.5g
礬石	fán shí	Alum	二分 2 fēn	1.5g
烏喙	wū huì	Main tuber of Aconitum carmichaeli	二分 2 fēn	1.5g
杏仁	xìng rén	Dried seed of Prunus armeniaca	二分 2 fēn	1.5g
乾薑	gān jiāng	Dried root of Zingiber officinale	二分 2 fēn	1.5g
桂心	guì xīn	Shaved inner bark of Cinnamomum cassia	二分 2 fēn	1.5g
巴豆	bā dòu	Seed of Croton tiglium	二分 2 fēn	1.5g
前胡	qián hú	Root of Peucedanum praeruptorum	四分 4 fēn	3g
人參	rén shēn	Root of Panax ginseng	四分 4 fēn	3g
代赭	dài zhě	Hematite	五分 5 fēn	3.75g
阿膠	ē jiāo	Gelatinous glue produced from Equus asinus	五分 6 fēn	4.5g
大黃	dà huáng	Root of Rheum palmatum	八分 8 fēn	6g

上十四味，為末，蜜丸如梧子。雞鳴時服一丸，日益一丸，至五丸止，仍從一起。下白者，風也；赤者，癥瘕也；青微黃者，心腹病。

Pulverize the above fourteen ingredients and mix with honey into pills the size of firmiana seeds. At the time of the cockcrow watch, take one pill. Daily increase [the dosage] by one pill up to five pills, then stop and begin again from one [pill a day]. If the discharge is white, it indicates wind;[2] if red, it indicates concretions and conglomerations; if green or slightly yellow, it indicates a disease of the heart or abdomen.

1. The name of the pills is related to the instructions below to take the pills at the time of the cockcrow watch, i.e., at 1-3 a.m.
2. This means that wind is identified as the etiological agent.

LINE 2.40

遼東都尉所上丸治臍下堅癖，無所不治方。

Pills Presented by the Commander-in-Chief of Liáo-Dōng treat hard aggregations below the navel. There are none that this prescription cannot treat.

Pills Presented by the Commander-in-Chief of Liáo-Dōng
遼東都尉所上丸 *liáo dōng dū wèi suǒ shàng wán*

恆山 大黃 巴豆（各一分）天雄（二枚）苦參 白薇 乾薑 人參 細辛 狼牙

龍膽 沙參 玄參 丹參（各三分） 芍藥 附子 牛膝 茯苓（各五分） 牡蒙（四分） 萑蘆（六分）。

恒山	héng shān	Root of Dichroa febrifuga	一分 1 fēn	.75g
大黃	dà huáng	Root of Rheum palmatum	一分 1 fēn	.75g
巴豆	bā dòu	Seed of Croton tiglium	一分 1 fēn	.75g
天雄	tiān xióng	Mature root of Aconitum carmichaeli	二枚 2 méi	2 pcs
苦參	kǔ shēn	Root of Sophora flavescens	三分 3 fēn	2.25g
白薇	bái wēi	Root of Cynanchum atratum	三分 3 fēn	2.25g
乾薑	gān jiāng	Dried root of Zingiber officinale	三分 3 fēn	2.25g
人參	rén shēn	Root of Panax ginseng	三分 3 fēn	2.25g
細辛	xì xīn	Complete plant including root of Asarum heteropoides	三分 3 fēn	2.25g
狼牙	láng yá	Root of Potentilla cryptotaenia	三分 3 fēn	2.25g
龍膽	lóng dǎn	Root and rhizome of Gentiana scabra	三分 3 fēn	2.25g
沙參	shā shēn	Root of Adenophora tetraphylla	三分 3 fēn	2.25g
玄參	xuán shēn	Root of Scrophularia ningpoensis	三分 3 fēn	2.25g
丹參	dān shēn	Root of Salvia miltiorrhiza	三分 3 fēn	2.25g
芍藥	sháo yào	Root of Paeonia albiflora	五分 5 fēn	3.75g
附子	fù zǐ	Lateral root of Aconitum carmichaeli	五分 5 fēn	3.75g
牛膝	niú xī	Root of Achyranthes bidentata	五分 5 fēn	3.75g
茯苓	fú líng	Dried fungus of Poria cocos	五分 5 fēn	3.75g
牡蒙	mǔ méng	Root of Paris quadrifolia	四分 4 fēn	3g
萑蘆	guàn lú	Guànlú fungus	五分 6 fēn[1]	4.5g

上二十味，為末，蜜丸。宿勿食，服五丸，日三。大羸瘦，月水不調，當二十五日服之，下長蟲，或下種種病，出二十五日服，中所苦悉愈，肌膚盛，五十日萬病除，斷緒者有子。

Pulverize the above twenty ingredients and [mix with] honey into pills [the size of firmiana seeds]. After fasting overnight, take five pills three times a day. In cases of extreme emaciation with menstrual irregularities, she should take it for twenty-five days. She will discharge long worms or all kinds of diseases. After taking it for more than twenty-five days, she will completely recover from what bothered her in the center [of the abdomen][2] and her flesh and skin will become exuberant. After fifty days, [all her] myriad illnesses will be eliminated, and, in cases of infertility, she will be with child.

1. 服中所苦 *fú zhōng suǒ kǔ*: My insertion is based on the version of this prescription in the *Qiān Jīn Yì Fāng*, which has 腹 *fù* (abdomen) instead of 服 *fú* "to take."
2. *Sòng* editors' note: "Another [version of this] prescription says 2 *liǎng* 3 *fēn* of *guàn lú* 藋蘆."

LINE 2.41

牡蠣丸治經閉不通 , 不欲飲食方。

Oyster Shell Pills treat menstrual block and stoppage with no desire for food and drink.

Oyster Shell Pills
牡蠣丸 *mǔ lì wán*

牡蠣 (四兩) 大黃 (一斤) 柴胡 (五兩) 乾薑 (三兩) 芎藭 茯苓 (各二兩半) 蜀椒 (十兩) 葶藶子 芒消 杏仁 (各五合) 水蛭 虻蟲 (各半兩) 桃仁 (七十枚)。

牡蠣	mǔ lì	Shell of Ostrea rivularis	四兩 4 liǎng	12g
大黃	dà huáng	Root of Rheum palmatum	一斤 1 jīn	48g
柴胡	chái hú	Root of Bupleurum chinense	五兩 5 liǎng	15g
乾薑	gān jiāng	Dried root of Zingiber officinale	三兩 3 liǎng	9g
川芎	chuān xiōng	Root of Ligusticum wallichii	二兩半 2.5 liǎng	7.5g
茯苓	fú líng	Dried fungus of Poria cocos	二兩半 2.5 liǎng	7.5g
蜀椒	shǔ jiāo	Seed capsules of Zanthoxylum bungeanum	十兩 10 liǎng	30g
葶藶子	tíng lì zǐ	Seed of Lepidium apetalum	五合 5 gě	35ml
硭硝	máng xiāo	Hydrated sodium sulfate	五合 5 gě	35ml
杏仁	xìng rén	Dried seed of Prunus armeniaca	五合 5 gě	35ml
水蛭	shuǐ zhì	Dried body of Whitmania pigra	半兩 0.5 liǎng	1.5g
虻蟲	méng chóng	Dried body of the female of Tabanus bivittatus	半兩 0.5 liǎng	1.5g
桃仁	táo rén	Seed of Prunus persica	七十枚 70 méi	70 pcs

上十三味 , 為末 , 蜜丸如梧子大。飲服七丸 , 日三。

Pulverize the above thirteen ingredients and mix with honey into pills the size of firmiana seeds. Take seven pills in fluid three times a day.

LINE 2.42

當歸丸治腰腹痛，月水不通利方。

Chinese Angelica Pills treat lumbar and abdominal pain and menstrual stoppage or inhibition.

Chinese Angelica Pills
當歸丸 *dāng guī wán*

當歸 芎藭（各四兩） 虻蟲 烏頭 丹參 乾漆（各一兩） 人參 牡蠣 土瓜根 水蛭（各二兩） 桃仁（五十枚）。

當歸	dāng guī	Root of Angelica polimorpha	四兩 4 liǎng	12g
川芎	chuān xiōng	Root of Ligusticum wallichii	四兩 4 liǎng	12g
虻蟲	méng chóng	Dried body of the female of Tabanus bivittatus	一兩 1 liǎng	3g
烏頭	wū tóu	Main tuber of Aconitum carmichaeli	一兩 1 liǎng	3g
丹參	dān shēn	Root of Salvia miltiorrhiza	一兩 1 liǎng	3g
乾漆	gān qī	Dried sap of Rhus verniciflua	一兩 1 liǎng	3g
人參	rén shēn	Root of Panax ginseng	二兩 2 liǎng	6g
牡蠣	mǔ lì	Shell of Ostrea rivularis	二兩 2 liǎng	6g
土瓜根	tǔ guā gēn	Root of Trichosanthes cucumerina	二兩 2 liǎng	6g
水蛭	shuǐ zhì	Dried body of Whitmania pigra	二兩 2 liǎng	6g
桃仁	táo rén	Seed of Prunus persica	五十枚 50 méi	50 pcs

上十一味，為末，以白蜜丸如梧子大。酒下三丸，日三服。

Pulverize the above eleven ingredients and mix with white honey into pills the size of firmiana seeds. Down three pills in liquor three times a day.

LINE 2.43

消石湯治血瘕，月水留，瘀血大不通，下病，散堅血方。

Niter Decoction treats blood conglomerations, retained menses, and static blood [causing] enlargement and stoppage, by precipitating the disease and dissipating the hardened blood.

Niter Decoction
硝石湯 *xiāo shí tāng*

消石 附子 虻蟲 (各三兩) 大黃 細辛 乾薑 黃芩 (各一兩) 芍藥 土瓜根 丹參 代赭 蠐螬 (各二兩) 大棗 (十枚) 桃仁 (二升) 牛膝 (一斤) 朴消 (四兩) 。

消石	xiāo shí	Niter	三兩 3 liǎng	9g
附子	fù zǐ	Lateral root of Aconitum carmichaeli	三兩 3 liǎng	9g
虻蟲	méng chóng	Dried body of the female of Tabanus bivittatus	三兩 3 liǎng	9g
大黃	dà huáng	Root of Rheum palmatum	一兩 1 liǎng	3g
細辛	xì xīn	Complete plant including root of Asarum heteropoides	一兩 1 liǎng	3g
乾薑	gān jiāng	Dried root of Zingiber officinale	一兩 1 liǎng	3g
黃芩	huáng qín	Root of Scutellaria baicalensis	一兩 1 liǎng	3g
芍藥	sháo yào	Root of Paeonia albiflora	二兩 2 liǎng	6g
土瓜根	tǔ guā gēn	Root of Trichosanthes cucumerina	二兩 2 liǎng	6g
丹參	dān shēn	Root of Salvia miltiorrhiza	二兩 2 liǎng	6g
代赭	dài zhě	Hematite	二兩 2 liǎng	6g
蠐螬	qí cáo	Dried larva of Holotrichia diomphalia	二兩 2 liǎng	6g
大棗	dà zǎo	Mature fruit of Ziziphus jujuba	十枚 10 méi	10 pcs
桃仁	táo rén	Seed of Prunus persica	二升 2 shēng	48g
牛膝	niú xī	Root of Achyranthes bidentata	一斤 1 jīn	48g
朴消	pò xiāo	Impure mirabilite	四兩 4 liǎng	12g

上十六味，㕮咀，以酒五升，水九升漬藥一宿，明旦煎取四升，去滓，下朴消，消石烊盡。分四服，相去如炊頃。去病後食黃鴨羹，勿見風。

Pound the above sixteen ingredients. Soak the drugs in five *shēng* of liquor and nine *shēng* of water overnight. On the next morning, simmer it to obtain four *shēng* and discard the dregs. Add the *pò xiāo* 朴消 and *xiāo shí* 消石 and let them melt completely. Divide it into four doses and separate them from each other by the time it takes to cook a meal. After the disease abates, eat yellow duck broth and avoid exposure to wind.

465

3. Red and White Vaginal Discharge, Center Flooding, and Vaginal Spotting
赤白帶下，崩中，漏下

Translator's note: The order of prescriptions in this section varies substantially between editions. The introductory essay and the following prescription are found in the middle of the section in the *Sūn Zhēn Rén* edition.

LINE 3.1

(一) 論曰：諸方說三十六疾者，十二癥，九痛，七害，五傷，三痼不通是也。(二) 何謂十二癥？是所下之物，一曰狀如膏，二曰如黑血，三曰如紫汁，四曰如赤肉，五曰如膿痂，六曰如豆汁，七曰如葵羹，八曰如凝血，九曰如清血，血似水，十曰如米泔，十一曰如月浣乍前乍卻，十二曰經度不應期也。(三) 何謂九痛？一曰陰中痛傷，二曰陰中淋瀝痛，三曰小便即痛，四曰寒冷痛，五曰經來即腹中痛，六曰氣滿痛，七曰汁出陰中，如有蟲嚙痛，八曰脅下分痛，九曰腰胯痛。(四) 何謂七害？一曰窮孔痛不利，二曰中寒熱痛，三曰小腹急堅痛，四曰藏不仁，五曰子門不端引背痛，六曰月浣乍多乍少，七曰害吐。(五) 何謂五傷？一曰兩脅支滿痛，二曰心痛引脅，三曰氣結不通，四曰邪思洩利，五曰前後痼寒。(六) 何謂三痼？一曰羸瘦不生肌膚，二曰絕產乳，三曰經水閉塞。(七) 病有異同，具治之方。

(1) Essay:[1]The "thirty-six diseases" referred to in the various prescription texts consist of the "twelve concretions," the "nine pains," the "seven injuries," the "five damages," and the "three intractable diseases of stoppage."

(2) What do the so-called "twelve concretions" refer to? These [are differentiated by] the substance that is discharged: The first one is called "resembling lard;"[2] the second, "resembling black blood;" the third, "resembling purple liquid;" the fourth, "resembling red flesh;" the fifth, "resembling scabby pus;" the sixth, "resembling bean juice;" the seventh, "resembling mallow broth;" the eighth, "resembling congealed blood;" the ninth, "resembling fresh, watery blood;" the tenth, "resembling rice water;" the eleventh, "resembling the monthly 'rinse,'[3] now early, now withheld;" the twelfth, "resembling the regular amount of her menses, but not corresponding to the proper time."

(3) What do the so-called "nine pains" refer to? The first one is called "pain from wounds

in the vagina;" the second, "dribbling and pain in the vagina;" the third, "pain upon urination;" the fourth, "coldness pain;" the fifth, "abdominal pain at the onset of menstruation;" the sixth, "*qì* fullness pain;" the seventh, "liquid discharge in the vagina with gnawing pain as if from worms;" the eighth, "pain in both rib-sides separately;" the ninth, "lumbar and hip pain."

(4) What do the so-called "seven injuries" refer to?[4] The first one is called "pain with inhibition of the orifices and holes;"[5] the second, "pain with cold or heat strike;" the third "pain with tension and hardness in the lower abdomen;" the fourth, "discomfort of the viscera;" the fifth, "a crooked infant's gate with pain stretching to the back;" the sixth, "a monthly 'rinse' that is now excessive now scanty;" the seventh, "injury from vomiting."[6]

(5) What do the so-called "five damages" refer to? The first one is called "propping fullness and pain in both rib-sides;" the second, "heart pain stretching to the rib-sides;" the third, "*qì* bind and stoppage;" the fourth, "evil thoughts diarrhea;"[7] the fifth, "intractable cold from beginning to end."

(6) What do the so-called "three intractable diseases" refer to? The first one is called "marked emaciation and failure to engender flesh and skin;" the second, "interruption of childbearing;" the third, "menstrual block."[8]

(7) Among [these] diseases, there are differences and commonalities. Here are prescriptions to treat them all.

1.   This entire essay is an almost literal quotation from the *Bìng Yuán Lùn* (《病源論》 38:50). The most relevant discrepancies are stated in the following notes. This essay is also quoted in the *Ishimpô* (《醫心方》 21:24) in a version that is much closer to the *Bìng Yuán Lùn* than to the *Qiān Jīn Fāng*, suggesting that the current *Bìng Yuán Lùn* version is one of the earliest sources for this categorization.

2.   膏 *gāo*: the soft fat rendered from horn-less animals such as pigs.

3.   月浣 *yuè huàn*: a reference to menstruation that apparently emphasizes the physiological function of flushing the uterus of stale blood. This is not a standard medical term.

4.   The following five names are found in the *Bìng Yuán Lùn* as the names of the five damages. The seven injuries are there listed as "first, injury from food; second, injury from *qì*; third, injury from cold; fourth, injury from taxation; fifth, injury from sexual activity; sixth, injury from pregnancy; and seventh, injury from sleep." (《病源論》 38:50). The names listed by Sūn Sī-Miǎo for the five damages are not found at all in the *Bìng Yuán Lùn* and are therefore most probably a later addition, whether by Sūn Sī-Miǎo himself or the editor of Sūn Sī-Miǎo's source. The alterations in the *Qiān Jīn Fāng* might seem minor, but do indicate an increase in medical knowledge about women's health and a greater awareness of and attention to the anatomical particularities of the female body. The *Bìng Yuán Lùn* list of the five damages, for example, is much less gender-specific and reminiscent of other, non-gendered lists such as the "five taxations and seven damages" found in the *Jīn Guì Yào Luè*. Sūn Sī-Miǎo's enumeration, in contrast, reflects a heightened awareness of the diagnostic and etiological subtleties specific to the treatment of women. This observation supports the argument that the *Qiān Jīn Fāng* represents a significant step in the creation of a full-fledged Chinese gynecology.

5.   竅孔 *qiào kǒng*: This expression could refer generally to the body's nine orifices (九竅 *jiǔ qiào*), i.e., the two ears, two eyes, two nostrils, mouth, anus and vagina. In the context

of this essay, however, it should probably be interpreted in a narrower sense as referring only to the lower orifices of the anus and vagina. This restricted sense is supported by the fact that the earlier version of this essay found in the *Bìng Yuán Lùn* has 窮孔 *qióng kǒng* (extremity hole) here. While this is not a standard expression, the character 窮 is used in several compounds to refer to the pelvic area, such as 窮骨 *qióng gǔ* (sacrum) and 窮端 *qióng duān* (coccyx). A modern commentary on the essay as it is cited in the *Ishimpô* paraphrases this term as 陰道口 *yīn dào kǒu* (entrance to the vagina) (《醫心方》21:24, p. 438, n. 7).

6. 害吐 *hài tù*. The *Sūn Zhēn Rén* edition has 喜吐 *xǐ tù* (tendency to vomit) instead, which does not substantially alter the meaning of the text.

7. 邪思洩利 *xié sī xiè lì*: This refers to diarrhea induced by evil thoughts. Alternatively, and perhaps more likely, the modern editors of the *Sūn Zhēn Rén* edition and the *Rén Mín* edition interpret this as a textual corruption and read 思 *sī* as 惡 *è*, based on the *Ishimpô* version of this essay. The meaning of the whole phrase would then be "malignity diarrhea."

8. The *Bìng Yuán Lùn* also cites the first name, but then continues: "As for the remaining two, the literature is deficient and does not record them." (《病源論》38:50). It concludes: "The thirty-six types of diseases mentioned by Zhāng Zhòng-Jǐng are all caused by cold and heat and taxation damage to the uterus, which is why women suffer from vaginal discharge..."

LINE 3.2

白堊丸治女人三十六疾方。

Chalk Pills treat women's thirty-six diseases.[1]

Chalk Pills
白堊丸 *bái è wán*

白堊 龍骨 芍藥（各十八銖）黃連 當歸 茯苓 黃芩 瞿麥 白薇 石韋 甘草 牡蠣 細辛 附子 禹餘糧 白石脂 人參 烏賊骨 藁本 甘皮 大黃（以上各半兩）。

白堊	bái è	Chalk	十八銖 18 zhū	2.25g
龍骨	lóng gǔ	Os draconis	十八銖 18 zhū	2.25g
芍藥	sháo yào	Root of Paeonia albiflora	十八銖 18 zhū	2.25g
黃連	huáng lián	Rhizome of Coptis chinensis	半兩 0.5 liǎng	1.5g
當歸	dāng guī	Root of Angelica polimorpha	半兩 0.5 liǎng	1.5g
茯苓	fú líng	Dried fungus of Poria cocos	半兩 0.5 liǎng	1.5g
黃芩	huáng qín	Root of Scutellaria baicalensis	半兩 0.5 liǎng	1.5g
瞿麥	qú mài	Entire plant, including flowers, of Dianthus superbus	半兩 0.5 liǎng	1.5g

白薟	bái liǎn	Root of Ampelopsis japonica	半兩	0.5 liǎng	1.5g
石韋	shí wéi	Foliage of Pyrrosia lingua	半兩	0.5 liǎng	1.5g
甘草	gān cǎo	Root of Glycyrrhiza uralensis	半兩	0.5 liǎng	1.5g
牡蠣	mǔ lì	Shell of Ostrea rivularis	半兩	0.5 liǎng	1.5g
細辛	xì xīn	Complete plant including root of Asarum heteropoides	半兩	0.5 liǎng	1.5g
附子	fù zǐ	Lateral root of Aconitum carmichaeli	半兩	0.5 liǎng	1.5g
禹餘糧	yǔ yú liáng	Limonite	半兩	0.5 liǎng	1.5g
白石脂	bái shí zhī	Kaolin	半兩	0.5 liǎng	1.5g
人參	rén shēn	Root of Panax ginseng	半兩	0.5 liǎng	1.5g
烏賊骨	wū zéi gǔ	Calcified shell of Sepiella maindroni	半兩	0.5 liǎng	1.5g
藁本	gǎo běn	Rhizome and root of Ligusticum sinense	半兩	0.5 liǎng	1.5g
甘皮	gān pí[2]	Bark of Saccharum sinensis	半兩	0.5 liǎng	1.5g
大黃	dà huáng	Root of Rheum palmatum	半兩	0.5 liǎng	1.5g

上二十一味，為末，蜜和丸如梧子大。空腹飲服十丸，日再，不知加之。二十日知，一月百病除。若十二癥，倍牡蠣，禹餘糧，烏賊骨，白石脂，龍骨；若九痛，倍黃連，白薟，甘草，當歸；若七害，倍細辛，藁本，甘皮，加椒，茱萸各一兩；若五傷，倍大黃，石韋，瞿麥；若三痼，倍人參，加赤石脂，礬石，巴戟天各半兩。合藥時隨病增減之。

Pulverize the above twenty-one ingredients and mix with honey into pills the size of firmiana seeds. On an empty stomach, take ten pills with fluid twice a day. If no effect is noticed, increase [the dosage]. In twenty days, you will notice [an effect], and after one month the myriad diseases will be expelled. For treating the twelve concretions, double the *mǔ lì* 牡蠣, *yǔ yú liáng* 禹餘糧, *wū zéi gǔ* 烏賊骨, *bái shí zhī* 白石脂, and *lóng gǔ* 龍骨. For the nine pains, double the *huáng lián* 黃連, *bái liǎn* 白薟, *gān cǎo* 甘草, and *dāng guī* 當歸. For the seven injuries, double the *xì xīn* 細辛, *gǎo běn* 藁本, and *gān pí* 甘皮, and add one *liǎng* each of *shǔ jiāo* (蜀椒 Seed capsules of Zanthoxylum bungeanum) and *wú zhū yú* (吳茱萸 Unripe fruit of Evodia rutaecarpa). For the five damages, double the *dà huáng* 大黃, *shí wéi* 石韋, and *qú mài* 瞿麥. For the three intractable diseases, double the *rén shēn* 人參 and add half a *liǎng* each of *chì shí zhī* (赤石脂 Halloysite), *fán shí* (礬石 Alum), and *bā jǐ tiān* (巴戟天 Root of Morinda officinalis). When compounding the medicine, increase or reduce the amount [of each ingredient] in accordance with the condition.

---

1. *Sòng* editors' note: "(For another prescription, see below.)" This refers to the prescription in Line 3.51 below with an almost identical prologue.
2. 甘皮 *gān pí*: Not attested in any materia medica literature. Most likely, this is a reference to 甘蔗皮 *gān zhè pí*, the bark of Saccharum sinensis or Chinese sugar cane (《中藥大辭典》 #1066).

LINE 3.3

治女人腹中十二疾，一曰經水不時，二曰經來如清水，三曰經水不通，四曰不周時，五曰生不乳，六曰絕無子，七曰陰陽減少，八曰腹苦痛如刺，九曰陰中寒，十曰子門相引痛，十一曰經來凍如葵汁狀，十二曰腰急痛。凡此十二病得之時，因與夫臥起，月經不去，或臥濕冷地，及以冷水洗浴，當時取快，而後生百疾，或瘡痍未瘥，便合陰陽，及起早作勞，衣單席薄，寒從下入方。

[The following] prescription treats women's twelve diseases in the abdomen. The first one is called "unpredictable menstrual flow;" the second, "menses arriving like fresh water;" the third, "menstrual stoppage;" the fourth, "[menstruation] not recurring in regular cycles;" the fifth, "failure to nurse after birth;"[1] the sixth, "interruption and lack of offspring;"[2] the seventh, "reduced *yīn* and *yáng*;"[3] the eighth, "bitter pain in the abdomen as if being stabbed;" the ninth, "cold in the vagina;"[4] the tenth, "pain from the [two sides of the] infant's gate pulling at each other;"[5] the eleventh, "arrival of the menses as if frozen and like mallow juice;" the twelfth, "lumbar tension and pain."[6] All these twelve diseases were contracted because [the woman] slept and rose with her husband and failed to [completely] eliminate her menses.[7] Alternatively, perhaps she slept in a damp or cool location or bathed herself in cold water, at that time contracting [the condition] quickly and subsequently generating the hundred diseases. Or perhaps, when she still had unhealed [vaginal] sores, she engaged in sexual intercourse or rose [from bedrest] prematurely and exerted herself,[8] or her clothes were unlined and her seating mat too thin, [allowing] cold to enter from below.

Formula

半夏 赤石脂（各一兩六銖） 蜀椒 乾薑 吳茱萸 當歸 桂心 丹參 白薇 防風（各一兩） 萑蘆（半兩）。

半夏	bàn xià	Rhizome of Pinellia ternata	一兩六銖 1 liǎng 6 zhū	3.75g
赤石脂	chì shí zhī	Halloysite	一兩六銖 1 liǎng 6 zhū	3.75g
蜀椒	shǔ jiāo	Seed capsules of Zanthoxylum bungeanum	一兩 1 liǎng	3g
乾薑	gān jiāng	Dried root of Zingiber officinale	一兩 1 liǎng	3g
吳茱萸	wú zhū yú	Unripe fruit of Evodia rutaecarpa	一兩 1 liǎng	3g
當歸	dāng guī	Root of Angelica polimorpha	一兩 1 liǎng	3g
桂心	guì xīn	Shaved inner bark of Cinnamomum cassia	一兩 1 liǎng	3g
丹參	dān shēn	Root of Salvia miltiorrhiza	一兩 1 liǎng	3g

白蘞	bái liǎn	Root of Ampelopsis japonica	一兩 1 liǎng	3g
防風	fáng fēng	Root of Ledebouriella divaricata	一兩 1 liǎng	3g
藋蘆	guàn lú	Guànlú fungus	半兩 0.5 liǎng	1.5g

上十一味，為末，蜜和丸如梧子大。每日空心酒服十丸，日三，不知稍加，以知為度。

Pulverize the above eleven ingredients and mix with honey into pills the size of firmiana seeds. Every day, take ten pills in liquor on an empty stomach three times a day. If no effect is noticed, increase [the dosage] gradually until you notice [a change].

1. 生不乳 *shēng bù rǔ*: This is a reference to agalactia. This condition occurs in this prescription for menstrual disorders because Chinese medical theory considers breast milk to be the transformed menstrual fluid after childbirth.

2. 絕無子 *jué wú zǐ*: This is not a standard term. It could be interpreted either as "total infertility" or as a compound of two technical terms, 絕產 *jué chǎn* (interruption of childbearing) and 無子 (lack of children, i.e., infertility). In that case, it refers specifically to temporary as well as permanent infertility.

3. 陰陽減少 *yīn yáng jiǎn shǎo*: The exact meaning of this phrase here is unclear. It could refer to a general shortage of *yīn* and/or *yáng* [*qì*] in the body, or to a simultaneous shortage of *yīn* and *yáng*, in the sense of a vacuity in the viscera and bowels, which is indeed a likely cause of female diseases. Alternatively, 陰陽 could also be interpreted as a reference to sexual activity, in which case this phrase would mean "reduced [interest in?] sexual intercourse." This is the way in which I read this term below in the phrase 陰陽患痛 *yīn yáng huàn tòng*: "pain during sexual intercourse," (lit. "*yīn yáng* discomfort and pain" (below in Line 3.6).

4. 陰中寒 *yīn zhōng hán*: The *Sūn Zhēn Rén* edition instead has 腹中冷熱不調 *fù zhōng lěng rè bù tiáo* (imbalance of hot and cold in the abdomen).

5. 子門相引痛 *zǐ mén xiāng yǐn tòng*. This refers to tightness in the cervix and inner part of the vagina. The above translation retains the concrete image, because this graphic description reflects the medieval male interpretation of the internal, and hence invisible, processes within the female body.

6. 腰急痛 *yāo jí tòng*: The *Sūn Zhēn Rén* edition instead has 腰背痛 *yāo bèi tòng* (lumbar and back pain).

7. 與夫臥起，月經不去 *yù fū wò qǐ, yuè jīng bù qù*: The meaning of this phrase is unclear. Interpreting "lying down with the husband" as a euphemism for sexual intercourse, it could refer to the notion that sexual intercourse during the menstrual period prevented the complete elimination of menstrual blood from the uterus. Alternatively, it could mean that her menstrual fluids were not eliminated completely because she engaged in strenuous daily activities that were too taxing for her body during menstruation, a time that required special care and extra rest.

8. Given the common use of this exact wording in explaining the etiologies of postpartum conditions, it is most likely a reference to observing the postpartum restrictions to ensure full recovery from the physical taxations and injuries of childbirth.

LINE 3.4

白石脂丸治婦人三十六疾，胞中痛，漏下赤白方。

Kaolin Pills treat women's thirty-six diseases with pain in the uterus and spotting of red or white vaginal discharge.

Kaolin Pills
白石脂丸 *bái shí zhī wán*

白石脂 烏賊骨 禹餘糧 牡蠣（各十八銖） 赤石脂 乾地黃 乾薑 龍骨 桂心 石韋 白蘞 細辛 芍藥 黃連 附子 當歸 黃芩 蜀椒 鍾乳 白芷 芎藭 甘草（各半兩）。

白石脂	bái shí zhī	Kaolin	十八銖 18 zhū	2.25g
烏賊骨	wū zéi gǔ	Calcified shell of Sepiella main-droni	十八銖 18 zhū	2.25g
禹餘糧	yǔ yú liáng	Limonite	十八銖 18 zhū	2.25g
牡蠣	mǔ lì	Shell of Ostrea rivularis	十八銖 18 zhū	2.25g
赤石脂	chì shí zhī	Halloysite	半兩 0.5 liǎng	1.5g
乾地黃	gān dì huáng	Dried root of Rehmannia glutinosa	半兩 0.5 liǎng	1.5g
乾薑	gān jiāng	Dried root of Zingiber officinale	半兩 0.5 liǎng	1.5g
龍骨	lóng gǔ	Os draconis	半兩 0.5 liǎng	1.5g
桂心	guì xīn	Shaved inner bark of Cinnamomum cassia	半兩 0.5 liǎng	1.5g
石韋	shí wéi	Foliage of Pyrrosia lingua	半兩 0.5 liǎng	1.5g
白蘞	bái liǎn	Root of Ampelopsis japonica	半兩 0.5 liǎng	1.5g
細辛	xì xīn	Complete plant including root of Asarum heteropoides	半兩 0.5 liǎng	1.5g
芍藥	sháo yào	Root of Paeonia albiflora	半兩 0.5 liǎng	1.5g
黃連	huáng lián	Rhizome of Coptis chinensis	半兩 0.5 liǎng	1.5g
附子	fù zǐ	Lateral root of Aconitum carmi-chaeli	半兩 0.5 liǎng	1.5g
當歸	dāng guī	Root of Angelica polimorpha	半兩 0.5 liǎng	1.5g
黃芩	huáng qín	Root of Scutellaria baicalensis	半兩 0.5 liǎng	1.5g
蜀椒	shǔ jiāo	Seed capsules of Zanthoxylum bungeanum	半兩 0.5 liǎng	1.5g
鍾乳	zhōng rǔ	Stalactite	半兩 0.5 liǎng	1.5g
白芷	bái zhǐ	Root of Angelica dahurica	半兩 0.5 liǎng	1.5g
川芎	chuān xiōng	Root of Ligusticum wallichii	半兩 0.5 liǎng	1.5g

| 甘草 | gān cǎo | Root of Glycyrrhiza uralensis | 半兩 0.5 liǎng | 1.5g |

上二十二味，為末，蜜和丸如梧子大。每日空心酒下十五丸，日再。

Pulverize the above twenty-two ingredients and mix with honey into pills the size of firmiana seeds. Every day, on an empty stomach down fifteen pills in liquor twice a day.*

---

*   *Sòng* editors' note: "Another [version of this] prescription includes half a *liǎng* of *huáng bò* (黃檗 Bark of Phellodendron amurense)."

LINE 3.5

小牛角鰓散治帶下五賁，一曰熱病下血；二曰寒熱下血；三曰經脈末斷為房事，則血漏；四曰經來舉重，傷任脈下血；五曰產後臟開經利。五賁之病，外實內虛方。

Minor Ox Horn Marrow Powder treats the five [types of] vaginal gushing.[1] The first one is called "heat disease with descent of blood;" the second, "[aversion to] cold and heat [effusion] with descent of blood;" the third, "vaginal spotting of blood due to sexual activity before the menstrual flow has stopped;" the fourth, "vaginal bleeding due to heavy lifting at the onset of menstruation and damage to the controlling vessel;" and the fifth, "disinhibited menstruation due to openness of the uterus after childbirth." The five gushing diseases are [characterized by] external repletion and internal vacuity.[2]

1.   賁 *bēn*: This character is used interchangeably with 奔 *bēn*, which, in a medical context, is used most commonly in the compound 奔豚 *bēn tún* (running piglet), a type of kidney accumulation characterized by a counterflow upward surge of *qì*.
2.   This and the following prescription for *Dragon Bone Powder* are missing in the *Sūn Zhēn Rén* edition, which instead cites two prescriptions for hemorrhoids.

Minor Ox Horn Marrow Powder
小牛角腮散 *xiǎo niú jiǎo sāi sǎn*

牛角鰓（一枚，燒令赤）鹿茸 禹餘糧 當歸 乾薑 續斷（各二兩）阿膠（三兩）烏賊骨 龍骨（各一兩）赤小豆（二升）。

牛角腮, 燒令赤	niú jiǎo sāi, shāo lìng chì	Ossified marrow in the center of the horn of Bos taurus domesticus, heated until red	一枚 1 méi	1 pc
鹿茸	lù róng	Pilose antler of Cervus nippon	二兩 2 liǎng	6g
禹餘糧	yǔ yú liáng	Limonite	二兩 2 liǎng	6g

當歸	dāng guī	Root of Angelica polimorpha	二兩 2 liǎng	6g
乾薑	gān jiāng	Dried root of Zingiber officinale	二兩 2 liǎng	6g
續斷	xù duàn	Root of Dipsacus asper	二兩 2 liǎng	6g
阿膠	ē jiāo	Gelatinous glue produced from Equus asinus	三兩 3 liǎng	9g
烏賊骨	wū zéi gǔ	Calcified shell of Sepiella maindroni	一兩 1 liǎng	3g
龍骨	lóng gǔ	Os draconis	一兩 1 liǎng	3g
赤小豆	chì xiǎo dòu	Fruit of Phaseolus calcaratus	二升 2 shēng	48g

上十味，治下篩。空腹以酒服方寸匕，日三。

Finely pestle and sift the above ten ingredients. On an empty stomach, take a square-inch spoon in liquor three times a day.[*]

---

[*]   Sòng editors' note: "The Qiān Jīn Yì Fāng does not use lù róng   鹿茸 and wū zéi
gǔ 烏賊骨."

LINE 3.6

龍骨散治淳下十二病絕產，一曰白帶，二曰赤帶，三曰經水不利，四曰陰胎，五曰子藏堅，六曰藏癖，七曰陰陽患痛，八曰內強，九曰腹寒，十曰藏閉，十一曰五藏酸痛，十二曰夢與鬼交，宜服之。

Dragon Bone Powder treats the twelve diseases of vaginal downpouring,[1] which interrupt her ability to bear children. The first one is called "white vaginal discharge;" the second, "red vaginal discharge;" the third, "inhibited menstrual flow;" the fourth, "*yīn* fetus;"[2] the fifth, "hardness of the uterus;" the sixth, "uterine aggregations;" the seventh, "*yīn yáng* discomfort and pain;"[3] the eighth, "internal rigidity;" the ninth, "abdominal coldness;" the tenth, "blockage of the uterus;" the eleventh, "aching and pain in the five viscera;" and the twelfth, "dreams of intercourse with ghosts."[4] It is suitable to take these [pills for the above conditions].[5]

Dragon Bone Powder
龍骨散 *lóng gǔ sǎn*

龍骨（三兩） 黃檗 半夏 竈中黃土 桂心 乾薑（各二兩） 石韋 滑石（各一兩） 烏賊骨 代赭（各四兩） 白殭蠶（五枚）。

| 龍骨 | lóng gǔ | Os draconis | 三兩 3 liǎng | 9g |
| 黃檗 | huáng bò | Bark of Phellodendron amurense | 二兩 2 liǎng | 6g |

半夏	bàn xià	Rhizome of Pinellia ternata	二兩 2 liǎng	6g
竈中黃土	zào zhōng huáng tǔ	Stove earth	二兩 2 liǎng	6g
桂心	guì xīn	Shaved inner bark of Cinnamomum cassia	二兩 2 liǎng	6g
乾薑	gān jiāng	Dried root of Zingiber officinale	二兩 2 liǎng	6g
石韋	shí wéi	Foliage of Pyrrosia lingua	一兩 1 liǎng	3g
槐實	huái shí	Fruit of Sophora japonica	一兩 1 liǎng	3g
烏賊骨	wū zéi gǔ	Calcified shell of Sepiella maindroni	四兩 4 liǎng	12g
代赭	dài zhě	Hematite	四兩 4 liǎng	12g
白僵蠶	bái jiāng cán	Dried 4th or 5th stage larva of the moth of Bombyx mori	五枚 5 méi	5 pcs

上十一味，治下篩。酒服方寸匕，日三。白多者，加烏賊骨，殭蠶各二兩；赤多者，加代赭五兩；小腹冷，加黃蘗二兩；子藏堅，加乾薑，桂心各二兩。以上各隨病增之。服藥三月，有子即住藥。藥太過多，生兩子。當審方取好藥。寡婦，童女不可妄服。

Finely pestle and sift the above eleven ingredients. Take a square-inch spoon in liquor three times a day. For predominantly white discharge, add two more *liǎng* each of *wū zéi gǔ* 烏賊骨 and *bái jiāng cán* 白僵蠶. For predominantly red discharge, add five more *liǎng* of *dài zhě* 代赭. For coolness in the lower abdomen, add two more *liǎng* of *huáng bò* 黃蘗. For hardness of the uterus, add two more *liǎng* each of *gān jiāng* 乾薑 and *guì xīn* 桂心. Increase the amount [of each ingredient] according to the [guidelines outlined] above, adapting it to the condition. After taking this medicine for three months, she will be with child and must then stop the medicine. If she takes an excessive amount of this medicine, she will give birth to twins. You must examine this prescription judiciously and choose high-quality drugs. Widows and virgins may not recklessly take it.[6]

1. 淳下 *zhūn xià*: The character 淳, which is more commonly read *chún* (concentrated/pure), can also be read *zhūn*, meaning "to irrigate, pour water." It is not a common technical term in a gynecological context.
2. 陰胎 *yīn tāi*: Most likely, 陰 should be read as 蔭 *yìn* (shaded, sheltered, covered). In later literature, 蔭胎 *yìn tāi* is a medical term denoting a fetus that has stopped growing in the uterus, due to the mother's physical weakness, insufficiency of *yīn* blood, and subsequent inability to nurture the fetus sufficiently. On a most literal level, the term suggests perhaps that a surplus of *yīn* in the mother's body affected the fetus negatively, stunting its growth and leading to a miscarriage.
3. 陰陽患痛 *yīn yáng huàn tòng*: On the possible interpretations of 陰陽, see Line 3.3, note 3, above. In this case, it most likely refers to discomfort and pain during sexual intercourse.
4. The connection between infertility and the etiological category of "dreams of intercourse with ghosts" is twofold: First, it might have caused a lack of offspring because the relationship with a ghost made the woman averse to engage in sexual intercourse with

mortals. Second, invasion by ghosts was explained as caused by an underlying vacuity of *qì* and blood. This resulted, on the one hand, in a weakening of the body's defenses and subsequent susceptibility to external evils like wind, cold, and ghosts and on the other, in a decline of the hold on the spirit (see 《病源論》 40.95 and 96). It serves therefore here as both a cause of infertility and as a symptom that is indicating an underlying etiology of blood and *qì* depletion.

5. *Sòng* editors' note: "Instead of 'vaginal downpouring' (淳下), another edition has 'below the abdomen' (腹下). This note, presumably inserted by the *Sòng* editors, is reflected, for example, in the *Sūn Zhēn Rén* edition.

6. The fact that Sūn Sī-Miǎo limits the suitability of this formula to sexually active women raises many interesting questions, which unfortunately transcend the limits of this study. At first sight, it conflicts with the fact that he lists "dreams of intercourse with ghosts" among the indications for this formula, a condition that was seen as related to a lack of sexual activity. See, for example, the explanation Péng Zǔ 彭祖 offers to Cǎi Nǚ 采女 in the *Yù Fáng Mì Jué* 玉房秘訣: "[The reason for the disease of intercourse with ghosts is] that *yīn* and *yáng* have no interaction (i.e., a woman suffers from lack of sexual intercourse) and her affects become deep-seated and serious. Then ghosts and goblins assume a false appearance and have intercourse with her. The way in which they have intercourse with her is superior to that of humans. If this goes on for a long time, she will be deluded and seduced and will conceal and hide it, unwilling to inform others, and herself considering it to be excellent. Consequently, it will cause her to die on her own (i.e., without ever having married) and no-one will be aware of [the reason]." (《醫心方》 21:30).

LINE 3.7

治女人帶下諸病方。

[The following] prescription treats women's various diseases of vaginal discharge.[1]

Formula

大黃（蒸三斗米下）附子 茯苓 牡蒙 牡丹 桔梗 葶藶（各三兩）厚朴 芎藭 人參 當歸 虻蟲 蜀椒 吳茱萸 柴胡 乾薑 桂心（各半兩）細辛（二兩半）。

大黃, 蒸三斗米下	dà huáng, zhēng sān dǒu mǐ xià	Root of Rheum palmatum, steamed under three dǒu of rice	三兩 3 liǎng	9g
附子	fù zǐ	Lateral root of Aconitum carmichaeli	三兩 3 liǎng	9g
茯苓	fú líng	Dried fungus of Poria cocos	三兩 3 liǎng	9g
牡蒙	mǔ méng	Root of Paris quadrifolia	三兩 3 liǎng	9g
桔梗	jié gěng	Root of Platycodon grandiflorum	三兩 3 liǎng	9g
葶藶	tíng lì	Seed of Lepidium apetalum	三兩 3 liǎng	9g

厚朴	hòu pò	Bark of Magnolia officinalis	一兩半 1.5 liǎng	4.5g
川芎	chuān xiōng	Root of Ligusticum wallichii	一兩半 1.5 liǎng	4.5g
人參	rén shēn	Root of Panax ginseng	一兩半 1.5 liǎng	4.5g
當歸	dāng guī	Root of Angelica polimorpha	一兩半 1.5 liǎng	4.5g
虻蟲	méng chóng	Dried body of the female of Tabanus bivittatus	一兩半 1.5 liǎng	4.5g
蜀椒	shǔ jiāo	Seed capsules of Zanthoxylum bungeanum	一兩半 1.5 liǎng	4.5g
吳茱萸	wú zhū yú	Unripe fruit of Evodia rutaecarpa	一兩半 1.5 liǎng	4.5g
柴胡	chái hú	Root of Bupleurum chinense	一兩半 1.5 liǎng	4.5g
乾薑	gān jiāng	Dried root of Zingiber officinale	一兩半 1.5 liǎng	4.5g
桂心	guì xīn	Shaved inner bark of Cinnamomum cassia	一兩半 1.5 liǎng	4.5g
細辛	xì xīn	Complete plant including root of Asarum heteropoides	二兩半 2.5 liǎng	7.5g

上十八味，為末，蜜和丸如梧子大。每日空心酒服二丸，不知加之，以腹中溫溫為度。

Pulverize the above eighteen ingredients and mix with honey into pills the size of firmiana seeds. Every day, take two pills in liquor on an empty stomach. Increase [the dosage] if you notice no effect, until the center of the abdomen feels warm.[2]

1. 帶下 *dài xià*: The *Sūn Zhēn Rén* edition instead has 臍下 *qí xià* (below the navel).
2. *Sòng* editors' note: "Another edition includes 3 *liǎng* of *má zǐ rén* (麻子 Seed of Cannabis sativa) and half a *liǎng* of *zé lán* (澤蘭 Foliage and stalk of Lycopus lucidus), but lacks *shǔ jiāo* 蜀椒 and *tíng lì* 葶藶."

LINE 3.8

治帶下百病，無子，服藥十四日下血，二十日下長蟲，及清黃汁出，三十日病除，五十日肥白方。

[The following] prescription treats the hundred diseases of vaginal discharge and infertility. After taking this medicine for fourteen days, she will discharge blood; after twenty days, long worms and a clear yellow liquid; after thirty days; she will expel the disease;

and after fifty days, she will be fat and white.[1]

Formula

大黃 (破如豆粒 , 熬令黑色) 柴胡 朴消 (各一斤) 芎藭 (五兩) 乾薑 蜀椒 (各一升) 茯苓 (如雞子大一枚) 。

大黃, 破如豆粒 , 熬令黑色	dà huáng, pò rú dòu lì, āo lìng hēi sè	Root of Rheum palmatum, broken into grain-sized pieces and roasted until black	一斤 1 jīn	48g
柴胡	chái hú	Root of Bupleurum chinense	一斤 1 jīn	48g
朴消	pò xiāo	Impure mirabilite	一斤 1 jīn	48g
川芎	chuān xiōng	Root of Ligusticum wallichii	五兩 5 liǎng	15g
乾薑	gān jiāng	Dried root of Zingiber officinale	一升 1 shēng	24g
蜀椒	shǔ jiāo	Seed capsules of Zanthoxylum bungeanum	一升 1 shēng	24g
茯苓	fú líng	Dried fungus of Poria cocos	如雞子大一枚 rú jī zǐ dà 1 méi	an amount the size of a chicken egg

上七味 , 為末 , 蜜丸如梧子大。先食米飲服七丸 , 不知加至十丸 , 以知為度。

Pulverize the above seven ingredients and mix with honey into pills the size of firmiana seeds. Before meals, take seven pills in rice soup. If no effect is noticed, increase [the dosage] to a maximum of ten pills, until an effect is noticed.

1. This prescription is missing in the *Sūn Zhēn Rén* edition.
2. 米飲 *mǐ yǐn*: This refers to water that rice has been cooked in, as opposed to 米汁 *mǐ zhī*, rice juice (obtained by grinding rice in water), and 米泔 *mǐ gān*, rice water (water that rice has been rinsed in).

LINE 3.9

治帶下方。

[The following] prescription treats vaginal discharge.

Formula

枸杞根（一斤）生地黃（五斤）。

枸杞根	gǒu qǐ gēn	Bark of the root of Lycium chinensis	一斤 1 jīn	48g
生地黃	shēng dì huáng	Fresh root of Rehmannia glutinosa	五斤 5 jīn	240g

上二味，㕮咀，以酒一斗煮取五升，分為三服。水煮亦得。

Pound the above two ingredients and decoct in one *dǒu* of liquor to obtain five *shēng*. Divide into three doses. Decocting the [drugs] in water is also possible.

LINE 3.10

治婦人及女子赤白帶方。

[The following] prescription treats red and white vaginal discharge in married women as well as girls.

Formula

禹餘糧 當歸 芎藭（各一兩半） 赤石脂 白石脂 阿膠 龍骨 石韋（一兩六銖） 烏賊骨 黃蘗 白薇 黃芩 續斷 桑耳 牡蠣（各一兩）。

禹餘糧	yǔ yú liáng	Limonite	一兩半 1.5 liǎng	4.5g
當歸	dāng guī	Root of Angelica polimorpha	一兩半 1.5 liǎng	4.5g
川芎	chuān xiōng	Root of Ligusticum wallichii	一兩半 1.5 liǎng	4.5g
赤石脂	chì shí zhī	Halloysite	一兩六銖 1 liǎng 6 zhū	3.75g
白石脂	bái shí zhī	Kaolin	一兩六銖 1 liǎng 6 zhū	3.75g
阿膠	ē jiāo	Gelatinous glue produced from Equus asinus	一兩六銖 1 liǎng 6 zhū	3.75g
龍骨	lóng gǔ	Os draconis	一兩六銖 1 liǎng 6 zhū	3.75g

石韋	shí wéi	Foliage of Pyrrosia lingua	一兩六銖 1 liǎng 6 zhū	3.75g
烏賊骨	wū zéi gǔ	Calcified shell of Sepiella maindroni	一兩 1 liǎng	3g
黃檗	huáng bò	Bark of Phellodendron amurense	一兩 1 liǎng	3g
白蘞	bái liǎn	Root of Ampelopsis japonica	一兩 1 liǎng	3g
黃芩*	huáng qín	Root of Scutellaria baicalensis	一兩 1 liǎng	3g
續斷	xù duàn	Root of Dipsacus asper	一兩 1 liǎng	3g
桑耳	sāng ěr	Mulberry wood ear	一兩 1 liǎng	3g
牡蠣	mǔ lì	Shell of Ostrea rivularis	一兩 1 liǎng	3g

上十五味，為末，蜜丸梧子大。空心飲下十五丸，日再，加至三十丸為度。

Pulverize the above fifteen ingredients and mix with honey into pills the size of firmiana seeds. On an empty stomach, down fifteen pills with fluid twice a day. Increase [the dosage] to a maximum of thirty pills.

* *Sòng* editors' note: "Another [version] uses *huáng lián* (黃連 Rhizome of Coptis chinensis)."

LINE 3.11

白馬蹄丸治女人下焦寒冷，成帶下赤白浣方。

White Horse's Hoof Pills treat women's coldness in the lower burner, causing the formation of vaginal discharge like a red or white flood.[1]

White Horse's Hoof Pills
白馬蹄丸 *bái mǎ tí wán*

白馬蹄 鱉甲 鯉魚甲 龜甲 蜀椒（各一兩） 磁石 甘草 杜仲 草薢 當歸 續斷 芎藭 禹餘糧 桑耳 附子（各二兩）。

白馬蹄	bái mǎ tí	Hoof of Equus caballus	一兩 1 liǎng	3g
鱉甲	biē jiǎ	Dorsal shell of Amyda sinensis	一兩 1 liǎng	3g
鯉魚甲	lǐ yú jiǎ	Scales of Cyprinus carpio	一兩 1 liǎng	3g
龜甲	guī jiǎ	Shell of Chinemys reevesii	一兩 1 liǎng	3g
蜀椒	shǔ jiāo	Seed capsules of Zanthoxylum bungeanum	一兩 1 liǎng	3g

磁石	cí shí	Loadstone	二兩 2 liǎng	6g
甘草	gān cǎo	Root of Glycyrrhiza uralensis	二兩 2 liǎng	6g
杜仲	dù zhòng	Bark of Eucommia ulmoidis	二兩 2 liǎng	6g
萆薢	bì xiè	Rhizome of Dioscorea hypoglauca	二兩 2 liǎng	6g
當歸	dāng guī	Root of Angelica polimorpha	二兩 2 liǎng	6g
續斷	xù duàn	Root of Dipsacus asper	二兩 2 liǎng	6g
川芎	chuān xiōng	Root of Ligusticum wallichii	二兩 2 liǎng	6g
禹餘糧	yǔ yú liáng	Limonite	二兩 2 liǎng	6g
桑耳	sāng ěr	Mulberry wood ear	二兩 2 liǎng	6g
附子	fù zǐ	Lateral root of Aconitum carmichaeli	二兩 2 liǎng	6g

上十五味，為末，蜜丸梧子大。以酒服十丸，加至三十丸，日三服。

Pulverize the above fifteen ingredients and mix with honey into pills the size of firmiana seeds. Take ten pills [per dose] in liquor, increasing [the dosage] to a maximum of thirty pills, three doses a day.[2]

1. 赤白浣 *chì bái huàn*: The *Sūn Zhēn Rén* edition instead has the two characters 去浣 *qù huàn* (running like a flood).
2. *Sòng* editors' note: "Another edition does not include *guī jiǎ* 龜甲."

LINE 3.12

白馬駼散治帶下方。
下白者，取白馬駼；下赤者，取赤馬駼；隨色取之。

White Horse's Mane Powder treats vaginal discharge.
For white discharge, use a white horse's mane; For red discharge, use a red horse's mane. Choose [the color of the mane] in accordance with the color [of the discharge].[1]

White Horse's Mane Powder
白馬毛散 *bái mǎ tuō sǎn*

白馬駼（二兩）龜甲（四兩）鱉甲（十八銖）牡蠣（一兩十八銖）。

白馬駼	bái mǎ tuō[2]	Mane of Equus caballus	二兩 2 liǎng	6g
龜甲	guī jiǎ	Shell of Chinemys reevesii	四兩 4 liǎng	12g
鱉甲	biē jiǎ	Dorsal shell of Amyda sinensis	十八銖 18 zhū	2.25g

| 牡蠣 | mǔ lì | Shell of Ostrea rivularis | 一兩十八銖 1 | 5.25g |
| | | | liǎng 18 zhū | |

上四味，治下篩。空心酒下方寸匕，日三服，加至一匕半。

Finely pestle and sift the above four ingredients. On an empty stomach, down a square-inch spoon in liquor three times a day. Increase [the dosage] to a maximum of one and a half spoons.

1. This sentence is marked as commentary in modern critical editions of this text, but the fact that it is also found in exactly the same wording in the *Sūn Zhēn Rén* edition strongly suggests that it was an integral part of the original instructions.

2. More commonly called 白馬鬃 *bái mǎ zōng*, as which it is listed in the Materia Medica Index.

LINE 3.13

治五色帶下方。

[The following] prescription treats vaginal discharge in the five colors.

服大豆紫湯，日三服。

Take *Soybean Purple Decoction* three times a day.*

* *Sòng* editors' note: "For the prescription, see volume three, chapter on Wind Strike." In the translation here, this is found in chapter three of volume three, Line 3.2 (p. 268 - 270).

LINE 3.14

又方

Another prescription:

燒馬左蹄為末，以酒服方寸匕，日三服。

Char and pulverize a horse's left hooves and take a square-inch spoon in liquor three times a day.

LINE 3.15

又方

Another prescription:

燒狗頭和毛皮骨為末，以酒服方寸匕。

Char and pulverize a dog's head, complete with hair, skin, and bones. Take a square-inch spoon in liquor.

LINE 3.16

又方

Another prescription:

煮甑帶汁，服一杯良。

Boil the cord handle of a steamer in liquid. Drinking one cup is good.

LINE 3.17

又方

Another prescription:

燒馬蹄底護，乾為末。以酒服方寸匕，日三。

Char, dry, and pulverize the protected underside of a horse's hoof. Take a square-inch spoon in liquor three times a day.

LINE 3.18

雲母芎藭散衛公治五崩，身瘦，欬逆，煩滿少氣，心下痛，面生瘡，腰痛不可俛仰，陰中腫如有瘡狀，毛中癢時痛與子藏相通，小便不利常拘急，頭眩，鵶項急痛，手足熱，氣逆衝急，心煩不得臥，腹中急痛，食不下，吞醋噫苦，上下腸鳴，漏下赤白青黃黑汁，大臭如膠污衣狀，皆是內傷所致。中寒即下白，熱即下赤，多飲即下黑，多食即下黃，多藥即下青，或喜或怒，心中常恐，或憂勞便發動，大惡風寒。

Muscovite and Chuānxiōng Powder is a prescription by the Duke of Wèi[1] for treating the five floodings,[2] generalized emaciation, counterflow cough, vexation fullness and shortage of *qì*, pain below the heart, formation of sores in the face, inability to bend and stretch in the lumbus and back, swelling in the vagina as if there were sores, itching in the [pubic] hair and occasional pain that penetrates to the uterus, inhibited urination with constant hypertonicity, dizziness in the head, tension and pain in the neck, heat in the hands and feet, *qì* counterflow surging and tension, heart vexation and inability to rest, tension and pain in the abdomen, inability to get down food, acid regurgitation with bitter belching, rumbling in the upper and lower intestines, vaginal spotting of red, white, blue-green, yellow, or black liquid, and severe body odor and stains on the clothing as if dirtied by glue. All these [symptoms] are caused by internal damage. In cases of wind strike, [she will present with] white vaginal discharge; in cases of heat, with red discharge; in cases of excessive fluid intake, with black discharge; in cases of excessive eating, with yellow discharge; and in cases of excessive [consumption of] medicines, with blue-green discharge. [She may also suffer from excessive] joy or anger, from constant fear in her heart, from anxiety taxation and subsequent arousal [of affects], and from severe aversion to wind and cold.

Muscovite and Chuānxiōng Powder
雲母芎藭散 *yún mǔ xiōng qióng sǎn*

雲母 芎藭 代赭 東門邊木（燒，各一兩） 白殭蠶 烏賊骨 白堊 蝟皮（各六銖） 鱉甲 桂心 伏龍肝 生鯉魚頭（各十八銖）。

雲母	yún mǔ	Muscovite	一兩 1 liǎng	3g
川芎	chuān xiōng	Root of Ligusticum wallichii	一兩 1 liǎng	3g
代赭	dài zhě	Hematite	一兩 1 liǎng	3g
東門邊木, 燒	dōng mén biān mù, shāo	Wood from the side of the eastern gate, charred	一兩 1 liǎng	3g
白僵蠶	bái jiāng cán	Dried 4th or 5th stage larva of the moth of Bombyx mori	六銖 6 zhū	0.75g
烏賊骨	wū zéi gǔ	Calcified shell of Sepiella maindroni	六銖 6 zhū	0.75g
白堊	bái è	Chalk	六銖 6 zhū	0.75g
蝟皮	wèi pí	Skin of Erinaceus europaeus	六銖 6 zhū	0.75g
鱉甲	biē jiǎ	Dorsal shell of Amyda sinensis	十八銖 18 zhū	2.25g
桂心	guì xīn	Shaved inner bark of Cinnamomum cassia	十八銖 18 zhū	2.25g
伏龍肝	fú lóng gān	Stove earth	十八銖 18 zhū	2.25g
生鯉魚頭	shēng lǐ yú tóu[3]	Fresh Cyprinus carpio head	十八銖 18 zhū	2.25g

上十二味，治下篩。酒服方寸匕，日三夜一。

Finely pestle and sift the above twelve ingredients. Take a square-inch spoon in liquor, three times during the day and once at night.[4]

1. 衛公 Wèi gōng: The duke of the state of Wèi, one of the Warring States (戰國 zhàn guó). The *Sūn Zhēn Rén* edition instead has: 此衛公方秘之 cǐ wèi gōng fāng mì zhī (This is the prescription of the Duke of Wèi. Keep it secret).
2. 五崩 wǔ bēng: heavy flow of vaginal discharge in the five colors, depending on the internal organs affected. It is more severe than the "five gushings," (五奔 wǔ bēn, see Line 3.5 above).
3. While it is not specifically mentioned, I assume that the carp head should be prepared by charring and pulverizing since this is the standard way of preparing carp head in prescriptions for similar symptoms. See (《本草綱目》44:1), entry "鯉魚" section "附方" (appended prescriptions).
4. *Sòng* editors' note: "Another [version] has *guī jiǎ* (龜甲 Shell of Chinemys reevesii) instead of *biē jiǎ* 鱉甲. Another [version of this] prescription contains *lóng gǔ* (龍骨 Os draconis) and *gān gé* [*gēn*] 乾葛[根] Dried root of Pueraria lobata)."

LINE 3.19

慎火草散治崩中漏下赤白青黑，腐臭不可近，令人面黑無顏色，皮骨相連，月經失度，往來無常，小腹弦急，或苦絞痛上至心，兩脅腫脹，食不生肌膚，令人偏枯，氣息乏少，腰背痛連脅，不能久立，每嗜臥困懶。（又方見後。）

Stonecrop Powder treats center flooding and spotting of red, white, blue-green, and black discharge that is so foul-smelling that no one can get near her, [disease that is] causing the patient's face to be black and without color, and her skin to stick to the bones, an excessive menstrual period that comes and goes without constancy, bow-string tension in the lower abdomen, possibly with discomfort from gripping pain ascending all the way to the heart, swelling and distention in both rib-sides, eating without engendering flesh, causing her to [suffer from] hemilateral withering, lack of *qi* and breath, lumbar and back pain connecting to the rib-sides, inability to stand for a long period of time, and pervasive somnolence, encumbrance, and laziness.
(See below for further prescriptions.)

Stonecrop Powder
慎火草散 *shèn huǒ cǎo sǎn*

慎火草 白石脂 禹餘糧 鱉甲 乾薑 細辛 當歸 芎藭 石斛 芍藥 牡蠣（各二兩）黃連 薔薇根皮 乾地黃（各四兩）熟艾 桂心（各一兩）。

慎火草	shèn huǒ cǎo	Entire plant of Sedum erythrosticum	二兩 2 liǎng	6g
白石脂	bái shí zhī	Kaolin	二兩 2 liǎng	6g
禹餘糧	yǔ yú liáng	Limonite	二兩 2 liǎng	6g
鱉甲	biē jiǎ	Dorsal shell of Amyda sinensis	二兩 2 liǎng	6g
乾薑	gān jiāng	Dried root of Zingiber officinale	二兩 2 liǎng	6g
細辛	xì xīn	Complete plant including root of Asarum heteropoides	二兩 2 liǎng	6g
當歸	dāng guī	Root of Angelica polimorpha	二兩 2 liǎng	6g
川芎	chuān xiōng	Root of Ligusticum wallichii	二兩 2 liǎng	6g
石斛	shí hú	Whole plant of Dendrobium nobile	二兩 2 liǎng	6g
芍藥	sháo yào	Root of Paeonia albiflora	二兩 2 liǎng	6g
牡蠣	mǔ lì	Shell of Ostrea rivularis	二兩 2 liǎng	6g
黃連	huáng lián	Rhizome of Coptis chinensis	四兩 4 liǎng	12g
薔薇根皮	qiáng wēi gēn pí	Bark of the root of Rosa multiflora	四兩 4 liǎng	12g
乾地黃	gān dì huáng	Dried root of Rehmannia glutinosa	四兩 4 liǎng	12g
熟艾	shú ài	Cooked foliage of Artemisia argyi	一兩 1 liǎng	3g
桂心	guì xīn	Shaved inner bark of Cinnamomum cassia	一兩 1 liǎng	3g

上十六味，治下篩。空腹酒服方寸匕，日三，稍加至二匕。若寒多者，加附子，椒；熱多者，加知母，黃芩各一兩；白多者，加乾薑，白石脂；赤多者，加桂心，代赭各二兩。

Finely pestle and sift the above sixteen ingredients. On an empty stomach, take a square-inch spoon in liquor three times a day, gradually increasing [the dosage] to a maximum of two spoons. For excessive cold, add [one *liǎng* each of] *fù zǐ* (附子Lateral root of Aconitum carmichaeli) and *shǔ jiāo* (蜀椒 Seed capsules of Zanthoxylum bungeanum). For excessive heat, add one *liǎng* each of *zhī mǔ* (知母 Root of Anemarrhena asphodeloides) and *huáng qín* (黃芩 Root of Scutellaria baicalensis). For excessive white discharge, add [two *liǎng* each of] *gān jiāng* 乾薑 and *bái shí zhī* 白石脂. For excessive red discharge, add two *liǎng* each of *guì xīn* (桂心 Shaved inner bark of Cinnamomum cassia) and *dài zhě* (代赭 Hematite).

LINE 3.20

禹餘糧丸治崩中，赤白不絕，困篤方。

Limonite Pills treat center flooding, incessant red and white [vaginal discharge], and critical encumbrance.

Limonite Pills
禹餘糧丸 *yǔ yú liáng wán*

禹餘糧（五兩） 白馬蹄（十兩） 龍骨（三兩） 鹿茸（二兩） 烏賊骨（一兩）。

禹餘糧	yǔ yú liáng	Limonite	五兩 5 liǎng	15g
白馬蹄	bái mǎ tí	Hoof of Equus caballus	十兩 10 liǎng	30g
龍骨	lóng gǔ	Os draconis	三兩 3 liǎng	9g
鹿茸	lù róng	Pilose antler of Cervus nippon	二兩 2 liǎng	6g
烏賊骨	wū zéi gǔ	Calcified shell of Sepiella maindroni	一兩 1 liǎng	3g

上五味，為末，蜜丸梧子大。以酒服二十丸，日再，以知為度。

Pulverize the above five ingredients and mix with honey into pills the size of firmiana seeds. Take twenty pills in liquor twice a day, until you notice an effect.

LINE 3.21

勞損禹餘糧丸治女人勞損因成崩中，狀如月經來去多不可禁止，積日不斷，五藏空虛，失色黃瘦，崩竭暫止，少日復發，不耐動搖，小勞輒劇。治法且宜與湯，未宜與此丸也。發時服湯，減退即與此丸。若是疾久，可長與此方。

Modified Limonite Pills treat women's center flooding due to taxation detriment that resembles a menstrual period, coming and going profusely, impossible to stop, and continuing incessantly for several days, emptiness vacuity in the five viscera, and loss of color, yellow complexion, and emaciation. When the flooding has exhausted itself, it stops temporarily, then erupts again after only a few days, with unbearable agitation and shaking and intensified by only minor taxation. Treatment method: You should always give a decoction first* before you give these pills. At the time of an attack, [make the patient] take a decoction, and then, when it recedes, give these pills. If the condition is chronic, you may give these pills over a long period of time.

Modified Limonite Pills
增損禹餘糧丸 *zēng sǔn yǔ yú liáng wán*

禹餘糧 龍骨 人參 桂心 紫石英 烏頭 寄生 杜仲 五味子 遠志（各二兩） 澤瀉 當歸 石斛 蓯蓉 乾薑（各三兩） 蜀椒 牡蠣 甘草（各一兩）。

禹餘糧	yǔ yú liáng	Limonite	二兩 2 liǎng	6g
龍骨	lóng gǔ	Os draconis	二兩 2 liǎng	6g
人參	rén shēn	Root of Panax ginseng	二兩 2 liǎng	6g
桂心	guì xīn	Shaved inner bark of Cinnamomum cassia	二兩 2 liǎng	6g
紫石英	zǐ shí yīng	Fluorite	二兩 2 liǎng	6g
烏頭	wū tóu	Main tuber of Aconitum carmichaeli	二兩 2 liǎng	6g
寄生	jì shēng	Branches and foliage of Viscum coloratum	二兩 2 liǎng	6g
杜仲	dù zhòng	Bark of Eucommia ulmoidis	二兩 2 liǎng	6g
五味子	wǔ wèi zǐ	Fruit of Schisandra chinensis	二兩 2 liǎng	6g
遠志	yuǎn zhì	Root of Polygala tenuifolia	二兩 2 liǎng	6g
澤瀉	zé xiè	Rhizome of Alisma plantago-aquatica	三兩 3 liǎng	9g
當歸	dāng guī	Root of Angelica polimorpha	三兩 3 liǎng	9g
石斛	shí hú	Whole plant of Dendrobium nobile	三兩 3 liǎng	9g
蓯蓉	cōng róng	Stalk of Cistanche salsa	三兩 3 liǎng	9g
乾薑	gān jiāng	Dried root of Zingiber officinale	三兩 3 liǎng	9g
蜀椒	shǔ jiāo	Seed capsules of Zanthoxylum bungeanum	一兩 1 liǎng	3g
牡蠣	mǔ lì	Shell of Ostrea rivularis	一兩 1 liǎng	3g
甘草	gān cǎo	Root of Glycyrrhiza uralensis	一兩 1 liǎng	3g

上十八味，為末，蜜丸梧子大。空心酒下十丸，漸加至二十丸，日三服。

Pulverize the above eighteen ingredients and mix with honey into pills the size of firmiana seeds. On an empty stomach, down ten pills in liquor, gradually increasing [the dosage] to a maximum of twenty pills, three doses a day.

*   It is unclear what decoction Sūn Sī-Miǎo is referring to here since the following and preceding prescriptions are also for pills. He does, however, record several decoction prescriptions for the treatment of center flooding in the following pages. Most likely, this refers to a decoction for dispersing any hardened blood. See a similar warning below in Line 3.50, (p. 508 - 509, and note 3).

LINE 3.22

治女人白崩及痔病方。

[The following] prescription treats women's white flooding, as well as hemorrhoid diseases.*

Formula

槐耳 白蘞 艾葉 蒲黃 白芷（各二兩） 黃芪 人參 續斷 當歸 禹餘糧 橘皮 茯苓 乾地黃 蝟皮（各三兩） 牛角䚡（四兩） 豬後懸蹄（二十個） 白馬蹄（四兩，酒浸一宿，熬）。

槐耳	huái ěr	Auricularia auricula (sophora wood ear)	二兩 2 liǎng	6g
白蘞	bái liǎn	Root of Ampelopsis japonica	二兩 2 liǎng	6g
艾葉	ài yè	Dry-roasted foliage of Artemisia argyi	二兩 2 liǎng	6g
蒲黃	pú huáng	Pollen of Typha angustata	二兩 2 liǎng	6g
白芷	bái zhǐ	Root of Angelica dahurica	二兩 2 liǎng	6g
黃芪	huáng qí	Root of Astragalus membranaceus	三兩 3 liǎng	9g
人參	rén shēn	Root of Panax ginseng	三兩 3 liǎng	9g
續斷	xù duàn	Root of Dipsacus asper	三兩 3 liǎng	9g
當歸	dāng guī	Root of Angelica polimorpha	三兩 3 liǎng	9g
禹餘糧	yǔ yú liáng	Limonite	三兩 3 liǎng	9g
橘皮	jú pí	Peel of Citrus reticulata	三兩 3 liǎng	9g
茯苓	fú líng	Dried fungus of Poria cocos	三兩 3 liǎng	9g
乾地黃	gān dì huáng	Dried root of Rehmannia glutinosa	三兩 3 liǎng	9g
蝟皮	wèi pí	Skin of Erinaceus europaeus	三兩 3 liǎng	9g
牛角䚡	niú jiǎo sāi	Ossified marrow in the center of the horn of Bos taurus domesticus	四兩 4 liǎng	12g
豬後懸蹄	zhū hòu xuán tí	Hind hooves of Sus scrofa domestica	二十個 20 gè	20 pcs
白馬蹄，酒浸一宿，熬	bái mǎ tí, jiǔ jìn yī xiǔ, āo	Hoof of Equus caballus, soaked in liquor overnight and heated slowly	四兩 4 liǎng	12g

上十七味，為末，蜜丸。每日空心酒下二十丸，日二，加之。

Pulverize the above seventeen ingredients and [mix with] honey into pills. Every day, down twenty pills in liquor on an empty stomach twice a day, increasing [the dosage].

---

* 痔 *zhì*: This disease category may be translated with the biomedical term "hemorrhoids" since its definition overlaps broadly with the Chinese term as explained in sources

roughly contemporaneous to the *Qiān Jīn Fāng*. The *Jīn Guì Yào Luè* describes it as suddenly appearing scrofula around the inside or outside of the anus, mostly caused by damp heat, overeating, constipation, sexual intercourse when intoxicated, — which caused a loss of essence and *qì* and allowed damp heat to enter,— by heavy lifting, or by excessive straining during childbirth (quoted in 《中華醫學大辭典》, pp. 1207-1208).

LINE 3.23

治婦人忽暴崩中，去血不斷，或如鵝鴨肝者方。

[The following] prescription treats women's sudden and fulminant center flooding and incessant loss of blood, possibly [of a consistency] like goose or duck liver.

Formula

小薊根（六兩） 當歸 阿膠 續斷 青竹茹 芎藭（各三兩） 生地黃（八兩） 地榆 釜月下土（各四兩，絹裏） 馬通（一升，赤帶用赤馬，白帶用白馬）。

小薊根	xiǎo jì gēn	Root of Cephalanopsis segetum	六兩 6 liǎng	18g
當歸	dāng guī	Root of Angelica polimorpha	三兩 3 liǎng	9g
阿膠	ē jiāo	Gelatinous glue produced from Equus asinus	三兩 3 liǎng	9g
續斷	xù duàn	Root of Dipsacus asper	三兩 3 liǎng	9g
青竹筎	qīng zhú rú	Shavings of Phyllostachys nigra	三兩 3 liǎng	9g
川芎	chuān xiōng	Root of Ligusticum wallichii	三兩 3 liǎng	9g
生地黃	shēng dì huáng	Fresh root of Rehmannia glutinosa	八兩 8 liǎng	24g
地榆	dì yú	Root of Sanguisorba officinalis	四兩 4 liǎng	12g
釜月下土，絹裏	fǔ yuè xià tǔ, juàn lǐ	Soot from the bottom of a pan, wrapped in silk	四兩 4 liǎng	12g
馬通	mǎ tōng*	Dung of Equus caballus	一升 1 shēng	24g

上十味，㕮咀，以水八升和馬通汁煮取三升。分三服，不止，頻服三四劑。未全止，續服後丸方。

Pound the above ten ingredients and decoct in eight *shēng* of water blended with the horse dung liquid, to obtain three *shēng*. Divide into three doses and, without stopping, take three or four preparations by sipping continuously. Before she has completely finished these and stops, continue [the treatment] by taking the following pills.

* *Sòng* editors' note: "For red discharge, use a red horse's [dung]; for white discharge, a white horse's [dung]."

Formula

續斷 甘草 地榆 鹿茸 小薊根 丹參（各三十銖） 乾地黃（二兩半） 芎藭 赤石脂 阿膠 當歸（各一兩半） 柏子仁（一兩，《集驗》作柏葉） 龜甲 秦牛角鰓（各三兩，剉，熬令黑）。

續斷	xù duàn	Root of Dipsacus asper	三十銖 30 zhū	3.75g
甘草	gān cǎo	Root of Glycyrrhiza uralensis	三十銖 30 zhū	3.75g
地榆	dì yú	Root of Sanguisorba officinalis	三十銖 30 zhū	3.75g
鹿茸	lù róng	Pilose antler of Cervus nippon	三十銖 30 zhū	3.75g
小薊根	xiǎo jì gēn	Root of Cephalanopsis segetum	三十銖 30 zhū	3.75g
丹參	dān shēn	Root of Salvia miltiorrhiza	三十銖 30 zhū	3.75g
乾地黃	gān dì huáng	Dried root of Rehmannia glutinosa	二兩半 2.5 liǎng	7.5g
川芎	chuān xiōng	Root of Ligusticum wallichii	一兩半 1.5 liǎng	4.5g
赤石脂	chì shí zhī	Halloysite	一兩半 1.5 liǎng	4.5g
阿膠	ē jiāo	Gelatinous glue produced from Equus asinus	一兩半 1.5 liǎng	4.5g
當歸	dāng guī	Root of Angelica polimorpha	一兩半 1.5 liǎng	4.5g
柏子仁*	bǎi zǐ rén	Seed of Platycladus orientalis	一兩 1 liǎng	3g
龜甲	guī jiǎ	Shell of Chinemys reevesii	三兩 3 liǎng	9g
蝟皮	wèi pí	Skin of Erinaceus europaeus	三兩 3 liǎng	9g
秦牛角鰓，剉，熬令黑	Qín niú jiǎo sāi, cuò āo lìng hēi	Ossified marrow in the center of the horn of Bos taurus domesticus, broken up and heated slowly until black	三兩 3 liǎng	9g

上十四味，為末，蜜丸梧子大。空心以酒服十丸，日再，後稍加至三十丸。

Pulverize the above fourteen ingredients and mix with honey into pills the size of firmiana seeds. On an empty stomach, take ten pills in liquor twice a day, later increasing [the dosage] gradually to a maximum of thirty pills.

* *Sòng* editors' note: "The *Jí Yàn Fāng* has *bǎi yè* (柏葉 Foliage of Platycladus orientalis)."

LINE 3.24

治女人崩中，去赤白方。

[The following] prescription treats women's center flooding with red or white [discharge].

Formula

白馬蹄（五兩）蒲黃 鹿茸 禹餘糧 白馬鬃毛 小薊根 白芷 續斷（各四兩）
人參 乾地黃 柏子仁 烏賊骨 黃芪 茯苓 當歸（各三兩）艾葉 蓯蓉 伏龍肝（
各二兩）。

白馬蹄	bái mǎ tí	Hoof of Equus caballus	五兩 5 liǎng	15g
蒲黃	pú huáng	Pollen of Typha angustata	四兩 4 liǎng	12g
鹿茸	lù róng	Pilose antler of Cervus nippon	四兩 4 liǎng	12g
禹餘糧	yǔ yú liáng	Limonite	四兩 4 liǎng	12g
白馬鬃毛	bái mǎ zōng máo	Mane of Equus caballus	四兩 4 liǎng	12g
小薊根	xiǎo jì gēn	Root of Cephalanopsis segetum	四兩 4 liǎng	12g
白芷	bái zhǐ	Root of Angelica dahurica	四兩 4 liǎng	12g
續斷	xù duàn	Root of Dipsacus asper	四兩 4 liǎng	12g
人參	rén shēn	Root of Panax ginseng	三兩 3 liǎng	9g
乾地黃	gān dì huáng	Dried root of Rehmannia glutinosa	三兩 3 liǎng	9g
柏子仁	bǎi zǐ rén	Seed of Platycladus orientalis	三兩 3 liǎng	9g
烏賊骨	wū zéi gǔ	Calcified shell of Sepiella maindroni	三兩 3 liǎng	9g
黃芪	huáng qí	Root of Astragalus membranaceus	三兩 3 liǎng	9g
茯苓	fú líng	Dried fungus of Poria cocos	三兩 3 liǎng	9g
當歸	dāng guī	Root of Angelica polimorpha	三兩 3 liǎng	9g
艾葉	ài yè	Dry-roasted foliage of Artemisia argyi	二兩 2 liǎng	6g
蓯蓉	cōng róng	Stalk of Cistanche salsa	二兩 2 liǎng	6g
伏龍肝	fú lóng gān	Stove earth	二兩 2 liǎng	6g

上十八味，為末，蜜丸如梧子大。空心飲服二十丸，日再，加至四十丸。

Pulverize the above eighteen ingredients and mix with honey into pills the size of firmiana seeds. On an empty stomach, take twenty pills in fluid twice a day, gradually increasing [the dosage] to a maximum of forty pills.

LINE 3.25

當歸湯治崩中，去血，虛羸方。

Chinese Angelica Decoction treats center flooding with hemorrhaging and vacuity emaciation.

Chinese Angelica Decoction
當歸湯 *dāng guī tāng*

當歸 芎藭 黃芩 芍藥 甘草（各二兩）生竹茹（二升）。

當歸	dāng guī	Root of Angelica polimorpha	二兩 2 liǎng	6g
川芎	chuān xiōng	Root of Ligusticum wallichii	二兩 2 liǎng	6g
黃芩	huáng qín	Root of Scutellaria baicalensis	二兩 2 liǎng	6g
芍藥	sháo yào	Root of Paeonia albiflora	二兩 2 liǎng	6g
甘草	gān cǎo	Root of Glycyrrhiza uralensis	二兩 2 liǎng	6g
生竹茹	shēng zhú rú	Fresh shavings of the stripped core Phyllostachys stalks	二升 2 shēng	48g

上六味，㕮咀，以水一斗煮竹茹取六升，去滓，內諸藥，煎取三升半，分三服。忌勞動，嗔怒，禁百日房事。

Pound the above six ingredients. Decoct the *zhú rú* 竹茹 in one *dǒu* of water to obtain six *shēng*. Discard the dregs and add all the drugs. Simmer to obtain three and a half *shēng* and divide into three doses. Avoid taxing physical labor and outbreaks of rage, and restrict sexual activities for one hundred days.

LINE 3.26

治崩中晝夜十數行，眾醫所不能瘥者方。

[The following] prescription treats center flooding with more than ten outbreaks day or night, which common physicians are unable to cure.

芎藭八兩，㕮咀，以酒五升煮取三升，分三服。不飲酒，水煮亦得。

Pound eight *liǎng* of *chuān xiōng* (川芎 Root of Ligusticum wallichii) and decoct it in five *shēng* of liquor to obtain three *shēng*. Divide into three doses. If she cannot drink liquor, decocting it in water is also possible.

LINE 3.27

治崩中下血 ，出血一斛 ，服之即斷 ，或月經來過多 ，及過期不來者 ，服之亦佳 ，方。

[The following] prescription treats center flooding with hemorrhaging of one *hú* of blood. Taking this [medicine] will make it stop. It is also excellent to take it for cases where the menstrual period arrives in excessive amounts or passes its normal time without arriving.*

Formula

吳茱萸 當歸（各三兩） 芎藭 人參 芍藥 牡丹 桂心 阿膠 生薑 甘草（各二兩） 半夏（八兩） 麥門冬（一升）。

吳茱萸	wú zhū yú	Unripe fruit of Evodia rutaecarpa	三兩 3 liǎng	9g
當歸	dāng guī	Root of Angelica polimorpha	三兩 3 liǎng	9g
川芎	chuān xiōng	Root of Ligusticum wallichii	二兩 2 liǎng	6g
人參	rén shēn	Root of Panax ginseng	二兩 2 liǎng	6g
芍藥	sháo yào	Root of Paeonia albiflora	二兩 2 liǎng	6g
牡丹	mǔ dān	Bark of the root of Paeonia suffruticosa	二兩 2 liǎng	6g
桂心	guì xīn	Shaved inner bark of Cinnamomum cassia	二兩 2 liǎng	6g
阿膠	ē jiāo	Gelatinous glue produced from Equus asinus	二兩 2 liǎng	6g
生薑	shēng jiāng	Fresh root of Zingiber officinale	二兩 2 liǎng	6g
甘草	gān cǎo	Root of Glycyrrhiza uralensis	二兩 2 liǎng	6g
半夏	bàn xià	Rhizome of Pinellia ternata	八兩 8 liǎng	24g
麥門冬	mài mén dōng	Tuber of Ophiopogon japonicus	一升 1 shēng	24g

上十二味 ，哎咀 ，以水一斗煮取三升 ，分為三服。

Pound the above twelve ingredients and decoct in one *dǒu* of water to obtain three *shēng*. Divide into three doses.

---

*　　月經來過多及過期不來者 *yuè jīng lái guò duō jí guò qī bù lái zhě*: This phrase is quite ambiguous. 月經來過多 could also be interpreted "a menstrual period that arrives too frequently and for an excessive period of time. In cases when it fails to arrive,. .." The *Sūn Zhēn Rén* edition only states, 月經來過期 *yuè jīng lái guò qī* (a menstrual period that arrives in excess of its time…). This prescription stands out here as the only one that treats a lack of or delayed menstruation in conjunction with treating hemorrhaging. The *Qiān Jīn Yì Fāng* does not contain any prescriptions either that address deficient menstruation with the same prescription as excessive bleeding.

LINE 3.28

治暴崩中 ，去血不止方。

[The following] prescription treats fulminant center flooding with incessant hemorrhaging.

Formula

牡蠣 兔骨 （各二兩半 ，炙 ）。

牡蠣	mǔ lì	Shell of Ostrea rivularis	二兩半 liǎng	2.5	7.5g
兔骨, 炙	tù gǔ, zhì	Bones of Oryctolagus domesticus, roasted	二兩半 liǎng	2.5	7.5g

上二味 ，治下篩。酒服方寸匕 ，日三。

Finely pestle and sift the above two ingredients. Take a square-inch spoon in liquor three times a day.

LINE 3.29

治女人白崩方。

[The following] prescription treats women's white flooding.

Formula

芎藭 桂心 阿膠 赤石脂 小薊根 （各二兩 ） 乾地黃 （四兩 ） 伏龍肝 （如雞子大七枚 ）。

川芎	chuān xiōng	Root of Ligusticum wallichii	二兩 2 liǎng	6g
桂心	guì xīn	Shaved inner bark of Cinnamomum cassia	二兩 2 liǎng	6g
阿膠	ē jiāo	Gelatinous glue produced from Equus asinus	二兩 2 liǎng	6g
楮實子	chǔ shí zǐ	Fruit of Broussonetia papyrifera	二兩 2 liǎng	6g
小薊根	xiǎo jì gēn	Root of Cephalanopsis segetum	二兩 2 liǎng	6g
乾地黃	gān dì huáng	Dried root of Rehmannia glutinosa	四兩 4 liǎng	12g
伏龍肝	fú lóng gān	Stove earth	如雞子大七枚 rú jī zǐ dà 7 méi	a piece as big as an egg

上七味，㕮咀，以酒六升，水四升合煮取三升，去滓，內膠令烊盡，分三服，日三。

Pound the above seven ingredients and decoct in a mix of six *shēng* of liquor and four *shēng* of water to obtain three *shēng*. Discard the dregs and add the *ē jiāo* 阿膠, letting it melt completely. Divide into three doses [and take] three times daily.[*]

---

[*]   *Sòng* editors' note: "The *Qiān Jīn Yì Fāng* stops after six ingredients, lacking *fú lóng gān* 伏龍肝."

LINE 3.30

伏龍肝湯治崩中，去赤白或如豆汁方。

Stove Earth Decoction treats center flooding with discharge of a red or white or bean juice-like fluid.

Stove Earth Decoction
伏龍肝湯 *fú lóng gān tāng*

伏龍肝（如彈丸七枚） 生地黃（四升） 生薑（五兩） 甘草 艾葉 赤石脂 桂心（各二兩）。

伏龍肝	fú lóng gān	Stove earth	如彈丸七枚 rú dàn wán 7 méi	7 pcs

生地黄	shēng dì huáng	Fresh root of Rehmannia glutinosa	四升 4 shēng[1]	96g
生薑	shēng jiāng	Fresh root of Zingiber officinale	五兩 5 liǎng	15g
甘草	gān cǎo	Root of Glycyrrhiza uralensis	二兩 2 liǎng	6g
艾葉	ài yè	Dry-roasted foliage of Artemisia argyi	二兩 2 liǎng	6g
楮實子	chǔ shí zǐ	Fruit of Broussonetia papyrifera	二兩 2 liǎng	6g
桂心	guì xīn	Shaved inner bark of Cinnamomum cassia	二兩 2 liǎng	6g

上七味，㕮咀，以水一斗煮取三升。分四服，日三夜一。

Pound the above seven ingredients and decoct in one *dǒu* of water to obtain three *shēng*. Divide into four doses [and take] three times during the day and once at night.[2]

1. *Sòng* editors' note: "Another [version of this] prescription has 5 *liǎng*."
2. After this sentence, the *Sūn Zhēn Rén* edition adds the following phrase: 數試有驗 *shù shì yǒu yàn* (It has achieved good results in numerous tests).

LINE 3.31

大牛角中仁散治積冷崩中，去血不止，腰背痛，四肢沈重，虛極方。

Major Ox Horn Marrow Powder treats accumulated cold, center flooding, incessant hemorrhaging, lumbar and back pain, heaviness of the four limbs, and extreme vacuity.

Major Ox Horn Marrow Powder
大牛角中仁散 *dà niú jiǎo zhōng rén sǎn*

牛角仁（一枚，燒）續斷 乾地黄 桑耳 白朮 赤石脂 礬石 乾薑附子 龍骨 當歸（各三兩）人參（一兩）蒲黄 防風 禹餘糧（各二兩）。

牛角仁，燒	niú jiǎo rén, shāo	Ossified marrow in the center of the horn of Bos taurus domesticus, charred	一枚 1 méi	1 pc
續斷	xù duàn	Root of Dipsacus asper	三兩 3 liǎng	9g
乾地黄	gān dì huáng	Dried root of Rehmannia glutinosa	三兩 3 liǎng	9g
桑耳	sāng ěr	Mulberry wood ear	三兩 3 liǎng	9g
白朮	bái zhú	Rhizome of Atractylodes macrocephala	三兩 3 liǎng	9g

赤石脂	chì shí zhī	Halloysite	三兩 3 liǎng	9g
礬石	fán shí	Alum	三兩 3 liǎng	9g
乾薑	gān jiāng	Dried root of Zingiber officinale	三兩 3 liǎng	9g
附子	fù zǐ	Lateral root of Aconitum carmichaeli	三兩 3 liǎng	9g
龍骨	lóng gǔ	Os draconis	三兩 3 liǎng	9g
當歸	dāng guī	Root of Angelica polimorpha	三兩 3 liǎng	9g
人參	rén shēn	Root of Panax ginseng	一兩 1 liǎng	3g
蒲黃	pú huáng	Pollen of Typha angustata	二兩 2 liǎng	6g
防風	fáng fēng	Root of Ledebouriella divaricata	二兩 2 liǎng	6g
禹餘糧	yǔ yú liáng	Limonite	二兩 2 liǎng	6g

上十五味，治下篩。以溫酒未食方寸匕，日三，不知稍加。

Finely pestle and sift the above fifteen ingredients. Take a square-inch spoon in heated liquor before meals three times a day. If you do not notice [an effect], gradually increase [the dosage].

* 牛角中仁 *niú jiǎo zhōng rén*: Although not attested elsewhere, I equate this with what is commonly termed 牛角䚡 *niú jiǎo sāi*, ox horn marrow, as a medicinal ingredient. This equation is supported by the fact that the *Sūn Zhēn Rén* edition has *niú jiǎo sāi*.

LINE 3.32

治崩中，去血積時不止，起死方。

[The following] prescription treats center flooding and chronic incessant hemorrhaging. It will raise the dead.

肥羊肉（三斤）乾薑 當歸（各三兩）生地黃（二升）。

肥羊肉	féi yáng ròu	Unrendered fat of Capra hircus	三斤 3 jīn	144g
乾薑	gān jiāng	Dried root of Zingiber officinale	三兩 3 liǎng	9g
當歸	dāng guī	Root of Angelica polimorpha	三兩 3 liǎng	9g
生地黃	shēng dì huáng*	Fresh root of Rehmannia glutinosa	二升 2 shēng	48g

上四味，㕮咀，以水二斗煮羊肉，取一斗三升，下地黃汁及諸藥，煮取三升，分四服，即斷。尤宜羸瘦人服之。

Pound the above four ingredients. Cook the sheep or goat's meat in two *dǒu* of water to obtain one *dǒu* and three *shēng*. Add the *shēng dì huáng zhī* 生地黃汁 and various [other] drugs and decoct it to obtain three *shēng*. Divide into four doses. [After taking it], [the flooding] will stop promptly. Taking this [prescription] is particularly suitable for patients with marked emaciation.

*   生地黃 *shēng dì huáng*: The *Sūn Zhēn Rén* edition has 地黃汁 *dì huáng zhī* (rehmannia juice) instead, which is supported by the instructions that accompany this prescription.

LINE 3.33

生地黃湯治崩中，漏下，日去數升方。

Fresh Rehmannia Decoction treats center flooding and spotting, losing several *shēng* of blood per day.

Fresh Rehmannia Decoction
生地黃湯 *shēng dì huáng tāng*

生地黃（一斤）細辛（三兩）。

| 生地黃 | shēng dì huáng[1] | Fresh root of Rehmannia glutinosa | 一斤 1 jīn | 48g |
| 細辛 | xì xīn | Complete plant including root of Asarum heteropoides | 三兩 3 liǎng | 9g |

上二味，㕮咀，以水一斗煮取六升。服七合，久服佳。

Pound the above two ingredients and decoct in one *dǒu* of water to obtain six *shēng*. Take seven *gě* [per dose]. It is excellent to take this for a long period of time.

LINE 3.34

治崩中，漏下，赤白不止，氣虛竭方。

[The following] prescription treats center flooding, spotting, incessant red and white [discharge], and qì exhaustion.

Formula

龜甲 牡蠣（各三兩）。

龜甲	guī jiǎ	Shell of Chinemys reevesii	三兩 3 liǎng	9g
牡蠣	mǔ lì	Shell of Ostrea rivularis	三兩 3 liǎng	9g

上二味，治下篩。酒服方寸匕，日三。

Finely pestle and sift the above two ingredients. Take a square-inch spoon in liquor three times a day.

LINE 3.35

又方

Another prescription:

燒亂髮，酒和服方寸匕，日三。

Char *luàn fà* (亂髮 Matted hair) and take a square-inch spoon mixed with liquor three times a day.

LINE 3.36

又方

Another prescription:*

Formula

桑耳（二兩半）鹿茸（十八銖）。

桑耳	sāng ěr	Mulberry wood ear	二兩半 2.5 liǎng	7.5g
鹿茸	lù róng	Pilose antler of Cervus nippon	十八銖 18 zhū	2.25g

上二味，以醋五升漬，炙燥，漬盡為度，治下篩。服方寸匕，日三。

Soak the above two ingredients in five *shēng* of vinegar, then fry and roast them until the soaking liquid is all gone. Finely pestle and sift [the drugs]. Take a square-inch spoon three times a day.

*   *Sòng* editors' note: "Instead of this prescription, the *Sūn Zhēn Rén* edition contains two prescriptions for taking *sāng ěr* 桑耳 and *lù róng* 鹿茸 as single medicinals, each charred and mixed into liquor."

LINE 3.37

又方

Another prescription:

燒鹿角為末，酒服方寸匕，日三。

Pulverize charred *lù jiǎo* (鹿角 Ossified antler or antler base of Cervus nippon). Take a square-inch spoon in liquor three times a day.

LINE 3.38

又方

Another prescription:

燒桃核為末，酒服方寸匕，日三。

Pulverize charred *táo hé* (桃核 Seed of Prunus persica).˙ Take a square-inch spoon in liquor three times a day.

*   桃核 *táo hé*: As a medicinal ingredient, usually called 桃仁 *táo rén*.

LINE 3.39

又方

Another prescription:

Formula

地榆 知母。

| 地榆 | dì yú | Root of Sanguisorba officinalis |
| 知母 | zhī mǔ | Root of Anemarrhena asphodelo-ides |

上二味，各指大長一尺者，㕮咀，以醋三升東向竈中治極濃，去滓，服
之。

Of each of the above two ingredients, take a piece as wide as a finger and one *chǐ* long. Pound them. Finely pestle [and decoct?] them in an east-facing stove with three *shēng* of vinegar to the consistency of an extremely concentrated thick liquid. Discard the dregs and take it.

LINE 3.40

又方

Another prescription:

桑木中蝎屎，燒灰，酒服方寸匕。

Char the excrement of mulberry wood scorpions˙ into ashes and take a square-inch spoon in liquor.

*   桑木中蝎 *sāng mù zhōng xiē*: In accordance with the *Sòng* edition, the *Huá Xià* edition has 蜴 *yì* (lizard) instead of 蝎, but I follow the *Huá Xià* edition, which considers this a textual corruption, based on the fact that the *Sūn Zhēn Rén* edition, as well as several related prescriptions in the *Wài Tái Mì Yào* and *Qiān Jīn Fāng* use 桑樹中蝎蟲屎 *sāng shù zhōng xiē chóng shǐ* or 桑蝎蟲屎 *sāng xiē chóng shǐ* (the excrement of mulberry wood scorpions) for stopping bleeding.

LINE 3.41

治崩中，下血，羸瘦少氣，調中補虛，止血方。

[The following] prescription treats center flooding, descent of blood, marked emaciation, and shortage of *qì*, by regulating the center, supplementing the vacuity, and stanching bleeding.

Formula

澤蘭 蜀椒（二兩六銖） 藁本 柏子仁 山茱萸 厚朴（各十八銖） 乾地黃 牡蠣（各一兩半） 代赭 桂心 防風 細辛 乾薑（各一兩） 甘草 當歸 芎藭（各一兩十八銖） 蕪荑（半兩）。

澤蘭	zé lán	Foliage and stalk of Lycopus lucidus	二兩六銖 2 liǎng 6 zhū	6.75g
蜀椒	shǔ jiāo	Seed capsules of Zanthoxylum bungeanum	二兩六銖 2 liǎng 6 zhū	6.75g
藁本	gǎo běn	Rhizome and root of Ligusticum sinense	十八銖 18 zhū	2.25g
柏子仁	bǎi zǐ rén	Seed of Platycladus orientalis	十八銖 18 zhū	2.25g
山茱萸	shān zhū yú	Fruit of Cornus officinalis	十八銖 18 zhū	2.25g
厚朴	hòu pò	Bark of Magnolia officinalis	十八銖 18 zhū	2.25g
乾地黃	gān dì huáng	Dried root of Rehmannia glutinosa	一兩半 1.5 liǎng	4.5g
牡蠣	mǔ lì	Shell of Ostrea rivularis	一兩半 1.5 liǎng	4.5g
代赭	dài zhě	Hematite	一兩 1 liǎng	3g
桂心	guì xīn	Shaved inner bark of Cinnamomum cassia	一兩 1 liǎng	3g
防風	fáng fēng	Root of Ledebouriella divaricata	一兩 1 liǎng	3g
細辛	xì xīn	Complete plant including root of Asarum heteropoides	一兩 1 liǎng	3g
乾薑	gān jiāng	Dried root of Zingiber officinale	一兩 1 liǎng	3g
甘草	gān cǎo	Root of Glycyrrhiza uralensis	一兩十八銖 1 liǎng 18 zhū	5.25g
當歸	dāng guī	Root of Angelica polimorpha	一兩十八銖 1 liǎng 18 zhū	5.25g
川芎	chuān xiōng	Root of Ligusticum wallichii	一兩十八銖 1 liǎng 18 zhū	5.25g
蕪荑	wú yí	Processed fruit of Ulmus macrocarpa	半兩 0.5 liǎng	1.5g

上十七味，治下篩。空心溫酒服方寸匕，日三，神良。

Finely pestle and sift the above seventeen ingredients. On an empty stomach, take a square-inch spoon in heated liquor three times a day. [This prescription] is divinely good.*

* *Sòng* editors' note: "Another [version of this] prescription adds 18 *zhū* each of *bái zhǐ* (白芷 Root of Angelica dahurica) and *lóng gǔ* (龍骨 Os draconis) and 1 *liǎng* and 18 *zhū* of *rén shēn* (人參 Root of Panax ginseng), making it a total of 20 ingredients."

LINE 3.42

治崩中方。

[The following] prescription treats center flooding.

Formula

白茅根（三斤） 小薊根（五斤）。

白茅根	bái máo gēn	Imperata cylindrica	三斤 3 jīn	144g
小薊根	xiǎo jì gēn	Root of Cephalanopsis segetum	五斤 5 jīn	240g

上二味，㕮咀，以水五斗煎取四斗，稍稍服之。

Pound the above two ingredients and decoct in five *dǒu* of water to obtain four *dǒu*. Take by sipping it slowly.*

* *Sòng* editors' note: "The *Wài Tái Mì Yào* uses liquor to decoct it."

LINE 3.43

丹參酒治崩中去血，及產餘疾方。

Salvia Liquor treats center flooding and bleeding, as well as residual diseases from childbirth.

Salvia Liquor
丹參酒 *dān shēn jiǔ*

丹參 艾葉 地黃 忍冬 地榆（各五斤）。

丹參	dān shēn	Root of Salvia miltiorrhiza	五斤 5 jīn	240g
艾葉	ài yè	Dry-roasted foliage of Artemisia argyi	五斤 5 jīn	240g
地黃	dì huáng	Root of Rehmannia glutinosa	五斤 5 jīn	240g
忍冬	rěn dōng	Different parts of Lonicera japonica	五斤 5 jīn	240g
地榆	dì yú	Root of Sanguisorba officinalis	五斤 5 jīn	240g

上五味，剉，先洗，臼熟舂，以水漬三宿，出滓，煮取汁，以黍米一斛炊飯釀酒，酒熟酢之。初服四合，後稍稍添之。

Break the above five ingredients into pieces. First wash and pestle [the drugs] thoroughly in a mortar. Then soak them in water for three nights, remove the dregs, and boil [the liquid]. Use it to steam one *hú* of millet and ferment it into liquor. When the liquor is finished, express the liquid. Initially, take four *gě* [per dose], later increase [the amount] very gradually.

LINE 3.44

牡丹皮湯治崩中血盛，併服三劑即瘥方。

Moutan Decoction treats center flooding and blood exuberance. Taking three preparations together causes prompt recovery.[1]

Moutan Decoction
牡丹皮湯 *mǔ dān pí tāng*

牡丹皮 乾地黃 斛脈（各三兩） 禹餘糧 艾葉 龍骨 柏葉 厚朴 白芷 伏龍肝 青竹茹 芎藭 地榆（各二兩） 阿膠（一兩） 芍藥（四兩）。

牡丹皮	mǔ dān pí	Bark of the root of Paeonia suffruticosa	三兩 3 liǎng	9g
乾地黃	gān dì huáng	Dried root of Rehmannia glutinosa	三兩 3 liǎng	9g
斛脈	hú mài[2]	unknown	三兩 3 liǎng	9g
柏葉	bǎi yè	Foliage of Platycladus orientalis	二兩 2 liǎng	6g
厚朴	hòu pò	Bark of Magnolia officinalis	二兩 2 liǎng	6g
白芷	bái zhǐ	Root of Angelica dahurica	二兩 2 liǎng	6g
伏龍肝	fú lóng gān	Stove earth	二兩 2 liǎng	6g
青竹茹	qīng zhú rú	Shavings of Phyllostachys nigra	二兩 2 liǎng	6g
川芎	chuān xiōng	Root of Ligusticum wallichii	二兩 2 liǎng	6g

地榆	dì yú	Root of Sanguisorba officinalis	二兩 2 liǎng	6g
阿膠	ē jiāo	Gelatinous glue produced from Equus asinus	一兩 1 liǎng	3g
芍藥	sháo yào	Root of Paeonia albiflora	四兩 4 liǎng	12g

上十五味 , 㕮咀 , 以水一斗五升煮取五升。分五服 , 相去如人行十里久再服。

Pound the above fifteen ingredients. Decoct in one *dǒu* and five *shēng* of water to obtain five *shēng*. Divide into five doses and take the doses separated by the length of time it takes a person to walk ten lǐ.

1. In the *Sūn Zhēn Rén* edition, the prescription is indicated for "extremely critical cases of center collapse" (崩中極重者 *bēng zhōng jí zhòng zhě*).
2. 斛脈 *hú mài*: Most probably an abbreviation for 槲葉脈 *hú yè mài* (oak leaf veins), which is what the *Sūn Zhēn Rén* edition has here.

LINE 3.45

治崩中單方。

[The following] single-ingredient prescription treats center flooding.

燒牛角末 , 以酒服方寸匕 , 日三服。亦治帶下。

Pulverize charred *niú jiǎo* (牛角 Ossified marrow in the center of the horn of Bos taurus domesticus). Take a square-inch spoon in liquor three times a day. It also treats vaginal discharge.

LINE 3.46

又方

Another prescription:

桑耳燒令黑 , 為末 , 酒服方寸匕 , 日二服。亦治帶下。

Char *sāng ěr* (桑耳 Mulberry wood ear) until black and pulverize it. Take a square-inch spoon in liquor twice a day. It also treats vaginal discharge.

LINE 3.47

又方

Another prescription:

生薊根一斤半，擣取汁，溫服。亦可酒煮服之。

Take one and a half *jīn* of fresh *jì gēn* (薊根 Root of Cirsium japonicum) and pound it to obtain the juice. Drink it heated. You may also decoct it in liquor and take it that way.

LINE 3.48

又方

Another prescription:

羊胰一具，以酢煮，去血服之，即止。忌豬，魚，酢滑物，犯之便死。亦治帶下。

Cook one complete sheep's or goat's pancreas in vinegar. Take it when bleeding and it will promptly stop. Avoid pork, fish, and sour or slippery foods. If she breaks [this prohibition], she will die. It also treats vaginal discharge.

LINE 3.49

治白崩方。

[The following] prescription treats white flooding.

Moxibustion Method

灸小腹橫文當臍孔直下百壯。
又，灸內踝上三寸，左右各百壯。

Burn 100 moxa cones directly below where the horizontal line of the lower abdomen meets the navel.

Another: Burn 100 moxa cones each on the point three *cùn* above the left and right inner ankle.

LINE 3.50

(一) 論曰：治漏血不止，或新傷胎，及產後餘血不消作堅，使胞門不閉，淋瀝去血，經逾日月不止者，未可以諸斷血湯。(二) 宜且與牡丹丸，散等，待血堅消便停也。(三) 堅血消者，所去淋瀝便自止，亦漸變消少也。(四) 此後有餘傷毀，不復處此，乃可作諸主治耳。(五) 婦人產乳去血多，傷胎去血多，崩中去血多，金瘡去血多，拔牙齒去血多，未止，心中懸虛，心悶眩冒，頭重目暗，耳聾滿，舉頭便悶欲倒，宜且煮當歸，芎藭各三兩，以水四升煮取二升，去滓，分二服，即定。(六) 展轉續次合諸湯治之。

(1) Essay: When treating incessant blood spotting, possibly from recent damage to the fetus, or failure to disperse residual postpartum blood so that it solidifies, prevents the uterus entrance from closing, and causes dribbling blood loss for days and months without stopping, you may not yet use the various decoctions for interrupting the blood flow.

(2) For the time being, you should administer *Moutan Pills* or *Powders*[1] until the solidified blood has dispersed, before stopping (the treatment).

(3) When the solidified blood is dissipated, the dribbling bleeding will then stop on its own [since it is] also gradually being transformed, dissipated, and reduced.

(4) And if afterwards there is further damage and destruction,[2] do not repeat this treatment. Now you can administer the various cures and treatments.[3]

(5) Women's excessive loss of blood from childbirth, damage to the fetus, center flooding, incised wounds, or dental extractions, that will not stop [and is accompanied by] suspension vacuity in the heart, heart oppression and veiling dizziness, heaviness of the head and dimmed vision, deafness and fullness in the ears, and oppression and tendency to faint when lifting the head should be treated by decocting three *liǎng* each of *dāng guī* (當歸 Root of Angelica polimorpha) and *chuān xiōng* (川芎 Root of Ligusticum wallichii) in four *shēng* of water to obtain two *shēng*. Discard the dregs and divide into two doses, then [the patient] will be promptly stabilized.

(6) Turn this over and over in your mind and follow the order [of medicines recommended above] when compounding the various decoctions to treat [these conditions].

1. 牡丹丸散 *mǔ dān wán sǎn*: Rather than referring to specific prescriptions, this most likely means to take moutan as a supplement in pill or powder form. In the *Shén Nóng Běn Cǎo Jīng*, moutan is classified as belonging to the middle category, which "are used primarily to nurture human nature, . . . are partially toxic,. . . and prevent disease by supplementing vacuity and emaciation" (《神農本草經》 1:1). The entry for moutan states that "it is acrid, cold, and non-toxic. It treats [aversion to] cold and heat [effusion], wind strike, . . . evil *qi*, eliminates concretions and hardness, and static blood lodging in the intestines and stomach. . . " (《神農本草經》 3:161). It was thus already in medieval times used as a gentle and supplementing medicinal for breaking up blood stagnation and eliminating evils, therefore being an ideal drug in the context discussed by Sūn Sī-Miǎo here.

2. 有餘傷毀 *yǒu yú shāng huǐ*: This refers to cases where the removal of the solidified blood has not completely cured the woman's problems.

3. This passage discusses the dangers of administering strong blood-stanching medicinals to treat bleeding in cases where the condition is caused by an underlying etiology of blood stagnation and solidification, because they would only exacerbate the root cause of inhibited blood flow. Thus, the careful physician needs to diagnose blood stagnation and first resolve this with a gentle and supplementing treatment with moutan, before he can proceed to treat other symptoms of bleeding with the customary blood-stanching medicinals. Sūn Sī-Miǎo here advocates the somewhat counterintuitive use of blood-moving drugs in the treatment of vaginal bleeding, based on an underlying etiology of postpartum retention of lochia. The choice of ingredients in the following prescriptions serve as a practical application of the theoretical explanation in this essay.

LINE 3.51

白聖丸治女人參十六疾，胞中病，漏下不絕方。

Chalk Pills treat women's thirty-six diseases [of vaginal discharge], diseases in the uterus, and incessant vaginal spotting.[1]

Chalk Pills
白堊丸 *bái è wán*

邯鄲白堊 禹餘糧 白芷 白石脂 乾薑 龍骨 桂心 瞿麥 大黃 石韋 白薟 細辛 芍藥 甘草 黃連 附子 當歸 茯苓 鍾乳 蜀椒 黃芩（各半兩）牡蠣 烏賊骨（各十八銖）。

邯鄲白堊	hán dān bái è	Chalk	半兩 0.5 liǎng	1.5g
禹餘糧	yǔ yú liáng	Limonite	半兩 0.5 liǎng	1.5g
白芷	bái zhǐ	Root of Angelica dahurica	半兩 0.5 liǎng	1.5g
白石脂	bái shí zhī	Kaolin	半兩 0.5 liǎng	1.5g
乾薑	gān jiāng	Dried root of Zingiber officinale	半兩 0.5 liǎng	1.5g
龍骨	lóng gǔ	Os draconis	半兩 0.5 liǎng	1.5g
桂心	guì xīn	Shaved inner bark of Cinnamomum cassia	半兩 0.5 liǎng	1.5g
瞿麥	qú mài	Entire plant, including flowers, of Dianthus superbus	半兩 0.5 liǎng	1.5g
大黃	dà huáng	Root of Rheum palmatum	半兩 0.5 liǎng	1.5g
石韋	shí wéi	Foliage of Pyrrosia lingua	半兩 0.5 liǎng	1.5g
白薟	bái liǎn	Root of Ampelopsis japonica	半兩 0.5 liǎng	1.5g

細辛	xì xīn	Complete plant including root of Asarum heteropoides	半兩 0.5 liǎng	1.5g
芍藥	sháo yào	Root of Paeonia albiflora	半兩 0.5 liǎng	1.5g
甘草	gān cǎo	Root of Glycyrrhiza uralensis	半兩 0.5 liǎng	1.5g
黃連	huáng lián	Rhizome of Coptis chinensis	半兩 0.5 liǎng	1.5g
附子	fù zǐ	Lateral root of Aconitum carmichaeli	半兩 0.5 liǎng	1.5g
當歸	dāng guī	Root of Angelica polimorpha	半兩 0.5 liǎng	1.5g
茯苓	fú líng	Dried fungus of Poria cocos	半兩 0.5 liǎng	1.5g
鐘乳	zhōng rǔ	Stalactite	半兩 0.5 liǎng	1.5g
蜀椒	shǔ jiāo	Seed capsules of Zanthoxylum bungeanum	半兩 0.5 liǎng	1.5g
黃芩	huáng qín	Root of Scutellaria baicalensis	半兩 0.5 liǎng	1.5g
牡蠣	mǔ lì	Shell of Ostrea rivularis	十八銖 18 zhū	2.25g
烏賊骨	wū zéi gǔ	Calcified shell of Sepiella maindroni	十八銖 18 zhū	2.25g

上二十三味，為末，蜜丸梧子大，空心酒服五丸，日再服，不知加至十丸。

Pulverize the above twenty-three ingredients and mix with honey into pills the size of firmiana seeds. On an empty stomach, take five pills in liquor twice a day. If you notice no effect, increase [the dosage] to a maximum of ten pills.

1. *Sòng* editors' note: "For another prescription, see above." This refers to the prescription on Line 3.2 above (pp. 468 - 469).
2. 邯鄲白堊 *hán dān bái è*: chalk from the region of Hán-Dān 邯鄲, located in modern Hé-Běi 河北 Province.

LINE 3.52

治女人漏下，或瘥或劇，常漏不止，身體羸瘦，飲食減少，或赤或白或黃，使人無子者方。

[The following prescription treats women's vaginal spotting that is now treated now aggravated, constant incessant spotting, marked emaciation of the body, reduced intake of food and drink, and red, white, or yellow vaginal discharge, all of which are preventing the patient from bearing children.

Formula

牡蠣 伏龍肝 赤石脂 白龍骨 桂心 烏賊骨 禹餘糧（各等分）。

牡蠣	mǔ lì	Shell of Ostrea rivularis	等分 děng fēn	Equal amounts
伏龍肝	fú lóng gān	Stove earth		
赤石脂	chì shí zhī	Halloysite		
白龍骨	bái lóng gǔ	Bleached fossilized vertebra and bone of mammals		
桂心	guì xīn	Shaved inner bark of Cinnamomum cassia		
烏賊骨	wū zéi gǔ	Calcified shell of Sepiella maindroni		
禹餘糧	yǔ yú liáng	Limonite		

上七味，治下篩。空心酒服方寸匕，日二。白多者，加牡蠣，龍骨，烏賊骨；赤多者，加赤石脂，禹餘糧；黃多者，加伏龍肝，桂心；隨病加之。

Finely pestle and sift the above seven ingredients. On an empty stomach, take a square-inch spoon in liquor twice a day. For mostly white discharge, increase the *mǔ lì* 牡蠣, *lóng gǔ* 龍骨, and *wū zéi gǔ* 烏賊骨. For mostly red discharge, increase the *chì shí zhī* 赤石脂 and *yǔ yú liáng* 禹餘糧. For mostly yellow discharge, increase the *fú lóng gān* 伏龍肝 and *guì xīn* 桂心. Increase the drugs in accordance with the [particular] condition.*

---

*   *Sòng* editors' note: "Zhāng Wén-zhòng [quotes] the same [prescription and states that] it treats center flooding. The *Zhǒu Hòu Fāng* does not include *bái lóng gǔ* 白龍骨 and [instructs] to drink it with gruel."

LINE 3.53

治婦人漏下不止，散方。

[The following] powder prescription treats women's incessant vaginal spotting.

Formula

鹿茸 阿膠（各三兩） 烏賊骨 當歸（各二兩） 蒲黃（一兩）。

鹿茸	lù róng	Pilose antler of Cervus nippon	三兩 3 liǎng	9g
阿膠	ē jiāo	Gelatinous glue produced from Equus asinus	三兩 3 liǎng	9g
烏賊骨	wū zéi gǔ	Calcified shell of Sepiella maindroni	二兩 2 liǎng	6g
當歸	dāng guī	Root of Angelica polimorpha	二兩 2 liǎng	6g
蒲黃	pú huáng	Pollen of Typha angustata	一兩 1 liǎng	3g

上五味，治下篩。空心酒服方寸匕，日三夜再服。

Finely pestle and sift the above five ingredients. On an empty stomach, take a square-inch spoon in liquor three times a day and twice at night.

LINE 3.54

治女人產後漏下，及痔病下血方。

[The following] prescription treats women's postpartum vaginal spotting as well as hemorrhoids and descent of blood.

Formula

礬石（一兩）附子（一枚）。

| 礬石 | fán shí | Alum | 一兩 1 liǎng | 3g |
| 附子 | fù zǐ | Lateral root of Aconitum carmichaeli | 一枚 1 méi | 1 pc |

上二味，為末，蜜丸如梧子大。空心酒下二丸，日三，稍加至五丸，數日瘥。能百日服之，永斷。

Pulverize the above two ingredients and mix with honey into pills the size of firmiana seeds. On an empty stomach, take two pills in liquor three times a day, increasing the dosage gradually to a maximum of five pills. She will recover in a number of days. If she is able to take it for one hundred days, she will stop [the condition] permanently.

LINE 3.55

芎藭湯治帶下漏血不止方。

Chuānxiōng Decoction treats incessant vaginal discharge and spotting of blood.

Chuānxiōng Decoction
芎藭湯 *xiōng qióng tāng*

芎藭 乾地黃 黃芪 芍藥 吳茱萸 甘草（各二兩） 當歸 乾薑（各三兩）。

川芎	chuān xiōng	Root of Ligusticum wallichii	二兩 2 liǎng	6g
乾地黃	gān dì huáng	Dried root of Rehmannia glutinosa	二兩 2 liǎng	6g
黃芪	huáng qí	Root of Astragalus membranaceus	二兩 2 liǎng	6g
芍藥	sháo yào	Root of Paeonia albiflora	二兩 2 liǎng	6g
吳茱萸	wú zhū yú	Unripe fruit of Evodia rutaecarpa	二兩 2 liǎng	6g
甘草	gān cǎo	Root of Glycyrrhiza uralensis	二兩 2 liǎng	6g
當歸	dāng guī	Root of Angelica polimorpha	三兩 3 liǎng	9g
乾薑	gān jiāng	Dried root of Zingiber officinale	三兩 3 liǎng	9g

上八味，哎咀，以水一斗煮取三升，分三服。若月經後，因有赤白不止者，除地黃，吳茱萸，加杜仲，人參各二兩。

Pound the above eight ingredients and decoct in one *dǒu* of water to obtain three *shēng*. Divide into three doses. For red and white incessant [discharge] after menstruation, take out the *[gān] dì huáng* [乾]地黃 and *wú zhū yú* 吳茱萸, and add two *liǎng* each of *dù zhòng* (杜仲 Bark of Eucommia ulmoidis) and *rén shēn* (人參 Root of Panax ginseng).

LINE 3.56

治漏下去血不止方。

[The following] prescription treats vaginal spotting and incessant bleeding.

取水蛭，治下篩。酒服一錢許，日二，惡血消即愈。

Take *shuǐ zhì* (水蛭 Dried body of Whitmania pigra) and finely pestle and sift them. Take about one *qián* in liquor twice a day. She will recover as soon as the malign blood is dispersed.

LINE 3.57

治漏下神方。

[The following] is a divine prescription for treating vaginal spotting.

取槐子燒末，酒服方寸匕，日三，立瘥。

Char and pulverize *huái zǐ* (槐子 Fruit of Sophora japonica). Take a square-inch spoon in liquor three times a day. It will cause immediate recovery.

LINE 3.58

治漏下去黑方。

[The following] prescription treats black vaginal spotting.[1]

Formula

乾漆 麻黃 細辛 桂心（各一兩） 甘草（半兩）。

乾漆	gān qī	Dried sap of Rhus verniciflua	一兩 1 liǎng	3g
麻黃	má huáng	Stalk of Ephedra sinica	一兩 1 liǎng	3g
細辛	xì xīn	Complete plant including root of Asarum heteropoides	一兩 1 liǎng	3g
桂心	guì xīn	Shaved inner bark of Cinnamomum cassia	一兩 1 liǎng	3g
甘草	gān cǎo	Root of Glycyrrhiza uralensis	半兩 0.5 liǎng	1.5g

上五味，治下篩。以指撮著米飲中服之。

Finely pestle and sift the above five ingredients. Take it by adding a finger pinch to rice soup.[2]

1. 漏下去黑 *lòu xià qù hēi*. In this and the following prescriptions with parallel wording in the other colors, the *Sūn Zhēn Rén* edition instead has 漏下黑血 *lòu xià hēi xuè* (vaginal leaking of black [or red, or yellow etc.] blood). Thereby, the vaginal discharge in all prescriptions in this chapter is identified as blood, specifically as the malign blood that has solidified in the uterus after childbirth.
2. The *Sūn Zhēn Rén* edition has instead: "Take a square-inch spoon in a bowl of rice water three times a day."

LINE 3.59

治漏下去赤方。

[The following] prescription treats red vaginal spotting.

Formula

白朮（二兩）白薇（半兩）黃蘗（二兩半）。

白朮	bái zhú	Rhizome of Atractylodes macro-cephala	二兩 2 liǎng	6g
白薇	bái wēi	Root of Cynanchum atratum	半兩 0.5 liǎng	1.5g
黃蘗	huáng bò	Bark of Phellodendron amurense	二兩半 2.5 liǎng	7.5g

上三味，治下篩。空心酒服方寸匕，日三。

Finely pestle and sift the above three ingredients. On an empty stomach, take a square-inch spoon in liquor three times a day.

LINE 3.60

治漏下去黃方。

[The following] prescription treats yellow vaginal spotting.

Formula

黃連 大黃 桂心（各半兩）黃芩 蟅蟲 乾地黃（各六銖）。

黃連	huáng lián	Rhizome of Coptis chinensis	半兩 0.5 liǎng	1.5g
大黃	dà huáng	Root of Rheum palmatum	半兩 0.5 liǎng	1.5g
桂心	guì xīn	Shaved inner bark of Cinnamomum cassia	半兩 0.5 liǎng	1.5g
黃芩	huáng qín	Root of Scutellaria baicalensis	六銖 6 zhū	0.75g
蟅蟲	zhè chóng	Entire dried body of the female of Eupolyphaga sinensis	六銖 6 zhū	0.75g
乾地黃	gān dì huáng	Dried root of Rehmannia glutinosa	六銖 6 zhū	0.75g

上六味，治下篩。空心酒服方寸匕，日三。

Finely pestle and sift the above six ingredients. On an empty stomach, take a square-inch spoon in liquor three times a day.

LINE 3.61

治漏下去青方。

[The following] prescription treats blue-green vaginal spotting.

Formula

大黃 黃芩 白薇（各半兩） 桂心 牡蠣（各六銖）。

大黃	dà huáng	Root of Rheum palmatum	半兩 0.5 liǎng	1.5g
黃芩	huáng qín	Root of Scutellaria baicalensis	半兩 0.5 liǎng	1.5g
白薇	bái wēi	Root of Cynanchum atratum	半兩 0.5 liǎng	1.5g
桂心	guì xīn	Shaved inner bark of Cinnamomum cassia	六銖 6 zhū	0.75g
牡蠣	mǔ lì	Shell of Ostrea rivularis	六銖 6 zhū	0.75g

上五味，治下篩。空心酒服方寸匕，日三。

Finely pestle and sift the above five ingredients. On an empty stomach, take a square-inch spoon in liquor three times a day.

LINE 3.62

治漏下去白方。

[The following] prescription treats white vaginal spotting.

Formula

鹿茸（一兩） 白薟（十八銖） 狗脊（半兩）。

鹿茸	lù róng	Pilose antler of Cervus nippon	一兩 1 liǎng	3g
白薟	bái liǎn	Root of Ampelopsis japonica	十八銖 18 zhū	2.25g
狗脊	gǒu jǐ	Rhizome of Cibotium barometz	半兩 0.5 liǎng	1.5g

上三味，治下篩。空心米飲服方寸匕，日三。

Finely pestle and sift the above three ingredients. Take a square-inch spoon in rice soup on an empty stomach three times a day.

LINE 3.63

治女子漏下，積年不斷，困篤方。

[The following] prescription treats vaginal spotting in girls* [that has persisted] for several years without interruption, causing critical encumbrance.

取鵲重巢柴燒灰，作末。服方寸匕，日三服，三十日愈，甚良。重巢者，鵲去年在巢中產，今年又在上作重巢產者是也。

Take twigs from a twice-used magpie's nest and char them into ashes. Pulverize them and take a square-inch spoon three times a day. After thirty days, she will recover. It is excellent. As for a "twice-used nest," it is a nest in which a magpie gave birth the previous year and in which she has given birth for the second time in the current year.

*   女子 *nǚ zǐ*. The *Sūn Zhēn Rén* edition has 女人 *nǚ rén* (women) instead. The use of the term *nǚ zǐ* here is likely intentional, indicating that this prescription refers to conditions of vaginal leaking that are unrelated to sexual activity and previous childbirth - and therefore, by implication, to the presence of "malign blood" left over from a pregnancy. When Sūn Sī-Miǎo refers to sexually active women in their childbearing years, he consistently uses the term 婦人 *fù rén* (lit. "wives"). This is also the term used by Sūn Sī-Miǎo throughout the other sections on his "prescriptions for women" (婦人方 *fù rén fāng*). Nevertheless, in rare exceptions, Sūn Sī-Miǎo uses the term *nǚ rén*, both in the *Sūn Zhēn Rén* edition and the *Sòng* revisions, to refer to what is clearly a married woman (see, for example, the prescription for "treating women who have sustained injury from their husband" in volume 3, Line 8.44. I therefore suspect that Sūn Sī-Miǎo's frequent use of *nǚ rén* instead of *fù rén* throughout this section might be coincidental, especially given the close etiological associations of vaginal discharge with previous failure to eliminate the "malign blood" after childbirth.

LINE 3.64

馬通湯治漏下血，積月不止方。

Horse Dung Decoction treats vaginal spotting of blood that has persisted incessantly for several months.

Horse Dung Decoction
馬通湯 *mǎ tōng tāng*

赤馬通汁（一升，取新馬屎絞取汁，乾者水浸絞取汁*）生艾葉 阿膠（各三兩）當歸 乾薑（各二兩）好墨（半丸）。

赤馬通汁	chì mǎ tōng zhī	Dung juice of red Equus caballus	一升 1 shēng	24g
生艾葉	shēng ài yè	Fresh foliage of Artemisia argyi	三兩 3 liǎng	9g
阿膠	ē jiāo	Gelatinous glue produced from Equus asinus	三兩 3 liǎng	9g
當歸	dāng guī	Root of Angelica polimorpha	二兩 2 liǎng	6g
乾薑	gān jiāng	Dried root of Zingiber officinale	二兩 2 liǎng	6g
好墨	hǎo mò	Good ink	半丸 0.5 wán	half a ball

上六味，㕮咀，以水八升，酒二升煮取三升，去滓，內馬通汁及膠，微火煎取二升，分再服，相去如人行十里久。

Of the six ingredients above, pound [the drugs] and decoct them in eight *shēng* of water and two *shēng* of liquor to obtain three *shēng*. Discard the dregs and add the *mǎ tōng zhī* 馬通汁 and *ē jiāo* 阿膠. Simmer it over a small flame to obtain two *shēng* and divide it into two doses. Separate the doses by the length of time it takes a person to walk ten *lǐ*.

*   Take fresh horse dung and wring it out to obtain the juice. When using dried dung, soak it in water, and then wring it out to obtain the juice.

LINE 3.65

馬蹄屑湯治白漏不絕方。

Horse's Hoof Flakes Decoction treats continuous white spotting.

Horse's Hoof Flakes Decoction
馬蹄屑湯 *mǎ tí xiè tāng*

白馬蹄 赤石脂（各五兩） 禹餘糧 烏賊骨 龍骨 牡蠣（各四兩） 附子 乾地黃 當歸（各三兩） 甘草（二兩） 白殭蠶（一兩）。

白馬蹄	bái mǎ tí	Hoof of Equus caballus	五兩 5 liǎng	15g
赤石脂	chì shí zhī	Halloysite	五兩 5 liǎng	15g
禹餘糧	yǔ yú liáng	Limonite	四兩 4 liǎng	12g
烏賊骨	wū zéi gǔ	Calcified shell of Sepiella maindroni	四兩 4 liǎng	12g
龍骨	lóng gǔ	Os draconis	四兩 4 liǎng	12g
牡蠣	mǔ lì	Shell of Ostrea rivularis	四兩 4 liǎng	12g
附子	fù zǐ	Lateral root of Aconitum carmichaeli	三兩 3 liǎng	9g
乾地黃	gān dì huáng	Dried root of Rehmannia glutinosa	三兩 3 liǎng	9g
當歸	dāng guī	Root of Angelica polimorpha	三兩 3 liǎng	9g
甘草	gān cǎo	Root of Glycyrrhiza uralensis	二兩 2 liǎng	6g
白僵蠶	bái jiāng cán	Dried 4th or 5th stage larva of the moth of Bombyx mori	一兩 1 liǎng	3g

上十一味，㕮咀，以水二斗煮取九升，分六服，日三。

Pound the above eleven ingredients and decoct in two *dǒu* of water to obtain nine *shēng*. Divide into six doses and take three times a day.

LINE 3.66

馬蹄丸治白漏不絕方。

Horse's Hoof Pills treat continuous white spotting.

Horse's Hoof Pills
馬蹄丸 *mǎ tí wán*

白馬蹄 禹餘糧（各四兩） 龍骨（三兩） 烏賊骨 白殭蠶 赤石脂（各二兩）

。

白馬蹄	bái mǎ tí	Hoof of Equus caballus	四兩 4 liǎng	12g
禹餘糧	yǔ yú liáng	Limonite	四兩 4 liǎng	12g
龍骨	lóng gǔ	Os draconis	三兩 3 liǎng	9g
烏賊骨	wū zéi gǔ	Calcified shell of Sepiella maindroni	二兩 2 liǎng	6g
白僵蠶	bái jiāng cán	Dried 4th or 5th stage larva of the moth of Bombyx mori	二兩 2 liǎng	6g

| 赤石脂 | chì shí zhī | Halloysite | 二兩 2 liǎng | 6g |

上六味，為末，蜜丸梧子大。酒服十丸，不知加至三十丸。

Pulverize the above six ingredients and mix with honey into pills the size of firmiana seeds. Take ten pills in liquor. If you notice no effect, increase [the dosage] to a maximum of thirty pills.

LINE 3.67

慎火草散治漏下方。

Stonecrop Powder treats vaginal spotting.[*]

Stonecrop Powder
慎火草散 *shèn huǒ cǎo sǎn*

慎火草（十兩，熬令黃）當歸 鹿茸 阿膠（各四兩）龍骨（半兩）。

慎火草, 熬令黃	shèn huǒ cǎo, āo lìng huáng	Entire plant of Sedum erythrosticum, toasted until yellow	十兩 10 liǎng	300g
當歸	dāng guī	Root of Angelica polimorpha	四兩 4 liǎng	12g
鹿茸	lù róng	Pilose antler of Cervus nippon	四兩 4 liǎng	12g
阿膠	ē jiāo	Gelatinous glue produced from Equus asinus	四兩 4 liǎng	12g
龍骨	lóng gǔ	Os draconis	半兩 0.5 liǎng	1.5g

上五味，治下篩。先食酒服方寸匕，日三。

Finely pestle and sift the above five ingredients. Before meals, take a square-inch spoon in liquor three times a day.

---

*   *Sòng* editors' note: "For another prescription, see above." This refers to a prescription with the identical title in Line 3.19 above (pp. 485 - 486).

LINE 3.68

蒲黃散治漏下不止方。

Typha Pollen Powder treats incessant vaginal spotting.

Typha Pollen Powder
蒲黃散 *pú huáng sǎn*

蒲黃（半升）鹿茸 當歸（各二兩）。

蒲黃	pú huáng	Pollen of Typha angustata	半升 0.5 shēng	12g
鹿茸	lù róng	Pilose antler of Cervus nippon	二兩 2 liǎng	6g
當歸	dāng guī	Root of Angelica polimorpha	二兩 2 liǎng	6g

上三味，治下篩。酒服五分匕，日三，不知稍加至方寸匕。

Finely pestle and sift the above three ingredients. Take a five-*fēn* spoon in liquor three times a day. If you notice no effect, increase [the dosage] gradually to a maximum of one square-inch spoon.

LINE 3.69

Moxibustion Methods (灸法 *jiǔ fǎ*)

Moxibustion Treatments

(一) 女人胞漏下血不可禁止：灸關元兩傍相去三寸。(二) 女人陰中痛引心下，及小腹絞痛，腹中五寒：灸關儀百壯，穴在膝外邊上一寸宛宛中是。(三) 女人漏下赤白及血：灸足太陰五十壯，穴在內踝上三寸，足太陰經內踝上三寸名三陰交。(四) 女人漏下赤白，月經不調：灸交儀三十壯，穴在內踝上五寸。(五) 女人漏下赤白：灸營池四穴三十壯，穴在內踝前後兩邊池中脈上，一名陰陽是。(六) 女人漏下赤白，四肢酸削：灸漏陰三十壯，穴在內踝下五分微動腳脈上。(七) 女人漏下赤白，泄注：灸陰陽隨年壯，三報，穴在足拇趾下屈裏表頭白肉際是。

(1) For [the treatment of] women with uterine spotting and unstoppable descent of blood: Burn moxa three *cùn* to each side of Pass Head.[1]

(2) For [the treatment of] women's pain in the vagina, stretching to below the heart, as well as for gripping pain in the lower abdomen and the five types of coldness[2] in the center of the abdomen: Burn 100 moxa cones at Pass Apparatus.[3] The point is located in the center of the depression one *cùn* above the outer side of the knee.

(3) For [the treatment of] women's spotting of red and white vaginal discharge or blood: Burn 50 moxa cones on the foot greater *yīn* [channel]. The point is located three *cùn*

above the inner side of the ankle. [The point] three *cùn* above the inner side of the ankle on the foot greater *yīn* channel is called Three Yīn Intersection.[4]

(4) For [the treatment of] women's red and white spotting and for irregular menstruation: Burn 30 moxa cones at Intersection Apparatus.[5] The point is located five *cùn* above the inner side of the ankle.

(5) For [the treatment of] women's red and white spotting: Burn 30 moxa cones at the four points of Construction Pool.[6] The points are located on top of the vessel in the depressions in both the front and the back of the inner side of the ankle. Another name for these points is *yīn yáng*.

(6) For [the treatment of] women's red and white spotting with aching and whittling in the four limbs: Burn 30 moxa cones at Leaky Yīn.[7] The point is located five *fēn* below the inner side of the ankle on the slightly moving foot vessel.

(7) For [the treatment of] women's red and white spotting and downpour diarrhea: Burn moxa at *yīn yáng*, the number of cones corresponding to her years of age. Repeat the treatment three times. This point is located under the big toe, at the edge of the white flesh on the surface of where the [flesh] curves and becomes thicker.

1. 關元 *guān yuán*: CV-4, a point of great importance for the treatment of women's reproductive problems.
2. 五寒 *wǔ hán*: Not a standard term.
3. 關儀 *guān yí*: Not a standard point and not attested elsewhere. The *Zhōng Yī Dà Cí Diǎn* merely quotes this passage and states that it is indicated for gripping pain in the lesser abdomen. See 李經緯, 主編. 《中醫大辭典》 p. 709.
4. 三陰交 *sān yīn jiāo*: SP-6.
5. 交儀 *jiāo yí*: LV-5.
6. 營池 *yíng chí*: not a standard point, but mentioned also in the *Qiān Jīn Yì Fāng* (volume 26), *Běn Cǎo Gāng Mù*, and other texts, as a treatment for red and white vaginal discharge and excessive menstrual flow. In contemporary TCM, identical with 陰陽 *yīn yáng* (木下晴都 《中國經絡學》 p. 43, and 李經緯, 主編. 《中醫大辭典》 p. 1548).
7. 漏陰 *lòu yīn*: KI-6.
8. 陰陽 *yīn yáng*: According to the statement by Sūn Sī-Miǎo above, this is an alternate name for 營池 *yíng chí*, but the description of the location here below the toe contradicts that identification. The *yīn yáng* point below the toe is mentioned also in the *Qiān Jīn Yì Fāng*, *Běn Cǎo Gāng Mù*, and other texts as indicated for red and white vaginal discharge (木下晴都 《中國經絡學》 p. 41). The *Sūn Zhēn Rén* edition has 陰陵 *yīn líng* (Yīn Mound) instead, but that seems to be a scribal error since that name is unattested elsewhere.

523

4. Menstrual Irregularities 月經不調

LINE 4.1

白堊丸治婦人月經一月再來，或隔月不來，或多或少，淋瀝不斷，或來而腰腹痛，噓吸不能食，心腹痛，或青黃黑色，或如水，舉體沈重方。

Chalk Pills treat women's menstrual period arriving twice in one month, or failing to arrive every other month, or of an excessive or scanty amount, or as incessant dribbling, possibly with lumbar and abdominal pain at the onset of menstruation; huffing and gasping, inability to eat, heart and abdominal pain, possibly [vaginal discharge of] blue-green, yellow, or black color, or like water, and heaviness when lifting the limbs.

Chalk Pills
白堊丸 *bái è wán*

白堊 白石脂 牡蠣 禹餘糧 龍骨 細辛 烏賊骨（各一兩半） 當歸 芍藥 黃連 茯苓 乾薑 桂心 人參 瞿麥 石韋 白芷 白薇 附子 甘草（各一兩） 蜀椒（半兩）。

白堊	bái è	Chalk	一兩半 1.5 liǎng	4.5g
白石脂	bái shí zhī	Kaolin	一兩半 1.5 liǎng	4.5g
牡蠣	mǔ lì	Shell of Ostrea rivularis	一兩半 1.5 liǎng	4.5g
禹餘糧	yǔ yú liáng	Limonite	一兩半 1.5 liǎng	4.5g
龍骨	lóng gǔ	Os draconis	一兩半 1.5 liǎng	4.5g
細辛	xì xīn	Complete plant including root of Asarum heteropoides	一兩半 1.5 liǎng	4.5g
烏賊骨	wū zéi gǔ	Calcified shell of Sepiella maindroni	一兩半 1.5 liǎng	4.5g
當歸	dāng guī	Root of Angelica polimorpha	一兩 1 liǎng	3g

芍藥	sháo yào	Root of Paeonia albiflora	一兩 1 liǎng	3g
黃連	huáng lián	Rhizome of Coptis chinensis	一兩 1 liǎng	3g
茯苓	fú líng	Dried fungus of Poria cocos	一兩 1 liǎng	3g
乾薑	gān jiāng	Dried root of Zingiber officinale	一兩 1 liǎng	3g
桂心	guì xīn	Shaved inner bark of Cinnamomum cassia	一兩 1 liǎng	3g
人參	rén shēn	Root of Panax ginseng	一兩 1 liǎng	3g
瞿麥	qú mài	Entire plant, including flowers, of Dianthus superbus	一兩 1 liǎng	3g
石韋	shí wéi	Foliage of Pyrrosia lingua	一兩 1 liǎng	3g
白芷	bái zhǐ	Root of Angelica dahurica	一兩 1 liǎng	3g
白蘞	bái liǎn	Root of Ampelopsis japonica	一兩 1 liǎng	3g
附子	fù zǐ	Lateral root of Aconitum carmichaeli	一兩 1 liǎng	3g
甘草	gān cǎo	Root of Glycyrrhiza uralensis	一兩 1 liǎng	3g
蜀椒	shǔ jiāo	Seed capsules of Zanthoxylum bungeanum	半兩 0.5 liǎng	1.5g

上二十一味，為末，蜜丸如梧子大。空心酒下二十丸，日三。至月候來時，日四五服為佳。

Pulverize the above twenty-one ingredients and mix with honey into pills the size of firmiana seeds. On an empty stomach, down twenty pills in liquor three times a day. It is excellent to take four or five doses a day at the onset of the menstrual period.

LINE 4.2

桃仁湯治產後及墮身，月水不調，或淋瀝不斷，斷後復來，狀如瀉水，四體噓吸，不能食，腹中堅痛，不可行動，月水或前或後，或經月不來，舉體沈重，惟欲眠臥，多思酸物方。

Peach Kernel Decoction treats menstrual irregularities after childbirth or miscarriage,[1] possibly dribbling incessantly or recurring after it has stopped or like watery diarrhea, with huffing and gasping [that strains] the entire body, inability to eat, hardness and pain in the abdomen, inability to actively move around,[2] a menstrual flow that is sometimes early and sometimes late or fails to arrive at all, heaviness when lifting the limbs, only wanting to rest and sleep, and excessive thought of sour foods.

Peach Kernel Decoction
桃仁湯 *táo rén tāng*

桃仁（五十枚） 澤蘭 甘草 芎藭 人參（各二兩） 牛膝 桂心 牡丹皮 當歸（各三兩） 芍藥 生薑 半夏（各四兩） 地黃（八兩） 蒲黃（七合）。

桃仁	táo rén	Seed of Prunus persica	五十枚 50 méi	50 pcs
澤蘭	zé lán	Foliage and stalk of Lycopus lucidus	二兩 2 liǎng	6g
甘草	gān cǎo	Root of Glycyrrhiza uralensis	二兩 2 liǎng	6g
川芎	chuān xiōng	Root of Ligusticum wallichii	二兩 2 liǎng	6g
人參	rén shēn	Root of Panax ginseng	二兩 2 liǎng	6g
牛膝	niú xī	Root of Achyranthes bidentata	三兩 3 liǎng	9g
桂心	guì xīn	Shaved inner bark of Cinnamomum cassia	三兩 3 liǎng	9g
牡丹皮	mǔ dān pí	Bark of the root of Paeonia suffruticosa	三兩 3 liǎng	9g
當歸	dāng guī	Root of Angelica polimorpha	三兩 3 liǎng	9g
芍藥	sháo yào	Root of Paeonia albiflora	四兩 4 liǎng	12g
生薑	shēng jiāng	Fresh root of Zingiber officinale	四兩 4 liǎng	12g
半夏	bàn xià	Rhizome of Pinellia ternata	四兩 4 liǎng	12g
地黃	dì huáng	Root of Rehmannia glutinosa	八兩 8 liǎng	24g
蒲黃	pú huáng	Pollen of Typha angustata	七合 7 gě	49ml

上十四味，咬咀，以水二斗煮取六升半，分六服。

Pound the above fourteen ingredients and decoct in two *dǒu* of water to obtain six and a half *shēng*. Divide into six doses.

1. 墮身 *duò shēn*: Based on context, I interpret this as identical to the more common term 墮胎 *duò tāi* (lit. dropping the fetus), which refers to miscarriage or abortion. Alternatively, it could also mean simply "fall of the body."
2. 不可行動 *bù kě xíng dòng*: Alternatively, this phrase could be linked to the previous one, meaning "hardness and pain in the abdomen that cannot be moved around." This is how the *Rén Mín* edition punctuates this sentence.

LINE 4.3

杏仁湯治月經不調，或一月再來，或兩月，三月一來，或月前或月後，閉塞不通方。

Apricot Kernel Decoction treats menstrual irregularities, possibly arriving twice in one month, or once in two or three months, or prematurely or delayed, or menstrual stoppage.

Apricot Kernel Decoction
杏仁湯 *xìng rén tāng*

杏仁（二兩） 桃仁（一兩） 大黃（三兩） 水蛭 虻蟲（各三十枚）。

杏仁	xìng rén	Dried seed of Prunus armeniaca	二兩 2 liǎng	6g
桃仁	táo rén	Seed of Prunus persica	一兩 1 liǎng	3g
大黃	dà huáng	Root of Rheum palmatum	三兩 3 liǎng	9g
水蛭	shuǐ zhì	Dried body of Whitmania pigra	三十枚 30 méi	30 pcs
虻蟲	méng chóng	Dried body of the female of Tabanus bivittatus	三十枚 30 méi	30 pcs

上五味，㕮咀，以水六升煮取二升，分三服。一服當有物隨大小便有所下；下多者，止之；少者，勿止，盡三服。

Pound the above five ingredients and decoct in six *shēng* of water to obtain two *shēng*. Divide into three doses. After one dose, she should discharge a substance after a bowel movement. If the discharge is copious, stop [taking the medicine]. If it is scanty, do not stop and use up all three doses.

LINE 4.4

大黃朴消湯治經年月水不利，胞中有風冷所致，宜下之。

Rhubarb and Impure Mirabilite Decoction treats inhibited menstrual flow for several consecutive years, caused by the presence of wind-cold in the uterus. [This decoction] is suitable for precipitating it.

Rhubarb and Impure Mirabilite Decoction
大黃朴硝湯 *dà huáng pò xiāo tāng*

大黃 牛膝（各五兩） 朴消 牡丹 甘草 紫菀（各三兩，《千金翼》作紫葳）代赭（一兩） 桃仁 虻蟲 水蛭 乾薑 細辛 芒消（各二兩） 麻仁（五合）。

大黃	dà huáng	Root of Rheum palmatum	五兩 5 liǎng	15g
牛膝	niú xī	Root of Achyranthes bidentata	五兩 5 liǎng	15g

朴消	pò xiāo	Impure mirabilite	三兩 3 liǎng	9g
牡丹	mǔ dān	Bark of the root of Paeonia suffruticosa	三兩 3 liǎng	9g
甘草	gān cǎo	Root of Glycyrrhiza uralensis	三兩 3 liǎng	9g
紫菀[1]	zǐ wǎn	Root and rhizome of Aster tataricus	三兩 3 liǎng	9g
代赭	dài zhě	Hematite	一兩 1 liǎng	3g
桃仁	táo rén	Seed of Prunus persica	二兩 2 liǎng	6g
虻蟲	méng chóng	Dried body of the female of Tabanus bivittatus	二兩 2 liǎng	6g
水蛭	shuǐ zhì	Dried body of Whitmania pigra	二兩 2 liǎng	6g
乾薑	gān jiāng	Dried root of Zingiber officinale	二兩 2 liǎng	6g
細辛	xì xīn	Complete plant including root of Asarum heteropoides	二兩 2 liǎng	6g
硭硝	máng xiāo	Hydrated sodium sulfate	二兩 2 liǎng	6g
麻仁	má rén	Seed of Cannabis sativa	五合 5 gě	35ml

上十四味，㕮咀，以水一斗五升煮取五升，去滓，內消令烊。分五服，五更為首，相去一炊頃，自下後將息，忌見風。

Pound the above fourteen ingredients and decoct in one *dǒu* and five *shēng* of water to obtain five *shēng*. Discard the dregs and add the mirabilite, letting it melt. Divide into five doses. Take the first [dose] during the fifth nightwatch,[2] and then separate the doses from each other by the length of time it takes to cook a meal. After she has spontaneously discharged something, she should rest. Avoid exposure to wind.

1.   *Sòng* editors' note: "The *Qiān Jīn Fāng* has *zǐ wēi* (紫葳 Flower of Campsis grandiflora)."
2.   五更 *wǔ gēng*: The time of the last nightwatch, i.e., right before dawn.

LINE 4.5

茱萸虻蟲湯治久寒月經不利，或多或少方。

Evodia and Tabanus Decoction treats chronic cold-related inhibited menstruation, whether profuse or scanty.

Evodia and Tabanus Decoction
茱萸虻蟲湯 *zhū yú méng chóng tāng*

吳茱萸（三升）虻蟲 水蛭 蟅蟲 牡丹（各一兩）生薑（一斤）小麥 半夏（

各一升）大棗（二十枚）桃仁（五十枚）人參 牛膝（各三兩）桂心（六兩）甘草（一兩半）芍藥（二兩）。

吳茱萸	wú zhū yú	Unripe fruit of Evodia rutaecarpa	三兩	3 liǎng	9g
虻蟲	méng chóng	Dried body of the female of Tabanus bivittatus	一兩	1 liǎng	3g
水蛭	shuǐ zhì	Dried body of Whitmania pigra	一兩	1 liǎng	3g
蟅蟲	zhè chóng	Entire dried body of the female of Eupolyphaga sinensis	一兩	1 liǎng	3g
牡丹	mǔ dān	Bark of the root of Paeonia suffruticosa	一兩	1 liǎng	3g
生薑	shēng jiāng	Fresh root of Zingiber officinale	一斤	1 jīn	48g
小麥	xiǎo mài	Seed of Triticum aestivum	一升	1 shēng	24g
半夏	bàn xià	Rhizome of Pinellia ternata	一升	1 shēng	24g
大棗	dà zǎo	Mature fruit of Ziziphus jujuba	二十枚	20 méi	20 pcs
桃仁	táo rén	Seed of Prunus persica	五十枚	50 méi	50 pcs
人參	rén shēn	Root of Panax ginseng	三兩	3 liǎng	9g
牛膝	niú xī	Root of Achyranthes bidentata	三兩	3 liǎng	9g
桂心	guì xīn	Shaved inner bark of Cinnamomum cassia	六兩	6 liǎng	18g
甘草	gān cǎo	Root of Glycyrrhiza uralensis	一兩半	1.5 liǎng	4.5g
芍藥	sháo yào	Root of Paeonia albiflora	二兩	2 liǎng	6g

上十五味，㕮咀，以酒一斗，水二斗煮取一斗，去滓，適寒溫，一服一升，日三。不能飲酒人，以水代之。湯欲成，乃內諸蟲。不耐藥者，飲七合。

Pound the fifteen ingredients and decoct in one *dǒu* of liquor and two *dǒu* of water to obtain one *dǒu*. Discard the dregs, adjust the temperature, and take one *shēng* per dose three times a day. For patients who cannot drink liquor, you may substitute water for it. Add the various insects only when the decoction is just about done. If she cannot bear [to take the full dose of] the medicine, make her drink seven *gě*.

LINE 4.6

抵党湯治月經不利，腹中滿時自減，並男子膀胱滿急方。

Tangut Resisting Decoction treats inhibited menstruation and fullness in the center of the abdomen that sometimes recedes spontaneously, as well as men's fullness and tension in the urinary bladder.

Tangut-Resisting Decoction
抵党湯 dǐ dǎng tāng[1]

虎掌 大黃（各二兩）桃仁（三十枚）水蛭（二十枚）。

虎掌[2]	hǔ zhàng	Arisaema	二兩 2 liǎng	6g
大黃	dà huáng	Root of Rheum palmatum	二兩 2 liǎng	6g
桃仁	táo rén	Seed of Prunus persica	三十枚 30 méi	30 pcs
水蛭	shuǐ zhì	Dried body of Whitmania pigra	二十枚 20 méi	20 pcs

上四味，以水三升煮取一升，盡服之，當下惡血為度。

Decoct the above four ingredients in three *shēng* of water to obtain one *shēng*. Consume the entire [decoction]. Take the discharge of malign blood as a measure [of the medicine's efficacy].

1. The name of this prescription does not make any sense in this context. It is most likely a scribal error for 虎掌 *hǔ zhǎng* (arisaema), since it is standard practice throughout the *Qiān Jīn Fāng* to name prescriptions after their first, or most prevalent, ingredient(s), or otherwise offer an explanation for the name. 党 *dǎng* refers to the Tanguts, a proto-Tibetan tribe at the Western borders of the *Táng* empire.
2. *Sòng* editors' note: "The *Qiān Jīn Fāng* has *hǔ zhàng* (虎杖 Root of Polygonum cuspidatum)."

LINE 4.7

七熬丸治月經不利，手足煩熱，腹滿，默默不欲寤，心煩方。

Seven Roasted [Ingredients] Pills treat inhibited menstruation, vexation and heat in the hands and feet, abdominal fullness, deep silence and unwillingness to wake up, and heart vexation.

Seven Roasted [Ingredients] Pills
七熬丸 qī āo wán

大黃（一兩半）前胡（一作柴胡）芒消（熬，各五兩）葶藶 蜀椒（並

熬，各六銖）生薑 芎藭（各十八銖）茯苓（十五銖）杏仁（九銖，熬）
桃仁（二十枚，熬）虻蟲（熬）水蛭（各半合，熬）。

大黃	dà huáng	Root of Rheum palmatum	一兩半 1.5 liǎng	4.5g
前胡[1]	qián hú	Root of Peucedanum praeruptorum	六銖 6 zhū	0.75g
硭硝, 熬	máng xiāo, āo	Hydrated sodium sulfate, roasted	六銖 6 zhū	0.75g
葶藶, 熬	tíng lì, āo	Seed of Lepidium apetalum, roasted	六銖 6 zhū	0.75g
蜀椒, 熬	shǔ jiāo, āo	Seed capsules of Zanthoxylum bungeanum, roasted	六銖 6 zhū	0.75g
生薑	shēng jiāng	Fresh root of Zingiber officinale	十八銖 18 zhū	2.25g
川芎	chuān xiōng	Root of Ligusticum wallichii	十八銖 18 zhū	2.25g
茯苓	fú líng	Dried fungus of Poria cocos	十五銖 15 zhū	1.88g
杏仁, 熬	xìng rén, āo	Dried seed of Prunus armeniaca, roasted	九銖 9 zhū	1.13g
桃仁, 熬	táo rén, āo	Seed of Prunus persica, roasted	二十枚 20 méi	20 pcs
虻蟲, 熬	méng chóng, āo	Dried body of the female of Tabanus bivittatus, roasted	半合 0.5 gě	3.5ml
水蛭, 熬	shuǐ zhì, āo	Dried body of Whitmania pigra, roasted	半合 0.5 gě	3.5ml

上十二味，為末，蜜丸梧子大。空腹飲服七丸，日三，不知加一倍。

Pulverize the above twelve ingredients and mix with honey into pills the size of firmiana seeds. On an empty stomach, take seven pills with fluid three times a day. If you notice no effect, double the dose.[2]

1. *Sòng* editors' note: "Another [version] has *chái hú* (柴胡 Root of Bupleurum chinense)."
2. *Sòng* editors' note: "The *Qiān Jīn Yì Fāng* lacks *chuān xiōng* 川芎. Another [version of this] prescription includes two *liǎng* each of *zhè chóng* (蟅蟲 Entire dried body of the female of Eupolyphaga sinensis) and *mǔ dān* (牡丹 Bark of the root of Paeonia suffruticosa), with a total of 14 ingredients."

LINE 4.8

桃仁散治月經來繞臍痛，上衝心胸，往來寒熱如瘧疰狀。

Peach Kernel Powder treats arrival of the menses with pain around the navel, upsurging to the heart and chest, and alternating [aversion to] cold and heat [effusion] as in malaria or infixation.*

Peach Kernel Powder
桃仁散 *táo rén sǎn*

桃仁（五十枚） 蟅蟲（二十枚） 桂心（五寸） 茯苓（一兩） 薏苡仁 牛膝
代赭（各二兩） 大黃（八兩）。

桃仁	táo rén	Seed of Prunus persica	五十枚 50 méi	50 pcs
蟅蟲	zhè chóng	Entire dried body of the female of Eupolyphaga sinensis	二十枚 20 méi	20 pcs
桂心	guì xīn	Shaved inner bark of Cinnamomum cassia	五寸 5 cùn	5 cm
茯苓	fú líng	Dried fungus of Poria cocos	一兩 1 liǎng	3g
薏苡仁	yì yǐ rén	Seed kernel of Coix lachryma-jobi	二兩 2 liǎng	6g
牛膝	niú xī	Root of Achyranthes bidentata	二兩 2 liǎng	6g
代赭	dài zhě	Hematite	二兩 2 liǎng	6g
大黃	dà huáng	Root of Rheum palmatum	八兩 8 liǎng	24g

上八味，治下篩。宿勿食，溫酒服一錢匕，日三。

Finely pestle and sift the above eight ingredients. After fasting overnight, take one *qián*-sized spoon in warm liquor three times a day.

* 疰 *zhù*: Infixation refers to diseases characterized by infections that become chronically lodged (such as summer infixation, 疰夏 *zhù xià*, or worm infixation, 疰蟲 *zhù chóng*). It is often used interchangeably with 注 *zhù* (influx) but also carries the connotation of 住 *zhù* (to lodge, stay). In its narrowest and most serious sense as "corpse influx" (尸注 *hù zhù*), it is described in the *Bìng Yuán Lùn* as a dreadful condition caused by externally contracted ghost evil, which leads to increasing suffering from intermittent cold and heat, urinary problems, general severe discomfort, confusion, panting, pain in the abdomen, heart, rib-side, lumbus, and back, and eventually causes the patient's death. Being highly contagious after death, it is likely to be passed on to other members of the family (《病源論》23:2:6). See also Wiseman and Féng, *Practical Dictionary*, p. 300, and 《中華醫學大辭典》 p. 1087. For a detailed analysis of 疰 by medieval medical writers, see Michel Strickman, *Chinese Magical Medicine*, pp. 23-34.

LINE 4.9

治月經往來，腹腫，腰腹痛方。

[The following] prescription treats intermittent menstruation with abdominal swelling and lumbar and abdominal pain.

Formula

虻蟲（四枚） 蜀椒 乾薑（各六銖） 大黃 女青 桂心 芎藭（各半兩）。

蟅蟲	zhè chóng	Entire dried body of the female of Eupolyphaga sinensis	四枚 4 méi	4 pcs
蜀椒	shǔ jiāo	Seed capsules of Zanthoxylum bungeanum	六銖 6 zhū	0.75g
乾薑	gān jiāng	Dried root of Zingiber officinale	六銖 6 zhū	0.75g
大黃	dà huáng	Root of Rheum palmatum	半兩 0.5 liǎng	1.5g
女青	nǚ qīng	unknown	半兩 0.5 liǎng	1.5g
桂心	guì xīn	Shaved inner bark of Cinnamomum cassia	半兩 0.5 liǎng	1.5g
川芎	chuān xiōng	Root of Ligusticum wallichii	半兩 0.5 liǎng	1.5g

上七味，治下篩。取一刀圭，先食酒服之，日三。十日微下，善養之。

Finely pestle and sift the above seven ingredients. Take one *dāo guī* [of the medicine] in liquor before meals three times a day. After ten days, she will have a slight discharge. Nurture her well.

---

*   刀圭: a unit of measurement for powders that is equivalent to one tenth of a square-inch spoon, according to the instructions on medicinals in volume 1 of the *Qiān Jīn Fāng* (《千金方》1:7).

LINE 4.10

治月經不調，或月頭，或月後，或如豆汁，腰痛如折，兩腳疼，胞中風寒，下之之方。

[The following] prescription treats menstrual irregularities, whether the period is occurring at the beginning of the month or at the end of the month, or resembling bean juice, accompanied by pain in the lumbus as if fit to break, aches in both legs, and wind-cold in the center of the uterus, which this prescription will precipitate.

Formula

大黃 朴消（各四兩） 牡丹（三兩） 桃仁（一升） 人參 陽起石 茯苓 甘草
水蛭 虻蟲（各二兩）。

大黃	dà huáng	Root of Rheum palmatum	四兩 4 liǎng	12g
朴消	pò xiāo	Impure mirabilite	四兩 4 liǎng	12g
牡丹	mǔ dān	Bark of the root of Paeonia suffruticosa	三兩 3 liǎng	9g
桃仁	táo rén	Seed of Prunus persica	一升 1 shēng	24g
人參	rén shēn	Root of Panax ginseng	二兩 2 liǎng	6g
陽起石	yáng qǐ shí	Actinolite	二兩 2 liǎng	6g
茯苓	fú líng	Dried fungus of Poria cocos	二兩 2 liǎng	6g
甘草	gān cǎo	Root of Glycyrrhiza uralensis	二兩 2 liǎng	6g
水蛭	shuǐ zhì	Dried body of Whitmania pigra	二兩 2 liǎng	6g
虻蟲	méng chóng	Dried body of the female of Tabanus bivittatus	二兩 2 liǎng	6g

上十味，㕮咀，以水九升煮取三升，去滓，內朴消令烊盡。分三服，相去
如一飯頃。

Pound the above ten ingredients and decoct in nine *shēng* of water to obtain three *shēng*. Discard the dregs and add the *pò xiāo* 朴消, letting it melt completely. Divide into three doses [and take them] separated from each other by the time [it takes to prepare] one meal.

LINE 4.11

陽起石湯治月水不調，或前或後，或多或少，乍赤乍白方。

Actinolite Decoction treats menstrual irregularities, early or late, profuse or scanty, or now red now white.

Actinolite Decoction
陽起石湯 *yáng qǐ shí tāng*

陽起石 甘草 續斷 乾薑 人參 桂心（各二兩） 附子（一兩） 赤石脂（三兩）
伏龍肝（五兩） 生地黃（一升）。

陽起石	yáng qǐ shí	Actinolite	二兩 2 liǎng	6g
甘草	gān cǎo	Root of Glycyrrhiza uralensis	二兩 2 liǎng	6g
續斷	xù duàn	Root of Dipsacus asper	二兩 2 liǎng	6g
乾薑	gān jiāng	Dried root of Zingiber officinale	二兩 2 liǎng	6g
人參	rén shēn	Root of Panax ginseng	二兩 2 liǎng	6g
桂心	guì xīn	Shaved inner bark of Cinnamomum cassia	二兩 2 liǎng	6g
附子	fù zǐ	Lateral root of Aconitum carmichaeli	一兩 1 liǎng	3g
赤石脂	chì shí zhī	Halloysite	三兩 3 liǎng	9g
伏龍肝	fú lóng gān	Stove earth	五兩 5 liǎng	15g
生地黃	shēng dì huáng	Fresh root of Rehmannia glutinosa	一升 1 shēng	24g

上十味，以水一斗煮取三升二合。分四服，日三夜一。

Decoct the above ten ingredients in one *dǒu* of water to obtain three *shēng* and two *gě*. Divide into four doses and take three times a day and once at night.

LINE 4.12

治婦人憂恚，心下支滿，膈中伏熱，月經不利，血氣上搶心，欲嘔，不可多食，懈怠不能動方。

[The following] prescription treats women's anxiety and rage, propping fullness below the heart, latent heat in the center of the diagphragm, inhibited menstruation, *qì* and blood ascending to prod the heart, tendency to vomit and inability to eat a lot, and fatigue and inability to move.

Formula

大黃 芍藥 虻蟲（各二兩） 土瓜根 蜀椒 黃芩 白朮 乾薑 地骨皮 芎藭（各一兩） 桂心 乾漆（各一兩半）。

大黃	dà huáng	Root of Rheum palmatum	二兩 2 liǎng	6g
芍藥	sháo yào	Root of Paeonia albiflora	二兩 2 liǎng	6g
虻蟲	méng chóng	Dried body of the female of Tabanus bivittatus	二兩 2 liǎng	6g
土瓜根	tǔ guā gēn	Root of Trichosanthes cucumerina	一兩 1 liǎng	3g
蜀椒	shǔ jiāo	Seed capsules of Zanthoxylum bungeanum	一兩 1 liǎng	3g

黃芩	huáng qín	Root of Scutellaria baicalensis	一兩 1 liǎng	3g
白术	bái zhú	Rhizome of Atractylodes macrocephala	一兩 1 liǎng	3g
乾薑	gān jiāng	Dried root of Zingiber officinale	一兩 1 liǎng	3g
地骨皮	dì gǔ pí	Bark of the root of Lycium chinensis	一兩 1 liǎng	3g
川芎	chuān xiōng	Root of Ligusticum wallichii	一兩 1 liǎng	3g
桂心	guì xīn	Shaved inner bark of Cinnamomum cassia	一兩半 1.5 liǎng	4.5g
乾漆	gān qī	Dried sap of Rhus verniciflua	一兩半 1.5 liǎng	4.5g

上十二味，為末，蜜丸如梧子。每服十丸，日三，不知加之。

Pulverize the above twelve ingredients and mix with honey into pills the size of firmiana seeds. Take ten pills per dose three times a day, increasing [the dosage] if you notice no effect.

LINE 4.13

牛膝丸治產後月水往來，乍多乍少，仍復不通，時時疼痛，小腹裏急，下引腰，身重方。

Achyranthes Pills treat intermittent menstruation after chidlbirth, abruptly fluctuating in the amount, then failing to flow when returning, constant pain, tension in the lower abdomen, downward pulling in the lumbus, and heaviness of the body.

Achyranthes Pills
牛膝丸 *niú xī wán*

牛膝 芍藥 人參 大黃（各三兩） 牡丹皮 甘草 當歸 芎藭（各二兩） 桂心（一兩） 蟅蟲 蠐螬 蜚蠊（各四十枚） 虻蟲 水蛭（各七十枚）。

牛膝	niú xī	Root of Achyranthes bidentata	三兩 3 liǎng	9g
芍藥	sháo yào	Root of Paeonia albiflora	三兩 3 liǎng	9g
人參	rén shēn	Root of Panax ginseng	三兩 3 liǎng	9g
大黃	dà huáng	Root of Rheum palmatum	三兩 3 liǎng	9g
牡丹皮	mǔ dān pí	Bark of the root of Paeonia suffruticosa	二兩 2 liǎng	6g
甘草	gān cǎo	Root of Glycyrrhiza uralensis	二兩 2 liǎng	6g
當歸	dāng guī	Root of Angelica polimorpha	二兩 2 liǎng	6g
川芎	chuān xiōng	Root of Ligusticum wallichii	二兩 2 liǎng	6g

桂心	guì xīn	Shaved inner bark of Cinnamomum cassia	一兩 1 liǎng	3g
蟅蟲	zhè chóng	Entire dried body of the female of Eupolyphaga sinensis	四十枚 40 méi	40 pcs
蠐螬	qí cáo	Dried larva of Holotrichia diomphalia	四十枚 40 méi	40 pcs
蜚蠊	fěi lián	Whole body of Blatta orientalis	四十枚 40 méi	40 pcs
虻蟲	méng chóng	Dried body of the female of Tabanus bivittatus	七十枚 70 méi	70 pcs
水蛭	shuǐ zhì	Dried body of Whitmania pigra	七十枚 70 méi	70 pcs

上十四味，為末，蜜丸如梧子。酒服五丸，日三，不知稍增。

Pulverize the above fourteen ingredients and mix with honey into pills the size of firmiana seeds. Take five pills in liquor three times a day, gradually increasing [the dosage] if you notice no effect.

LINE 4.14

又方

Another prescription:

鹿角末服之。

Pulverize *lù jiǎo* (鹿角 Ossified antler or antler base of Cervus nippon) and take [a square-inch spoon in liquor].*

---

*   This addition of the measurement comes from the *Sūn Zhēn Rén* edition, but is missing in the other editions.

LINE 4.15

又方

Another prescription:

生地黃汁三升，煮取二升，服之。

Decoct three *shēng* of *shēng dì huáng zhī* (生地黃汁 Juice from the fresh root of Rehmannia glutinosa) to obtain two *shēng* and take it.

LINE 4.16

又方

Another prescription:

飲人乳汁三合。

Drink three *gě* of human breast milk.

LINE 4.17

又方

Another prescription:

燒月經衣，井花水服之。

Char menstrual cloth and take it in well-flower water.

LINE 4.18

又方

Another prescription:

燒白狗糞焦，作末，酒服方寸匕，日三。

Char a white dog's feces˙ until scorched, make a powder, and take a square-inch spoon in liquor three times a day.

*   The *Sūn Zhēn Rén* edition has 白狗莖 *bái gǒu jīng* (white dog's penis), instead, which most likely is a scribal error, as even the *Běn Cǎo Gāng Mù* quotes the prescription above in the entry on "white dog's feces" as an example for its use in the treatment of menstrual irregularities (《本草綱目》50:, p. 18)

LINE 4.19

又方

Another prescription:

取白馬尿，服一升，良。

Taking a white horse's urine and taking one *shēng* is good.

LINE 4.20

治月經不斷方。

[The following] prescription treats incessant menstrual flow.

船茹一斤，淨洗，河水四升半煮取二升，分二服。

Wash one *jīn* of *chuán rú* (船茹 Shavings of entangled Phyllostachys bambusoides roots) and decoct in four and a half *shēng* of river water to obtain two *shēng*. Divide into two doses.

LINE 4.21

又方

Another prescription:

服地黃酒良。

Taking rehmannia wine is good.

LINE 4.22

又方

Another prescription:

服大豆酒亦佳。

Taking soybean wine is also good.

LINE 4.23

又方

Another prescription:

燒箕舌灰，酒服之。

Char a winnowing basket tongue* into ashes and take it in liquor.

---

* 箕舌 *jī shé*: Lit. "the tongue of a winnowing basket." As a medicinal ingredient, it is explained in the *Běn Cǎo Gāng Mù* as a "basket for winnowing" (簸揚之箕 *bǒ yáng zhī jī*), in the South made of bamboo, in the North made of willow (《本草綱目》 38:1442). According to the *Dà Hàn Hé Cí Diǎn*, 箕舌 is the widened area in the front of the winnowing basket (諸橋轍次, 主編《大漢和辭典》 8:26143).

LINE 4.24

又方

Another prescription:

灸內踝下白肉際青脈上，隨年壯。

Burn moxa on top of the green-blue vessel at the edge of the white flesh below the inner side of the ankle, the number of cones corresponding to her age.

Appendix A: Sūn Sī-Miǎo's Biography in the *Jiù Táng Shū* 舊唐書

Background: This text was completed in 945, in the Latter Jìn 後晉 Period by Liú Xù 劉昫 et al. Originally entitled "Táng History" (*Táng Shū* 唐書), the name was altered in order to distinguish it from the *Xīn Táng Shū* 新唐書 (New Táng History) composed by Ōu-Yáng Xiū 歐陽修 et al. in 1060. The comparative merits and demerits of both texts as sources of biographical information on Sūn Sī-Miǎo are the subject of debate.[1] In regard to the *Jiù Táng Shū*, its sources of information are often questioned because it was composed during times of unrest and general upheaval. Nevertheless, Gān Zǔ-Wàng, for example, considers it to be more reliable than the *Xīn Táng Shū* because it is more explicit and concrete. Nathan Sivin, on the other hand, criticizes both texts extensively and considers the biographical information as mostly hagiographical since it cannot be substantiated with other primary sources. In general, he considers the *Xīn Táng Shū* information to be more reliable because it was composed in a time of greater peace and social stability when more extensive historical information was available to the editors. He does admit, however, that stylistic concerns motivated the latter's editors to exclude some significant material and also that "there is not a single discrepancy in the two biographies of such a nature as to suggest that the HTS [sic. *Xīn Táng Shū*] editors had access to new archival material."[2]

Translation of *Jiù Táng Shū* 舊唐書191, pp. 5094-5097

Sūn Sī-Miǎo was from Huá-Yuán 華原 in Jīng-Zhào 京兆.[3] At age seven, he took up studying, daily reciting thousands of characters. In his twenties, he excelled at discussing the theories of the *Zhuāng Zǐ*, the *Lǎo Zǐ*, and the Hundred Schools [of classical philosophy], and was equally skilled in Buddhist literature. When the governor of Luò-Zhōu 洛州,[4] Dú-Gū Xìn 獨孤信,[5] saw him, he said with a sigh: "This is a sagely youth. But regrettably his talent is so great that his suitability is diminished and he will be difficult to employ." At the time of Emperor Xuān of Zhōu [578-579], when the ruling house was embroiled in frequent upheavals, Sūn lived in retreat on Mount Tài-Bó 太白山.[6] When Emperor Wén 文 of the *Suí* 隋 dynasty was regent of the government [580-589],

---

1. See, for example, 干祖望《孫思邈評傳》pp.3-4, and Sivin, *Chinese Alchemy,* pp. 87-89.
2. Nathan Sivin, *Chinese Alchemy*, p. 99, n. 31
3. Location in present-day Yào County in Shǎn-Xī Province 陝西耀縣 in the vicinity of the Western capital Cháng-Ān.
4. County in modern Shǎn-Xī Province, located in modern Fū-Zhōu Prefecture 鄜州 in Fù County 富縣.
5. According to his biographies in the *Zhōu Shū* 周書 and *Běi Shǐ* 北史, a famous military man whose encounter with Sūn would have had to have occurred between 537 and 540, according to the rank mentioned. This leads Sivin to judge the entire encounter as fictitious, invented to increase Sūn's fame. See Nathan Sivin, *Chinese Alchemy*, p. 91.
6. Modern Zhōng-Nán Mountain 終南山, located in Shǎn-Xī Province in the South of Zhōu-Wǔ County 盩屋縣. It is the highest peak of the Wǔ-Gōng mountain range 武功山 and is also known as Tài-Yī 太一 or Tài-Yǐ 太乙.

he was summoned to become an Erudite of the National University 國子博士, but he declined under the pretext of illness. Addressing a close friend, he said: "After 50 years have passed, there should be a sage emerging [as ruler] and I will assist him with my prescriptions in saving people."

When [*Táng* Emperor] Tài-Zōng 太宗 ascended the throne [in 627], he summoned Sūn to the metropolitan area. Stunned by the great youthfulness of his appearance, [the emperor] addressed him saying: "Thus I know that there are people who have obtained the *Dào* and can be sincerely revered. How could talk about *Xiàn Mén* 羡門[7] and *Guāng Chéng* 光成[8] be empty words!" When [Sūn] was about to be conferred the rank of a noble, he firmly refused and did not accept. In the fourth year of Xiǎn-Qìng 顯慶 [659], emperor Gāo-Zōng 高宗 summoned him to an audience, appointing him Grand Master of Remonstrance,[9] and again he firmly refused and did not accept. In the first year of Shàng-Yuán 上元 [674], he requested to return home on the grounds of illness. He was presented with a horse of exceptional quality and with the administrative office of Princess Pó-Yáng's 鄱陽 estate for his residence.[10]

At that time, well-known scholars such as Sòng Lìng-Wén 宋令文,[11] Mèng Shēn 孟詵,[12] and Lú Zhào-Lín 盧照鄰[13] treated him with the decorum accorded a teacher in order to serve him. Sī-Miǎo once followed in the Emperor's retinue to Jiǔ-Chéng Palace 九成宮[14] and Zhào-Lín stayed behind in his house. At that time, there was a diseased pear tree in front of the main hall. Zhào-Lín made a poem about it, its preface saying: "In the year Guǐ-Yǒu 癸酉, I lay down with illness at an official building in the Guāng-Dé Precinct 光德坊 in Cháng-Ān. An elder said: 'This is the administrative office of Princess Pó-Yáng's estate. Long ago, the princess died before getting married, and her estate has fallen into disrepair.' Currently, the hermit Sūn Sī-Miǎo is in residence there. Miǎo's way harmonizes the past with the present, and he has studied the arts of calculation[15] to the extreme. His eminent discussion of Orthodox Oneness[16] is on a par with the ancient Zhuāng-Zǐ. His deep penetration of non-duality is on a par with the contemporary Vimalakirti. His astrological prognostications and measurements of the masculine and feminine[17] are on a par with Luò-Xià

---

7. An ancient immortal who was famous for his medicinal prescriptions and is said to have lived in the Warring States to Qín period. The First Qín emperor sent an expedition to find him.

8. Guāng Chéng-Zǐ 廣成子, another famous immortal. According to Lǎo-Zǐ's biography in the *Shén Xiān Zhuàn*, a name for Lǎo-Zǐ during the time of the Yellow Emperor. According to the *Zhuāng Zǐ*, the Yellow Emperor went to visit him on Kōng-Tóng Mountain 崆峒山.

9. 諫議大夫 *jiàn yì dà fū*: See Charles O. Hucker, *A Dictionary of Official Titles in Imperial China*, p. 148: "...one of the category of prestigious officials called Remonstrance Officials or Speaking Officials whose principal function was to attend and advise the emperor, and especially to remonstrate him with what they considered improper conduct or policy..."

10. Also a place name referring to a district in modern northeastern Jiāng-Xī 江西 Province.

11. Recorded in his son's biography as having occupied the position of "Literatus Reviser and Corrector in the Imperial Chancellery during the reign of Gāo-Zōng (Nathan Sivin, *Chinese Alchemy*, p. 101).

12. Famous physician and alchemist of the early *Táng*, estimated by Sivin to have lived ca. 621- ca. 713 (*Chinese Alchemy*, p. 101).

13. One of the "Four Heroes [of Prose Writing] of the Early Táng" (初唐四傑 *chū táng sì jié*), because of his literary accomplishments. According to his biography in the *Jiù Táng Shū*, he retired from his official career because of severe illness, withdrew to the mountains, and eventually drowned himself. Sivin estimates his dates as ca. 641-ca. 680 (*Chinese Alchemy*, p. 101).

14. Emperor's summer retreat in Shǎn-Xī Province, in the west of Lín-Yóu County 麟遊縣. Originally built in the *Suí*, Táng Tài-Zōng had it restored in 631.

15. I.e., hemerology.

16. A branch of religious Daoism that combined the Celestial Master tradition with the Shàng-Qīng and Líng-Bǎo traditions. In medieval Daoism, this term was used as a reference to Orthodox Daoist practices, as opposed to the unorthodox practices of the "masters of prescriptions," local cults and popular religion.

17. A reference to his alchemical skills?

18. According to the *Hàn Shū*, a *Hàn* dynasty hermit and famous astrologer and geographer who served as astrologer during the reign of Hàn Wǔ-Dì. His last name is also written with the character 落.

19. Master of [medicinal and macrobiotic] prescriptions from the *Qín* period.

Hóng 洛下閎[18] and Ān-Qī Shēng 安期生."[19]

Zhào-Lín had a malignant illness which physicians were unable to cure, so he went and asked Sī-Miǎo, "What principles do the famous physicians employ to cure illness?" Sī-Miǎo answered: "I have heard that if one is skilled at talking about Heaven, one must substantiate it in the human realm; if one is skilled at talking about humans, one must also root it in Heaven. In Heaven, there are four seasons and five phases; winter cold and summer heat alternate with each other. When this cyclical revolution is harmonious, it forms rain; when it is angry, wind; when it congeals, frost and snow; when it stretches out, rainbows. These are the constancies of Heaven and Earth.

"Humans have four limbs and five internal organs. They alternate between being awake and sleeping. In exhaling and inhaling, spitting out and sucking in,[20] essence and *qì* leave and come. In their flow, they constitute the constructive and protective [energies of the body], they manifest as facial color, and they erupt as sound. These are the constancies of humanity. *Yáng* employs the form, *yīn* employs the essence. This is where Heaven and humanity are identical."[21]

"When [the constancies] are lost, if [*qì* and essence] steam upward, they cause heat [in the body];[22] if they are blocked, they cause cold; if they are bound, tumors and excrescences; if they sink, abscesses; if they scatter wildly, panting and dyspnea; and if they are exhausted, scorching and withering. Their symptoms arise on the face, and their transformations move around in the body."

"When one extends this analogy to apply to Heaven and Earth, it is also likewise. Thus the waxing and waning of the Five Planets, the irregular motions of the constellations, the eclipses of the sun and moon, the flight of shooting stars, these are Heaven and Earth's symptoms of danger. Unseasonable winter cold and summer heat are the ascent or blockage [of *qì* and essence] in Heaven and Earth. Uprighted boulders and thrust-up earth are the tumors and excrescences of Heaven and Earth. Collapsing mountains and caved-in ground are the abscesses of Heaven and Earth. Scattered winds and violent rain are the panting and dyspnea of Heaven and Earth. Dried-up streams and parched marshes are the scorching and withering of Heaven and Earth. An excellent physician guides [*qì* and essence] with medicines and [lancing] stones and rescues them with needles and prescriptions. A sage[ly ruler] harmonizes them in order to perfect his power and uses them as support in order to manage the affairs of humanity. Thus, the human body has illnesses that can be cured, and Heaven and Earth have calamities that can be dispersed."[23]

Again, he said: "Wish for a gallbladder that is large, and a heart that is small, for knowledge that is round, and for action that is square. The *Shǐ Jīng* passage, "like approaching a deep abyss or treading on thin ice," refers to a small heart. "The elegant warrior, he is a protection and wall to

---

20. Daoist breathing exercise, also called "spitting out the old and sucking in the new" (吐故納新 *tǔ gù nà xīn*).

21. This entire quotation is based broadly on *Sù Wén* 5, 陰陽應象大論 *yīn yáng yīng xiang dà lùn*.

22. "Heat" and "cold" are here to be read as pathological conditions, parallel to the following lists of tumors etc.

23. While Sivin argues convincingly that this quotation probably does not reflect Sūn's own words (*Chinese Alchemy*, pp. 112-114), for the purpose of characterizing Sūn's thought and intellectual background, it is a highly significant passage. It situates him plainly in the midst between the ideal Confucian sage-ruler who rules by harmonizing human society with the cosmos and the physician who applies these intuitive insights to the physical body in his medical practice. As we can see in Sūn's life, the foundation for both of these skills is found in the practice of retreating to the mountains to engage in philosophical and religious speculations as well as practicing alchemical and calendrical arts. Sūn is powerful proof that simplistic distinctions between "Confucian" and "Daoist" (or for that matter, "Daoist" and "Buddhist") figures in medieval China need to be revised in light of the information found in their biographies.

the prince," refers to a large gallbladder. "He does not take a crooked course for gain, nor does he consider acting in righteousness a distress," refers to action that is square. "He perceives the first signs and immediately takes action; he does not wait even a whole day," refers to knowledge that is rounded.[24]

Sī-Miǎo himself said that he was born in the Xīn-Yǒu 辛酉 year of the Kāi-Huáng 開皇 period [581-600], and that he was presently 93 years old.[25] When inquiries were made in his home village, people unanimously stated that he had been a person of several hundred years of age.[26] When he spoke of affairs during the [Northern] Zhōu [557-581] and Qí [550-577] periods, it was as vivid as from an eye witness. Considering this, he cannot have been a person of a mere hundred years. But nevertheless, his sight and hearing were not weakened, and his spirit flourishing. He can be called one of the extensively illuminated immortals of ancient times.

Previously, Wèi Wēi 魏微 et al. received an imperial order to compile the histories of the Five Dynasties, of Qí 齊, Liáng 梁, Chén 陳, Zhōu 周, and Suí 隋.[27] Fearful of leaving out anything, they paid frequent calls to him. Among Sī-Miǎo's oral transmissions, there were some that were [as vivid] as if he had seen them with his own eyes.[28]

When the Vice Director of the Chancellery, Sūn Chǔ-Yuē 孫處約,[29] presented his five sons Tǐng 侹, Jǐng 儆, Jùn 俊, Yòu 佑, and Quán 佺 to Sī-Miǎo, Sī-Miǎo said: "Jùn will be the first to obtain high office, Yòu will reach it later, Quán will be the most famous and important, but disaster will strike when he serves in the military."[30] Afterwards, all this occurred as he had said.

When the Supervisor of the Household of the Heir Apparent, Lú Qí-Qīng 盧齊卿, was in his youth, he requested to inquire about his prospects[31] and Sī-Miǎo said: "Fifty years from now, you will have risen to the post of Regional Inspector and my grandson will serve as your subordinate. You will personally be able to protect him."[32] Subsequently, when Qí-Qīng was serving as head of

---

24. These quotations are found in 《詩經》195, 《詩經》7, 《左傳》31st year of Duke Zhao, and 《易經》 "繫詞" B.5 (see Nathan Sivin, *Chinese Alchemy*, p. 114, n. 61).

25. Since his conversation with Lú supposedly took place in 673, it would put his birth date at 581 or 582, the date most commonly accepted by current scholarship. This is in accordance with the previous statement if one accepts the claim of the *Sì Kù Quán Shū* editors that his birth year should be read as Xīn-Chǒu 辛丑 (i.e., the 38th year of the cycle) rather than Xīn-Yǒu 辛酉.

26. 數百歲 *shù bǎi suì* 數百歲. This is not a translation error and should not be read as "more than a hundred years." While it could be argued by a critical Western mind that this might be the result of a scribal error and should be understood as 數十百歲 *shù shí bǎi suì* (more than a hundred years), I find it much more likely that the authors of this biography were indeed convinced of—or at least faithfully recorded the villagers of his hometown as believing in—his great age of over two hundred years.

27. According to the *Jiù Táng Shū*, the project was initiated in 629. Wèi Wēi was indeed active as supervisor in particular of the history of the Suí dynasty, and the completed project was submitted to the Emperor in 636. Taking Sūn's birth date as 581, this would put him only in his early fifties. This relatively young age would make it slightly questionable that they would have consulted him. Sivin claims that "it is not patently absurd, so long as Wèi and his associates believed that Sūn was, despite his appearance, a very old man, and providing that Sūn was a very skilled liar" (*Chinese Alchemy*, p. 126). I would rather argue either for an earlier birth date or take into consideration the possibility that his fame as a clairvoyant and sage had made him a likely consultant for this type of inquiry.

28. 口以傳授有如目睹 *kǒu yǐ chuán shòu yǒu rú mù dǔ*: Alternatively, this could mean, "his oral record was so good that he must have observed it with his own eyes."

29. According to Sivin, Sūn Chǔ-Yuè never filled that position, but was a high-ranking official in such functions as Vice President of the Grand Imperial Secretariat and Vice Rector of the National University. Sivin suggests that the incident mentioned here took place in the sixth decade of the seventh century since his final appointment and retirement are recorded to have occurred in 664 (*Chinese Alchemy*, pp. 127-128, n. 83, and *Jiù Táng Shū* 81.11a-b).

30. According to the *Xīn Táng Shū*, Sūn Quán did indeed become Governor-General, but perished in the war in Manchuria.

31. 請問人倫 *qǐng wèn rén lún*: While this can literally simply refer to "human interrelationships," it most likely refers to physiognomy in this context.

Xú Prefecture 徐州,[33] Sī-Miǎo's grandson Pú 溥 was indeed employed as an aid in Xiāo County 蕭縣 in Xú-Zhōu. When Sī-Miǎo had initially talked to Qí-Qīng, Pú had not even been born yet, and still he had known of this affair in advance. In all cases, the various traces of marvel stories are mostly of this kind.

Sī-Miǎo died in the first year of *Yǒng-Chún* 永淳 [682]. He left behind orders for a simple funeral, to not be buried with any funerary objects, and to worship the spirits without sacrificing any animals. After more than a month had passed, his outward appearance was unchanged and when lifting the corpse, it was stiff as wood as if it were merely empty clothes. His contemporaries regarded this as a miracle.

He wrote commentaries on the *Lǎo Zǐ* and *Zhuāng Zǐ* and composed the *Qiān Jīn Fāng*, which has been circulated through the generations. He also composed the *Fú Lù Lùn* 福祿論 in three volumes, the *Shè Shēng Zhēn Lù* 攝生真錄, the *Zhěn Zhōng Sù Shū* 枕中素書, and the *Huì Sān Jiào Lùn* 會三教論, each in one volume.

His son Xíng 行 held the post of Vice Director of the Imperial Secretariat in the reign period Tiān-Shòu 天授 [690-692].[34]

---

32. 可自保 *kě zì bǎo*: Sivin renders this as, "take care of yourself." My version seems more likely when one considers a more elaborate version of the story, found in the *Dìng Mìng Lù* 定命錄, composed between 827 and 835 by Lǚ Dào-Shēng 呂道生, where Sūn is recorded to have made a similar prognostication to a man called Gāo Zhòng-Shū 高仲舒, warning that " 'although he [i.e., Sūn's grandson or in this case son] will incur a beating, I hope that you will remember the words of an old man and let him go.' Afterward, it happened as he said. Only after [Gāo had had Sūn's son] stripped did he suddenly remember and pardon him" (quoted in Sivin, *Chinese Alchemy*, p. 130). According to the *Jiù Táng Shū*, Lú Qí-Qīng did serve as prefect sometime between 713 and 730, but not in Xú Prefecture.
33. Located in modern Jiāng-Sū 江蘇.
34. 鳳閣侍郎 *fèng gé shì láng*: According to Charles Hucker, "the second executive post in the Secretariat and... included among the officials serving as Grand Councilors" (*Dictionary of Official Titles*, pp. 426-427). This information is significant since it clearly marks the Sūn family as part of the high-ranking elite with close connections to the court.

Appendix B: Materia Medica with excerpts from the Shén Nóng Běn Cǎo Jīng

The following appendix consists of a complete list of the medicinal ingredients used in the formulas above, alphabetized by pinyin. For each entry, we give the Chinese characters and pinyin pronunciation, botanical identification, English common name, additional information about relevant aspects such as the plant itself, the medicinal preparation, and related substances, and the entry number in the *Zhōng Yī Dà Cí Diǎn* 中藥大辭典 for readers literate in Chinese who want more medicinal information. This information is included as "Translator's Notes."

Most importantly, however, we have translated the complete entries, whenever available, from the *Shén Nóng Běn Cǎo Jīng* 神農本草經, arguably the most important materia medica text in early medieval China that dates back to the *Hàn* period. Our rationale for including an original translation of this material was to enlighten readers on how physicians viewed and utilized a certain substance in the clinical context during Sūn Sī-Miǎo's time - as opposed to its contemporary usage. This information can serve as a guide to analyzing the medicinal composition of the formulas translated above and thereby to understanding the intended effect of each medicinal individually and of all ingredients in a formula in combination. It is our sincere hope that this partial translation of the *Shén Nóng Běn Cǎo Jīng* will stimulate readers' interest in and appreciation of this important text and result in the publication of a complete translation of the *Shén Nóng Běn Cǎo Jīng* in the near future.

In its original version, the *Shén Nóng Běn Cǎo Jīng* discusses 365 medicinal substances that are ranked in three hierarchical grades, corresponding to the trinity of Heaven, Humanity, and Earth.

According to the preface, the highest-ranking drugs, which are called "sovereigns" (君 *jūn*), "nourish life" 養命 *yǎng mìng*, correspond to Heaven, are non-toxic (無毒 *wú dú*), are to be taken over for a long time, and are used to lighten the body, boost *qì*, and prolong life. The "ministers" (臣 *chén*) of the middle grade "nourish [human] nature" 養性 *yǎng xìng*, correspond to humanity, are partly toxic, partly non-toxic, and are used to prevent illness and supplement vacuity and emaciation. In the lowest category, the "assistants" (佐 *zuǒ*) and "couriers" (使 *shǐ*) "treat disease," correspond to earth, are toxic and cannot be taken over a long period of time, and are used to "expel the evil *qì* of cold or heat, break up accumulations, and cure disease."

艾葉 *ài yè*
Dry-roasted foliage of Artemisia argyi

Translator's note:
Common name: Mugwort.
Family: Aster (Asteraceae).
Other species used: Artemisia vulgaris.
《中藥大辭典》#1591.

菴䕡子 *ān lǘ zǐ*
Fruit of Artemisia keiskeana
Vol. 1, line 47 Highest Grade

味苦，微寒，無毒。主五臟瘀血，腹中水氣，臚張，留熱，風寒濕痹，身體諸痛。久服，輕身、延年、不老。生川谷及道邊。

Flavor: Bitter
Nature: Slightly cold
Toxicity: Non-toxic
Alt. names: n/a

Actions and Indications:
Indicated for static blood in the five viscera, water *qì* in the abdomen, extended belly, lodged heat, wind-cold-damp impediment, and all pains in the body.

Additional Information:
Taken over a long time, it lightens the body, extends the years, and prevents aging.
Grows in valleys with streams and alongside roads.

Translator's note:
Common name: Keiske artemisia fruit.
Family: Aster (Asteraceae).
This needs to be distinguished from several other species of artemisia used medicinally, especially 艾葉 *ài yè*.
《中藥大辭典》#3966.

巴豆 *bā dòu*
Seed of Croton tiglium
Vol. 3, line 59 Lowest Grade

味辛，溫，有大毒。主傷寒、溫瘧、寒熱，破症
瘕、結聚堅積，留飲、痰癖。大腹水脹，蕩滌五
臟六腑，開通閉塞，利水谷道，去惡肉，除鬼
毒、蠱注、邪物，殺蟲魚。生川谷。

Flavor: Acrid
Nature: Warm
Toxicity: Greatly toxic
Alt. names: 巴叔

Actions and Indications:
Indicated for cold damage, warm malaria, [aversion to]
cold and heat [effusion], and for breaking up concretions and conglomerations, binds and gatherings,
hardenings and accumulations, lodged rheum, and
phlegm aggregations.
[Treats] greater abdominal water distention, flushes
the five viscera and six bowels, opens blockages,
disinhibits the pathways of water and grain, removes
malign flesh, expels ghost toxin and *gǔ* infixation and
evil things, and kills worms and fish.

Additional Information:
Grows in valleys with streams.

Translator's note:
Common name: Croton seed.
Family: Spurge (Euphorbiaceae).
《中藥大辭典》#0656.

巴戟天 *bā jǐ tiān*
Root of Morinda officinalis
Vol. 1, line 43 Highest Grade

味辛，微溫，無毒。主大風邪氣，陰痿不起，強
筋骨，安五臟，補中，增志，益氣。生山谷。

Flavor: Bitter
Nature: Warm
Toxicity: Non-toxic
Alt. names: n/a

Actions and Indications:
Indicated for the evil *qì* of great wind, and *yīn* wilting
with inability to raise [the penis].
Strengthens the sinews and bones, quiets the five
viscera, supplements the center, increases the will,
and boosts *qì*.

Additional Information:
Grows in mountain valleys.

Translator's note:

Common name: Morinda root.
Family: Madder (Rubiaceae).
《中藥大辭典》#0662.

白艾 *bái ài*
Foliage of Crossostephium chinense

Translator's note:
Common name: Crossostephium leaf.
Family: Aster (Asteraceae).
Other species used: Crossostephium artemisiodes
A close relative of the more commonly used 艾葉 *ài yè*.
《中藥大辭典》#2730, where it is listed as 香菊 *xiāng
jú*.

白堊 *bái è*
Chalk
Vol. 3, line 7 Lowest Grade

味苦，溫，無毒。主女子寒热、症瘕、月闭、积
聚，陰腫痛，漏下，無子。生山谷。

Flavor: Bitter
Nature: Warm
Toxicity: Non-toxic
Alt. names: n/a

Actions and Indications:
Indicated for women's [aversion to] cold and heat [ef-
fusion], concretions and conglomerations, menstrual
block, accumulations and gatherings, swelling and
pain in the genitals, vaginal spotting, and sterility.

Additional Information:
Grows in mountain valleys.

Translator's note:
《中藥大辭典》#1094.

白狗糞 *bái gǒu fèn*
Feces of Canis familiaris

Translator's note:
Common Name: White dog's feces,
Family: Canine (Canidae).
Not specifically listed in the *Zhōng Yào Dà Cí Diǎn*.
For information on the medical use of other parts of
Canis familiaris, see 《中藥大辭典》#2020 and the
following entries. 《本草綱目》50:1017 discusses the

various uses of dog; white dog feces are specifically described there.

白芨 *bái jí*
Rhizome of Bletilla striata
Vol. 3, line 32 Lowest Grade

味苦，平，無毒。主癰腫、惡創、敗疽，傷陰，死肌，胃中邪氣，賊風，鬼擊，痱緩不收。生川谷。

Flavor: Bitter
Nature: Neutral
Toxicity: Non-toxic
Alt. names: 甘根、連及草

Actions and Indications:
Indicated for welling-abscess swelling, malign wounds, vanquished flat-abscesses, damage to the genitals, dead flesh, evil *qi* in the stomach, bandit wind, attacks by ghosts, and disablement and slackness with failure to contract.

Additional Information:
Grows in valleys with streams.

Translator's note:
Common name: Bletilla rhizome.
Family: Orchid (Orchidaceae).
《中藥大辭典》#1083.

白僵蠶 *bái jiāng cán*
Dried 4th or 5th stage larva of the moth of Bombyx mori

Translator's note:
Common name: Infected silkworm larva.
Family: Silkworm (Bombycidae).
Used after the moth larvae have been killed by infection of the fungus Beauveria bassiana. This state of the silkworm moth is commonly referred to as "bombyx batryticatus" in a medicinal context. Also called 殭蠶 *jiāng cán*.
《中藥大辭典》#1160.

白膠 *bái jiāo*
Glue produced from Cervus nippon
Vol. 1, line 117 Highest Grade

The info here may also apply for 鹿角.

味甘，平，無毒。主傷中勞絕，腰痛，羸瘦，補中益氣，女人血閉無子，止痛、安胎。久服，輕身、延年。

Flavor: Sweet
Nature: Neutral
Toxicity: Non-toxic
Alt. names: 鹿角膠

Actions and Indications:
Indicated for damage to the center and taxation expiry, lumbar pain, and marked emaciation.
Supplements the center and boosts *qi*.
[Treats] women's blood blockage and infertility, relieves pain, and quiets the fetus.

Additional Information:
Taken for a long time, it lightens the body and extends the years.

Translator's note:
Common Name: Deerhorn glue.
Family: Deer (Cervidae).
Other species used: Cervus elaphus
The gelatinous glue produced from the horn of Cervus nippon, collected in the seventh lunar month. Deerhorn glue is also called 鹿角膠 *lù jiǎo jiāo*. Note that 鹿角 *lù jiǎo* must be distinguished from 鹿茸 *lù róng*, velvet deerhorn.
《中藥大辭典》#3703.

白薟 *bái liǎn*
Root of Ampelopsis japonica
Vol. 3, line 29 Lowest Grade

味苦，平，無毒。主癰腫疽創，散結氣，止痛，除熱，目中赤，小兒惊癇，溫瘧，女子陰中腫痛。生山谷。

Flavor: Bitter
Nature: Neutral
Toxicity: Non-toxic
Alt. names: 兔核、白草

Actions and Indications:
Indicated for welling-abscess swelling, flat-abscesses, and wounds.
Dissipates bound *qi*, relieves pain, eliminates heat with redness in the eyes, and [treats] small children's fright epilepsy, warm malaria, and women's genital swelling and pain.

Additional Information:
Grows in mountain valleys.

Translator's note:
Common name: Ampelopsis root.
Family: Grape (Vitaceae).
《中藥大辭典》#1103.

白龍骨 *bái lóng gǔ*
Bleached fossilized vertebrae and bone of mammals

Translator's note:
Common name: White dragon bone.
Other species used: Elephants or oxen.
While 龍骨 *lóng gǔ* can also refer to two other drugs, namely 接骨草 *jiē gǔ cǎo* (gyrating desmodium, Steward's elastostema, elder, or Formosan elder, 《中藥大辭典》#3297) or 鹿茸草 *lù róng cǎo* (monochasma, 《中藥大辭典》#3722), given the significance and specificity of colors in other drug names used by Sūn, I read it literally as "white dragon bones," not an uncommon medicinal ingredient.
《中藥大辭典》#5053.
For the medicinal properties of 龍骨 *lóng gǔ* in the *Shén Nóng Běn Cǎo Jīng*, see entry on 龍骨 *lóng gǔ* below.

白馬尿 *bái mǎ niào*
Urine of white Equus caballus

Translator's note:
Common name: White horse's urine.
Family: Horse (Equidae).
《中藥大辭典》#3139 (on 馬肉 *mǎ ròu*, "horse meat") contains a general description of the medicinal uses of the animal, but does not mention horse's urine specifically. The *Běn Cǎo Gāng Mù* 本草綱目 covers the medicinal use of various parts of the horse, including an entry on white horse urine (《本草綱目》50:1780). For more information on horse dung in general, see the entry on 馬通 *mǎ tōng* below.

白馬蹄 *bái mǎ tí*
Hoof of white Equus caballus

Translator's note:
Common name: White horse's hooves

Family: Horse (Equidae).
For more information, and the translation of the entry from the *Shén Nóng Běn Cǎo Jīng* on "hair, hooves, and nails of the six domestic animals," see the entry below on 馬蹄底護乾 *mǎ tí dǐ hù gān* (Desiccated protected underside of a Equus caballus's hoof).

白馬駝 *bái mǎ tuō*
Mane of white Equus caballus

Translator's note:
Common Name: White horse's mane.
Family: Horse (Equidae).
More commonly called 白馬鬃 *bái mǎ zōng*. For more information and the translation of the *Shén Nóng Běn Cǎo Jīng* entry on "hair, hooves, and nails of the six domestic animals," see the entry below on (馬蹄底護乾 *mǎ tí dǐ hù gān* Desiccated protected underside of a Equus caballus's hoof).

白馬鬃 *bái mǎ zōng*
Mane of white Equus caballus

Translator's note:
Common Name: White horse's mane.
Family: Horse (Equidae).
《中藥大辭典》#3148 lists only 馬鬃 *mǎ zōng* (horse's mane) in general and states that both the mane and tail hair are used. For more information and the translation from the *Shén Nóng Běn Cǎo Jīng* on "hair, hooves, and nails of the six domestic animals," see the entry below on 馬蹄底護乾 *mǎ tí dǐ hù gān* (Desiccated protected underside of a Equus caballus's hoof).

白茅根 *bái máo gēn*
Root of Imperata cylindrica

Translator's note:
Common Name: Imperata root.
Family: Grass (Poaceae).
This plant is also called cogon grass. Its flower is also used medicinally (《中藥大辭典》#1136).
For the root and description of the plant, see 《中藥大辭典》#1137.

白蜜 *bái mì*
Honey of Apis cerana
Vol. 1, line 121 Highest Grade

味甘，平，無毒。主心腹邪氣，諸惊痙癎，安五臟，諸不足，益氣補中，止痛解毒，除眾病，和百藥。久服，強志、輕身、不飢、不老。生山谷。

Flavor: Sweet
Nature: Neutral
Toxicity: Non-toxic
Alt. names: 石飴

Actions and Indications:
Indicated for evil *qì* in the heart and abdomen and for all fright, tetany, and epilepsy.
Quiets the five viscera and [treats] all insufficiencies, boosts *qì* and supplements the center, relieves pain and resolves toxin, eliminates the multitudes of diseases, and harmonizes the hundred medicinals.

Additional Information:
Taken for a long time, it strengthens the will, lightens the body, and prevents hunger and aging
Grows in mountain valleys.

Translator's note:
Common Name: Honey.
Family: Bee (Apidae).
Honey is more commonly called 蜂蜜 *fēng mì*.
《中藥大辭典》#4352.

白前 *bái qián*
Root and rhizome of Cynanchum stauntoni

Translator's note:
Common Name: Willowleaf swallowwort root and rhizome.
Family: Dogbane (Apocynaceae).
Other species used: Cynanchum glaucescens
《中藥大辭典》#1091.

白石英 *bái shí yīng*
White quartz
Vol. 1, line 14 Highest Grade

味甘，微溫，無毒。主消渴，陰痿不足，咳逆，胸膈間久寒，益氣，除風濕痹。久服，輕身、長年。生山谷。

Flavor: Sweet
Nature: Slightly warm

Toxicity: Non-toxic
Alt. names: n/a

Actions and Indications:
Indicated for dispersion thirst, *yīn* wilt (i.e. impotence) and [sexual] insufficiency, cough with counterflow, and chronic cold in the area of the chest and diaphragm.
Boosts *qì*, and eliminates wind-damp impediment.

Additional Information:
Taken for a long time, it lightens the body and lengthens the years.
Grows in mountain valleys.

Translator's note:
《中藥大辭典》#1115.

白石脂 *bái shí zhī*
Kaolin

Translator's note:
Common Name: China clay.
《中藥大辭典》#1116.

白頭翁 *bái tóu wēng*
Root of Pulsatilla chinensis
Vol. 3, line 44 Lowest Grade

味苦，溫，有毒。主溫瘧，狂易寒熱，症瘕積聚，癭氣，逐血，止痛，療金瘡。生山谷及田野。

Flavor: Bitter
Nature: Warm
Toxicity: Toxic
Alt. names: 野丈人，胡王使者

Actions and Indications:
Indicated for warm malaria, mania with tendency to [aversion to] cold and heat [effusion], concretions, conglomerations, accumulations, and gatherings, and goiter *qì*.
Expels blood, relieves pain, and treats incised wounds.

Additional Information:
Grows in mountain valleys and open fields.

Translator's note:
Common Name: Pulsatilla/ anemone root.
Family: Buttercup (Ranunculaceae).
Other species used: Pulsatilla dahurica, P. koreana, P. turczaninovii, or P. ambigua.
《中藥大辭典》#1164.

白薇 *bái wēi*
Root of Cynanchum atratum
Vol. 2, line 46 Middle Grade

味苦，平，無毒。主暴中風，身熱，肢滿，忽忽
不知人，狂惑邪氣，寒熱酸疼，溫瘧洒洒，發作
有時。生平原川谷。

Flavor: Bitter
Nature: Neutral
Toxicity: Non-toxic
Alt. names: n/a

Actions and Indications:
Indicated for fulminant wind strike, generalized fever,
fullness in the limbs, sudden inability to recognize
people, mania and confusion and evil *qì*, [aversion
to] cold and heat [effusion] with soreness and pain,
and warm malaria with shivering that erupts in regular
attacks.

Additional Information:
Grows in flatlands and valleys with streams.

Translator's note:
Common Name: Black swallowwort root.
Family: Dogbane family (Apocynacea).
Other species used: Cynanchum versicolor
《中藥大辭典》#1100.

白楊皮 *bái yáng pí*
Bark of Populus davidiana

Translator's note:
Common Name: David's poplar bark.
Family: Willow family (Salicaceae).
《中藥大辭典》#1208.

白玉 *bái yù*
Fine slivers of white jade

Translator's note:
《中藥大辭典》#1035, where it is listed as 玉屑 *yù xiè*
(jade slivers).

白芷 *bái zhǐ*
Root of Angelica dahurica
Vol. 2, line 31 Middle Grade

味辛，溫，無毒。主女人漏下赤白，血閉，陰
腫，寒熱風頭侵目淚出。長肌膚，潤澤。可作面
脂。生川谷下澤。

Flavor: Acrid
Nature: Warm
Toxicity: Non-toxic
Alt. names: 芳香

Actions and Indications:
Indicated for women's vaginal spotting of red or white
discharge, for blocked blood and genital swelling, and
for [aversion to] cold and heat [effusion] with wind in
the head invading the eyes and causing tearing.
Makes the skin and flesh grow and moisturizes it.

Additional Information:
Can be made into a salve for the face.
Grows in valleys with streams and low-lying marshes.

Translator's note:
Common Name: Dahurican angelica root.
Family: Carrot (Apiaceae).
A species related to 當歸 *dāng guī* (Root of Angelica
polimorpha) and 獨活 *dú huó* (Root and rhizome of
Angelica pubescens).
《中藥大辭典》#1090.

[白]朮 *[bái] zhú*
Rhizome of Atractylodes macrocephala
Vol. 1, line 25 Highest Grade

味苦，溫，無毒。主風寒濕痺、死肌、痙、疸。
止汗，除熱，消食。作煎餌。久服，輕身、延
年、不飢。生山谷。

Flavor: Bitter
Nature: Warm
Toxicity: Non-toxic
Alt. names: 山薊

Actions and Indications:
Indicated for wind-cold-damp impediment, dead flesh,
tetany, and jaundice.
Checks sweating, eliminates heat, and disperses
food.

Additional Information:
To take medicinally, prepare as a concentrated brew.
Taken over a long time, it lightens the body, extends
the years, and prevents hunger.
Grows in mountain valleys.

Translator's note:
Common Name: Atractylodes rhizome.
Family: Aster family (Asteraceae).
《中藥大辭典》#1085.

柏葉 *bǎi yè*
Foliage of Platycladus orientalis

Translator's note:
Common Name: Arborvitae/ Biota needles.
Family: Cypress (Cupressaceae).
Other species used: Biota/ Thuja orientalis
《中藥大辭典》#3251, where it is listed as 側柏葉 *cè bǎi yè*.

柏子仁 *bǎi zǐ rén*
Seed of Platycladus orientalis
Vol. 1, line 97 Highest Grade

In the *Shén Nóng Běn Cǎo Jīng*, under the entry for 柏實.

味甘，平，無毒。主惊悸，安五臟，益氣，除濕痹。久服，令人悅澤美色，耳目聰明，不飢、不老，輕身、延年。生山谷。

Flavor: Sweet
Nature: Neutral
Toxicity: Non-toxic.
Alt. names: n/a

Actions and Indications:
Indicated for fright palpitations.
Quiets the five viscera, boosts *qì*, and eliminates damp impediment.

Additional Information:
Taken for a long time, it gives the person joy and a shiny and a beautiful complexion, sharpens the ears and eyes, prevents hunger and aging, lightens the body, and extends the years.
Grows in mountain valleys.

Translator's note:
Common Name: Arborvitae/ Biota seed.
Family: Cypress (Cupressaceae).
Other species used: Thuja orientalis.
《中藥大辭典》#2379.

敗船茹 *bài chuán rú*
Shavings of entangled Phyllostachys bambusoides roots

Translator's note:
Common Name: Rotten bamboo shavings.
According to Táo Hóng-Jīng, these are shavings of entangled bamboo roots (most likely mostly of the species Phyllostachys bambusoides), which were once used to fix leaky boats. By Lǐ Shí-Zhēn's time, they had been replaced by hemp fiber and putty, which might explain why this ingredient is not listed in the *Zhōng Yào Dà Cí Diǎn* (《本草綱目》38:1431). In the *Qiān Jīn Fāng*, it is also called 故舡上竹茹 *gù chuán shàng zhú rú*. For the medicinal qualities of bamboo, see the entry below on 竹 *zhú*.

敗鼓皮 *bài gǔ pí*
Skin of Bos taurus domesticus

Translator's note:
Common name: Rotten drum skin.
According to Kòu Zōng-Shì 寇宗奭, a medical writer of the early 12th century, any hide such as horse or donkey is acceptable for medicinal efficacy, but cow hide (from 黃牛 *huáng niú*, Bos taurus domesticus) is best. By Lǐ Shí-Zhēn's time, it had mostly fallen out of use as a medicinal ingredient (《本草綱目》50:1797). Not listed in the *Zhōng Yào Dà Cí Diǎn*.

敗醬 *bài jiàng*
Whole plant with root of Patrinia villosa
Vol. 2, line 39 Middle Grade

味苦，平，無毒。主暴熱，火創、赤氣，疥瘙，疽痔，馬鞍熱氣。生川谷。

Flavor: Bitter
Nature: Neutral
Toxicity: Non-toxic
Alt. names: 鹿腸

Actions and Indications:
Indicated for fulminant heat, fire wounds and red qì, scabs and itches, flat-abscesses and hemorrhoids, and hot qì from saddle sores.

Additional Information:
Grows in valleys with streams.

Translator's note:
Common name: Patrinia plant.
Family: Valerian (Valerianaceae).

Other species used: Patrinia scabiosaefolia.
《中藥大辭典》#3306.

班蝥 *bān māo*
Dried body of Mylabris phalerata
Vol. 3, line 87 Lowest Grade

味辛，寒，有毒。主寒熱、鬼注、蠱毒、鼠瘻、
惡創、疽蝕、死肌，破石癃。生川谷。

Flavor: Acrid
Nature: Cold
Toxicity: Toxic
Alt. names: 龍尾

Actions and Indications:
- Indicated for [aversion to] cold and heat [effusion],
ghost infixation, *gǔ* toxin, mouse fistulas, malign
wounds, flat-abscesses with erosion, and dead flesh,
and for breaking up urinary stones and dribbling
block.

Additional Information:
Lives in valleys with streams.

Translator's note:
Common Name: Mylabris.
Family: Blister Beetle (Meloidae).
Other species used: Mylabris cichorii
A close relative of Epicauta gorhami, mylabris is the
most common origin of the skin irritant cantharidin.
See entry below on 葛上亭長 *gé shàng tíng cháng* for
Epicauta gorhami.
《中藥大辭典》#3789.

半夏 *bàn xià*
Rhizome of Pinellia ternata
Vol. 3, line 13 Lowest Grade

味辛，平，有毒。主傷寒寒熱，心下堅，下氣，
喉咽腫痛，頭眩，胸脹，咳逆，腸鳴，止汗。生
川谷。

Flavor: Acrid
Nature: Neutral
Toxicity: Toxic
Alt. names: 地文，水玉

Actions and Indications:
Indicated for cold damage with [aversion to] cold
and heat [effusion], hardenings below the heart, for
precipitating *qì*, for swelling and pain in the throat,
dizziness in the head, distention in the chest, cough
with counterflow, rumbling intestines, and checking
sweating.

Additional Information:
Grows in valleys with streams.

Translator's note:
Common Name: Pinellia rhizome.
Family: Arum (Araceae).
《中藥大辭典》#0981.

貝齒 *bèi chǐ*
Shell of Monetaria moneta
Vol. 3, line 88 Lowest Grade

In the *Shén Nóng Běn Cǎo Jīng*, under the entry for 貝子.

味咸，平，有毒。主目翳、鬼注蟲毒、腹痛、下
血、五癃，利水道。燒用之，良。生東海池澤。

Flavor: Salty
Nature: Neutral
Toxicity: Toxic
Alt. names: 貝齒

Actions and Indications:
Indicated for eye screens, ghost infixation and worm
toxin, abdominal pain, precipitation of blood, the five
types of dribbling urinary block, and for disinhibiting
the water ways.

Additional Information:
Using it burnt is excellent.
Lives in the ponds and marshes of Dōng-Hǎi.

Translator's note:
Common Name: Cowrie shell.
Family: Cowrie (Cypraeidae).
Other species used: Monetaria (Cypraea) moneta or
M. annulus.
《中藥大辭典》#1789, where it is listed as 貝子 *bèi zǐ*.

貝母 *bèi mǔ*
Bulb of Fritillaria cirrhosa
Vol. 2, line 30 Middle Grade

味辛，平，無毒。主傷寒煩熱，淋瀝邪氣，疝
瘕，喉痹，乳難，金創，風痙。

Flavor: Acrid
Nature: Neutral
Toxicity: Non-toxic
Alt. names: 空草

Actions and Indications:

Indicated for cold damage with vexing heat, dribbling urination with evil *qì*, mounting conglomerations, throat impediment, lactation difficulties, incised wounds, and wind tetany.

Translator's note:
Common Name: Fritillaria bulb.
Family: Lily (Liliaceae).
Other species used: Fritillaria delavayi, F. przewalskii, F. ussuriensis, F. pallidiflora, or P. maximowiczii. These species are usually more specifically referred to as 川貝母 *chuān bèi mǔ* (Sichuan fritillaria). Another species, F. verticillata, is also used medicinally and is called 浙貝母 *zhè bèi mǔ* (Zhè-Jiāng fritillaria 《中藥大辭典》#2880).
《中藥大辭典》#0543.

萆薢 *bì xiè*
Rhizome of Dioscorea hypoglauca
Vol. 2, line 45 Middle Grade

味苦，平，無毒。主腰背痛，強骨節，風寒濕周痹，惡創不瘳，熱氣。生山谷。

Flavor: Bitter
Nature: Neutral
Toxicity: Non-toxic
Alt. names: n/a

Actions and Indications:
Indicated for pain in the lumbus and back, for strengthening the bones and joints, for generalized wind-cold-damp impediment, for malign wounds that won't heal, and for hot *qì*.

Additional Information:
Grows in mountain valleys.

Translator's note:
Common Name: Fish poison yam.
Family: Yam (Dioscoreaceae).
Other species used: Dioscorea collettii, D. tokoro, or D. gracillima.
Distinguish from 薯蕷 *shǔ yù*, dioscorea (Dioscorea opposita/batatas, the common potato yam).
《中藥大辭典》#3968.

弊帚頭 *bì zhǒu tóu*
Old broom top

Translator's note:
According to Lǐ Shí-Zhēn, this refers to a broom made of bamboo. (《本草綱目》38:1441). Not listed in the *Zhōng Yào Dà Cí Diǎn*. For information on the

medicinal properties of bamboo, see the entry on 竹 *zhú* below.

蝙蝠刺 *biān fú cì*
Fruit of Arctium lappa

Translator's note:
Common Name: Burdock fruit.
Family: Aster (Asteraceae).
Literally translated "bat stinger," it is more commonly called 牛蒡子 *niú bàng zǐ*. The root of this plant, 牛蒡根 *niú bàng gēn*, is more frequently used medicinally. (See entry below on 牛蒡 *niú bàng*.)
《中藥大辭典》#0927.

鱉甲 *biē jiǎ*
Dorsal shell of Amyda
(Trionyx) sinensis
Vol. 2, line 91 Middle Grade

味咸，平，無毒。主心腹症瘕堅積、寒熱，去痞、息肉、陰蝕、痔、惡肉。生池澤。

Flavor: Salty
Nature: Neutral
Toxicity: Non-toxic
Alt. names: n/a

Actions and Indications:
Indicated for concretions, conglomerations, hardenings and gatherings in the heart and abdomen, and for [aversion to] cold and heat [effusion].
Removes glomus, polyps, genital erosion, hemorrhoids, and malign flesh.

Additional Information:
Lives in ponds and marshes.

Translator's note:
Common Name: Turtle shell.
Family: Softshell Turtle (Trionychidae).
《中藥大辭典》#5661.

鱉頭 *biē tóu*
Dried head of Amyda (Trionyx) sinensis

Translator's note:
Common Name: Turtle's head.

Family: Softshell Turtle (Trionychidae).
《中藥大辭典》#5666.

檳榔 *bīng láng*
Fruit of Areca catechu

Translator's note:
Common Name: Betel nut.
Family: Palm (Arecaceae).
《中藥大辭典》#5203.

蠶子 *cán zǐ*
Eggs of Bombyx mori

Translator's note:
Common Name: Silkworm eggs.
Family: Silkworm family (Bombycidae).
More commonly called 原蠶子 *yuán cán zǐ*.
《中藥大辭典》#2776.

柴胡 *chái hú*
Root of Bupleurum chinense
Vol. 1, line 31 Highest Grade

味苦，平，無毒。主心腹，去腸胃中結氣，飲食
積聚，寒熱邪氣，推陳致新。久服，輕身、明
目、益精。

Flavor: Bitter
Nature: Neutral
Toxicity: Non-toxic
Alt. names: 地熏

Actions and Indications:
Indicated for the heart and abdomen.
Removes bound *qì* in the intestines and stomach, ac-
cumulations and gatherings of food and drink, and evil
qì of cold and heat.
Pushes out the old to institute the new.

Additional Information:
Taken over a long time, it lightens the body, brightens
the eyes, and boosts essence.

Translator's note:
Common Name: Bupleurum root.
Family: Carrot (Apiaceae).
Other species used: Bupleurum scorzonerifolium and
several related species.

《中藥大辭典》#2422.

蟬殼 *chán ké*
Moulted shell of Cryptotympana atrata
Vol. 2, line 93 Middle Grade

In the *Shén Nóng Běn Cǎo Jīng*, under the entry for
柞蟬.

味咸，寒，無毒。主小儿惊癎、夜啼，癲病，寒
熱。生楊柳上。

Flavor: Salty
Nature: Cold
Toxicity: Non-toxic
Alt. names: n/a

Actions and Indications:
Indicated for small children's fright epilepsy, crying at
night, withdrawal disease, and [aversion to] cold and
heat [effusion].

Additional Information:
Lives in the canopy of willows.

Translator's note:
Common Name: Cicada moulting.
Family: Cicada (Cicadidae).
《中藥大辭典》#5253, where it is listed as 蟬蛻 *chán
tuì*.

菖蒲 *chāng pú*
Rhizome of Acorus gramineus
Vol. 1, line 19 Highest Grade

味辛，溫，無毒。主風寒濕痹，咳逆上氣，開心
孔，補五臟，通九竅，明耳目，出聲音。久服，
輕身、不忘、不迷或，延年。生池澤。

Flavor: Acrid
Nature: Warm
Toxicity: Non-toxic
Alt. names: 昌陽

Actions and Indications:
Indicated for wind-cold-damp impediment and cough
with counterflow ascent of *qì*.
Opens the holes of the heart, supplements the five
viscera, frees the nine orifices, brightens the ears and
eyes, and makes [mutes] emit sound.

Additional Information:
Taken over a long time, it lightens the body, prevents
forgetfulness and confusion, and extends the years.

Grows in ponds and marshes.

Translator's note:
Common Name: Acorus rhizome.
Family: Arum (Araceae).
Sweet flag. Most often called 石菖蒲 *shí chāng pǔ*.
《中藥大辭典》#1281.

常山 *cháng shān*
Root of Dichroa febrifuga
Vol. 3, line 26 Lowest Grade

味苦，寒，有毒。主傷寒，寒熱，發溫瘧，鬼毒，胸中痰結，吐逆。生川谷。

Flavor: Bitter
Nature: Cold
Toxicity: Toxic
Alt. names: 玄草

Actions and Indications:
Indicated for cold damage with [aversion to] cold and heat [effusion], outbreaks of warm malaria, ghost toxin, phlegm bind in the chest, and counterflow vomiting.

Additional Information:
Grows in valleys with streams.

Translator's note:
Common Name: Dichroa root.
Family: Hydrangea family (Hydrangeaceae). See also the entry below on 蜀漆 *shǔ qī*, which refers to the foliage of the same plant.
《中藥大辭典》#3282.

車釭脂 *chē gōng zhī*
Cart axle grease

Translator's note:
In the *Qiān Jīn Fāng*, more often called 車軸脂 *chē zhóu zhī*. See that entry below.

車前子 *chē qián zǐ*
Seed of Plantago asiatica
Vol. 1, line 34 Highest Grade

味甘，寒，無毒。主氣癃，止痛，利水道小便，除濕痺。久服，輕身、耐老。生平澤，丘陵阪道中。

Flavor: Sweet
Nature: Cold
Toxicity: Non-toxic
Alt. names: 當道

Actions and Indications:
Indicated for *qì* dribbling urinary block.
Relieves pain, disinhibits urine in the water ways, and eliminates damp impediment.

Additional Information:
Taken over a long time, it lightens the body and allows the person to endure aging.
Grows in flatlandss and marshes, on hills, and on sloped pathways.

Translator's note:
Common Name: Plantago seed.
Family: Plantain (Plantagonaciae).
Other species used: Plantago depressa.
《中藥大辭典》#1817.

車軸脂 *chē zhóu zhī*
Cart axle grease

Translator's note:
The oil used to grease the metal parts in the axle. See 《本草綱目》38:1430, where it is listed as 車脂 *chē zhī* (cart grease). Also called 車釭脂 *chē gōng zhī*. Not listed in the *Zhōng Yào Dà Cí Diǎn*.

陳廩米 *chén lǐn mǐ*
Seed of Oryza sativa

Translator's note:
Common Name: Old rice.
Family: True Grass (Poaceae).
This is common household rice (粳米 *jīng mǐ*) that has been stored for several years. See entry below on 粳米 *jīng mǐ*.
《中藥大辭典》# 3649, where it is listed as 陳倉米 *chén cāng mǐ*.

陳麴 *chén qū*
Old leaven

Translator's note:
Common Name: Medicated leaven.
More commonly called 神麴 *shén qū* (spirit leaven), it is a leavened preparation made from wheat flour, bran,

and various herbs like 杏仁 *xìng rén* (Dried seed of Prunus armeniaca), 青蒿 *qīng hāo* (Foliage of Artemisiae Apiacceae), 蒼耳 *cāng ěr* (Fruit of Xanthium), and 赤小豆 *chì xiǎo dòu* (Fruit of Phaseolus calcaratus). 《中藥大辭典》#3007, which includes two detailed recipes. For the significance of the name, see the entry below on 神麴 *shén qū*.

秤錘 *chèng zhōng*
Steelyard weight

Translator's note:
As a medicinal ingredient, it is heated until glowing red and tempered in liquor, which is then ingested. Various iron implements are used in this way in gynecological prescriptions, most commonly for treating childbirth complications such as breech presentation, stalled labor, or retained placenta. In the *Běn Cǎo Gāng Mù*, they are conflated into the category of "Various Iron Implements" (諸鐵器 *zhū tiě qì*, see 《本草綱目》 8:143).
Not listed in the *Zhōng Yào Dà Cí Diǎn*.

赤芍 *chì sháo*
Root of Paeonia rubra

Translator's note:
Common Name: Red peony root.
Family: Buttercup (Ranunculaceae).
Other species used: Paeonia albiflora Pall. var. Trichocarpa, P. obovata, or P. veitchii.
It needs to be distinguished from the related species 牡丹 *mǔ dān*, moutan (P. suffruticosa, P. officinalis or P. fruticosa), and 白芍 *bái sháo*, white peony (P. albiflora and P. lactiflora, which is also called 芍藥 *sháo yào*). 《中藥大辭典》#1799.

赤石脂 *chì shí zhī*
Halloysite

Translator's note:
《中藥大辭典》#1796.

赤小豆 *chì xiǎo dòu*
Fruit of Phaseolus calcaratus

Translator's note:
Common Name: Azuki bean, rice bean.
Family: Pea family (Fabaceae).
Other species used: Phaseolus angularis (sometimes called Vigna angularis). For more information and the entry in the *Shén Nóng Běn Cǎo Jīng* on beans in general, see entry below on 大豆黃卷 *dà dòu huáng juǎn*.
《中藥大辭典》#1795.

楮實子 *chǔ shí zǐ*
Fruit of Broussonetia papyrifera

Translator's note:
Common Name: Paper mulberry fruit.
Family: Mulberry family (Moraceae).
According to the *Zhōng Yào Dà Cí Diǎn*, this drug is called 穀子 *gǔ zǐ* elsewhere in the *Qiān Jīn Fāng*.
《中藥大辭典》#4235.

川芎 *chuān xiōng*
see *xiōng qióng* 芎藭

炊蔽 *chuī bì*
Steaming basket

Translator's note:
Not listed in the *Zhōng Yào Dà Cí Diǎn* or *Běn Cǎo Gāng Mù*. The term refers to a woven screen made from bamboo or rushes that is used for steaming food. The *Běn Cǎo Gāng Mù* does have an entry for 炊單布 *chuī dān bù* (cloth used for steaming food), in which Lǐ Shí-Zhēn explains the rationale behind its medicinal use: A cloth that has been used for steaming food for a long time has absorbed the *qì* emitted by the hot liquids. Therefore it can be used to draw out the "toxin" of hot liquids (such as in burns from steam). See 《本草綱目》 38:1439.

醇酒 *chún jiǔ*
Pure grain spirit

Translator's note:
According to a commentary in the *Hàn Shū* 漢書, this refers to "undiluted, concentrated liquor" (cited in 楊吉成《中國飲食辭典》 p. 624).
Not listed in the *Zhōng Yào Dà Cí Diǎn* or *Běn Cǎo Gāng Mù.*

雌黃 *cī huáng*
Orpiment
Vol. 2, line 3 Middle Grade

味辛，平，有毒。主惡創，頭禿，痂疥，殺毒
蟲、虱，身痒，邪氣、諸毒。煉之。久服，輕
身、增年、不老。生山谷。

Flavor: Acrid
Nature: Neutral
Toxicity: Toxic
Alt. names: n/a

Actions and Indications:
Indicated for malign sores and for balding and scabbing of the head.
Kills toxic worms, lice, generalized itch, evil *qì*, and all toxins.

Additional Information:
Concentrate it.
Taken for a long time, it lightens the body, increases the years, and prevents aging.
Grows in mountain valleys.

Translator's note:
A transparent yellow mineral that is extremely toxic. It usually appears together with another arsenic sulfide, realgar (雄黃 *xióng huáng*), which is originally of a deep ruby-red color. The Chinese names, lit. "female yellow" and "male yellow" stem from the fact that they were believed to originate on the shady and sunny side of the mountains. According to the *Běn Cǎo Gāng Mù*, "With insufficient *yáng qì*, orpiment is formed; with sufficient *yáng qì*, realgar." See 《本草綱目》9:165.
《中藥大辭典》#4403.

雌雞肝 *cī jī gān*
Liver of female Gallus gallus domesticus

Translator's note:
Common Name: Hen liver

《中藥大辭典》#5549 concerns the medicinal uses of chicken liver (雞肝 *jī gān*). For more information see the entry on 雄雞 *xióng jī* (Complete body of male Gallus gallus domesticus) below, which includes a translation of the *Shén Nóng Běn Cǎo Jīng* entry.

磁石 *cí shí*
Loadstone
Vol. 2, line 6 Middle Grade

味辛，寒，無毒。主周痹風濕，肢節中痛，不可
持物，洒洒酸疼，除大熱煩滿，及耳聾。生川谷
及山陰，有鐵處，則生其陽。

Flavor: Acrid
Nature: Cold
Toxicity: Non-toxic
Alt. names: 元石, 玄石

Actions and Indications:
Indicated for generalized impediment from wind and dampness, pain in the joints of the limbs to the point of being unable to hold things, and shivering with soreness and pain.
Eliminates great heat with vexation and fullness, and [treats] deafness.

Additional Information:
Grows in valleys with streams on the shady side of mountains.
In locations with iron, it is formed on the sunny side [of the mountain].

Translator's note:
Common Name: Magnetite or magnetic iron ore.
《中藥大辭典》#4731.

蔥白 *cōng bái*
Stalk of Allium fistulosum
Vol. 2, line 111 Middle Grade

In the *Shén Nóng Běn Cǎo Jīng*, under the entry for 蔥實.

味辛，溫，無毒。主明目，補中不足。其莖可作
湯，主傷寒寒熱，出汗，中風面目腫。生平澤。

Flavor: Acrid
Nature: Warm
Toxicity: Non-toxic
Alt. names: n/a

Actions and Indications:
Indicated for brightening the eyes and supplementing

insufficiencies in the center.

Additional Information:
The stalk can be prepared as a decoction and is indicated for cold damage with [aversion to] cold and heat [effusion], sweating, and wind strike with swelling in the face and eyes.
Grows in flatlandss and marshes.

Translator's note:
Common Name: Scallion white.
Family: Lily (Liliaceae).
Aalso known as Japanese bunching onion.
《中藥大辭典》#4337.

菘蓉 *cōng róng*
Stalk of Cistanche salsa

Translator's note:
Common Name: Cistanche stalk.
Family: Broomrape (Orobanchaceae).
Other species used: Cistanche deserticola, or C. ambigua. For more information and a translation of the relevant passage from the *Shén Nóng Běn Cǎo Jīng*, see the entry below on 肉菘蓉 *ròu cōng róng*, a more common name for this medicinal.
《中藥大辭典》#1583.

醋 *cù*
Vinegar

Translator's note:
Made from rice, wheat, sorghum, liquor, or liquor dregs.
《中藥大辭典》#4812.

酢漿水 *cù jiāng shuǐ*
Fermented millet drink

Translator's note:
This is the literal translation of this term, which is not attested elsewhere as a medicinal ingredient. See the entry on 漿 *jiāng* (Sour millet water) below. Depending on context, it could also be related to the medicinal herb 酢漿草 *cù jiāng cǎo* (entire plant of Oxalis corniculata (creeping oxalis) in the Wood Sorrel family), which was already recorded in *Táng* materia medica literature (《本草綱目》20:702,《中藥大辭典》#4003).

大豆黃卷 *dà dòu huáng juǎn*
Sprouted seed of Glycine max
Vol. 2, line 107 Middle Grade

味甘，平，無毒。主濕痹，筋攣，膝痛。生大豆塗癰腫，煮汁飲，殺鬼毒，止痛。赤小豆 主下水，排癰腫膿血。生平澤。

Flavor: Sweet
Nature: Neutral
Toxicity: Non-toxic
Alt. names: n/a

Actions and Indications:
Indicated for damp impediment, hypertonicity of the sinews, and knee pain.

Additional Information:
Fresh soybean can be spread on welling-abscess swelling. Boiled, the juice can be drunk to kill ghost toxin and relieve pain.
Aduki bean is indicated for precipitating water and expelling pus and blood from welling-abscess swellings.
Grows in flatlandss and marshes.

Translator's note:
Common Name: Dried soybean sprouts.
Family: Pea family (Fabaceae).
大豆黃卷 *Dà dòu huáng juǎn* is prepared by first being sundried, then simmered with 淡竹葉 *dàn zhú yè* (Leaves of Lopatherum gracile) and 燈心草 *dēng xīn cǎo* (Pith of Junci Medulla) until the fluid has evaporated, then sun-dried again.
《中藥大辭典》#0253.

大黃 *dà huáng*
Root of Rheum palmatum
Vol. 3, line 16 Lowest Grade

味苦，寒，無毒。主下瘀血、血閉寒熱，破症瘕積聚，留飲，宿食，蕩滌腸胃，推陳致新，通利水穀，調中化食，安和五臟。生山谷。

Flavor: Bitter
Nature: Cold
Toxicity: Non-toxic
Alt. names: n/a

Actions and Indications:
Indicated for precipitating static blood, blocked blood with [aversion to] cold and heat [effusion], and for breaking up concretions and conglomerations, accumulations and gatherings, lodged rheum, and abiding food.
Flushes the intestines and stomach, removes the old and institutes the new, disinhibits water and grain, regulates the center and transforms food, and quiets

and harmonizes the five viscera.

Additional Information:
Grows in mountain valleys.

Translator's note:
Common Name: Rhubarb root
Family: Knotweed family (Polygonaceae).
Other species used: Rheum tanguticum, or R. officinale.
《中藥大辭典》 #0197.

大薊根 *dà jì gēn*
Root of Cirsium japonicum

Translator's note:
Common Name: Japanese thistle root.
Family: Aster (Asteraceae).
Sometimes abbreviated as 薊根 *jì gēn*.
《中藥大辭典》 #0200.

大麻仁 *dà má rén*
Seed of Cannabis sativa

Translator's note:
Common Name: Cannabis fruit.
Family: Hemp (Cannabaceae).
Also called 火麻仁 *huǒ má rén*.
《中藥大辭典》 #0873.

大麥 *dà mài*
Seed of Hordeum vulgare

Translator's note:
Common Name: Barley.
Family: Grass family (Poaceae).
《中藥大辭典》 #0194.

大麥麴 *dà mài qū*
Barley leaven

Translator's note:
Not listed in the *Zhōng Yào Dà Cí Diǎn* or *Běn Cǎo Gāng Mù*, but it is most likely a variety of 陳麴 *chén*

qū (Medicated leaven) that is made with barley rather than wheat. See the entry above on 陳麴 *chén qū*.

大青 *dà qīng*
Indigo-colored foliage of Isatis tinctoria

Translator's note:
Common Name: Isatis leaf.
Family: Mustard (Brassicaceae), Verbena (Verbenacea), Knotweed (Polygonaceae), or Acanthus (Acanthaceae).
Other species used: Isatis indigotica, Clerodendron cyrtophyllum (glory-bowers), Polygonum tinctorium (dyer's knotweed), and Baphicacanthus cusia (Strobilanthes flaccidifolia or Assam indigo).
Note that 大青 *dà qīng* is sometimes erroneously referred to in English as "indigo," which is the common English name for a variety of species of Indigofera in the Pea family. None of these are used for this medicinal. In addition, 大青 *dà qīng*, more properly called 大青葉 *dà qīng yè*, needs to be distinguished from 大青草 *dà qīng cǎo* (Hygrophila salicifolia, willow-leafed hygrophila of the Acanthus family, 《中藥大辭典》 #0212).
《中藥大辭典》 #0213.

大棗 *dà zǎo*
Mature fruit of Ziziphus jujuba
Vol. 1, line 132 Highest Grade

味甘，平，無毒。主心腹邪氣，安中養脾，助十二經，平胃氣，通九竅，補少氣、少津液、身中不足，大惊，四肢重，和百藥。久服，輕身、長年。葉覆麻黃，能令出汗。生平澤。

Flavor: Sweet
Nature: Neutral
Toxicity: Non-toxic
Alt. names: n/a

Actions and Indications:
Indicated for evil *qì* in the heart and abdomen.
Quiets the center and nourishes the spleen, assists the twelve channels, calms stomach *qì*, frees the nine orifices, supplements shortage of *qì*, shortage of fluids, and insufficiencies in the center of the body, [treats] great fright and heaviness of the four limbs, and harmonizes the hundred medicinals.

Additional Information:
Taken for a long time, it lightens the body and lengthens the years.
The leaves covered with 麻黃 *má huáng* can induce sweating.

Grows in flatlands and marshes.

Translator's note:
Common Name: Jujube.
Family: Buckthorn (Rhamnaceae).
《中藥大辭典》#0196.

代赭 *dài zhě*
Hematite
Vol. 3, line 5 Lowest Grade

味苦，寒，無毒。主鬼注、賊風、蠱毒，殺精物惡鬼，腹中毒，邪氣，女子赤沃漏下。生山谷。

Flavor: Bitter
Nature: Cold
Toxicity: Non-toxic
Alt. names: 须丸

Actions and Indications:
Indicated for ghost infixation, bandit wind, *gǔ* toxin, for killing specters and malign ghosts, for toxin in the abdomen, evil *qì*, and for women's vaginal spotting of red moisture.

Additional Information:
Grows in mountain valleys.

Translator's note:
《中藥大辭典》#0961.

丹沙 *dān shā*
Mercuric sulfide
Vol. 1, line 1 Highest Grade

味甘，微寒，无毒。主身体五脏百病，养精神，安魂魄，益氣，明目，杀精魁邪恶鬼。久服，通神明，不老。能化为汞，生山谷。

Flavor: Sweet
Nature: Slightly cold.
Toxicity: Non-toxic
Alt. names: n/a

Actions and Indications:
Indicated for the hundred diseases in the body and [especially] in the five viscera.
Nourishes the essence spirit, quiets the ethereal and corporeal souls, boosts *qì*, brightens the eyes, kills specters, goblins and evil and malign ghosts.
Taken for a long time, it frees the spirit light and prevents aging.

Additional information:

Can be transformed into mercury.
Grows in mountain valleys.

Translator's note:
Common Name: Cinnabar.
More commonly called 朱砂 *zhū shā*.
《中藥大辭典》#1435.

丹參 *dān shēn*
Root of Salvia miltiorrhiza
Vol. 1, line 68 Highest Grade

味苦，微寒，無毒。主心腹邪氣，腸鳴幽幽如走水，寒熱積聚，破症除瘕，止煩滿，益氣。生川谷。

Flavor: Bitter
Nature: Slightly cold
Toxicity: Non-toxic
Alt. names: 卻蟬草

Actions and Indications:
Indicated for evil *qì* in the heart and abdomen, subtle rumbling in the intestines like running water, and [aversion to] cold and heat [effusion] with accumulations and gatherings.
Breaks concretions and eliminates conglomerations.
Relieves vexation and fullness and boosts the *qì*.

Additional Information:
Grows in valleys with streams.

Translator's note:
Common Name: Salvia root.
Family: Mint (Lamiaceae).
Other species used: Salvia przewalskii or S. yunnanensis.
《中藥大辭典》#0594.

淡竹 *dàn zhú*
Lopatherum gracile

Translator's note:
Common Name: Bland bamboo.
Family: Grass (Poaceae).
Other species used: Phyllostachys or Lophatherum. In early literature, this term was used to refer to different genera of bamboo. The leaves (淡竹葉 *dàn zhú yè*), roots (淡竹根 *dàn zhú gēn*), sap (淡竹瀝 *dàn zhú lì*), and shavings (淡竹茹 *dàn zhú rú*) are used medicinally. For a description of the varieties of bamboo, see the entry below on 竹 *zhú*. In contemporary clinical literature, 淡竹葉 *dàn zhú yè* is identified as Lopatherum gracile (see 《中藥大辭典》#3360). While

Lophatherum and Phyllostachys are often confused in clinical practice, Sūn Sī-Miǎo differentiates between the two and uses 淡竹葉 dàn zhú yè in close proximity to 甘竹葉 gān zhú yè (sweet bamboo leaves) as well as to 淡竹根 dàn zhú gēn and 甘竹根 gān zhú gēn (see for example several prescriptions in the second chapter of volume 3 (p. 258) on "vacuity vexation." The Běn Cǎo Gāng Mù describes 淡竹 dàn zhú as either a synonym for or close relative of 甘竹 gān zhú and 苦竹 kǔ zhú (bitter bamboo). See 《本草綱目》 37:1343. I translate these terms literally to reflect most closely the intention —and confusion— of the materia medica literature during Sūn Sī-Miǎo's time. See the entry below on 竹 zhú for a translation of the relevant passage on bamboo from the Shén Nóng Běn Cǎo Jīng. 《中藥大辭典》 #1471 is an entry on 竹茹 zhú rú, which simply equates 甘竹 gān zhú and 淡竹 dàn zhú.

當歸 dāng guī
Root of Angelica polimorpha
Vol. 2, line 20 Middle Grade

味甘，溫，無毒。主咳逆上氣，溫瘧、寒熱洒洒在皮膚中，婦人漏下，絕子，諸惡創瘍、金創。煮飲之。生川谷。

Flavor: Sweet
Nature: Warm
Toxicity: Non-toxic
Alt. names: 干歸

Actions and Indications:
Indicated for cough with counterflow and ascent of qì, warm malaria, [aversion to] cold and heat [effusion] with shivering inside the skin, for women's vaginal spotting and interruption of childbearing, for all malign wounds and sores, and for incised wounds.

Additional Information:
Boil and then drink it.
Grows in valleys with streams.

Translator's note:
Common Name: Chinese angelica root.
Family: Carrot (Apiaceae).
This herb is commonly sold under the name don quai in the United States. Note that it needs to be distinguished from a related species of angelica, namely 白芷 bái zhǐ (Root of Angelica dahurica), which has different medicinal properties.
《中藥大辭典》 #4259.

稻 dào
Seed of Oryza sativa

Translator's note:
Common Name: Glutinous rice.
Family: Grass (Poaceae).
Now used as a general term for rice, including both glutinous rice (糯米 nuò mǐ) and non-glutinous rice (粳米 jīng mǐ). Until the Sòng dynasty, 稻 dào referred specifically to glutinous rice, and was only afterwards used also for the non-glutinous variety (楊吉成，編者《中國飲食辭典》p. 386).

地膚子 dì fū zǐ
Fruit of Kochia scoparia
Vol. 1, line 75 Highest Grade

味苦，寒，無毒。主膀胱熱，利小便，補中，益精氣。久服，耳目聰明、輕身、耐老。生平澤及田野。

Flavor: Bitter
Nature: Cold
Toxicity: Non-toxic
Alt. names: 地葵

Actions and Indications:
Indicated for heat in the bladder.
Disinhibits urine, supplements the center, and boosts essential qì.

Additional Information:
Taken over a long time, it sharpens the ears and eyes, lightens the body, and allows the person to endure aging.
Grows in flatlands and marshes and open fields.

Translator's note:
Common Name: Kochia /summer cypress fruit.
Family: Amaranth (Amaranthaceae).
In the South and East, the fruit of goosefoot (Chenopodium album) may be substituted. It is also called 地麥 dì mài.
《中藥大辭典》 #1403.

地骨皮 dì gǔ pí
Bark of the root of Lycium chinensis
Vol. 1, line 96 Highest Grade

味苦，寒，無毒。主五內邪氣，熱中，消渴，周痺。久服，堅筋骨，輕身，不老。生平澤。

Flavor: Bitter

Nature: Cold
Toxicity: Non-toxic
Alt. names: 杞根, 地骨, 枸忌, 地輔

Actions and Indications:
Indicated for evil *qì* inside the five viscera, heat in the center, dispersion thirst, and generalized impediment.

Additional Information:
Taken for a long time, it hardens the sinews and bones, lightens the body, and prevents aging.
Grows in flatlands and marshes.

Translator's note:
Common Name: Lycium bark.
Family: Nightshade (Solanaceae).
Other species used: Lycium barbaritum (Chinese wolfsberry or matrimony vine, also called 枸杞根 *gǒu qǐ gēn*). The most frequently used part of this plant is the fruit, called 枸杞子 *gǒu qǐ zǐ* (《中藥大辭典》#2369).
For the bark of the root, see 《中藥大辭典》#1388.

地黃 *dì huáng*
Root of Rehmannia glutinosa

Translator's note:
Common Name: Rehmannia root.
Family: Figwort (Scrophulariaceae).
It is used fresh (生 *shēng*), cooked (熟 *shú*), or dried (乾 *gān*). See the entry below on 乾地黃 *gān dì huáng* for a translation of the *Shén Nóng Běn Cǎo Jīng* entry on the dried root.
《中藥大辭典》#3221.

地麥 *dì mài*
Fruit of Kochia scoparia

Translator's note:
Common Name: Kochia /summer cypress fruit.
Family: Amaranth (Amaranthaceae).
In the South and East, goosefoot (Chenopodium album) fruit may be substituted. More commonly called 地膚子 *dì fū zǐ*. See entry on that term above for the translation of the *Shén Nóng Běn Cǎo Jīng* entry.
《中藥大辭典》#1403

地榆 *dì yú*
Root of Sanguisorba officinalis
Vol. 2, line 49 Middle Grade

味苦，微寒，無毒。主婦人乳痙痛，七傷、帶下病，止痛，除惡肉，止汗，消酒，明目，療金創。生山谷。

Flavor: Bitter
Nature: Slightly cold
Toxicity: Non-toxic
Alt. names: n/a

Actions and Indications:
Indicated for women's spasms and pain in the breasts, for the seven damages and vaginal discharge disease.
Relieves pain, eliminates malign flesh, checks sweating, disperses liquor, brightens the eyes, and heals incised wounds.

Additional Information:
Grows in mountain valleys.

Translator's note:
Common Name: Sanguisorba root.
Family: Rose (Rosaceae).
《中藥大辭典》#1364.

丁香 *dīng xiāng*
Flower bud of Syzygium aromaticum

Translator's note:
Common Name: Clove.
Family: Myrtle (Myrtaceae).
Other species used: Eugenia aromatica, Caryophyllus aromaticus.
《中藥大辭典》#0020.

冬瓜練 *dōng guā liàn*
Pulp of Benincasa hispida

Translator's note:
Common Name: Wax gourd flesh.
Family: Gourd (Cucurbitaceae)
Now commonly called 冬瓜瓤 *dōng guā ráng*.
《中藥大辭典》#0967.

東流水 *dōng liú shuǐ*
Water from an east-flowing source

Translator's note:
According to the *Běn Cǎo Gāng Mù*, it is similar in action to 千里水 *qiān lǐ shuǐ* (thousand-mile water) in being "suitable for cleansing away evil and filth; when preparing the various medicinal decoctions, it will restrain and exorcise spirits and ghosts." It shares the characteristics of all types of 流水 *liú shuǐ* (running water) to "move on the outside, but have a still nature, and to be of a soft consistency, but hard *qì*." See 《本草綱目》 5:14 for 流水.
Not listed in 《中藥大辭典》.

東門邊木 *dōng mén biān mù*
Wood from the side of the eastern gate

Translator's note:
Not listed in the *Zhōng Yào Dà Cí Diǎn* or *Běn Cǎo Gāng Mù*. The *Běn Cǎo Gāng Mù* does, however, contain an entry on 東壁土 *dōng bì tǔ* (dirt from the eastern wall): According to Kòu Zōng-Shì's 寇宗奭 commentary, the eastern direction ensures that the "dirt has first been baked by the true fire of the sun. It is therefore indicated for the treatment of seasonal epidemics. Use dirt from an east-facing wall rather than a south-facing wall since the *qì* of the newly emerging lesser fire [i.e., the weaker morning sun] is strong, but the *qì* of the strong fire at noon is weak." See 《本草綱目》 7:306.

東門上雄雞頭
dōng mén shàng xióng jī tóu
Head of a male Gallus gallus domesticus from above the eastern gate

Translator's note:
Common Name: Head of a rooster from above the eastern gate.
Not listed in the *Zhōng Yào Dà Cí Diǎn* or *Běn Cǎo Gāng Mù*. For the magical significance of the eastern direction, see the entry above on 東門邊木 *dōng mén biān mù* (Wood from the side of the eastern gate).

豆豉 *dòu chǐ*
Preparation of Glycine max

Translator's note:
Common Name: Fermented soybean.
Family: Pea (Fabaceae).
Soybeans are most commonly simmered in an infusion of 桑葉 *sāng yè* (Leaf of Mori) and 青蒿 *qīng hāo* (Foliage of Artemisiae Apiacceae) until evaporated, then steamed, fermented, and finally sun-dried. Depending on the intended effect, other herbs can be substituted. 《中藥大辭典》 #3361, where it is listed as 淡豆豉 *dàn dòu chǐ*.

獨活 *dú huó*
Root and rhizome of Angelica pubescens
Vol. 1, line 33 Highest Grade

味苦，平，無毒。主風寒所擊，金瘡，止痛，貫豚，癇，痓，女子疝瘕。久服，輕身、耐老。生川谷。

Flavor: Bitter
Nature: Neutral
Toxicity: Non-toxic
Alt. names: 羌活，羌青，護羌使

Actions and Indications:
Indicated for attacks by wind and cold, and incised wounds.
Relieves pain, [and treats] running piglet, epilepsy, tetany, and women's mounting conglomerations.

Additional Information:
Taken over a long time, it lightens the body and allows the person to endure aging.
Grows in valleys with streams.

Translator's note:
Common Name: Pubescent angelica root and rhizome.
Family: Parsley (Apiaceae) or Ivy (Araliaceae).
Other species used: Angelica porphyrocaulis, or A. dahurica (which is more properly called 白芷 *bái zhǐ*), Heracleum hemsleyanum, H. lanatum (cow parsnip), or of Aralia cordata (wild sasparilla).
《中藥大辭典》 #4896.

杜蘅 *dù héng*
Rhizome and root, or whole plant of Asarum forbesii
Vol. 1, line 78 Highest Grade

In the *Shén Nóng Běn Cǎo Jīng*, under the entry for 杜若.

味辛，微溫，無毒。主胸脅下逆氣，溫中，風入腦戶，頭腫痛，多涕淚出。久服，益精、明目、輕身。生川澤。

Flavor: Acrid
Nature: Slightly warm
Toxicity: Non-toxic
Alt. names: 杜衡

Actions and Indications:
Indicated for counterflow *qì* below the chest and rib-side, for warming the center, for wind entering the gate of the brain, swelling and pain in the head, and for increased snivel and tearing.

Additional Information:
Taken for a long time, it boosts essence, brightens the eyes, and lightens the body.
Grows in streams and marshes.

Translator's note:
Common Name: Forbes' asarum.
Family: Birthwort (Aristolochiaceae).
Closely related to 細辛 *xì xīn* (Asarum heteropoides and several other genera of asarum, sometimes called Chinese wild ginger). 杜蘅 *dù héng* is also called 南細辛 *nán xì xīn* (Southern asarum), 馬蹄細辛 *mǎ tí xì xīn* (horsehoof asarum), or 土細辛 *tǔ xì xīn* (local asarum).
《中藥大辭典》#1696.

杜仲 *dù zhòng*
Bark of Eucommia ulmoidis
Vol. 1, line 107 Highest Grade

味辛，平，無毒。主腰脊痛，補中，益精氣，堅筋骨，強志，除陰下痒濕，小便餘瀝。久服，輕身、耐老。生山谷。

Flavor: Acrid
Nature: Neutral
Toxicity: Non-toxic
Alt. names: 思仙

Actions and Indications:
Indicated for pain in the lumbus and spine.
Supplements the center, boosts essential *qì*, hardens the sinews and bones, strengthens the will, and eliminates itching and dampness below the genitals and

residual trickling of urine.

Additional Information:
Taken for a long time, it lightens the body and allows the person to endure aging.
Grows in mountain valleys.

Translator's note:
Common Name: Eucommia bark.
Family: Eucommia (Eucommiaceae).
《中藥大辭典》#1695.

阿膠 *ē jiāo*
Gelatinous glue produced from Equus asinus
Vol. 1, line 118 Highest Grade

味甘，平，無毒。主心腹內崩，勞极，洒洒如瘧狀，腰腹痛，四肢酸疼，女子下血，安胎。久服，輕身、益氣。

Flavor: Sweet
Nature: Neutral
Toxicity: Non-toxic
Alt. names: 傅致膠

Actions and Indications:
Indicated for flooding inside the heart or abdomen, taxation extreme, shivering like in malaria, lumbar and abdominal pain, soreness and pain in the four limbs, and women's vaginal bleeding.
Quiets the fetus.

Additional Information:
Taken for a long time, it lightens the body and boosts *qì*.

Translator's note:
Common name: Ass hide glue.
《中藥大辭典》#2225.

礬石 *fán shí*
Alum
Vol. 1, line 5 Highest Grade

味酸，寒，無毒。主寒熱泄利，白沃陰蝕，惡創，目痛，堅筋骨齒。煉餌服之，輕身、不老、增年。生山谷。

Flavor: Sour
Nature: Cold
Toxicity: Non-toxic
Alt. names: 羽涅

Actions and Indications:
Indicated for [aversion to] cold and heat [effusion], diarrhea, white foam [i.e. a type of anal discharge] and genital erosion, malign wounds, and eye pain.
Hardens the sinews, bones, and teeth.

Additional Information:
When taken as a concentrated alchemical preparation, it lightens the body, prevents aging, and increases the years.
Grows in mountain valleys.

Translator's note:
More commonly referred to as 白礬 *bái fán* or 明礬 *míng fán*.
《中藥大辭典》#1102.

防風 *fáng fēng*
Root of Ledebouriella divaricata
Vol. 1, line 60 Highest Grade

味甘，溫，無毒。主大風、頭眩痛，惡風，風邪，目盲無所見，風行周身，骨節疼痹，煩滿。久服，輕身。生川澤。

Flavor: Sweet
Nature: Warm
Toxicity: Non-toxic
Alt. names: 銅芸

Actions and Indications:
Indicated for great wind, dizziness and pain in the head, aversion to wind, wind evil, blindness so that the eyes don't see anything, wind moving all around the body, pain and impediment in the bones and joints, and vexation and fullness.

Additional Information:
Taken for a long time, it lightens the body.
Grows in streams and marshes.

Translator's note:
Common Name: Saposhnikovia root.
Family: Carrot (Apiaceae).
Other species used: Ledebouriella seseloides or Saposhnikovia divaricata.
《中藥大辭典》#1825.

防己 *fáng jǐ*
Root of Aristolochia fangchi
Vol. 2, line 52 Middle Grade

味辛，平，無毒。主風寒，溫瘧熱氣，諸癇，除

邪，利大小便，通腠理，利九竅。生川谷。

Flavor: Acrid
Nature: Neutral
Toxicity: Non-toxic
Alt. names: 解離

Actions and Indications:
Indicated for wind-cold, hot *qì* of warm malaria, and all epilepsy.
Eliminates evil, disinhibits urine and stool, frees the interstices, and disinhibits the nine orifices.

Additional Information:
Grows in valleys with streams.

Translator's note:
Common Name: Fángjǐ /birthwort root.
Family: Birthwort (Aristolochiacea).
Other species used: Aristolochia heterophylla (漢中防己 *hàn zhōng fáng jǐ*), Stephania tetranda (漢防己 *hàn fáng jǐ*) or Cocculus trilobus (木防己 *mù fáng jǐ*) of the Moonseed family (Menispermaceae).
Aristolochia fangchi is sometimes referred to in Chinese specifically as 廣防己 *guǎng fáng jǐ*.
《中藥大辭典》#1824.

防葵 *fáng kuí*
fáng kuí
Vol. 1, line 30 Highest Grade

味辛，寒，無毒。主疝瘕腸泄，膀胱熱結，溺不下，咳逆，溫瘧，癲癇，惊邪，狂走。久服，堅骨髓、益氣、輕身。生川谷。

Flavor: Acrid
Nature: Cold
Toxicity: Non-toxic
Alt. names: 梨蓋

Actions and Indications:
Indicated for mounting-conglomeration, intestinal diarrhea, heat bind in the bladder, inability to precipitate urine, cough with counterflow, warm malaria, epilepsy, fright evil, and manic wandering.

Additional Information:
Taken for a long time, it hardens the bones and marrow, boosts *qì*, and lightens the body.
Grows in valleys with streams.

Translator's note:
Common Name: n/a
A plant of unknown identity, it is not listed in the *Zhōng Yào Dà Cí Diǎn*. Most likely, it is a variety of Peucedanum of the Carrot Family (Apiaceae). In the *Běn Cǎo Gāng Mù*, it is listed under poisonous herbs. It is described as resembling 葵花 *kuí huā* (in the shape

of the leaves and stalkes, and resembling 防風 *fáng fēng* (Root of Ledebouriella divaricata) in the taste of the root, hence the name. Regarding the medicinal use of the root, Táo Hóng-Jǐng stated that it was interchangeable with 狼毒 *láng dú* (Root of Stellera chamaejasme) (《本草綱目》 17:532). None of its many synonyms are found in the *Zhōng Yào Dà Cí Diǎn*, except for 利如 *lì rú*, which is there identified as a rare synonym for 桔梗 *jié gěng* (Root of Platycodon grandiflorum) (《中藥大辭典》 #2877). However, this identification seems unlikely since Sūn Sī-Miǎo does refer to that medicinal by the proper name. Paul U. Unschuld also describes it as "identity uncertain" (*A History of Pharmaceutics*, p. 353). Bernard Read, *Chinese Materia Medica,* vol. 5, p. 61, as well as Rev. Stuart, *Chinese Materia Medica* (Shanghai, 1911, 1987 reprint, Taipei p. 315) identify it as Peucedanum japonicum. The *Zhōng Huá Běn Cǎo* 中華本草 (Shanghai, 1999), vol. 5, #5191, lists it as a synonym for 濱海前胡 *bīn hǎi qián hú* ("coastal peucedanum").

蜚蠊 *fěi lián*
Whole body of Blatta orientalis
Vol. 2, line 103 Middle Grade

味咸，寒，有毒。主血瘀、症堅、寒熱，破積聚，喉咽痹，內寒，無子。生川澤及人家屋間。

Flavor: Salty
Nature: Cold
Toxicity: Toxic
Alt. names: n/a

Actions and Indications:
Indicated for blood stasis, concretions and hardenings, and [aversion to] cold and heat [effusion]. Breaks up accumulations and gatherings, and [treats] throat impediment, internal cold, and infertility.

Additional Information:
Lives in streams and marshes and in the roofs of people's houses.

Translator's note:
Common Name: Cockroach.
Family: Cockroach (Blattidae).
This refers to the oriental cockroach, more commonly called 蟑螂 *zhāng láng* in modern Chinese.
《中藥大辭典》 #5153.

夫尿 *fū niào*
Husband's urine

Translator's note:

Not listed in the *Zhōng Yào Dà Cí Diǎn* or *Běn Cǎo Gāng Mù* specifically. However, human urine, especially from young boys under the age of ten, in which case it is usually referred to as 童便 *tóng biàn*, is still used medicinally (《中藥大辭典》 #0060).

夫靴 *fū xuē*
Husband's leather boots

Translator's note:
Not listed in the *Zhōng Yào Dà Cí Diǎn*, but the *Běn Cǎo Gāng Mù* has an entry on leather boots, (《本草綱目》 38:1391).

夫陰毛 *fū yīn máo*
Husband's pubic hair

Translator's note:
Not listed in *Zhōng Yào Dà Cí Diǎn*, but the *Běn Cǎo Gāng Mù* has is an entry on 陰毛 *yīn máo* (pubic hair) (《本草綱目》 52:1886).

茯苓 *fú líng*
Dried fungus of Poria cocos

Translator's note:
Common Name: Poria.
Family: Bracket Fungus (Polyporaceae).
Also known as Indian Bread. For information on root poria and the translation of the *Shén Nóng Běn Cǎo Jīng* entry for that medicinal, see the entry below on 茯神 *fú shén*.
《中藥大辭典》 #3064.

伏龍肝 *fú lóng gān*
Stove earth

Translator's note:
According to Táo Hóng-Jǐng, this refers to "dirt inside the stove beneath pots" (《本草綱目》 7:97). Since its medicinal efficacy is due to the *qì* of fire that it has absorbed, it needs to come from stoves that are at least ten years old. "Crouching Dragon" 伏龍 refers to the stove god who resides inside the stove. This medicinal ingredient is also called 灶中黃土 *zào zhōng*

huáng tǔ (yellow dirt from inside the stove).
《中藥大辭典》#1309.

茯神 *fú shén*
Sclerotium of Poria cocos
Vol. 1, line 98　Highest Grade

味甘，平，無毒。主胸脅逆氣，憂恚，惊邪，恐悸，心下結痛，寒熱，煩滿，咳逆，口焦舌干，利小便。久服，安魂、養神，不飢、延年。生山谷大松下。

Flavor: Sweet
Nature: Neutral
Toxicity: Non-toxic
Alt. names: 茯菟

Actions and Indications:
Indicated for counterflow *qì* in the chest and rib-sides, anxiety and hatred, fright evil and fear palpitations, binding pain below the heart, [aversion to] cold and heat [effusion], vexation and fullness, cough with counterflow, and parched mouth and dry tongue.
Disinhibits urine.

Additional Information:
Taken for a long time, it quiets the ethereal soul, nourishes the spirit, prevents hunger, and extends the years.
Grows in mountain valleys below pine trees.

Translator's note:
Common Name: Root poria.
Family: Bracket Fungus (Polyporaceae).
Sclerotium (i.e., white, hardened core in the center) of Poria cocos. For Poria cocos, see entry above on *fú líng* 茯苓.
《中藥大辭典》#3065.

釜底墨 *fǔ dǐ mò*
Pot soot

Translator's note:
Soot adhering to the bottom of a pan after dry-roasting various herbs.
《中藥大辭典》#3133, where it is listed as 釜臍墨 *fǔ qí mò.*

覆盆子 *fù pén zǐ*
Fruit of Rubus chingii
Vol. 1, line 134　Highest Grade

In the *Shén Nóng Běn Cǎo Jīng*, under the entry for 蓬蘽.

味酸，平，無毒。主安五臟，益精氣，長陰令堅，強志倍力，有子。久服，輕身、不老。生平澤。

Flavor: Sour
Nature: Neutral
Toxicity: Non-toxic
Alt. names: 覆盆

Actions and Indications:
Indicated for quieting the five viscera, boosting essential *qì*, lengthening the penis and making it hard, strengthening the will and doubling strength, and for fertility.

Additional Information:
Taken for a long time, it lightens the body and prevents aging.
Grows in flatlands and marshes.

Translator's note:
Common Name: Rubus berry.
Family: Rose (Rosaceae).
Other species used: Rubus officinalis
《中藥大辭典》#5260.

附子 *fù zǐ*
Lateral root of Aconitum carmichaeli
Vol. 3, line 10　Lowest Grade

味辛，溫，有大毒。主風寒，咳逆邪氣，溫中，金創，破症堅積聚，血瘕，寒濕，痿躄，拘攣，膝痛不能行步。生山谷。

Flavor: Acrid
Nature: Warm
Toxicity: Greatly toxic
Alt. names: 茛

Actions and Indications:
Indicated for wind-cold, counterflow cough with evil *qì*, warming the center, and incised wounds.
Breaks up concretions and hardenings, accumulations and gatherings, blood conglomerations, cold and dampness, crippling wilt, hypertonicity, and pain in the knee and inability to walk.

Additional Information:
Grows in mountain valleys.

Translator's note:
Common Name: Aconite.
Family: Buttercup (Ranunculaceae).
This refers to the processed lateral root of aconite (also called monkshood or wolfsbane in English), which is prepared by soaking it with different substances for different lengths of time. Plants from the Aconitum genus are extremely toxic, particularly in the root. A related species, Aconitum ferox is considered the most poisonous plant in the world (Thomas J. Elpel, *Botany in a Day*, p. 44). The main root of monkshood is used in the drug *wū tóu*.
《中藥大辭典》#0545.

甘草 *gān cǎo*
Root of Glycyrrhiza uralensis
Vol. 1, line 23 Highest Grade

味甘，平，無毒。主五臟六腑寒熱邪氣。堅筋骨，長肌肉，倍力，金創，重𤵺，解毒。久服，輕身、延年。生川谷。

Flavor: Sweet
Nature: Neutral
Toxicity: Non-toxic
Alt. names: 美草，密甘

Actions and Indications:
Indicated for evil *qi* of cold and heat in the five viscera and six bowels.
Hardens the sinews and bones, grows flesh, doubles the strength, treats incised wounds and swellings, and resolves toxin.

Additional Information:
Taken over a long time, it lightens the body and extends the years.
Grows in valleys with streams.

Translator's note:
Common Name: Licorice.
Family: Pea (Fabaceae).
Other species used: Glycyrrhiza glabra, G. kansuensis, or G. inflata.
《中藥大辭典》#1058.

乾地黃 *gān dì huáng*
Dried root of Rehmannia glutinosa
Vol. 1, line 24 Highest Grade

味甘，寒，無毒。主折跌絕筋，傷中。逐血痹，填骨髓，長肌肉。作湯，除寒熱、積聚。除痹。生者尤良。久服，輕身、不老。生川澤。

Flavor: Sweet
Nature: Cold
Toxicity: Non-toxic
Alt. names: 地髓

Actions and Indications:
Indicated for fractures and falls and severed sinews, and damage to the center.
Expels blood impediment, replenishes the bones and marrow, and grows flesh.

Additional Information:
Made into a decoction, it eliminates cold and heat, and accumulations and gatherings. Eliminates impediment.
Used fresh, it is particularly excellent.
Taken over a long time, it lightens the body and prevents aging.
Grows in streams and marshes.

Translator's note:
Common Name: Dried Rehmannia root.
Family: Figwort (Scrophulariaceae).
It is used fresh (生 *shēng*), cooked (熟 *shú*), or dried (乾 *gān*).
《中藥大辭典》#3221.

干姜 *gān jiāng*
Dried root of Zingiber officinale
Vol. 2, line 15 Middle Grade

味辛，溫，無毒。主胸滿，咳逆上氣，溫中，止血，出汗，逐風，濕痹，腸澼，下利。生者，尤良。味辛，微溫。久服，去臭氣、通神明。生川谷。

Flavor: Acrid
Nature: Warm
Toxicity: Non-toxic
Alt. names: n/a

Actions and Indications:
Indicated for fullness of the chest, cough with counterflow and ascent of *qi*.
Warms the center, stanches bleeding, makes the sweat come out, and expels wind.
[Treats] damp impediment, intestinal afflux, and diarrhea.

Additional Information:
The fresh one is particularly good. Its flavor is acrid and it is slightly warm.
Taken for a long time, it removes bad smells and frees the spirit light.
Grows in valleys with streams.

Translator's note:

Common Name: Dried Ginger.
Family: Ginger (Zingiberaceae).
Ginger is used fresh (生 shēng) or dried (乾 gān).
《中藥大辭典》#1073.

甘皮 gān pí
Bark of Saccharum sinensis

Translator's note:
Common Name: Sugar cane skin (Sweet bark).
Family: Grass (Poaceae).
As this term is not attested in the Shén Nóng Běn Cǎo Jīng, Běn Cǎo Gāng Mù, or Zhōng Yào Dà Cí Diǎn, I translate it literally, and assume that it is a synonym for 甘蔗皮 gān zhè pí.
For that medicinal, see 《中藥大辭典》#1066.

干漆 gān qī
Dried sap of Rhus verniciflua
Vol. 1, line 102 Highest Grade

味辛，溫，無毒。主絕傷，補中，續筋骨，填髓腦，安五臟，五緩六急，風寒濕痹。生漆，去長蟲。久服，輕身、耐老。生川谷。

Flavor: Acrid
Nature: Warm
Toxicity: Non-toxic
Alt. names: n/a

Actions and Indications:
Indicated for damage from severance.
Supplements the center, joins sinews and bones, replenishes the marrow and brain, quiets the five viscera, and [treats] the five types of retardation and six types of hypertonicity, and wind-cold-damp impediment.

Additional Information:
Fresh lacquer removes long worms.
Taken over a long time, it lightens the body and allows the person to endure aging.
Grows in valleys with streams.

Translator's note:
Common Name: Lacquer.
Family: Sumac (Anacardiaceae).
Other species used: Toxicodendron verniciluum
《中藥大辭典》#3218.

甘竹 gān zhú
Phyllostachys

Translator's note:
Common Name: Sweet bamboo.
Family: Grass (Poaceae).
The leaves (甘竹葉 gān zhú yè), roots (甘竹根 gān zhú gēn), sap (甘竹瀝 gān zhú lì), and shavings (甘竹茹 gān zhú rú) are used medicinally. For a description of the varieties of bamboo used medicinally and translation of the relevant passage from the Shén Nóng Běn Cǎo Jīng, see the entry below on zhú 竹 (bamboo). See also the entry above on 淡竹 dàn zhú (sweet bamboo).
《中藥大辭典》#1471 is an entry on 竹茹 zhú rú, which simply equates 甘竹 and 淡竹.

膏 gāo
Lard

Translator's note:
Soft fat from animals without horns, most commonly pigs. According to a Hàn period dictionary, "[Fat from animals] with horns is called 脂 zhī [see entry below]; [fat from animals] without horns is called 膏 gāo" (《說文解字》4:36). Lǐ Zhōng-Wén 李鍾文 has shown that the two terms are used consistently according to this definition in the Mǎ-Wáng-Duī medical material (李鍾文《五十二病方中膏脂類藥物的探討》, cited in Harper, Early Chinese Medical Literature, p. 223, n. 1).
《中藥大辭典》#4969 is an entry on 豬脂膏 zhū zhī gāo (the lard of Sus scrofa domestica).

藁本 gǎo běn
Rhizome and root of Ligusticum sinense
Vol. 2, line 43 Middle Grade

味辛，溫，無毒。主婦人疝瘕，陰中寒腫痛，腹中急，除風頭痛，長肌膚，悅顏色。生山谷。

Flavor: Acrid
Nature: Warm
Toxicity: Non-toxic
Alt. names: 鬼卿, 地新

Actions and Indications:
Indicated for women's mounting-conglomerations, for cold, swelling, and pain inside the genitals, and tension in the abdomen.
Eliminates wind with head ache, makes the skin and flesh grow, and [causes] a joyful complexion.

Additional Information:
Grows in mountain valleys.

Translator's note:
Common Name: Chinese lovage root and rhizome.
Family: Carrot (Apiaceae).
Other species used: Ligusticum jeholense, or L. tenuissimum.
《中藥大辭典》#5357.

葛根 *gé gēn*
Root of Pueraria lobata
Vol. 2, line 17 Middle Grade

味甘，平，無毒。主消渴，身大熱，嘔吐，諸痺，起陰氣，解諸毒。葛谷，主下利十歲以上。生川谷。

Flavor: Sweet
Nature: Neutral
Toxicity: Non-toxic
Alt. names: 雞齊根

Actions and Indications:
Indicated for dispersion thirst, generalized severe fever, vomiting, and all impediments.
Raises *yīn qì* and resolves all toxins.

Additional Information:
The fruit is indicated for diarrhea that has lasted for more than ten years.
Grows in valleys with streams.

Translator's note:
Common Name: Pueraria root.
Family: Pea (Fabaceae).
Other species used: Pueraria thomsanii, P. omeiensis, or P. phaseoloides).
《中藥大辭典》#4321.

葛上亭長 *gé shàng tíng cháng*
Dried body of Epicauta Gorhami

Translator's note:
Common Name: Epicauta.
Family: Blister Beetle (Meloidae).
The medicinally active ingredient is cantharidin, a skin irritant also found in the related species Mylabris and Lytta viesicatoria (commonly called Spanish fly). The substance was a common ingredient in European aphrodisiacs and is also used for wart treatments.
Sometimes, 葛上亭長 *gé shàng tíng cháng* is abbreviated as 亭長 *gé cháng*.
《中藥大辭典》#4328.

弓弩弦 *gōng nǔ xián*
Crossbow string

Translator's note:
Not listed in the *Zhōng Yào Dà Cí Diǎn*. According to Lǐ Shí-Zhēn, it is usually made from silk (《本草綱目》38:1415).

狗脊 *gǒu jǐ*
Rhizome of Cibotium barometz
Vol. 2, line 34 Middle Grade

味苦，平，無毒。主腰背強，關機緩急，周痺寒濕，膝痛。頗利老人。生川谷。

Flavor: Bitter
Nature: Neutral
Toxicity: Non-toxic
Alt. names: 百枝

Actions and Indications:
Indicated for stiffness in the lumbus and back, for slackening and stiffness in the joints, generalized impediment with cold-damp, and pain in the knees. Particularly benefits the elderly.

Additional Information:
Grows in valleys with streams.

Translator's note:
Common Name: Cibotium rhizome/ Scythian lamb rhizome.
Family: Tropical Tree Fern (Cyatheaceae).
《中藥大辭典》#2023.

枸杞 *gǒu qǐ*
Fruit of Lycium chinensis

Translator's note:
Common Name: Lycium, wolfsberry, or matrimony vine berry.
Family: Nightshade (Solanaceae).
Other species used: Lycium barbaritum.
《中藥大辭典》#2369. For the medicinal use of Lycium bark, see the following entry on *gǒu qǐ gēn* 枸杞根.

枸杞根 *gǒu qǐ gēn*
Bark of the root of Lycium chinensis

Translator's note:
Common Name: Lycium, wolfsberry, or matrimony vine root bark.
Family: Nightshade (Solanaceae).
Other species used: Lycium barbaritum.
Also referred to as 地骨皮 *dì gǔ pi* (see entry on that term above). The most frequently used part of this plant is the fruit (see preceding entry on *gǒu qǐ* 枸杞).
《中藥大辭典》#1388, where it is listed as 地骨皮 *dì gǔ pí*.

羖羊角 *gǔ yáng jiǎo*
Horn of the male Capra hircus
Vol. 2, line 83 Middle Grade

味咸，溫，無毒。主青盲，明目，殺疥蟲，止寒泄，辟惡鬼、虎、狼，止驚悸。久服，安心、益氣、輕身。生川谷。

Flavor: Salty
Nature: Warm
Toxicity: Non-toxic
Alt. names: n/a

Actions and Indications:
Indicated for clear-eye blindness.
Brightens the eyes, kills scabs and worms, checks cold diarrhea, repels malign ghosts, tigers, and wolves, and checks fright palpitations.

Additional Information:
Taken for a long time, it quiets the heart, boosts *qi*, and lightens the body.
Lives in valleys with streams.

Translator's note:
Common Name: Sheep's or goat's horn.
Family: Bovid (Bovidae).
Other species used: Ovis aries (domestic sheep).
《中藥大辭典》#3028.

瓜瓣 *guā bàn*
Seed of Benincasa hispida
Vol. 1, line 141 Highest Grade

In the *Shén Nóng Běn Cǎo Jīng*, under the entry for for 瓜子.

味甘，平，無毒。主令人悅澤，好顏色，益氣不飢。久服，輕身、耐老。生平澤。

Flavor: Sweet
Nature: Neutral
Toxicity: Non-toxic
Alt. names: 水芝

Actions and Indications:
Indicated for making people joyful and giving a shiny and beautiful complexion.
Boosts *qi* and prevents hunger.

Additional Information:
Taken for a long time, it lightens the body and allows the person to endure aging.
Grows in flatlands and marshes.

Translator's note:
Common Name: Wax gourd seed.
Family: Gourd (Cucurbitaceae).
《中藥大辭典》#0963, where it is listed as 冬瓜子 *dōng guā zǐ*.

栝蔞根 *guā lóu gēn*
Root of Trichosanthes kirilowii
Vol. 2, line 18 Middle Grade

味苦，寒，無毒。主消渴，身熱，煩滿，大熱，補虛，安中，續絕傷。生川谷及山陰。

Flavor: Bitter
Nature: Cold
Toxicity: Non-toxic
Alt. names: 地樓

Actions and Indications:
Indicated for dispersion thirst, generalized heat, vexation and fullness, and severe heat.
Supplements vacuity, quiets the center, and joins damage from severance.

Additional Information:
Grows in rivers with streams and on the shady side of mountains.

Translator's note:
Common Name: Trichosanthes root.
Family: Gourd (Cucurbitaceae).
Other species used: Trichosanthes hylonoma or T. sinopunctata.
This needs to be distinguished from the closely related 土瓜 *tǔ guā* (T. cucumerina or snake gourd, a term that is sometimes falsely used to refer to 栝蔞 *guā lóu*), which is used medicinally as an abortifacient. For the fruit and plant 栝蔞 *guā lóu* in general, see 《中藥大辭典》#2818. Trichosanthes root is more commonly known in a medicinal context as 天花粉 *tiān huā fěn*. 《中藥大辭典》#0632.

栝樓實 *guā lóu shí*
Fruit of Trichosanthes kirilowii

Translator's note:
Common Name: Trichosanthes fruit.
Family: Gourd (Cucurbitaceae).
See entry above on 栝蔞根 *guā lóu gēn* for the root, translation of the entry from the *Shén Nóng Běn Cǎo Jīng*, and general information.
《中藥大辭典》#2818.

冠纓 *guān yīng*
Cap tassel

Translator's note:
I translate this term literally, as it is not listed in the *Zhōng Yào Dà Cí Diǎn*, *Běn Cǎo Gāng Mù*, or any of the other major materia medica works. Alternatively, it could refer to the comb and wattle of a rooster, which are usually called 冠緌 *guān ruí*. This is, however, not a common medicinal. Based on the context of its occurrence in the *Qiān Jīn Fāng*, where it is charred and where animals are usually prepared by drying but clothing by charring, I prefer a literal reading of this term.

雚蘆 *guàn lú*
Guànlú fungus
Vol. 3, line 31 Lowest Grade

In the *Shén Nóng Běn Cǎo Jīng*, under the entry for 灌菌.

味鹹 ，平 ，有小毒。主心痛，溫中，去長蟲、白癬、蟯蟲、蛇螫毒，症瘕、諸蟲。生東海池澤及渤海。

Flavor: Salty
Nature: Neutral
Toxicity: Slightly toxic

Actions and Indications:
Indicated for heart pain, for warming the center, and for removing long worms, white lichen, pinworm, snake bite toxin, concretions and conglomerations, and all worms.

Additional Information:
Grows in Dōng-Hǎi in ponds and marshes, and in the Bó-Hǎi sea.

Translator's note:
Fungus of unknown identity. It is not found in the

Zhōng Yào Dà Cí Diǎn, but is listed in the *Běn Cǎo Gāng Mù* in the section on "vegetables," subsection "fungi," as 萑菌 *guàn jūn*. It is there described as a type of fungus growing underneath the plant 蘆葦 *lú wěi* (Phragmites communis or common reed).

貫眾 *guàn zhòng*
Rhizome of Aspidium crassirhizoma
Vol. 3, line 36 Lowest Grade

味苦 ，微寒 ，有毒。主腹中邪熱氣 ，諸毒 ，殺三蟲。生山谷。

Flavor: Bitter
Nature: Slightly cold
Toxicity: Toxic
Alt. names: 貫節 ，貫渠 ，百頭 ，虎卷 ，扁符

Actions and Indications:
Indicated for evil heat *qì* in the abdomen, all toxins, and killing the three types of worms.

Additional Information:
Grows in mountain valleys.

Translator's note:
Common Name: Aspidium rhizome.
Family: Wood Fern (Dryopteridaceae), Chain Fern (Polypodiaceae), Osmunda (Osmundaceae).
Other species used: Dryopteris crassirhizoma, also Woodwardia unigemmata (chain fern), Osmunda japonica (royal fern), and Matteuccia struthiopteris (ostrich fern).
《中藥大辭典》#3520.

龜甲 *guī jiǎ*
Shell of Chinemys reevesii
Vol. 1, line 125 Highest Grade

味鹹 ，平 ，無毒。主漏下赤白，破症瘕、瘭疢 ，五痔 、陰蝕 ，濕痺 ，四肢重弱 ，小儿囟不合。久服 ，輕身、不飢。生池澤。

Flavor: Salty
Nature: Neutral
Toxicity: Non-toxic
Alt. names: 神屋

Actions and Indications:
Indicated for vaginal spotting with red or white discharge, for breaking concretions and conglomerations, for malaria, the five types of hemorrhoids, genital erosion, damp impediment, heaviness and weakness of the four limbs, and nonconforming fonta-

nels in small children.

Additional Information:
Taken for a long time, it lightens the body and prevents hunger.
Lives in ponds and marshes.

Translator's note:
Common Name: Tortoise plastron.
Family: Geoemydidae.
This medicinal comes from Reeve's turtle, (syn. Geoclemys), a type of fresh-water turtle. The medicinal ingredient is also called 龜版 *guī bǎn*.
《中藥大辭典》#5088.

鬼箭 *guǐ jiàn*
Branch or plumes of Euonymus alatus
Vol. 2, line 78 Middle Grade

In the *Shén Nóng Běn Cǎo Jīng*, under the entry for 衛矛.

味苦，寒，無毒。主女子崩中下血、腹滿、汗出，除邪，殺鬼毒、蠱注。生山谷。

Flavor: Bitter
Nature: Cold
Toxicity: Non-toxic

Actions and Indications:
Indicated for women's flooding of the center with precipitation of blood, abdominal fullness, and sweating. Eliminates evil and kills ghost toxin and *gǔ* infixation.

Additional Information:
Grows in mountain valleys.

Translator's note:
Common Name: Spindle tree wings.
Family: Staff Vine (Celastraceae).
The plant is also called Winged spindle or burning bush.
《中藥大辭典》#3212.

鬼臼 *guǐ jiù*
Root of Dysosma versipellis
Vol. 3, line 45 Lowest Grade

味辛，溫，有毒。主殺蠱毒、鬼注、精物，辟惡氣不祥，逐邪，解百毒。生山谷。

Flavor: Acrid
Nature: Warm
Toxicity: Toxic

Alt. names: 爵犀，馬目毒公，九臼

Actions and Indications:
Indicated for killing *gǔ* toxin, ghost infixation, and spectral things, for repelling malign *qì* and inauspicious events, for expelling evil, and for resolving the hundred toxins.

Additional Information:
Grows in mountain valleys.

Translator's note:
Common Name: Common dysosma root.
Family: Barberry (Berberidaceae).
《中藥大辭典》#3206.

桂心 *guì xīn*
Shaved inner bark of Cinnamomum cassia

Translator's note:
Common Name: Shaved cinnamon bark.
Family: Laurel (Lauraceae).
《中藥大辭典》#1579, where it is listed as 肉桂 *ròu guì*. More specifically, 桂心 *guì xīn* refers to the inner bark, after the dark outer bark has been shaved off. For a translation from the *Shén Nóng Běn Cǎo Jīng*, see following entry on 桂枝 *guì zhī*.

桂枝 *guì zhī*
Twigs of Cinnamonum cassia
Vol. 1, line 92 Highest Grade

In the *Shén Nóng Běn Cǎo Jīng*, under the entry for 牡桂.

味辛，溫，無毒。主上氣咳逆，結氣，喉痹吐吸。利關節，補中益氣。久服，通神、輕身、不老。生山谷。

Flavor: Acrid
Nature: Warm
Toxicity: Non-toxic
Alt. names: 肉桂

Actions and Indications:
Indicated for ascent of *qì* with cough and counterflow, bound *qì*, and throat impediment during inhalation and exhalation.
Disinhibits the joints, supplements the center, and boosts *qì*.

Additional Information:

Taken over a long time, it frees the spirit, lightens the body, and prevents aging.
Grows in mountain valleys.

Translator's note:
Common Name: Cinnamon twig.
Family: Laurel (Lauraceae).
《中藥大辭典》#2828.

蝦蟆 *há má*
Whole body of Rana limnocharis
Vol. 3, line 80 Lowest Grade

味辛，寒，有毒。主邪氣，破症、堅血、癥腫、陰創。服之，不患熱病。生池澤。

Flavor: Acrid
Nature: Cold
Toxicity: Toxic
Alt. names: n/a

Actions and Indications:
Indicated for evil *qi*, breaking concretions and hardened blood, and for [treating] welling-abscess swelling and genital wounds.

Additional Information:
Taking [this medicinal], you will not be troubled by heat disease.
Lives in ponds and marshes.

Translator's note:
Common Name: Frog.
Family: True Frog (Ranidae).
The source of this medicinal is called rice or bog frog in English.
《中藥大辭典》#4785.

海藻 *hǎi zǎo*
Whole plant of Sargassum fusiforme
Vol. 2, line 50 Middle Grade

味苦，寒，無毒。主癭瘤氣，頸下核，破散結氣、癥腫、症瘕、堅氣，腹中上下鳴，下十二水腫。生東海池澤。

Flavor: Bitter
Nature: Cold
Toxicity: Non-toxic
Alt. names: 落首

Actions and Indications:
Indicated for goiter *qi* and nodes below the neck.
Breaks and dissipates bound *qi*, [treats] welling-

abscess swelling, concretions and conglomerations, hardened *qi*, and rumbling in the middle of and above and below the abdomen, and precipitates the twelve types of water swelling.

Additional Information:
Grows in Dōng-Hǎi in ponds and marshes.

Translator's note:
Common Name: Sargassum.
Family: Sargassum (Sargassaceae).
Other species used: Sargassum pallidum, S. tortile, S. Kjellmanianum, or S. thunbergii, hijiki).
Also called gulfweed or rockweed, it is a free-floating type of brown algae.
《中藥大辭典》#2900.

寒水石 *hán shuǐ shí*
Sodium calcium sulfate
Vol. 2, line 7 Middle Grade

In the *Shén Nóng Běn Cǎo Jīng*, under the entry for 凝水石.

味辛，寒，無毒。主身熱，腹中積聚、邪氣，皮中如火燒，煩滿。水飲之。久服，不飢。生山谷。

Flavor: Acrid
Nature: Cold
Toxicity: Non-toxic
Alt. names: 白水石

Actions and Indications:
Indicated for generalized fever, accumulations and gatherings and evil *qi* in the abdomen, a sensation like fire burning in the skin, and vexation and fullness.

Additional Information:
Drink it in water.
Taken for a long time, it prevents hunger.
Grows in mountain valleys.

Translator's note:
Common Name: Glauberite.
《中藥大辭典》#3776.

恒山 *héng shān*
Root of Dichroa febrifuga

Translator's note:
Common Name: Dichroa root.
Family: Hydrangea (Hydrangeaceae).
More commonly known as 常山 *cháng shān* (see

entry above).
《中藥大辭典》#3282.

A secondary mineral of lead, formed by the chemical action of carbonated water on the mineral galena. More commonly called 鉛粉 *qiān fěn*.
《中藥大辭典》#4389.

厚朴 *hòu pò*
Bark of Magnolia officinalis
Vol. 2, line 69 Middle Grade

味苦，溫，無毒。主中風、傷寒、頭痛、寒熱，惊悸，氣血痹，死肌，去三蟲。

Flavor: Bitter
Nature: Warm
Toxicity: Non-toxic
Alt. names: n/a

Actions and Indications:
Indicated for wind strike, cold damage, head ache, [aversion to] cold and heat [effusion], fright palpitations, *qì* and blood impediment, dead flesh, and removing the three types of worms.

Translator's note:
Common Name: Officinal magnolia bark.
Family: Magnolia (Magnoliaceae).
Other species used: Magnolia biloba.
Note that these are different species of magnolia from the ones used for the medicinal 辛夷 *xīn yí* (flower of magnolia liliflora, see entry for that term below).
《中藥大辭典》#2315.

狐莖 *hú jīng*
Penis of Vulpes vulpes

Translator's note:
Common Name: Fox penis.
Family: Canine (Canidae).
Not listed in the *Zhōng Yào Dà Cí Diǎn*, but in the *Běn Cǎo Gāng Mù* described as one of the parts of the fox that are used in medicine (《本草綱目》51:1827). Indicated for infertiliy, genital sores, swollen genitals in children, uterine prolapse and similar conditions. For the medicinal use of the fox in general, see 《中藥大辭典》#2011.

胡粉 *hú fěn*
Lead carbonite or cerrusite

Translator's note:
Common Name: Processed galenite.

胡麻 *hú má*
Black seed of Sesamum indicum
Vol. 1, line 136 Highest Grade

味甘，平，無毒。主傷中虛羸，補五內，益氣力，長肌肉，填髓腦。久服，輕身、不老。生川澤。

Flavor: Sweet
Nature: Neutral
Toxicity: Non-toxic
Alt. names: 巨勝, leaves: 青蘘

Actions and Indications:
Indicated for damage to the center and vacuity emaciation.
Supplements the five [viscera] inside, boosts *qì* and strength, grows flesh, and replenishes the marrow and brain.

Additional Information:
Taken for a long time, it lightens the body and prevents aging.
Grows in streams and marshes.

Translator's note:
Common Name: Black sesame seed.
Family: Sesame (Pedaliaceae).
Other species used: Sesamum orientale.
More often called 黑芝麻 *hēi zhī má*, the *Zhōng Yào Dà Cí Diǎn* also lists 胡麻 *hú má* as a synonym for 亞麻 *yà má*, the root, stalk, and leaves of Linum usitatissimum (flax, linseed) of the Flax family (《中藥大辭典》#1832). Nevertheless, I identify it as sesame since it is also called 胡麻 *hú má* in the *Shén Nóng Běn Cǎo Jīng*.
《中藥大辭典》#4164.

胡燕巢中草 *hú yàn cháo zhōng cǎo*
Straw from a swallow's nest
Vol. 2, line 87 Middle Grade

In the *Shén Nóng Běn Cǎo Jīng*, under the entry for 燕屎.

味辛，平，有毒。主蟲毒鬼注，逐不祥邪氣，破五癃，利小便。生高山平谷。

Flavor: Acrid

Nature: Neutral
Toxicity: Toxic
Alt. names: n/a

Actions and Indications:
Indicated for *gǔ* toxin and ghost infixation.
Expels inauspicious things and evil *qì*, breaks up the
five types of dribbling urinary block, and disinhibits
urine.

Additional Information:
Lives in high mountains, flatlandss, and valleys.

Translator's note:
Not listed in the *Zhōng Yào Dà Cí Diǎn*. Nevertheless,
in the entry on 胡燕卵 *hú yàn luǎn* (swallow's eggs),
胡燕 *hú yàn* is identified as Hirundo daurica japonica
(red-rumped swallow) of the Swallow and Martin family (Hirundinidae). See 《中藥大辭典》 #2601. According to Táo Hóng-Jīng, the swallow used medicinally
is 胡燕 *hú yàn* ("Western swallow"), which is identifiable by black spots on the chest and a loud voice, as
opposed to the "Southern swallow," 越燕 *yuè yàn*, of
smaller size with a purple chest, which is unsuited for
medicinal use. The *Běn Cǎo Gāng Mù* lists 胡燕巢土
hú yàn cháo tǔ (swallow's nest detritus) in the section
on soils (《本草綱目》7:73).

斛脈 *hú mài*
Húmài

Translator's note:
Substance of uncertain identity, not listed in any major
materia medica texts. It is possibly an abbreviation
for 槲葉脈 *hú yè mài* (jagged-leaved oak leaf veins),
the veins in the leaf of Quercus dentata (daimyo,
Mongolian, or jagged-leaved oak) of the Beech family
(Fagaceae). 槲葉 *hú yè* (jagged-leaved oak leaf) is
a common medicinal ingredient, as are the bark and
seed of this plant. During the *Táng* period, 槲葉 *hú
yè* was known to treat hemorrhoids, stop blood and
bloody diarrhea, and quench thirst. See 《中藥大辭
典》 #4710 and 《本草綱目》30:1110, for 槲實 *hú shí*
jagged-leaved oak seed, for 槲若 *hú ruò*.

虎杖 *hǔ zhàng*
Polygonum cuspidatum
Vol. 3, line 14 Lowest Grade

味苦 ，溫 ，有大毒。主心痛 ，寒熱 ，結氣、積
聚、伏梁、傷筋、瘻、拘緩 ，利水道。生山谷。

Flavor: Bitter
Nature: Warm

Toxicity: Greatly toxic
Alt. names: n/a

Actions and Indications:
Indicated for heart pain, [aversion to] cold and heat
[effusion], bound *qì*, accumulations and gatherings,
deep-lying beam disease, damaged sinews, wilting,
hypertonicity and slackening, and for disinhibiting the
water-ways.

Additional Information:
Grows in mountain valleys.

Translator's note:
Common Name: Bushy knotweed.
Family: Knotweed (Polygonaceae).
Also called fleeceflower or smartweed.
《中藥大辭典》 #2109.

滑石 *huá shí*
Talcum
Vol. 1, line 8 Highest Grade

味甘 ，寒 ，無毒。主身熱泄 ，女子乳難 ，癃閉。
利小便 ，蕩胃中積聚寒熱 ，益精氣。久服 ，輕
身、耐飢、長年。生山谷。

Flavor: Sweet
Nature: Cold
Toxicity: Non-toxic
Alt. names: n/a

Actions and Indications:
Indicated for generalized heat [effusion] and diarrhea, women's breastfeeding difficulties, and dribbling
urinary block.
Disinhibits urine, flushes out accumulations, and gatherings with [aversion to] cold and heat [effusion] from
inside the stomach, and boosts essential *qì*.

Additional Information:
Taken over a long time, it lightens the body, allows the
person to endure hunger, and lengthens the years.
Grows in mountain valleys.

Translator's note:
《中藥大辭典》 #4250.

樺 *huà*
Bark of Betula platyphylla

Translator's note:
Common Name: Chinese white birch bark.
Family: Birch (Betulaceae).

《中藥大辭典》#4852 on 樺木皮 *huà mù pí* for the bark, and 《中藥大辭典》#4854 on 樺樹液 *huà shù yè* for the sap.

槐耳 *huái ěr*
Wood ear that grows on the stem Sophora japonica

Translator's note:
Common Name: Sophora wood ear.
Family: Auriculariaceae.
A type of 木耳 *mù ěr* (Auricularia auricula) that grows on the stem of 槐樹 *huái shù* (Sophora japonica, also called pagoda tree, of the Pea family, Fabaceae).
For a general description of 木耳 *mù ěr*, see 《中藥大辭典》#0682. For the medicinal use of sophora, see the following entry in this index on 槐實 *huái shí* (fruit of sophora japonica) and 《中藥大辭典》#4487, which contains a description of the plant in general as well as of the flowers.
《中藥大辭典》#4477.

槐實 *huái shí*
Fruit of Sophora japonica
Vol. 1, line 95 Highest Grade

味苦，寒，無毒。主五內邪氣熱，止涎唾，補絕傷，五痔，火創，婦人乳瘕，子藏急痛。生平澤。

Flavor: Bitter
Nature: Cold
Toxicity: Non-toxic
Alt. names: n/a

Actions and Indications:
Indicated for evil *qì* and heat inside the five [viscera]. Checks drool and spittle, supplements damage from severance, and [treats] the five types of hemorrhoids, fire wounds, and women's breast conglomerations and tension and pain in the uterus.

Additional Information:
Grows in flatlands and marshes.

Translator's note:
Common Name: Sophora fruit.
Family: Pea (Fabaceae).
Also called Pagoda tree or Chinese scholar tree. In a medicinal context, the fruit is also called 槐子 *huái zǐ*, but is most often referred to as 槐角 *huái jiǎo*, under which name it is listed in the *Zhōng Yào Dà Cí Diǎn*.
《中藥大辭典》#4478.

槐枝 *huái zhī*
Tender branches of Sophora japonica

Translator's note:
Common Name: Sophora twig.
Family: Pea (Fabaceae).
The tree is also called pagoda tree or Chinese scholar tree. For more information on the medicinal uses of the fruit, as well as the translation of the *Shén Nóng Běn Cǎo Jīng*, see the preceding entry on 槐實 *huái shí*.
《中藥大辭典》#4479.

黃柏/檗 *huáng bǎi/bò*
Bark of Phellodendron amurense
Vol. 1, line 101 Highest Grade

In the *Shén Nóng Běn Cǎo Jīng*, under the entry 檗木.

味苦，寒，無毒。主五臟、腸胃中結熱，黃膽，腸痔，止泄利，女子漏下赤白，陰傷蝕創。生山谷。

Flavor: Bitter
Nature: Cold
Toxicity: Non-toxic
Alt. names: n/a

Actions and Indications:
Indicated for heat bind in the five viscera, intestines, and stomach, for jaundice, and for intestinal hemorrhoids.
Checks diarrhea and [treats] women's vaginal spotting of red or white discharge, and wounds from damage and erosion in the genitals.

Additional Information:
Grows in mountain valleys.

Translator's note:
Common Name: Phellodendron bark.
Family: Rue (Rutaceae).
Other species used: Phellodendron chinense .
This tree is also called amur or Chinese cork-tree. 檗 *bò* is the more formal name for the tree, but 柏 *bǎi* is ordinarily used for the medicinal.
《中藥大辭典》#4030 and 《本草綱目》35:1228.

黃連 *huáng lián*
Rhizome of Coptis chinensis
Vol. 1, line 55 Highest Grade

味苦，寒，無毒。主熱氣目痛、眥傷泣出，明

目，腸澼，腹痛下利，婦人陰中腫痛。久服，令
人不忘。生川谷。

Flavor: Bitter
Nature: Cold
Toxicity: Non-toxic
Alt. names: 王連

Actions and Indications:
Indicated for heat *qi* with eye pain, damage to the
corners of the eyes, and tearing.
Brightens the eyes.
[Treats] washed out intestines, abdominal pain and di-
arrhea, and women's swelling and pain in the genitals.

Additional Information:
Taken for a long time, it prevents forgetfulness.
Grows in valleys with streams.

Translator's note:
Common Name: Coptis rhizome.
Family: Buttercup (Ranunculaceae).
Other species used: Coptis deltoidea, C. omeiensis,
C. teetoides or C. quinquesecta.
《中藥大辭典》#4033.

黃芪 *huáng qí*
Root of Astragalus membranaceus
Vol. 1, line 58 Highest Grade

味甘，微溫，無毒。主癰疽，久敗創，排膿止
痛，大風癩疾，五痔鼠瘻，補虛，小儿百病。生
山谷。

Flavor: Sweet
Nature: Slightly warm
Toxicity: Non-toxic
Alt. names: 戴糝

Actions and Indications:
Indicated for welling-abscesses and flat-abscesses
and chronically vanquished wounds.
Expels pus, relieves pain, and [treats] great wind epi-
lepsy, and the five types of hemorrhoids and mouse
fistulas.
Supplements vacuity.
[Treats] the hundred diseases of small children.

Additional Information:
Grows in mountain valleys.

Translator's note:
Common Name: Astragalus, vetch root.
Family: Pea (Fabaceae).
Other species used: Astragalus mongholicus, A.
chrysopterus, A. floridus, and A. tongolensis.
The American varieties are known as "locoweed"
because of the plant's toxicity to livestock.

《中藥大辭典》#4031.

黃芩 *huáng qín*
Root of Scutellaria baicalensis
Vol. 2, line 33 Middle Grade

味苦，平，無毒。主諸熱黃疸，腸澼泄利，逐
水，下血閉，惡創，疽蝕火瘍。生川谷。

Flavor: Bitter
Nature: Neutral
Toxicity: Non-toxic
Alt. names: 腐腸

Actions and Indications:
Indicated for all heat-related jaundice and intestinal
afflux diarrhea.
Expels water, precipitates blood blockage, and [treats]
malign wounds, flat-abscesses, erosion, and fire
sores.

Additional Information:
Grows in valleys with streams.

Translator's note:
Common Name: Scutellaria, skullcap root.
Family: Mint (Lamiaceae).
Other species used: Scutellaria viscidula, S. amoena,
S. rehderiana, S. ikonnikovii, S. likiangensis or S.
hypericifolia.
《中藥大辭典》#4029.

雞腸 *jī cháng*
Intestine of Gallus gallus domesticus

Translator's note:
Common Name: Chicken intestine.
Family: Pheasant (Phasianidae).
《中藥大辭典》#5553. For more information on the
medicinal qualities of chickens and a translation of the
relevant *Shén Nóng Běn Cǎo Jīng* passage, see the
entry on 雄雞 *xióng jī* (Complete body of male Gallus
gallus domesticus) below.
《中藥大辭典》#5547.

雞糞 *jī fèn*
Excrement of Gallus gallus domesticus

Translator's note:

Common Name: Chicken droppings.
Family: Pheasant (Phasianidae).
《中藥大辭典》#5577, where it is listed as 雞屎 jī shǐ.
For more information on the medicinal qualities of
chickens and a translation of the relevant *Shén Nóng
Běn Cǎo Jīng* passage, see the entry on 雄雞 *xióng
jī* (Complete body of male Gallus gallus domesticus)
below.

雞毛 jī máo
Feathers of Gallus gallus domesticus

Translator's note:
Common Name: Chicken feathers.
Family: Pheasant (Phasianidae).
Not listed in the *Zhōng Yào Dà Cí Diǎn*. For more
information on the medicinal qualities of chickens and
a translation of the relevant *Shén Nóng Běn Cǎo Jīng*
passage, see the entry on 雄雞 *xióng jī* (Complete
body of male Gallus gallus domesticus) below.
《中藥大辭典》#5547.

雞膍膣 jī pí zhì
Dried skin from the inside the gizzard of Gallus gallus domesticus

Translator's note:
Common Name: Chicken gizzard lining.
Family: Pheasant (Phasianidae).
In medical literature, more commonly referred to as 雞
內金 *jī nèi jīn*. For more information on the medicinal
qualities of chickens and a translation of the relevant
Shén Nóng Běn Cǎo Jīng passage, see the entry on
雄雞 *xióng jī* (Complete body of male Gallus gallus
domesticus) below.
《中藥大辭典》#5560.

箕舌 jī shé
Winnowing basket tongue

Translator's note:
The tongue-shaped opening in the front of a bamboo
winnowing basket. Not listed in the *Zhōng Yào Dà Cí
Diǎn* or *Běn Cǎo Gāng Mù*.

雞子 jī zǐ
Egg of Gallus gallus domesticus

Translator's note:
Common Name: Chicken egg.
Family: Pheasant (Phasianidae).
For more information on the medicinal qualities of
chickens and a translation of the relevant *Shén Nóng
Běn Cǎo Jīng* passage, see the entry on 雄雞 *xióng
jī* (Complete body of male Gallus gallus domesticus)
below.
《中藥大辭典》#5546.

薊根 jì gēn
Root of Cirsium japonicum

Translator's note:
Common Name: Japanese thistle root.
Family: Aster (Asteraceae).
More commonly called 大薊根 *dà jì gēn*, as which it is
listed in *Zhōng Yào Dà Cí Diǎn*.
《中藥大辭典》#0200

寄生 jì shēng
Branches and foliage of Viscum coloratum

Translator's note:
Common Name: Mistletoe.
Family: Milstletoe (Santhalaceae).
Other species used: Loranthus parasiticus, Taxillus
chinensis, T. sutchuensensis, Loranthus gracilifolius,
or L. yadoriki.
Most commonly, it is specifically called 桑寄生 *sāng jì
shēng* (mulberry mistletoe). For more information and
a translation of the relevant passage from the *Shén
Nóng Běn Cǎo Jīng*, see that entry below.
《中藥大辭典》2871.

鯽魚 jì yú
Meat or whole body of Carassius auratus

Translator's note:
Common Name: Golden carp.
Family: Minnow (Cyprinidae).
《中藥大辭典》#5454.

繭絮 *jiǎn xù*
Silk made from the cocoon of the moth of Bombyx mori

Translator's note:
Common Name: Silkworm moth cocoon, Cocoon silk.
Family: Silkworm (Bombycidae).
《中藥大辭典》 #5689, where it is listed as 蠶繭 *cán jiǎn*.

薑 *jiāng*
Root of Zingiber officinale

Translator's note:
Common Name: Ginger.
Family: Ginger (Zingiberaceae).
Used fresh (生 *shēng*) or dried (乾 *gān*). For a translation of the *Shén Nóng Běn Cǎo Jīng* entry on the dried root, see the entry on 乾薑 *gān jiāng* above.
《中藥大辭典》 #1073.

漿 *jiāng*
Sour millet water

Translator's note:
A fermented alcoholic beverage, made by soaking heated millet in water for five to six days. It is most often called 漿水 *jiāng shuǐ*. See 楊吉成, 編者 《中國飲食辭典》, pp. 270 and 619, and 《本草綱目》 5:33.

殭蠶 *jiāng cán*
Dried 4th or 5th stage larva of the moth of Bombyx mori
Vol. 2, line 96 Middle Grade

味鹹 , 平 , 無毒。主小儿惊癇 , 夜啼 , 去三蟲 ,
滅黑皯 , 令人面色好 , 男子陰瘍病。生平澤。

Flavor: Salty
Nature: Neutral
Toxicity: Non-toxic
Alt. names: n/a

Actions and Indications:
Indicated for small children's fright epilepsy and crying at night.
Removes the three types of worms, eliminates black spots, improves a person's facial complexion, and

[treats] men's pudendal itch.

Additional Information:
Lives in flatlandss and marshes.

Translator's note:
Common Name: Infected silkworm larva.
Family: Silkworm (Bombycidae).
This state of the silkworm moth is commonly referred to as "bombyx batryticatus" in a medicinal context.
See the entry above on 白僵蠶 *bái jiāng cán*, a common synonym.
《中藥大辭典》 # 1160.

膠飴 *jiāo yí*
Malt candy

Translator's note:
A jelly-like confection made from malt syrup (飴 *yí*). In the *Zhōng Yào Dà Cí Diǎn*, it is listed as 飴糖 *yí táng* (entry #4663). See the entry below on 飴 *yí* for more information on malt syrup.

桔梗 *jié gěng*
Root of Platycodon grandiflorum
Vol. 3, line 18 Lowest Grade

味辛 , 微溫 , 有小毒。主胸脅痛如刀刺 , 腹滿 ,
腸鳴幽幽 , 惊恐悸氣。生山谷。

Flavor: Acrid
Nature: Slightly warm
Toxicity: Slightly toxic
Alt. names: n/a

Actions and Indications:
Indicated for pain in the chest and rib-sides like being stabbed by a knife, abdominal fullness, intestinal dark rumbling, and fright and fear palpitations.

Additional Information:
Grows in mountain valleys.

Translator's note:
Common Name: Balloon flower root, Chinese bellflower root.
Family: Bellflower (Campanulaceae).
《中藥大辭典》 #2877.

粳米 *jīng mǐ*
Grain of the non-glutinous variety of Oryza sativa

Translator's note:
Common Name: Non-glutinous rice, common household rice.
Family: True Grass (Poaceae).
《中藥大辭典》#4277.

井底泥 *jǐng dǐ ní*
Well-bottom mud

Translator's note:
Mud from the bottom of a well.
《中藥大辭典》#0549.

井花水 *jǐng huā shuǐ*
Well-flower water

Translator's note:
The first water drawn from a well at dawn. In the *Běn Cǎo Gāng Mù*, it is listed as 井泉水 *jǐng quán shuǐ* ("well springwater"), and 井花水 *jǐng huā shuǐ* is given as a synonym (《本草綱目》5:15). A common ingredient in Daoist alchemy, this medicinal has many medicinal applications. The best grade comes from deep wells that tap the veins in the earth, rather than from nearby rivers or lakes. According to Yú Tuán 虞摶, a physician active in the early 16th century, it is ideal for decocting medicines that replenish *yīn* and for smelting alchemical preparations since it contains the first true *qì* of Heaven that floats on the water's surface (quoted in 《本草綱目》5:15).

井中黃土 *jǐng zhōng huáng tǔ*
Dirt from inside a well

Translator's note:
Not listed in the *Zhōng Yào Dà Cí Diǎn*, but see above for the closely related 井底泥 *jǐng dǐ ní* (well-bottom mud).

韭 *jiǔ*
Foliage of Allium tuberosum

Translator's note:
Common Name: Chinese leek.
Family: Lily (Liliaceae).
《中藥大辭典》#2704, where it is listed as 韭菜 *jiǔ cài*.

菊花 *jú huā*
Flower of Chrysanthemum morafolii
Vol. 1, line 20 Highest Grade

味苦，平，無毒。主風頭，頭眩腫痛，目欲脫，淚出，皮膚死肌，惡風，濕痹。久服，利血氣，輕身、耐老、延年。生川澤及田野。

Flavor: Bitter
Nature: Neutral
Toxicity: Non-toxic
Alt. names: 節華

Actions and Indications:
Indicated for wind in the head, [causing] dizziness, swelling, and pain in the head, eyes about to fall out, tearing, dead flesh in the skin, aversion to wind, and damp impediment.

Additional Information:
Taken over a long time, it disinhibits blood and *qì*, lightens the body, allows the person to endure aging, and extends the years.
Grows in streams and marshes, and in open fields.

Translator's note:
Common Name: Chrysanthemum flower.
Family: Aster (Asteraceae).
《中藥大辭典》#3925.

橘皮 *jú pí*
Peel of Citrus reticulata
Vol. 1, line 111 Highest Grade

In the *Shén Nóng Běn Cǎo Jīng*, under the entry for 橘柚.

味辛，溫，無毒。主胸中瘕熱逆氣，利水谷。久服，去臭、下氣、通神。生川谷。

Flavor: Acrid
Nature: Warm
Toxicity: Non-toxic

Actions and Indications:

Indicated for conglomerations in the chest with heat [effusion] and counterflow *qì*.
Disinhibits water and grain.

Additional Information:
Taken for a long time, it removes malodor, precipitates *qì*, and frees the spirit.
Grows in valleys with streams.

Translator's note:
Common Name: Tangerine peel.
Family: Rue (Rutaceae).
Other species used: Citrus erythrosa or other citrus species.
It is also commonly called 陳皮 *chén pí*.
《中藥大辭典》 #4861.

櫸皮 *jǔ pí*
Bark of Zelkova schneideriana

Translator's note:
Common Name: Zelkova bark.
Family: Elm family (Ulmaceae).
《中藥大辭典》 #5468, where it is listed as 櫸樹皮 *jǔ shù pí*. The leaves are also used medicinally.

具齒 *jù chǐ*
Set of teeth

Translator's note:
Not listed in the *Zhōng Yào Dà Cí Diǎn*. The *Běn Cǎo Gāng Mù* has an entry on 牙齒 *yá chǐ* (《本草綱目》 52:1867).

卷柏 *juǎn bǎi*
Entire plant of Selaginella tamariscina
Vol. 1, line 51 Highest Grade

味辛，溫，無毒。主五臟邪氣，女子陰中寒熱痛，症瘕、血閉、絕子。久服，輕身、和顏色。生山谷石間。

Flavor: Acrid
Nature: Warm
Toxicity: Non-toxic
Alt. names: 萬歲

Actions and Indications:
Indicated for evil *qì* in the five viscera and women's

and girl's cold and heat pain in the genitals, concretions and conglomerations, blood blockage, and infertility.

Additional Information:
Taken over a long time, it lightens the body and harmonizes the complexion.
Grows in mountain valleys between rocks.

Translator's note:
Common Name: Selaginella.
Family: Spikemoss (Selaginellaceae).
《中藥大辭典》 #1896.

苦瓠 *kǔ hù*
Fruit of Lagenaria siceraria var. gourda
Vol. 3, line 101 Lowest Grade

味苦，寒，有毒。主大水，面目四肢浮腫，下水，令人吐。生川澤。

Flavor: Bitter
Nature: Cold
Toxicity: Toxic
Alt. names: n/a

Actions and Indications:
Indicated for severe water with puffy swelling in the face, eyes, and four limbs.
Precipitates water and induces vomiting.

Additional Information:
Grows in streams and marshes.

Translator's note:
Common Name: Bitter calabash.
Family: Gourd (Cucurbitaceae).
Also called 苦葫蘆 *kǔ hú lú*.
《中藥大辭典》 #2653.

苦參 *kǔ shēn*
Root of Sophora flavescens
Vol. 2, line 19 Middle Grade

味苦，寒，無毒。主心腹結氣，症瘕積聚，黃膽，溺有餘瀝。逐水，除癰腫，補中，明目，止淚。生山谷及田野。

Flavor: Bitter
Nature: Cold
Toxicity: Non-toxic
Alt. names: 水槐

Actions and Indications:

Indicated for bound *qì* in the heart and abdomen, for concretions, conglomerations, accumulations, and gatherings, for yellow jaundice, and for urinating with residual trickling.
Expels water, eliminates swollen welling-abscesses, supplements the center, brightens the eyes, and stops tearing.

Additional Information:
Grows in mountain valleys and open fields.

Translator's note:
Common Name: Flavescent sophora.
Family: Pea (Fabiaceae).
A close relative of Sophora japonica (pagoda tree, 槐樹 *huái shù*. See entry on 槐實 *huái shí* above).
《中藥大辭典》#2629.

苦竹 *kǔ zhú*
Arundinaria amabilis

Translator's note:
Common Name: Bitter bamboo.
Family: Grass (Poaceae).
Also called Tongking cane. The leaf (苦竹葉 *kǔ zhú yè*), root (苦竹根 *kǔ zhú gēn*), sap (苦竹瀝 *kǔ zhú lì*), and shavings (苦竹茹 *kǔ zhú rú*) are used medicinally. For a description of the varieties of bamboo, see entry below on 竹 *zhú* (bamboo).
《中藥大辭典》#2646.

款冬花 *kuǎn dōng huā*
Flower of Tussilago farfara
Vol. 2, line 53 Middle Grade

味辛，溫，無毒。主咳逆上氣，善喘、喉痹，諸驚癇，寒熱邪氣。生山谷及水傍。

Flavor: Acrid
Nature: Warm
Toxicity: Non-toxic
Alt. names: 橐吾、顆東、虎須、兔奚

Actions and Indications:
Indicated for cough and counterflow with ascent of *qì*, tendency to belching, throat impediment, all fright epilepsy, and evil *qì* of cold and heat.

Additional Information:
Grows in mountain valleys and alongside water.

Translator's note:
Common Name: Coltsfoot flower.
Family: Aster (Asteraceae).

《中藥大辭典》#3833.

葵根莖 *kuí gēn jīng*
Rhizome of Malva verticillata

Translator's note:
Common Name: Mallow rhizome
Family: Mallow (Malvaceae).
This medicinal comes from a type of mallow called "curved mallow" in English and 冬葵 *dōng kuí* ("winter mallow") in Chinese. The plant is described in the *Zhōng Yào Dà Cí Diǎn* under the entry for the seed (《中藥大辭典》#0971, see the entry on 葵子 *kuí zǐ* below). The character 葵 *kuí* can also refer to other related plants, such as 蜀葵 *shǔ kuí* (《中藥大辭典》#4347, Althaea rosa, hollyhock), of which the foliage and stalk are used medicinally, or to 向日葵 *xiàng rì kuí* (《中藥大辭典》#1346, Helianthus annuus, sunflower), of which the seeds are used medicinally. Nevertheless, I identify 葵根 *kuí gēn* with 冬葵 *dōng kuí* because only the root of this species is used medicinally and because 葵 *kuí* is a common abbreviation for 冬葵 *dōng kuí* in early medical literature, such as the *Běn Cǎo Jīng Jí Zhù*, the *Jīn Guì Yào Lüè*, and the *Fù Rén Dà Quán Liáng Fāng*. For a translation of the *Shén Nóng Běn Cǎo Jīng* passage on the seed, see the following entry on 葵子 *kuí zǐ*.
《中藥大辭典》#0972, where it is listed under 冬葵根 *dōng kuí gēn*.

葵子 *kuí zǐ*
Seed of Malva verticillata
Vol. 1, line 138 Highest Grade

In the *Shén Nóng Běn Cǎo Jīng*, under the entry for 冬葵子.

味甘，寒，無毒。主五臟六腑，寒熱、羸瘦、五癃，利小便。久服，堅骨、長肌肉、輕身、延年。

Flavor: Sweet
Nature: Cold
Toxicity: Non-toxic
Alt. names: n/a

Actions and Indications:
Indicated for the five viscera and six bowels, [aversion to] cold and heat [effusion], marked emaciation, and the five types of dribbling urinary block.
Disinhibits urine.

Additional Information:
Taken for a long time, it hardens the bones, grows the

flesh, lightens the body, and extends the years.

Translator's note:
Common Name: Mallow seed.
Family: Mallow (Malvaceae). For a discussion of the plant identification, see the preceding entry on 葵根莖 *kuí gēn jīng*.
《中藥大辭典》 #0971, where it is listed under 冬葵子 *dōng kuí zǐ*.

昆布 *kūn bù*
Leaf-shaped body of Laminaria japonica

Translator's note:
Common Name: Kelp.
Family: Laminariaceae
Other species used: Ecklonia kurome (kombu) or Undaria pinnatifida (wakame) of the family Alariaceae.
《中藥大辭典》 #1925.

蠟 *là*
Secretion of Apis cerana
Vol. 1, line 123 Highest Grade

In the *Shén Nóng Běn Cǎo Jīng*, under the entry for 蜜蠟.

味甘，微溫，無毒。主下利膿血，補中，續絕傷金創。益氣、不飢、耐老。生山谷。

Flavor: Sweet
Nature: Slightly warm
Toxicity: Non-toxic
Alt. names: n/a

Actions and Indications:
Indicated for diarrhea with pus and blood.
Supplements the center and joins damage from severance and incised wounds.
Boosts *qì*, prevents hunger, and allows the person to endure aging.

Additional Information:
Grows in mountain valleys.

Translator's note:
Common Name: Beeswax.
Family: Bee (Apidae).
《中藥大辭典》 #4606.

藍青 *lán qīng*
Dye produced from the foliage of Isatis tinctoria

Translator's note:
Common Name: Indigo residue.
Family: Mustard (Brassicaceae), Pea (Fabaceae), Acanthus (Acanthaceae), Knotweed (Polygonaceae).
Other species used: Isatis indigotica, Baphicacanthus cusia (Assam indigo), and Polygonum tinctorium (knotweed).
The foliage of some of these plants is also used medicinally and referred to as 大青葉 *dà qīng yè* (see entry above on *dà qīng* 大青).
《中藥大辭典》 #5240, where it is listed as 藍靛 *lán diàn*.

狼毒 *láng dú*
Root of Stellera chamaejasme
Vol. 3, line 43 Lowest Grade

味辛，平，有大毒。主咳逆上氣，破積聚、飲食寒熱，水氣、惡創，鼠瘻、疽蝕，鬼精、蠱毒，殺飛鳥、走獸。生山谷。

Flavor: Acrid
Nature: Neutral
Toxicity: Greatly toxic
Alt. names: 續毒

Actions and Indications:
Indicated for counterflow cough with ascent of *qì*, for breaking up accumulations and gatherings, for cold and heat from food and drink, water *qì*, malign wounds, mouse fistulas, flat-abscesses with erosion, ghosts and specters, and *gǔ* toxin.

Additional Information:
Kills flying birds and running beasts.
Grows in mountain valleys.

Translator's note:
Common Name: Chinese wolfsbane root.
Family: Mezereum (Thymelaeaceae).
Other species used: Euphorbia fischeriana or E. ebiacteolata.
《中藥大辭典》 #2977.

狼牙 *láng yá*
Root of Potentilla cryptotaenia
Vol. 3, line 38 Lowest Grade

Entry for 牙子.

味苦，寒，有毒。主邪氣、熱氣，疥瘙、惡瘍、創、痔，去白蟲。生川谷。

Flavor: Bitter
Nature: Cold
Toxicity: Toxic
Alt. names: 狼牙

Actions and Indications:
Indicated for evil *qì*, heat *qì*, scabs and itching, malign sores, wounds, and hemorrhoids.
Removes whiteworm.

Additional Information:
Grows in valleys with streams.

Translator's note:
Common Name: Cinquefoil root.
Family: Rose (Roasaceae).
Other species used: Agrimonia pilosa (downy agrimony or cocklebur).
In the *Shén Nóng Běn Cǎo Jīng*, Táo Hóng-Jǐng offers 狼牙 *láng yá* as a synonym for 牙子 *yǎ zǐ*. The *Běn Cǎo Gāng Mù* lists it as 狼牙 and gives several synonyms, none of which are found in the *Zhōng Yào Dà Cí Diǎn* (《本草綱目》17:533). Mǎ Jì-Xìng offers two possible identifications of 狼牙 *láng yá*, as it occurs in the Mǎ-Wáng-Duī material, namely either Potentilla cryptotaenia or a relative with similar characteristics, Agrimonia pilosa (as which it is identified in 《中華本草》4, #2545). See 馬繼興，主編《馬王堆古醫書考釋》p. 605, n. 2. For information on the medicinal use of agrimony root, see 《中藥大辭典》#0960, where it is listed as 仙鶴草根芽 *xiān hè cǎo gēn yá*. The possibility that it could literally refer to the teeth of Canis lupus, listed in the *Běn Cǎo Gāng Mù* as a medicinally useful substance under its entry on wolf (vol. 51:1833), seems unlikely, given that the the plant medicinal is identified in the Mǎ-Wáng-Duī manuscripts (MS1.E.239) as 狼牙根 *láng yá gēn* ("root of lángyá," see Harper, *Early Chinese Medical Literature*, p. 295), and that the description of the medicinal use of the herb 狼牙 in the *Běn Cǎo Gāng Mù* fits the usage in Sūn Sī-Miǎo's prescriptions so well.

酪 *lào*
Koumiss

Translator's note:
Fermented drink made from the milk of cows, goats, sheeps, water buffaloes, horses, camels, and other species of the Bovid family (Bovidae), similar to other fermented dairy products like yoghurt or kefir. According to Lǐ Shí-Zhēn, cow's milk koumiss is the most suitable for medicinal use. It is made by heating the milk, bringing it to a rolling boil ten times while stirring frequently, letting it cool, removing the skin on top (which can be used to make butter 酥 *sū*), adding some old koumiss culture, sealing it and letting it ferment (《本草綱目》50:1784).

藜蘆 *lí lú*
Root and rhizome of Veratrum nigrum
Vol. 3, line 22 Lowest Grade

味辛，寒，有毒。主蠱毒，咳逆，泄利，腸澼，頭瘍疥瘙，惡瘡，殺諸蟲毒，去死肌。生山谷。

Flavor: Acrid
Nature: Cold
Toxicity: Toxic
Alt. names: 蔥苒

Actions and Indications:
Indicated for *gǔ* toxin, cough with counterflow, diarrhea, intestinal afflux, sores, scabs, and itching on the head, and malign wounds.
Kills all worm toxins and removes dead flesh.

Additional Information:
Grows in mountain valleys.

Translator's note:
Common Name: Black hellebore root and rhizome.
Family: Lily family (Liliaceae).
Other species used: Veratrum maackii, V. puberulum, V. dahuricum, V. schindleri, V. grandiflorum, or V. mengtzeanum.
《中藥大辭典》#5345.

李根白皮 *lǐ gēn bái pí*
Shavings from the bark of the root of Prunus salicina

Translator's note:
Common Name: Plum root bark.
Family: Rose (Roasaceae).
《中藥大辭典》#1684, where it is listed as 李根皮 *lǐ gēn pí*. See also entry below on 生李根白皮 *shēng lǐ gēn bái pí* (fresh White bark of the root of Prunus salicina).

理石 *lǐ shí*
Fibrous gypsum
Vol. 2, line 12 Middle Grade

味辛，寒，無毒。主身熱，利胃，解煩，益精，
明目，破積聚，去三蟲。生山谷。

Flavor: Acrid
Nature: Cold
Toxicity: Non-toxic
Alt. names: 立制石

Actions and Indications:
Indicated for generalized fever, disinhibiting the stomach, resolving vexation, boosting essence, brightening the eyes, breaking up accumulations and gatherings, and removing the three types of worms.

Additional Information:
Grows in mountain valleys.

Translator's note:
The term 理石 *lǐ shí* is sometimes incorrectly applied to 礬石 *fán shí* (alunite, see entry above), but since Sūn Sī-Miǎo uses both terms repeatedly, I see no reason to suspect an inaccuracy on his part.
《中藥大辭典》#3368.

鯉魚 *lǐ yú*
Meat or whole body of Cyprinus carpio
Vol. 1, line 130 Highest Grade

In the *Shén Nóng Běn Cǎo Jīng*, under the entry for 鯉魚膽 (gallbladder) only.

味苦，寒，無毒。主目熱赤痛，青盲明目。久
服，強悍、益志氣。生池澤。

Flavor: Bitter
Nature: Cold
Toxicity: Non-toxic
Alt. names: n/a

Actions and Indications:
Indicated for heat, redness, and pain in the eyes and for green-blue blindness.
Brightens the eyes.

Additional Information:
Taken for a long time, it makes the person strong and brave and boosts the will and *qì*.
Lives in ponds and marshes.

Translator's note:
Common Name: Carp.
Family: Carp (Cyprinidae). The teeth (齒 *chǐ*, 《中藥大辭典》#5285) or scales (甲 *jiǎ*, 《中藥大辭

典》#5287, where they are called 鱗 *lín*) are also used as individual ingredients.
《中藥大辭典》#5287.

梁上塵 *liáng shàng chén*
Roofbeam dust

Translator's note:
Not listed in the *Zhōng Yào Dà Cí Diǎn*, but found in 《本草綱目》7:108.

羚羊角 *líng yáng jiǎo*
Horn of the male Saiga tatarica
Vol. 2, line 85 Middle Grade

味咸，寒，無毒。主明目，益氣，起陰，去惡血
注下，辟蠱毒、惡鬼、不祥，安心氣，常不厭
寐。久服強筋骨，輕身。生川谷。

Flavor: Salty
Nature: Cold
Toxicity: Non-toxic
Alt. names: n/a

Actions and Indications:
Indicated for brightening the eyes, boosting *qì*, and raising the penis.
Removes malign blood, [treats] downpour diarrhea, and repels *gǔ* poison, malign ghosts, and inauspicious events.
Quiets heart *qì* and makes the person not have nightmares.

Additional Information:
Taken for a long time, it strengthens the sinews and bones and lightens the body.
Lives in valleys with streams.

Translator's note:
Common Name: Antelope horn.
Family: Bovid (Bovidae).
《中藥大辭典》#3465

硫磺 *liú huáng*
Sulphur

Translator's note:
More completely called 石硫 *shí liú*. See the entry below on *shí liú huáng* 石硫磺, which includes a trans-

lation of the relevant passage from the *Shén Nóng Běn Cǎo Jīng*.
《中藥大辭典》#1278 where it is listed as 石硫磺 *shí liú huáng*.

柳絮 *liǔ xù*
Seed of Salix babylonica
Vol. 3, line 62 Lowest Grade

In the *Shén Nóng Běn Cǎo Jīng*, under the entry for 柳花.

味苦，寒，無毒。主風水，黃膽，面熱黑。葉，主馬疥，痂創。實，主潰癰，逐膿血。子汁，療渴。生川澤。

Flavor: Bitter
Nature: Cold
Toxicity: Non-toxic
Alt. names: 柳絮

Actions and Indications:
Indicated for wind water, jaundice, and heat and blackness of the face.

Additional Information:
Leaves: Indicated for horse scabs and sores.
Seeds: Indicated for ruptured welling-abscesses and for expelling pus and blood.
Juice from the seeds: Cures thirst.
Grows in streams and marshes.

Translator's note:
Common Name: Peking willow seed.
Family: Willow (Salicaceae). See 《中藥大辭典》#2414 for information on the plant.
《中藥大辭典》#2418.

龍膽 *lóng dǎn*
Root and rhizome of Gentiana scabra
Vol. 1, line 40 Highest Grade

味苦，寒，無毒。主骨間寒熱，惊癇，邪氣，續絕傷，定五臟，殺蠱毒。久服，益智、不忘、輕身、耐老。生山谷。

Flavor: Bitter
Nature: Cold
Toxicity: Non-toxic
Alt. names: 陵游

Actions and Indications:
Indicated for cold or heat between the bones, fright

epilepsy, and evil *qì*.
Joins damage from severance, settles the five viscera, and kills *gǔ* toxin.

Additional Information:
Taken over a long time, it boosts wisdom, prevents forgetfulness, lightens the body, and makes the person endure aging.
Grows in mountain valleys.

Translator's note:
Common Name: Gentian root and rhizome.
Family: Gentian (Gentianaceae).
Other species used: Gentiana triflora.
《中藥大辭典》#5056.

龍骨 *lóng gǔ*
Os draconis
Vol. 1, line 113 Highest Grade

味甘，平，無毒。主心腹鬼注，精物老魅，咳逆，泄利膿血，女子漏下、症瘕、堅結，小儿熱氣、惊癇。齒:主小儿、大人惊癇，癲疾狂走，心下結氣，不能喘息，諸痙，殺精物。久服，輕身、通神明、延年。生山谷。

Flavor: Sweet
Nature: Neutral
Toxicity: Non-toxic

Actions and Indications:
Indicated for ghost influx in the heart and abdomen, for spectral things and old demons, for cough with counterflow, for diarrhea with pus and blood, for girl's and women's vaginal spotting, for concretions and conglomerations, hardness and binding, and for heat *qì* and fright epilepsy in small children.

Additional Information:
Teeth: Indicated for fright epilepsy in small children and adults, withdrawal disease and manic running, bound *qì* below the heart, inability to pant and breathe, and all tetany. Kills spectral things.
Taken for a long time, [*lóng gǔ*] lightens the body, frees the spirit light, and extends the years.
Grows in mountain valleys.

Translator's note:
Fossilized vertebrae and bones of ancient mammals such as elephant or rhinoceros.
《中藥大辭典》#5053.

漏蘆 lòu lú
Root of Rhaponticum uniflorum
Vol. 1, line 64 Highest Grade

味苦咸，寒，無毒。主皮膚熱、惡創、疽痔、濕
痹，下乳汁。久服，輕身、益氣、耳目聰明、不
老、延年。生山谷。

Flavor: Bitter and salty
Nature: Cold
Toxicity:Non-toxic
Alt. names: 野蘭

Actions and Indications:
Indicated for heat in the skin, malign wounds, flat-abscesses and hemorrhoids, and damp impediment. Precipitates breastmilk.

Additional Information:
Taken over a long time, it lightens the body, boosts qì, sharpens the ears and eyes, prevents aging, and extends the years.
Grows in mountain valleys.

Translator's note:
Common Name: Globe thistle root.
Family: Aster (Asteraceae).
Other species used: Echinops latifolius.
The plant is also called Stemmacantha uniflora.
《中藥大辭典》#4501.

蘆根 lú gēn
Rhizome of Phragmites communis

Translator's note:
Common Name: Reed rhizome.
Family: True Grass (Poaceae).
《中藥大辭典》#5418.

露蜂房 lù fēng fáng
Nest of Polistes mandarinus
Vol. 2, line 90 Middle Grade

味苦，平，有毒。主惊癇，瘈瘲，寒熱邪氣，癲
疾，鬼精蠱毒，腸痔。火熬之，良。生山谷。

Flavor: Bitter
Nature: Neutral
Toxicity: Toxic
Alt. names: 蜂腸

Actions and Indications:
Indicated for fright epilepsy, tugging and slackening, evil qì of cold and heat, withdrawal disorder, ghosts and specters, gǔ toxin, and intestinal hemorrhoids.

Additional Information:
Roasting it in fire is excellent.
Lives in mountain valleys.

Translator's note:
Common Name: Wasp nest.
Family: Wasp (Vespidae).
Other species used: Polistes olivaceus, Parapolybia varia).
 In English TCM literature, it is sometimes rendered as "hornet's nest."
《中藥大辭典》#5448.

鹿角 lù jiǎo
Ossified antler or antler base of Cervus nippon

Translator's note:
Common Name: Deerhorn glue.
Family: Deer (Cervidae).
Other species used: Cervus elaphus
Collected in the seventh lunar month. Note that 鹿角 lù jiǎo must be distinguished from 鹿茸 lù róng, velvet deerhorn (see following entry). Moreover, the gelatinous glue produced from deerhorn, which is also an important medicinal ingredient, is usually called 白膠 bái jiāo, but also sometimes referred to as 鹿角膠 lù jiǎo jiāo. See entry on 白膠 bái jiāo above for information on that substance and the translation of the relevant passage from the Shén Nóng Běn Cǎo Jīng. See following entry on 鹿茸 lù róng for a translation of the relevant passage from the Shén Nóng Běn Cǎo Jīng.
《中藥大辭典》#3703.

鹿茸 lù róng
Pilose antler of Cervus nippon
Vol. 2, line 81 Middle Grade

味甘，溫，無毒。主漏下，惡血，寒熱，惊癇，
益氣，強志，生齒，不老。角，主惡創，癰腫，
逐邪惡氣，留血在陰中。

Flavor: Sweet
Nature: Warm
Toxicity: Non-toxic
Alt. names: n/a

Actions and Indications:
Indicated for vaginal spotting, malign blood, [aversion to] cold and heat [effusion], and fright epilepsy.

Boosts *qì*, strengthens the will, makes the teeth grow, and prevents aging.

Additional Information:
Antlers: Indicated for malign wounds and welling-abscess swelling. Expels evil malign *qì* and abiding blood in the genitals.

Translator's note:
Common Name: Velvet deerhorn.
Family: Deer (Cervidae).
Other species used: Cervus elaphus.
For this medicinal, the horn has not yet become ossified, and is collected in the fourth and fifth lunar month. Distinguish from 鹿角 *lù jiăo*, deerhorn, which is collected in the seventh lunar month (see preceding entry).
《中藥大辭典》#3706.

鹿肉 *lù ròu*
Meat of Cervus nippon

Translator's note:
Common Name: Venison of Sika or Red deer.
Family: Deer (Cervidae).
Other species used: Cervus elaphus.
《中藥大辭典》#3700.

亂髮 *luàn fà*
Matted hair
Vol. 1, line 112 Highest Grade

In the *Shén Nóng Běn Căo Jīng*, under the entry for 髮髲.

味苦，溫，無毒。主五癃，關格不通，利小便水道，療小儿瘤、大人痙，仍自還神化。

Flavor: Bitter
Nature: Warm
Toxicity: Non-toxic
Alt. names: n/a

Actions and Indications:
Indicated for the five types of dribbling urinary block, and block and repulsion with lack of free flow.
Disinhibits urine and the water ways, treats epilepsy in small children and tetany in adults, and allows for spontaneous return and spirit transformation.

Translator's note:
Not listed in the *Zhōng Yào Dà Cí Diăn*. The *Běn Căo Gāng Mù* explains that hair is related to the circulation and flourishing of vital fluids, *qì*, and blood, and quotes

the *Sù Wèn*: "The kidney's bloom is in the hair." Lǐ Shí-Zhēn himself explains that hair is the excess of blood and thus suitable for the treatment of blood-related illnesses, for supplementing *yīn*, and for treating fright (《本草綱目》52:1862).

麻布叩幎頭 *má bù kòu fù tóu*
Hempen kòufùtóu

Translator's note:
Not listed in the *Zhōng Yào Dà Cí Diăn*. The exact meaning of the term 叩幎頭 is unknown, but it is clearly a medicinal ingredient made out of hemp cloth. This is most probably related to such characters as 袚 *fú* (knee pad), 複 *fù* (doubled), or 補 *bǔ* (to patch, mend clothes). 叩幎頭 *kòu fù tóu* might therefore refer to some type of padded head covering.

麻黃 *má huáng*
Stalk of Ephedra sinica
Vol. 2, line 21 Middle Grade

味苦，溫，無毒。主中風，傷寒，頭痛，溫瘧，發表出汗，去邪熱氣，止咳逆上氣，除寒熱，破症堅積聚。生川谷。

Flavor: Bitter
Nature: Warm
Toxicity: Non-toxic
Alt. names: 龍沙

Actions and Indications:
Indicated for wind strike, cold damage, headache, and warm malaria.
Effuses the exterior, promotes sweating, removes evil heat *qì*, stops cough with counterflow and ascent of *qì*, eliminates [aversion to] cold and heat [effusion], and breaks up concretions, hardenings, accumulations, and gatherings.

Additional Information:
Grows in valleys with streams.

Translator's note:
Common Name: Ephedra, also called Mormon Tea.
Family: Ephedra (Ephedraceae).
Other species used: Ephedra equisetina or E. intermedia.
《中藥大辭典》#3744.

麻油 *má yóu*
Oil extracted from the seeds of Sesamum indicum

Translator's note:
Common Name: Sesame oil.
Family: Pedalium (Pedaliaceae).
For sesame, most often called 胡麻 *hú má* or 脂麻, 芝麻 *zhī má*, see 《中藥大辭典》#3740 and the entry above on 胡麻 *hú má*, which includes a translation of the relevant passage from the *Shén Nóng Běn Cǎo Jīng*.

麻子仁 *má zǐ rén*
Seed of Cannabis sativa
Vol. 1, line 137 Highest Grade

In the *Shén Nóng Běn Cǎo Jīng*, under the entry for 麻蕡, which according to the commentary is the flower of the plant.

味辛，平，無毒。主五勞七傷，利五臟，下血寒氣。多食，令人見鬼狂走。久服，通神明、輕身。麻子:味甘，平。主補中益氣，肥健、不老、神仙。生川谷。

Flavor: Acrid
Nature: Neutral
Toxicity: Non-toxic
Alt. names: 麻勃

Actions and Indications:
Indicated for the five taxations and seven damages.
Disinhibits the five viscera and precipitates blood and cold *qì*.

Additional Information:
Eaten in profusion, it makes the person see ghosts and run manically.
Taken for a long time, it frees the spirit light and lightens the body.
Hemp seeds: Sweet flavor, neutral nature. Indicated for supplementing the center and boosting *qì*, making the person fat and healthy, preventing aging, and turning the person into a spirit immortal.
Grows in valleys with streams.

Translator's note:
Common Name: Cannabis seed.
Family: Hemp (Cannabaceae).
The plant is more commonly called 大麻 *dà má*.
《中藥大辭典》#0873, where it is listed under 火麻仁 *huǒ má rén*.

馬蹄 *mǎ tí*
Hoof of Equus caballus
Vol. 2, line 80 Middle Grade

In the *Shén Nóng Běn Cǎo Jīng*, under the entry for 白馬莖 (white horse penis).

味咸，平，無毒。主傷中脈絕，陰不起，強志，益氣，長肌肉，肥健，生子。眼，主驚癇，腹滿，瘧疾。懸蹄，主驚邪，瘈瘲，乳難，辟惡氣、鬼毒、蠱注、不祥。生平澤。

Flavor: Salty
Nature: Neutral
Toxicity: Non-toxic
Alt. names: n/a

Actions and Indications:
Indicated for damage to the center, expiry of the pulse, and impotence.
Strengthens the will, boosts *qì*, makes the flesh grow, makes the person fat and healthy, and engenders offspring.

Additional Information:
Eyes: Indicated for fright epilepsy, abdominal fullness, and malaria.
Dewclaws: Indicated for fright evil, tugging and slackening, and lactation difficulties. Repels malign *qì*, ghost toxin, *gǔ* infixation, and inauspicious events.
Lives in flatlandss and marshes.

Translator's note:
Common Name: Horse hoof.
Family: Horse (Equidae).
For the properties of horse in general, see 《中藥大辭典》#3139 on 馬肉 *mǎ ròu*. See also the following entry on 馬蹄底護乾 *mǎ tí dǐ hù gān* (Desiccated protected underside of a horse's hoof), which contains the translation of the *Shén Nóng Běn Cǎo Jīng* passage on "hair, hooves, and nails of the six domestic animals." The *Běn Cǎo Gāng Mù* states that, depending on the condition to be treated, the hooves of both red and white horses are used, e.g. hooves from a red horse for red vaginal discharge and from a white horse for white discharge (《本草綱目》50:1780). 馬蹄 *mǎ tí* is sometimes used as a synonym for 荸薺 *bí qí* (Heleocharis dulcis or water chestnut), but that is highly unlikely given the context here.
《中藥大辭典》#3167, where it is listed as 馬蹄甲 *mǎ tí jiǎ*.

馬蹄底護乾 *mă tí dǐ hù gān*
Desiccated protected underside of the hoof of Equus caballus
Vol. 3, line 79 Lowest Grade

In the *Shén Nóng Běn Căo Jīng*, under the entry for 六畜毛蹄甲 ["hair, hooves, nails of the six domestic animals", i.e. horse, cow, sheep/goat, pig, dog, and chicken].

味咸，平，無毒。主鬼注、蠱毒，寒熱、惊癇，瘈瘲、狂走。駱駝毛，尤良。

Flavor: Salty
Nature: Neutral
Toxicity: Non-toxic
Alt. names: n/a

Actions and Indications:
Indicated for ghost infixation, *gŭ* toxin, [aversion to] cold and heat [effusion], fright epilepsy, derangement, and manic running. Camel hair is particularly good.

Translator's note:
Common Name: Desiccated protected underside of a horse's hoof.
Family: Horse (Equidae).
This is not a common medicinal ingredient and recorded in neither the *Zhōng Yào Dà Cí Diăn* nor the *Běn Căo Gāng Mù*. The entry on horse-based medicinals in the *Běn Căo Gāng Mù* lists "dirt from under the hoof of an east-running horse," which is used in magical prescriptions for finding out a woman's "outside emotions" (i.e., attachments to other men). See 《本草綱目》50:1780.

馬通[汁] *mă tōng [zhī]*
Dung (juice) of Equus caballus

Translator's note:
Common Name: Horse dung (juice).
Family: Horse (Equidae).
《中藥大辭典》#3139 (entry on 馬肉 *mă ròu*) contains a general description of the medicinal uses of Equus caballus of the Horse family (Equidae), but does not mention 馬通 *mă tōng*. The *Běn Căo Gāng Mù* covers the medicinal use of various parts of the horse, including 白馬通 *bái mă tōng* (white horse dung). In general, many parts of the horse, such as the liver, placenta, hoof, hide, mane, and tail, are used for gynecological problems, in particular those from horses of pure white color or from the Northwest. See 《本草綱目》50:1780.

買麻藤 *măi má téng*
Stalk and foliage or root of Gnetum parvifolium

Translator's note:
Common Name: Joint fir.
Family: Gnetum (Gnetaceae).
Other species used: Gnetum montanum 《中藥大辭典》#3993.

麥門冬 *mài mén dōng*
Tuber of Ophiopogon japonicus
Vol. 1, line 32 Highest Grade

味甘，平，無毒。主心腹結氣，傷中、傷飽，胃絡脈絕，羸瘦、短氣。久服，輕身、不老、不飢。生川谷及堤坂肥地石間久廢處。

Flavor: Sweet
Nature: Neutral
Toxicity: Non-toxic
Alt. names: In *Qín* 秦, called 羊韭; In *Qí* 齊, called 愛韭; In *Chŭ* 楚, called 馬韭; In *Yuè* 越, called 羊薺.

Actions and Indications:
Indicated for bound *qì* in the heart and abdomen, damage to the center, damage from overeating, expiry of the stomach channels and network vessels, marked emaciation, and shortness of breath.

Additional Information:
Taken over a long time, it lightens the body and prevents aging and hunger.
Grows in valleys with streams, as well as on embankments, in fertile soil, between rocks and in old wastelands.

Translator's note:
Common Name: Japanese hyacinth tuber.
Family: Lily (Liliaceae).
Other species used: Ophiopogon intermedius as well as several species of Liriope.
《中藥大辭典》#3734.

麥蘗 *mài niè*
Shoots of Hordeum vulgare

Translator's note:
Common Name: Barley sprout.
Family: True Grass (Poaceae).
《中藥大辭典》#3732, where it is listed as 麥芽 *mài yá*.

蔓菁根 *màn jīng gēn*
Root of Brassica rapa

Translator's note:
Common Name: Turnip root.
Family: Mustard (Brassicaceae).
It is more commonly known as 蕪菁 *wú jīng*, under which name it is listed in the *Zhōng Yào Dà Cí Diǎn*, where the tuber as well as the leaves are used. This medicinal needs to be distinguished from 蔓荊子 *màn jīng zǐ*, the fruit of Vitex rotundifolia or V. trifolia of the Mint family (Lamiaceae). See entries on 蕪菁 *wú jīng* and 蕪菁根 *wú jīng gēn* below.
《中藥大辭典》#4933.

硭硝 *máng xiāo*
High-grade hydrated sodium sulfate

Translator's note:
Common Name: Pure mirabilite.
The high-grade processed form of a naturally oc-curing sulfate mineral. It needs to be distinguished from a lower-grade product called 朴硝 *pò xiāo* low-grade sodium sulfate or impure mirabilite, 《中藥大辭典》#1440), as well as the natural unprocessed product, called 寒水石 *hán shuǐ shí* (glauberite). See the entry below on 朴硝 *pò xiāo* for information on that substance as well as for a translation of the relevant entry in the *Shén Nóng Běn Cǎo Jīng*. 硭硝 *máng xiāo* is also commonly called 消石 *xiāo shí* as which it is listed in the *Shén Nóng Běn Cǎo Jīng*. See the entry below on that term for more information, as well as a translation of the relevant passage from the *Shén Nóng Běn Cǎo Jīng*.
《中藥大辭典》#1761, where it is written as 芒消 *máng xiāo*.

梅核仁 *méi hé rén*
Fruit of Prunus mume
Vol. 2, line 106 Middle Grade

In the *Shén Nóng Běn Cǎo Jīng*, under the entry for 梅實.

味酸，平，無毒。主下氣，除熱、煩、滿，安心，止肢体痛，偏枯不仁，死肌，去青黑痣，惡疾。能益氣、不飢。生川谷。

Flavor: Sour
Nature: Neutral
Toxicity: Non-toxic
Alt. names: n/a

Actions and Indications:
Indicated for precipitating *qi*, eliminating heat with vexation and fullness, quieting the heart, and relieving pain in the limbs and trunk.
[Treats] one-sided withering and numbness, and dead flesh, removes green-blue and black hemorrhoids, and malignity disorders.

Additional Information:
Is able to boost *qi* and prevent hunger.
Grows in valleys with streams.

Translator's note:
Common Name: Japanese apricot.
Family: Rose (Rosaceae).
《中藥大辭典》#3328.

虻蟲 *méng chóng*
Dried body of the female of Tabanus bivittatus
Vol. 2, line 102 Middle Grade

In the *Shén Nóng Běn Cǎo Jīng*, under the entry for 蜚虻.

味苦，微寒，有毒。主逐瘀血，破下血積、堅痞症瘕、寒熱，通利血脈及九竅。生川谷。

Flavor: Bitter
Nature: Slightly cold
Toxicity: Toxic
Alt. names: n/a

Actions and Indications:
Indicated for expelling static blood, breaking and pre-cipitating blood accumulations, hardenings, glomus, concretions and conglomerations, for [aversion to] cold and heat [effusion], and for freeing and disinhibit-ing the blood in the channels and the nine orifices.

Additional Information:
Lives in valleys with streams.

蘼蕪 *mí wú*
Foliage and sprout of Ligusticum wallichii
Vol. 1, line 54 Highest Grade

味辛，溫，無毒。主咳逆，定驚氣，辟邪惡，除蠱毒鬼注，去三蟲。久服，通神。生川澤。

Flavor: Acrid
Nature: Warm

Toxicity: Non-toxic
Alt. names: 薇蕪

Actions and Indications:
Indicated for cough with counterflow.
Settles fright *qì*, repels evil and malignity, eliminates *gǔ* toxin and ghost infixation, and removes the three [types of] worms.

Additional Information:
Taken over a long time, it frees the spirit.
Grows in streams and marshes.

Translator's note:
Common Name: Lovage.
Family: Carrot (Apiaceae).
The plant is called 芎藭 *xiōng qióng* or 川芎 *chuān xiōng*. For the root and description of the plant, see 《中藥大辭典》#0540 and the entry on 芎藭 *xiōng qióng* below, which also gives the translation of the *Shén Nóng Běn Cǎo Jīng* entry.
《中藥大辭典》#5651.

米 *mǐ*
Grain of Oryza sativa

Translator's note:
Common Name: Rice.
Family: True Grass (Poaceae).
Common household rice.
In various forms, rice is used as a common medium for ingesting medicine, as in the following compounds: 米粉 *mǐ fěn* (rice flour), 米泔 *mǐ gān* (rice water, i.e., water that rice has been washed in), 米飲 *mǐ yǐn* (rice soup, that is, water in which rice has been cooked), and 米汁 *mǐ zhī* (rice juice, that is, liquid obtained by grinding rice in water).
《中藥大辭典》#4277.

墨 *mò*
Ink

Translator's note:
Manufactured from pine soot, glue, and various additives, its medicinal properties increase with age.
《中藥大辭典》#4699.

牡丹 *mǔ dān*
Bark of the root of Paeonia suffruticosa
Vol. 2, line 54 Middle Grade

味辛，寒，無毒。主寒熱，中風、瘈瘲痙，惊癇邪氣，除症堅，瘀血留舍腸胃，安五臟，療癰創。生山谷。

Flavor: Acrid
Nature: Cold
Toxicity: Non-toxic
Alt. names: 鹿韭, 鼠姑

Actions and Indications:
Indicated for [aversion to] cold and heat [effusion], wind strike, tugging, slackening, and tetany, and evil *qì* of fright epilepsy.
Eliminates concretions and hardenings, and static blood that is lodged in the intestines and stomach, quiets the five viscera, and heals welling-abscess wounds.

Additional Information:
Grows in mountain valleys.

Translator's note:
Common Name: Tree peony root bark.
Family: Buttercup (Ranunculaceae).
Other species used: Paeonia officinalis, P. fruticosa.
It needs to be distinguished from such related species as 白芍 *bái sháo* or 芍藥 *sháo yào* (Paeonia lactiflora/albiflora, white or herbaceous peony), and 赤芍 *chì sháo* (P. rubrae, red peony), each of which have distinct medicinal applications. See respective entries above and below for 芍藥 *sháo yào* and 赤芍 *chì sháo*.
《中藥大辭典》#1729.

牡荊子 *mǔ jīng zǐ*
Fruit of Vitex negundo L. var. cannabifolia
Vol. 1, line 104 Highest Grade

In the *Shén Nóng Běn Cǎo Jīng*, the entry is for 蔓荊實, which is a different, but related medicinal.

味苦，微寒，無毒。主筋骨間寒熱痹、拘攣，明目，堅齒，利九竅，去白蟲。久服，輕身、耐老。小荊實亦等。生山谷。

Flavor: Bitter
Nature: Slightly cold
Toxicity: Non-toxic

Actions and Indications:
Indicated for cold and heat impediment between the sinews and bones, and hypertonicity.
Brightens the eyes, hardens the teeth, disinhibits the

nine orifices, and removes whiteworms.

Additional Information:
Taken for a long time, it lightens the body and allows the person to endure aging.
Small *jīng zǐ* is also equal.
Grows in mountain valleys.

Translator's note:
Common Name: Hemp-leaved vitex seed.
Family: Mint (Laminaceae).
牡荊子 *mǔ jīng zǐ* is related to the chaste tree (Vitex agnus) and to be distinguished from 蔓荊子 *màn jīng zǐ* (Vitex rotundifolia or V. trifolia), a common herb for treating colds and flues in modern TCM that is usually translated as vitex.
《中藥大辭典》#1732.

牡蛎 *mǔ lì*
Shell of Ostrea rivularis
Vol. 1, line 124 Highest Grade

味咸，平，無毒。主傷寒寒熱，溫瘧洒洒，惊恚
怒氣，除拘緩鼠瘻，女子帶下赤白。久服，強骨
節、殺邪氣、延年。生池澤。

Flavor: Salty
Nature: Neutral
Toxicity: Non-toxic
Alt. names: 蠣蛤

Actions and Indications:
Indicated for cold damage with [aversion to] cold and heat [effusion], warm malaria with shivering, and for fright, hate, and anger *qì*.
Eliminates hypertonicity and slackening, mouse fistula, and women's vaginal discharge in red or white.

Additional Information:
Taken for a long time, it strengthens the bones and joints, kills evil *qì*, and extends the years.
Grows in ponds and marshes.

Translator's note:
Common Name: Oyster shell.
Family: Oyster (Ostreidae).
Other species used: Ostrea gigas, O. talienwhanensis.
《中藥大辭典》#1728.

牡蒙 *mǔ méng*
Root of Paris quadrifolia
Vol. 2, line 42 Middle Grade

In the *Shén Nóng Běn Cǎo Jīng*, under the entry for 紫参.

味苦，辛，寒，無毒。主心腹積聚，寒熱邪氣，
通九竅，利大小便。治牛病。生山谷。

Flavor: Bitter, acrid
Nature: Cold
Toxicity: Non-toxic
Alt. names: 牡蒙

Actions and Indications:
Indicated for accumulations and gatherings in the heart and abdomen, and for evil *qì* of cold or heat.
Frees the nine orifices and disinhibits urination and defecation.

Additional Information:
Treats cattle diseases.
Grows in mountain valleys.

Translator's note:
Common Name: Four-leaved paris root.
Family: Lily (Liliaceae).
Other species used: Paris verticillata.
In modern TCM, it is usually called 王孫 *wáng sūn*, but it was in earlier times often called 牡蒙 *mǔ méng*, including by such authorities as Táo Hóng-Jǐng.
《中藥大辭典》#0947.

木防己 *mù fáng jǐ*
Root of Cocculus trilobus

Translator's note:
Common Name: Southeast Asian fish berry.
Family: Moonseed (Menispermaceae).
Sometimes used in place of 防己 *fáng jǐ* (Root of Aristolochia fangchi) (《中藥大辭典》#1824).

牛旁 *niú bàng*
Root of Arctium lappa

Translator's note:
Common Name: Burdock root.
Family: Aster (Asteraceae). For information on the fruit, see the entry on 蝙蝠刺 *biān fú cì* (Fruit of Arctium lappa) above. The root is also called 黍粘根 *shǔ nián gēn* (see entry below).
《中藥大辭典》#0928.

牛角䰓 *niú jiǎo sāi*
Ossified marrow in the center of the horn of Bos taurus domesticus
Vol. 2, line 82 Middle Grade

溫，無毒。下閉血，瘀血疼痛，女人帶下血。
髓，補中，填骨髓，久服，增年。膽，治驚，寒
熱。可丸藥。

Flavor: n/a
Nature: Warm
Toxicity: Non-toxic
Alt. names: n/a

Actions and Indications:
Precipitates blocked blood, static blood with pain, and women's vaginal discharge and bleeding.

Additional Information:
Marrow: Supplements the center and banks up the bones and marrow. Taken for a long time, in increases the years.
Gallbladder: Treats fright and [aversion to] cold and heat [effusion]. It can be prepared as pill medicine.

Translator's note:
Common Name: Ox horn marrow.
Family: Bovine (Bovidae).
Other species used: Bubalus bubalis (water buffalo).
For a description of the animal, see 《中藥大辭典》 #0881 (entry on 牛肉 *niú ròu*, beef). According to Táo Hóng-Jīng, marrow being the essence of the horn, it is appropriate for conditions of *yīn* shortage and women's vaginal bleeding. In one instance, Sūn Sī-Miǎo refers to it also as 牛角中仁 *niú jiǎo zhōng rén* (ox horn core).
《中藥大辭典》 #0921.

牛乳 *niú rǔ*
Milk of Bos taurus domesticus

Translator's note:
Common Name: Cow's milk.
Family: Bovine (Bovidae).
Other species used: Bubalus bubalis (water buffalo).
Not listed in the Zhōng Yào Dà Cí Diǎn, Běn Cǎo Gāng Mù or Shén Nóng Běn Cǎo Jīng.
《中藥大辭典》 #0885.

牛屎 *niú shǐ*
Excrement of Bos taurus domesticus

Translator's note:
Common Name: Cow dung.
Family: Bovine (Bovidae).
Other species used: Bubalus bubalis (water buffalo).
Not listed in the Zhōng Yào Dà Cí Diǎn, Běn Cǎo Gāng Mù or Shén Nóng Běn Cǎo Jīng.

牛膝 *niú xī*
Root of Achyranthes bidentata
Vol. 1, line 27 Highest Grade

味苦，平，無毒。主寒濕痿痹，四肢拘攣，膝痛
不可屈伸。逐血氣，傷熱，火爛，墮胎。久服，
輕身、耐老。生川谷。

Flavor: Bitter
Nature: Neutral
Toxicity: Non-toxic
Alt. names: 百倍

Actions and Indications:
Indicated for wind-damp wilting and impediment, hypertonicity of the four extremities, and knee pain and inability to bend or stretch the knees.
Expels blood and *qì* [and treats] heat damage, fire erosion, and miscarriage.

Additional Information:
Taken over a long time, it lightens the body and allows the person to endure aging.
Grows in valleys with streams.

Translator's note:
Common Name: Achyranthes root.
Family: Amaranth (Amaranthaceae).
《中藥大辭典》 #0897.

女青 *nǚ qīng*
Unknown
Vol. 3, line 47 Lowest Grade

味辛，平，有毒。主蠱毒，逐邪惡氣，殺鬼，溫
瘧，辟不祥。生山谷。

Flavor: Acrid
Nature: Neutral
Toxicity: Toxic
Alt. names: 雀瓢

Actions and Indications:
Indicated for *gǔ* toxin, expelling evil and malign *qì*, killing ghosts, warm malaria, and for repelling inauspicious things.

Additional Information:
Grows in mountain valleys.

Translator's note:
Plant of unknown identity, but most likely a close relative of or synonym for 蘿藦 *luó mó* (Metaplexis japonica of the Milkweed family, Asclepiadaceae, which is now often subsumed under the Dogbane family. This plant is also called 白環藤 *bái huán téng* and is listed in 《中藥大辭典》 #5653. According to the *Shén Nóng Běn Cǎo Jīng*, 女青 *nǚ qīng* is also called 雀藤 *què téng* ("sparrow vine"), but the identity of this plant was debated already during Táo Hóng-Jīng's time. He cites three theories: 1. that it is identical with 蘿藦 *luó mó*, 2. that it is a plant very similar to 蘿藦 *luó mó*, and 3. that it is a name for the root of 蛇含 *shé hán* (Potentilla kleiniana of the Rose family, Rosaceae; 《中藥大辭典》 #3498). According to Táo, the description of the plant, however, contradicts any identification with 蛇含 *shé hán*, both in terms of the appearance of the plant, as well as the growing area and the plant parts used medicinally. Moreover, its offensive odor again strongly suggests a close relation with other plants of the Milkweed family, many of which produce offensive odors, such as carrion flower (Stapelia or Huernia). It is probably for this reason that the *Zhōng Yào Dà Cí Diǎn* lists it as a synonym for 雞屎藤 *jī shǐ téng* (Paederia scandens, a type of liana with a fecal smell, of the Madder family; 《中藥大辭典》 #5578). Lǐ Shí-Zhēn diplomatically explains that 女青 *nǚ qīng* refers to two plants, either a vine similar to 蘿藦 *luó mó*, or the root of 蛇含 *shé hán* (《本草綱目》 16:489, where it is listed right after 蛇含). Both Read and the *Zhōng Huá Běn Cǎo* list it as either Cynanchum sibiricum or Paederia tomentosa/scandens (Read, *Chinese Medicinal Plants, Botanical, Chemical and Pharmacological Reference List*, #164 and #87; 《中華本草》 #5818 and #5668).

女萎 *nǚ wěi*
Stalk of Clematis apiifolia
Vol. 1, line 29 Highest Grade

味甘，平，無毒。主中風暴熱，不能動搖，跌筋結肉，諸不足。久服，去面黑，好顏色、潤澤、輕身、不老。生山谷及丘陵。

Flavor: Sweet
Nature: Neutral
Toxicity: Non-toxic
Alt. names: 左眄，玉竹

Actions and Indications:
Indicated for wind strike with fulminant heat, inability to move and shake, bound flesh from falling on the sinews, and all insufficiencies.

Additional Information:
Taken over a long time, it removes blackness in the face, improves facial complexion by making it moist and lustrous, lightens the body, and prevents aging. Grows in mountain valleys and on hills.

Translator's note:
Common Name: October clematis stalk.
Family: Buttercup (Ranunculaceae).
《中藥大辭典》 #0314.

弩弦 *nǔ xián*
Bowstring

Translator's note:
Not listed in the *Zhōng Yào Dà Cí Diǎn*. The *Běn Cǎo Gāng Mù* explains that the string is made from silk and is used for stalled labor because of its association with speed, to stop bleeding by breaking the bow and string, and to ensure male offspring because of its association with maleness (《本草綱目》 38:1415, where it is listed as 弓弩弦 *gōng nǔ xián*).

糯米 *nuò mǐ*
Grain of Oryza glutinosa

Translator's note:
Common Name: Glutinous rice.
Family: True Grass (Poaceae).
Not listed in the *Zhōng Yào Dà Cí Diǎn*.

藕 *ǒu*
Large rhizome of Nelumbo nucifera
Vol. 1, line 131 Highest Grade

In the *Shén Nóng Běn Cǎo Jīng*, the entry is for 藕實莖 (stalk of the lotus fruit).

味甘，平，無毒。主補中養神，益氣力，除百疾。久服，輕身、耐老、不飢、延年。生池澤。

Flavor: Sweet
Nature: Neutral
Toxicity: Non-toxic

Alt. names: 水芝丹

Actions and Indications:
Indicated for supplementing the center and nourishing the spirit, boosting *qì* and strength, and eliminating the hundred diseases.

Additional Information:
Taken for a long time, it lightens the body, allows the person to endure aging, prevents hunger, and extends the years.
Grows in ponds and marshes.

Translator's note:
Common Name: Rhizome of Egyptian bean, sacred lotus or Chinese arrowroot.
Family: Lotus (Nelumbonaceae).
Used fresh (生 *shēng*) or cooked (熟 *shú*).
《中藥大辭典》#5339.

砒石 *pī shí*
Arsenic

Translator's note:
《中藥大辭典》#2469.

砒霜 *pī shuāng*
Sublimed arsenic

Translator's note:
《中藥大辭典》#2470.

朴消 *pò xiāo*
Low-grade hydrated sodium sulfate
Vol. 1, line 7 Highest Grade

味苦，寒，無毒。主百病，除寒熱邪氣，逐六腑積聚，結固留癖，能化七十二种石。煉餌服之，輕身神仙。生山谷。

Flavor: Bitter
Nature: Cold
Toxicity: Non-toxic
Alt. names: n/a

Actions and Indications:
Indicated for the hundred diseases.
Eliminates the evil *qì* of cold and heat, expels accumulations and gatherings in the six bowels, and bound,

fixed, abiding aggregations.

Additional Information:
It is able to transform the 72 types of stones.
Taken as an alchemical preparation, it lightens the body and turns the person into a spirit immortal.
Grows in mountain valleys.

Translator's note:
Common Name: Impure mirabilite.
This is the low-grade processed form of a naturally occuring sulfate mineral. It needs to be distinguished from the high-grade refined product called 砭硝 *máng xiāo*, as well as from 寒水石 *hán shuǐ shí* (glauberite, sodium calcium sulfate). Note the pronunciation of 朴 as *pò* in a medicinal context.
《中藥大辭典》#1440.

蒲黃 *pú huáng*
Pollen of Typha angustata
Vol. 1, line 61 Highest Grade

味甘，平，無毒。主心腹膀胱寒熱，利小便，止血，消瘀血。久服，輕身、益氣力，延年、神仙。生池澤。

Flavor: Sweet
Nature: Neutral
Toxicity: Non-toxic
Alt. names: n/a

Actions and Indications:
Indicated for cold or heat in the heart, abdomen, and bladder.
Disinhibits urine, stanches bleeding, and disperses static blood.

Additional Information:
Taken over a long time, it lightens the body, boosts *qì* and strength, extends the years, and [turns the person into] a spirit immortal.
Grows in ponds and marshes.

Translator's note:
Common Name: Typha pollen.
Family: Bulrush (Typhaceae).
Other species used: Typha angustifolia.
《中藥大辭典》#4568.

蠐螬 *qí cáo*
Dried larva of Holotrichia diomphalia
Vol. 2, line 94 Middle Grade

味咸，微溫，有毒。主惡血、血瘀，痹氣，破折，血在脅下堅滿痛，月閉，目中淫膚，青翳白膜。生平澤及人家積糞草中。

Flavor: Salty
Nature: Slightly warm
Toxicity: Toxic
Alt. names: 蟦蠐

Actions and Indications:
Indicated for malign blood, blood stasis, impediment *qi*, breaks and fractures, blood below the rib-side with hardenings, fullness, and pain, menstrual block, and for oozing skin, green-blue screens, and opaque films in the eyes.

Additional Information:
Lives in flatlands and marshes and in grass growing on people's night soil piles.

Translator's note:
Common Name: Korean black chafer.
Family: Scarab Beetle (Scarabaeidae).
In English, 蠐螬 *qí cáo* is often referred to as June beetle grub, but June beetle should more correctly refer to several species of Phyllophagon.
《中藥大辭典》 #5442.

牽牛子 *qiān niú zǐ*
Seed of Pharbitis nil

Translator's note:
Common Name: Morning glory seed.
Family: Morning Glory (Convolvulaceae).
Other species used: Pharbitis purpurea, Ipomoea nil.
《中藥大辭典》 #3366.

前胡 *qián hú*
Root of Peucedanum praeruptorum

Translator's note:
Common Name: Peucedanum root.
Family: Carrot (Apiaceae).
Other species used: Peucedanum decursivum.
Closely related to Foeniculum vulgare, (common fennel), this plant is also called hog fennel or sulfurweed.
《中藥大辭典》 #2287.

薔薇根皮 *qiáng wēi gēn pí*
Bark of the root of Rosa multiflora

Translator's note:
Common Name: Multiflora rose root bark.
Family: Rose (Rosaceae). For a description of the plant, see 《中藥大辭典》 #5138 on 薔薇花 *qiáng wēi huā* (multiflora rose).
《中藥大辭典》 #5139.

秦艽 *qín jiāo*
Root of Gentiana macrophylla
Vol. 2, line 27 Middle Grade

味苦，平，無毒。主寒熱邪氣，寒濕風痺，肢節痛，下水，利小便。生山谷。

Flavor: Bitter
Nature: Neutral
Toxicity: Non-toxic
Alt. names: 秦瓜

Actions and Indications:
Indicated for evil *qi* from cold and heat, for cold-damp-wind impediment, and for pain in the joints of the limbs.
Precipitates water and disinhibits urine.

Additional Information:
Grows in mountain valleys.

Translator's note:
Common Name: Large gentian root.
Family: Gentian (Gentianaceae).
Other species used: Gentiana crassicaulis, G. tibetica.
《中藥大辭典》 #3015.

秦椒 *qín jiāo*
Seed capsule of Zanthoxylum bungeanum
Vol. 2, line 71 Middle Grade

味辛，溫，有毒。主風邪氣，溫中，除寒痺，堅齒髮、明目。久服，輕身、好顏色、耐老、增年、通神。生川谷。

Flavor: Acrid
Nature: Warm
Toxicity: Toxic
Alt. names: n/a

Actions and Indications:
Indicated for wind evil *qi*, warming the center, and

eliminating cold impediment.
Hardens the teeth and hair of the head and brightens the eyes.

Additional Information:
Taken for a long time, it lightens the body, improves facial complexion, allows the person to endure aging, increases the years, and frees the spirit.
Grows in valleys with streams.

Translator's note:
Common Name: Shǎn-Xī zanthoxylum seed.
Family: Rue (Rutaceae).
More commonly referred to as 花椒 *huā jiāo*. Since Z. bungeanum grows in western China, it seems likely that Sūn Sī-Miǎo was referring to this species. In modern usage, 秦椒 *qín jiāo* mostly refers to a completely different plant, Capsicum frutescens of the Nightshade family (Solanaceae), the hot garden pepper native to the Americas, which is also referred to as 辣椒 *là jiāo* (《中藥大辭典》# 4624). Moreover, 秦椒 *qín jiāo* needs to be distinguished from 蜀椒 *shǔ jiāo* (Sì-Chuān zanthoxylum), which is also used by Sūn Sī-Miǎo and probably refers to another species of prickly ash that is native to Sì-Chuān. The *Zhōng Yào Dà Cí Diǎn* gives both 蜀椒 *shǔ jiāo* and 秦椒 *qín jiāo* as synonyms for 花椒 *huā jiāo*, which it identifies as Zanthoxylum bungeanum.
《中藥大辭典》#2084.

犊牛屎 *qín niú shǐ*
Qín buffalo dung

Translator's note:
Not listed in the *Zhōng Yào Dà Cí Diǎn*. The *Běn Cǎo Gāng Mù* explains in the entry on buffalo: "The Southern buffalo is called 㹀 *wú* and the Northern buffalo 秦 *qín*." It further explains: "There are two types of buffalo, the *qín* and the water buffalo. The *qín* buffalo is small and the water buffalo is big" (《本草綱目》50:1779).

秦皮 *qín pí*
Bark of the trunk of Fraxinus rhunchophylla
Vol. 2, line 70 Middle Grade

味苦，微寒，無毒。主風寒濕痹，洒洒寒氣，除熱，目中青翳、白膜。久服，頭不白、輕身。生川谷。

Flavor: Bitter
Nature: Slightly cold
Toxicity: Non-toxic
Alt. names: n/a

Actions and Indications:
Indicated for wind-cold-damp impediment, shivering with cold *qì*, for eliminating heat, and for green-blue screens and opaque films in the eyes.

Additional Information:
Taken for a long time, it prevents balding of the head and lightens the body.
Grows in valleys with streams.

Translator's note:
Common Name: Ash bark.
Family: Olive (Oleaceae).
Other species used: Fraxinus bungeana or F. paxiana.
《中藥大辭典》#3014.

清酒 *qīng jiǔ*
Clear liquor

Translator's note:
A pure aged liquor, traditionally used for sacrificing to the spirits (楊吉成, 編者《中國飲食辭典》p. 260).

青牛膽 *qīng niú dǎn*
Green cow bile

Translator's note:
According to the *Zhōng Yào Dà Cí Diǎn*, it is either prepared by drying the gallbladder after butchering the cow, or by removing the liquid from the gallbladder and storing it in a tightly sealed container. Alternatively, the gallbladder can be dry-roasted over heat.
《中藥大辭典》#0900 on 牛膽 *niú dǎn*.

青竹 *qīng zhú*
Phyllostachys

Translator's note:
Common Name: Green bamboo.
Family: True Grass (Poaceae).
The bark (青竹皮 *qīng zhú pí*) and shavings (青竹茹 *qīng zhú rú*) are used medicinally. 青竹 *qīng zhú* is apparently used interchangeably with 淡竹 *dàn zhú* (bland bamboo), but needs to be distinguished from 甘竹 *gān zhú* (sweet bamboo). For a description of the

varieties of bamboo, see the entry below on 竹 *zhú*.

瞿麥 *qú mài*
Entire plant, including flowers, of Dianthus superbus
Vol. 2, line 25 Middle Grade

味苦，寒，無毒。主關格，諸癃結，小便不通，
出刺，決癰腫，明目去翳，破胎墮子，下閉血。
生川谷。

Flavor: Bitter
Nature: Cold
Toxicity: Non-toxic
Alt. names: 巨句麥

Actions and Indications:
Indicated for block and repulsion, all urinary dribbling
block and binding, and stopped urination.
Removes thorns, bursts welling-abscesses, brightens
the eyes and removes screens, breaks the fetus and
aborts the child, and precipitates blocked blood.

Additional Information:
Grows in valleys with streams.

Translator's note:
Common Name: Dianthus.
Family: Pink (Caryophyllaceae).
Other species used: Dianthus chinensis (rainbow, or
China pink).
《中藥大辭典》#5220.

犬卵 *quǎn luǎn*
Testicles of Canis familiaris
Vol. 2, line 84 Middle Grade

In the *Shén Nóng Běn Cǎo Jīng*, under the entry for
牡狗阴莖 ("male dog's penis").

味咸，平，無毒。主傷中，陰痿不起，令強、
熱、大、生子，除女子帶下十二疾。膽主明目。

Flavor: Salty
Nature: Neutral
Toxicity: Non-toxic
Alt. names: 狗精

Actions and Indications:
Indicated for damage of the center and *yīn* wilt and
impotence.
Causes strength, heat, and largeness, and engenders
children.

Expels women's twelve disorders of vaginal discharge.

Additional Information:
The gallbladder is indicated for brightening the eyes.

Translator's note:
Common Name: Dog testicles.
Family: Canine (Canidae).
Listed in the *Zhōng Yào Dà Cí Diǎn* as 牧狗陰莖 *mù
gǒu yīn jīng*. For a description of the medicinal properties of dog in general, see 《中藥大辭典》#2020.
《中藥大辭典》#1741

鵲重巢柴 *què chóng cháo chái*
Twigs from a nest of Pica pica serica

Translator's note:
Common Name: Twigs from a twice-used magpie
nest.
Family: Crow (Corvidae).
Chinese magpie nest that has been used for two
years in a row. Not listed in the *Zhōng Yào Dà Cí
Diǎn*, but entry #5382 on 鵲肉 *què ròu* (magpie meat)
gives a description of the animal. The *Běn Cǎo Gāng
Mù* explains 重巢 *chóng cháo* as a nest in which
birds have repeatedly raised offspring (《本草綱
目》49:1756). See also Sūn Sī-Miǎo's explanation
in the Qiān Jīn Fāng: "A twice-used nest is a nest
in which a magpie gave birth the year before and in
which she has given birth again in the current year" (
《千金方》4.3.63).

人參 *rén shēn*
Root of Panax ginseng
Vol. 1, line 21 Highest Grade

味甘，微寒，無毒。主補五臟，安精神，定魂
魄，止惊悸，除邪氣，明目、開心、益智。久
服，輕身、延年。生山谷。

Flavor: Sweet
Nature: Slightly cold
Toxicity: Non-toxic
Alt. names: 人銜，鬼蓋

Actions and Indications:
Indicated for supplementing the five viscera, quieting
the essence spirit, settling the ethereal and corporeal
souls, checking fright palpitations, eliminating evil *qì*,
brightening the eyes, opening the heart, and boosting
wisdom.

Additional Information:

Taken over a long time, it lightens the body and extends the years.
Grows in mountain valleys.

Translator's note:
Common Name: Ginseng root.
Family: Ivy (Araliaceae).
《中藥大辭典》#1496.

人屎 *rén shǐ*
Human feces

Translator's note:
Not listed in the *Zhōng Yào Dà Cí Diǎn*. See 《本草綱目》52:1868.

人乳汁 *rén rǔ zhī*
Human breast milk

Translator's note:
《中藥大辭典》#0064 and 《本草綱目》52:1875.

戎鹽 *róng yán*
Halite
Vol. 3, line 6 Lowest Grade

主明目、目痛，益氣、堅肌骨，去毒蠱。大鹽，
令人吐。鹵鹽，味苦，寒，主大熱，消渴狂煩，
除邪及下蠱毒，柔肌膚。生鹽澤。

Toxicity: n/a
Alt. names: 寒石

Actions and Indications:
Indicated for brightening the eyes, eye pain, for boosting *qì*, hardening the flesh and bones, and removing toxic *gǔ*.

Additional Information:
Crude salt makes a person vomit.
Alkali is bitter in flavor and cold in nature. It is indicated for great heat, for dispersion thirst with mania and vexation, for eliminating evil and precipitating *gǔ* toxin, and for softening the flesh and skin.
Grows in salt flats.

Translator's note:
Common Name: Common or rock salt.
《中藥大辭典》#1430.

肉蓯蓉 *ròu cōng róng*
Fleshy stalk of Cistanche salsa
Vol. 1, line 59 Highest Grade

味甘，微溫，無毒。主五勞七傷，補中，除莖中
寒熱痛，養五臟，強陰，益精氣，多子，婦人症
瘕。久服，輕身。生山谷。

Flavor: Sweet
Nature: Slightly warm
Toxicity: Non-toxic
Alt. names: n/a

Actions and Indications:
Indicated for the five taxation and seven damages. Supplements the center, eliminates cold and heat pain inside the penis, nourishes the five viscera, strengthens *yīn*, boosts essence *qì*, increases fertility, and [treats] women's concretions and conglomerations.

Additional Information:
Taken for a long time, it lightens the body.
Grows in mountain valleys.

Translator's note:
Common Name: Cistanche.
Family: Broomrape (Orobanchaceae).
Other species used: Cistanche deserticola, C. ambigua. See also the entry on 蓯蓉 *cōng róng* above.
《中藥大辭典》#1583.

乳床 *rǔ chuáng*
Rǔchuáng

Translator's note:
No similar medicinal is found in any major materia medica work. My best guess is that it might be a scribal error, possibly for 乳香 *rǔ xiāng*, frankincense, the fragrant rosin from Boswellia carterii of the Torchwood family (Burseraceae). This identification seems particularly likely in the current context since frankincense is classified as warming and is known, among other effects, to harmonize *qì*, enliven blood, expel toxins, and treat congealed and stopped *qì* and blood, swellings, painful menstruation, and postpartum blocked blood with stabbing pain.
《中藥大辭典》#1829 for 乳香 *rǔ xiāng*.

桑白皮 *sāng bái pí*
Bark of the root of Morus alba

Translator's note:
Common Name: Mulberry root bark.

Family: Mulberry (Moraceae).
For a general description of mulberry, see 《中藥大辭典》#2863 on 桑葉 *sāng yè*.
《中藥大辭典》 #2868.

桑耳 *sāng ěr*
Auricularia auricula, growing on Morus alba
Vol. 2, line 63 Middle Grade

In the *Shén Nóng Běn Cǎo Jīng*, under the entry for 桑根白皮 (white bark of mulberry root).

味甘，寒，無毒。主傷中、五勞六极、羸瘦，崩中，脈絕，補虛益氣。葉主除寒熱出汗。桑耳黑者主女子漏下赤白汁，血病，症瘕積聚，陰痛，陰瘍寒熱，無子。五木耳名檽，益氣、不飢、輕身、強志。生山谷。

Flavor: Sweet
Nature: Cold
Toxicity: Non-toxic
Alt. names: n/a

Actions and Indications:
Indicated for damage to the center, the five taxations and six extremes, marked emaciation, center flooding, and expiry of the pulse.
Supplements vacuity and boosts *qì*.

Additional Information:
Leaves: Indicated for eliminating cold and heat by inducing sweating.
Black mulberry wood ear: Indicated for women's vaginal spotting of red and white fluid, diseases of the blood, concretions, conglomerations, accumulations, and gatherings, genital pain, genital sores with [aversion to] cold and heat [effusion], and infertility.
The five types of wood ear are called *rú* and boost *qì*, prevent hunger, lighten the body, and strengthen the will.
Grows in mountain valleys.

Translator's note:
A type of wood ear (木耳 *mù ěr*, Auricularia auricula, also called tree ear) that grows on the stem of the mulberry tree (Morus alba of the Mulberry family, Moraceae).
For a general description of 木耳 *mù ěr*, see 《中藥大辭典》 #0682.
《中藥大辭典》 #2857.

桑寄生 *sāng jì shēng*
Branches and foliage of Viscum coloratum
Vol. 1, line 106 Highest Grade

In the *Shén Nóng Běn Cǎo Jīng*, under the entry for 桑上寄生.

味苦，平，無毒。主腰痛，小儿背強，癰腫，安胎，充肌膚，堅發齒，長須眉。其實，明目、輕身、通神。生川谷。

Flavor: Bitter
Nature: Neutral
Toxicity: Non-toxic
Alt. names: 寄屑，寓木，宛童

Actions and Indications:
Indicated for lumbar pain, small children's rigidity in the back, and welling-abscess swelling.
Quiets the fetus, fills the flesh, hardens the hair on the head and teeth, and makes the beard and eyebrows grow long.

Additional Information:
The fruit brightens the eyes, lightens the body, and frees the spirit.
Grows in valleys with streams.

Translator's note:
Common Name: Mistletoe.
Family: Sandalwood (Santalaceae).
Other species used: Loranthus parasiticus (Taxillus chinensis), L. gracilifolius, or L. yadoriki (T. sutchuensensis).
Literally "mulberry parasite."
《中藥大辭典》 #2871.

桑螵蛸 *sāng piāo xiāo*
Cocoon-like egg capsules of Paratenodera sinensis
Vol. 1, line 126 Highest Grade

味咸，平，無毒。主傷中，疝瘕，陰痿，益精生子，女子血閉腰痛，通五淋，利小便水道。生桑枝上。采，蒸之。

Flavor: Salty
Nature: Neutral
Toxicity: Non-toxic
Alt. names: 蝕疣

Actions and Indications:
Indicated for damage to the center, mounting-conglomerations, and *yīn* wilt.
Boosts essence and fertility, [treats] women's and girls blood blockage with lumbar pain, frees the five types

of strangury, and disinhibits urine and the water ways.

Additional Information:
Lives on top of mulberry branches.
After picking, steam it.

Translator's note:
Common Name: Mantis eggcase.
Family: Praying Mantis (Mantidae).
Other species used: Statilia maculata, Mantis religiosa, Hierodula patellifera, or Paratenodera augustipennis. 《中藥大辭典》#2875.

桑蝎蟲矢 *sāng xiē chóng shǐ*
Mulberry worm excrement

Translator's note:
Not listed in the *Zhōng Yào Dà Cí Diǎn* or *Běn Cǎo Gāng Mù*. Both sources do, however, list 桑蠹蟲 *sāng dù chóng*, the larvae of such wood-boring beetles as Anoplophora chinensis or Apriona germari of the Longhorn beetles family (Cerambycidae). This substance is also called 桑木中蝎屎 *sāng mù zhōng yì shǐ*. See 《中藥大辭典》#2876, which gives 桑蝎蟲 *sāng xiē chóng* as a synonym.

沙參 *shā shēn*
Root of Adenophora tetraphylla
Vol. 1, line 79 Highest Grade

味苦，微寒，無毒。主血積惊氣，除寒熱，補中，益肺氣。久服，利人。生川谷。

Flavor: Bitter
Nature: Slightly cold
Toxicity: Non-toxic
Alt. names: 知母

Actions and Indications:
Indicated for blood accumulations and fright *qì*.
Eliminates cold and heat, supplements the center, and boosts lung *qì*.

Additional Information:
Taken for a long time, it benefits/disinhibits the person. Grows in valleys with streams.

Translator's note:
Common Name: Adenophora root.
Family: Bellflower (Campanulaceae).
Other species used: Adenophora axilliflora and several other related species.
It is commonly called 南沙參 *nán shā shēn* ("southern adenophora") in order to distinguish it from 北沙參

běi shā shēn ("northern adenophora"), which refers to glehnia root of the Carrot family (Apiaceae). In English, 沙參 *shā shēn* is sometimes erroneously translated as "glehnia root" or read as a reference to either of these plants. Nevertheless, in the *Zhōng Yào Dà Cí Diǎn*, 沙參 *shā shēn* is used only as a reference to adenophora, while glehnia is always referred to with the prefix 北 *běi* (northern). For 北沙參 *běi shā shēn*, see 《中藥大辭典》#0980. In addition, the root of adenophora is sometimes incorrectly called 知母 *zhī mǔ*, which should refer to Anemarrhena asphodeloides of the Lily family (Liliaceae) instead (see 《中藥大辭典》#2052 and entry on 知母 *zhī mǔ* in this appendix). 《中藥大辭典》#2300.

山驢角 *shān lǘ jiǎo*
Horn of Capricornis sumatraensis

Translator's note:
Common Name: Serow's horn.
Family: Bovine (Bovidae).
According to the *Zhōng Yào Dà Cí Diǎn*, it is sometimes erroneously identified with 山羊 *shān yáng* (Naemorhedus, Goral). The *Běn Cǎo Gāng Mù* notes that 山驢 *shān lǘ* is a wild donkey with horns similar to antelope horns that may be used as a substitute for the more expensive 羚羊 *líng yáng*, antelope horn (《本草綱目》 51:, entry on 羚羊). 《中藥大辭典》#0510.

山茱萸 *shān zhū yú*
Fruit of Cornus officinalis
Vol. 2, line 72 Middle Grade

味酸，平，無毒。主心下邪氣，寒熱，溫中，逐寒濕痹，去三蟲。久服，輕身。生山谷。

Flavor: Sour
Nature: Neutral
Toxicity: Non-toxic
Alt. names: 蜀棗

Actions and Indications:
Indicated for evil *qì* below the heart, [aversion to] cold and heat [effusion], for warming the center, expelling cold-damp impediment, and removing the three types of worms.

Additional Information:
Taken for a long time, it lightens the body.
Grows in mountain valleys.

Translator's note:
Common Name: Japanese cornel, cornus, dogwood

fruit.
Family: Dogwood (Cornaceae).
《中藥大辭典》#0469.

商陸 *shāng lù*
Root of Phytolacca acinosa
Vol. 3, line 40 Lowest Grade

味辛，平，有毒。主水脹、疝瘕、痺，熨除癰
腫，殺鬼精物。生川谷。

Flavor: Acrid
Nature: Neutral
Toxicity: Toxic
Alt. names: 葛根, 夜呼

Actions and Indications:
Indicated for water distention, mounting-conglomerations, and impediment.
As a hot compress, it eliminates welling-abscess
swelling and kills ghost and spectral things.

Additional Information:
Grows in valleys with streams.

Translator's note:
Common Name: Phytolacca root.
Family: Pokeweed (Phytolaccaceae).
In the *Ishimpô*, this drug is called 常陸根 *cháng lù
gēn*.
《中藥大辭典》#3263.

芍藥 *sháo yào*
Root of Paeonia albiflora
Vol. 2, line 23 Middle Grade

味苦，平，有小毒。主邪氣腹痛，除血痺，破堅
積、寒熱、疝瘕，止痛，利小便，益氣。生川谷
及丘陵。

Flavor: Bitter
Nature: Neutral
Toxicity: Slightly toxic.
Alt. names: n/a

Actions and Indications:
Indicated for evil *qi* with abdominal pain.
Eliminates blood impediment, breaks hard accumulations, cold and heat, and mounting-conglomerations,
relieves pain, disinhibits urine, and boosts *qi*.

Additional Information:
Grows in valleys with streams and on hills.

Translator's note:
Common Name: Peony root.
Family: Buttercup (Ranunculaceae).
Other species used: Paeonia lactiflora.
Also known as 白芍 *bái sháo*.
It needs to be distinguished from the related species
牡丹 *mǔ dān* (moutan, Paeonia suffruticosa) and 赤芍
chì sháo (red peony, Paeonia rubrae).
《中藥大辭典》#1118.

蛇床子 *shé chuáng zǐ*
Fruit of Cnidium monnieri
Vol. 1, line 74 Highest Grade

味苦，平，無毒。主婦人陰中腫痛，男子陰痿、
濕痒，除痺氣，利關節，癲癇惡創。久服，輕
身。生川谷及田野。

Flavor: Bitter
Nature: Neutral
Toxicity: Non-toxic
Alt. names: 蛇米

Actions and Indications:
Indicated for women's swelling and pain in the genitals and men's *yīn* wilt (i.e. impotence) and damp itch.
Eliminates impediment *qi*, disinhibits the joints, and
[treats] withdrawal and epilepsy and malign wounds.

Additional Information:
Taken for a long time, it lightens the body.
Grows in valleys with streams and open fields.

Translator's note:
Common Name: Cnidium seed.
Family: Carrot (Apiaceae).
Other species used: Ligusticum monnieri or Selinum
monnieri.
《中藥大辭典》#3507.

蛇蛻皮 *shé tuì pí*
Sloughed snake skin from
Elaphe taeniurus
Vol. 3, line 82 Lowest Grade

味鹹，平，無毒。主小兒百二十种惊癇、瘛瘲、
癲疾，寒熱、腸痔，蟲毒、蛇癇。火熬之，良。
生川谷及田野。

Flavor: Salty
Nature: Neutral
Toxicity: Non-toxic
Alt. names: 龍子衣, 蛇符, 龍子單衣, 弓皮

Actions and Indications:
Indicated for small children's 120 types of fright epilepsy, tugging and slackening, and withdrawal disease, for [aversion to] cold and heat [effusion], intestinal hemorrhoids, worm toxin, and snake epilepsy.

Additional Information:
Roasting it over the fire is excellent.
Lives in valleys with streams and open fields.

Translator's note:
Common Name: Sloughed snake skin.
Family: Colubrid (Colubridae).
Other species used: Elaphe carinata or Zaocys dhumnades.
《中藥大辭典》#3502, where it is listed under 蛇蛻 shé tuì.

射干 *shè gān*
Rhizome of Belamcanda chinensis
Vol. 3, line 24 Lowest Grade

味苦，平，有毒。主咳逆上氣，喉痹，咽痛，不得消息，散急氣，腹中邪逆，食飲大熱。生川谷田野。

Flavor: Bitter
Nature: Neutral
Toxicity: Toxic
Alt. names: 烏扇，烏蒲

Actions and Indications:
Indicated for cough with counterflow and ascent of *qì*, throat impediment, sore throat, and inability to breathe. Dissipates tension and *qì*, evil counterflow in the abdomen, and great heat from food and drink.

Additional Information:
Grows in valleys with streams and open fields.

Translator's note:
Common Name: Blackberry/leopard lily rhizome.
Family: Iris (Iridaceae).
《中藥大辭典》#2788.

麝香 *shè xiāng*
Dried secretion from the musk pod of Moschus moschiferus
Vol. 1, line 114 Highest Grade

味辛，溫，無毒。主辟惡氣，殺鬼精物，溫瘧，蠱毒，癇痙，去三蟲。久服，除邪，不夢寤厭

寐。生川谷。

Flavor: Acrid
Nature: Warm
Toxicity: Non-toxic
Alt. names: n/a

Actions and Indications:
Indicated for repelling malign *qì*.
Kills ghosts and spectral things, [treats] warm malaria, *gǔ* toxin, epilepsy, and tetany, and removes the three types of worms.

Additional Information:
Taken for a long time, it eliminates evil and prevents dreaming, awakening, and loathing sleep.
Grows in valleys with streams.

Translator's note:
Common Name: Musk.
Family: Musk Deer (Moschidae).
Dried secretion from the musk pod, a preputial gland in a sac under the skin of the abdomen, of the male Moschus moschiferus (musk deer).
《中藥大辭典》#5600.

神麴 *shén qū*
Medicated leaven

Translator's note:
A fermented mixture of various grains, beans, and medicinal plants. For more information, see the entry above on 陳麴 *chén qū* (Medicated leaven). Regarding the name "spirit leaven," the *Běn Cǎo Gāng Mù* gives specific instructions on making it: "On the fifth day of the fifth month, or the sixth day of the sixth month, or the days of 三伏 *sān fú* [i.e., the last ten days of the hot season], mix a hundred *jīn* of white flour with...." Lǐ Shí-Zhēn himself states that "one should use the day on which the various spirits gather and congregate to prepare it. For this reason, it has received the name 'spirit leaven.'" See 《本草綱目》25:947.
《中藥大辭典》#3007, which is the entry on 陳麴 *chén qū*, and includes two detailed recipes.

慎火草 *shèn huǒ cǎo*
Entire plant of Sedum erythrosticum
Vol. 1, line 76 Highest Grade

In the *Shén Nóng Běn Cǎo Jīng*, under the entry for 景天.

味苦，平，無毒。主大熱、火創、身熱煩，邪惡氣。花，主女人漏下赤白，輕身、明目。生川

谷。

Flavor: Bitter
Nature: Neutral
Toxicity: Non-toxic
Alt. names: 戒火, 水母

Actions and Indications:
Indicated for great heat, fire wounds, heat and vexation of the body, and evil and malign *qì*.

Additional Information:
The flowers are indicated for women's vaginal spotting of red or white discharge, for lightening the body, and for brightening the eyes.
Grows in valleys with streams.

Translator's note:
Common Name: Variegated sedum.
Family: Orpine (Crassulaceae).
《中藥大辭典》#3800, where it is listed under its more common name, 景天 *jǐng tiān*.

生李根白皮 *shēng lǐ gēn bái pí*
Fresh White bark of the root of Prunus salicina

Translator's note:
Common Name: Fresh Japanese plum root bark
Family: Rose (Rosaceae).
For a description of the plant, see 《中藥大辭典》#1681, entry on 李子 *lǐ zǐ*. See also the entry above on 李根白皮 *lǐ gēn bái pí*.
《中藥大辭典》#1684, where it is listed as 李根皮 *lǐ gēn pí*.

升麻 *shēng má*
Rhizome of Cimifuga foetida
Vol. 1, line 86 Highest Grade

味甘，辛，平，無毒。主解百毒，殺百老物殃鬼，辟溫疫、瘴氣、邪氣，蠱毒。久服，不夭。生山谷。

Flavor: Sweet, acrid
Nature: Neutral
Toxicity: Non-toxic
Alt. names: 周升麻

Actions and Indications:
Indicated for resolving the hundred toxins, killing the calamitous ghosts of the hundred old things, and repelling warm epidemics, miasmic *qì*, evil *qì*, and *gǔ*

toxin.

Additional Information:
Taken for a long time, it prevents premature death.
Grows in mountain valleys.

Translator's note:
Common Name: Rhizome of Cimicifuga, bugbane, or rattletop.
Family: Buttercup (Ranunculaceae).
Other species used: Cimifuga dahurica, C. heracleifolia (close relatives of black cohosh, Cimifuga racemosa).
《中藥大辭典》#0603.

石膏 *shí gāo*
Gypsum
Vol. 2, line 5 Middle Grade

味辛，微寒，無毒。主中風寒熱，心下逆氣，惊喘，口干舌焦，不能息，腹中堅痛，除邪鬼產乳，金創。生山谷。

Flavor: Acrid
Nature: Slightly cold
Toxicity: Non-toxic
Alt. names: n/a

Actions and Indications:
Indicated for wind strike with [aversion to] cold and heat [effusion], counterflow *qì* below the heart, fright and panting, dry mouth and scorched tongue, inability to breathe, and hardness and pain in the abdomen. Eliminates evil ghosts in childbearing and [treats] incised wounds.

Additional Information:
Grows in mountain valleys.

Translator's note:
《中藥大辭典》#1238.

石斛 *shí hú*
Whole plant of Dendrobium nobile
Vol. 1, line 42 Highest Grade

味甘，平，無毒。主傷中，除痹，下氣，補五臟虛勞、羸瘦、強陰。久服，厚腸胃、輕身、延年。生山谷。

Flavor: Sweet
Nature: Neutral

Toxicity: Non-toxic
Alt. names: 林蘭

Actions and Indications:
Indicated for damage to the center.
Eliminates impediment, precipitates *qì*, supplements vacuity taxation in the five viscera and marked emaciation.
Strengthens *yīn*.

Additional Information:
Taken for a long time, it thickens the stomach and intestines, lightens the body, and extends the years.
Grows in mountain valleys.

Translator's note:
Common Name: Dendrobium.
Family: Orchid (Orchidaceae).
Other species used: Dendrobium fimbriatum hook var. oculatum Hook, D. loddigesii, or D. chrysantum.
《中藥大辭典》#1235.

石灰 *shí huī*
Limestone
Vol. 3, line 1 Lowest Grade

味辛，溫，有毒。主疽瘍、疥瘙、熱氣，惡創、癩疾、死肌，墮眉，殺痔蟲，去黑子、息肉。生山谷。

Flavor: Acrid
Nature: Warm
Toxicity: Toxic
Alt. names: 惡灰

Actions and Indications:
Indicated for flat-abscesses and sores, scabs and itches, hot *qì*, and malign wounds, for *lài* disease, dead flesh, and drooping eyebrows.
Kills hemorrhoid worms and removes black spots and polyps.

Additional Information:
Grows in mountain valleys.

Translator's note:
Used medicinally either in its raw form or heat-processed.
《中藥大辭典》#1231.

石硫磺 *shí liú huáng*
Sulphur
Vol. 2, line 2 Middle Grade

味酸，溫，有毒。主婦人陰蝕，疽痔，惡血，堅筋骨，除頭禿，能化金銀銅鐵奇物。青白色，主益肝明目。生東海、山谷中。

Flavor: Sour
Nature: Warm
Toxicity: Toxic
Alt. names: n/a

Actions and Indications:
Indicated for women's genital erosion, flat-abscesses, hemorrhoids, and malign blood.
Hardens the sinews and bones and eliminates balding.

Additional Information:
Can transform gold, silver, bronze, and iron into marvelous things.
When green-glue and white in color, it is indicated for boosting the liver and brightening the eyes.
Grows in Dōng Hǎi, in mountain valleys.

Translator's note:
Also called 硫磺 *liú huáng*.
《中藥大辭典》#1278.

石榴皮 *shí liú pí*
Rind of the fruit of Punica granatum

Translator's note:
Common Name: Pomegranate rind.
Family: Loosestrife (Lythraceae).
This medicinal is also called 酸石榴皮 *suān shí liú pí*.
《中藥大辭典》#1283.

石楠葉 *shí nán yè*
Dry-roasted foliage of Photinia serrulata
Vol. 3, line 69 Lowest Grade

味辛，平，有毒。主養腎氣、內傷、陰衰，利筋骨皮毛。實殺蠱毒，破積聚，逐風痹。生山谷。

Flavor: Acrid
Nature: Neutral
Toxicity: Toxic
Alt. names: 鬼目

Actions and Indications:
Indicated for nourishing kidney *qì*, internal damage, *yīn* debilitation, and for benefiting the sinews, bones, skin, and body hair.

Additional Information:
The seeds kill *gǔ* toxin, break up accumulations and gatherings, and expel wind impediment.
Grows in mountain valleys.

Translator's note:
Common Name: Photinia leaf.
Family: Rose (Rosaceae).
《中藥大辭典》#1261.

石韋 *shí wéi*
Foliage of Pyrrosia lingua
Vol. 2, line 44 Middle Grade

味苦，平，無毒。主勞熱邪氣，五癃閉不通，利
小便水道。生山谷石上。

Flavor: Bitter
Nature: Neutral
Toxicity: Non-toxic
Alt. names: n/a
Actions and Indications:
Indicated for taxation heat and evil *qì* and for the five types of dribbling urinary block, causing stoppage. Disinhibits urine and the water ways.

Additional Information:
Grows in mountain valleys on top of rocks.

Translator's note:
Common Name: Pyrrosia leaf.
Family: Polypod Fern (Polypodiaceae).
Other species used: Pyrrosia sheareri, P. drakeana, P. petiolosa, P. davidii, or P. gralla.
《中藥大辭典》#1234.

石鐘乳 *shí zhōng rǔ*
Stalactite
Vol. 1, line 4 Highest Grade

味甘，溫，無毒。主咳逆上氣，明目益精，安五
臟，通百節，利九竅，下乳汁。生山谷。

Flavor: Sweet
Nature: Warm
Toxicity: Non-toxic
Alt. names: 留公乳

Actions and Indications:

Indicated for cough with counterflow and ascent of *qì*. Brightens the eyes, boosts essence, quiets the five viscera, frees the hundred joints, disinhibits the nine orifices, and precipitates breast milk.

Additional Information:
Grows in mountain valleys.

Translator's note:
Also called 鍾乳 *zhōng rǔ*.
《中藥大辭典》#5444.

食茱萸 *shí zhū yú*
Fruit of Zanthoxylum ailanthoides

Translator's note:
Common Name: Japanese prickly-ash fruit.
Family: Rue (Rutaceae).
Sometimes also called 辣子 *là zǐ*. However, that term also refers to the fruit of Capsicum or garden pepper, which is more often called 辣椒 *là jiāo*. This is a completely different plant, native to the Americas. 食茱萸 *shí zhū yú* further needs to be distinguished from 蜀椒 *shǔ jiāo*, Sì-Chuān zanthoxylum and 秦椒 *qín jiāo*, Shǎn-Xī zanthoxylum, two varieties of Zanthoxylum bungeanum, of which the seed capsules are used medicinally.
《中藥大辭典》#2725.

秫米 *shú mǐ*
Seed of the glutinous variety of
Panicum miliaceum

Translator's note:
Also known as broomcorn, which however refers strictly speaking to 高粱 *gāo liáng* (Sorghum vulgare, sorghum) of the True Grass family (Poaceae). In the *Zhōng Yào Dà Cí Diǎn*, this is listed as one of the synonyms for rice, but from the context it is clear that Sūn Sī-Miǎo distinguishes between glutinous rice (糯米 *nuò mǐ*), non-glutinous rice (粳米 *jīng mǐ*), non-glutinous broomcorn millet (黍米 *shǔ mǐ*), and glutinous millet (秫米 *shú mǐ*). See the following entry on 黍米 *shú mǐ* for a translation of the relevant passage from the *Shén Nóng Běn Cǎo Jīng*.

鼠婦 *shǔ fù*
Dried body of Armadillidium vulgare
Vol. 3, line 95 Lowest Grade

味酸，溫，無毒。主氣癃不得小便，女人月閉、血症，癇、痙、寒熱，利水道。生平谷及人家地上。

Flavor: Sour
Nature: Warm
Toxicity: Non-toxic
Alt. names: 負蟠

Actions and Indications:
Indicated for *qì* dribbling urinary block with inability to urinate, for women's menstrual block, and for blood concretions, epilepsy, tetany, and [aversion to] cold and heat [effusion].
Disinhibits the water ways.

Additional Information:
Lives in flat valleys and on the ground in people's houses.

Translator's note:
Common Name: Pill bug.
Family: Pill Bug (Armadillidiidae).
《中藥大辭典》# 4420.

蜀椒 *shǔ jiāo*
Seed capsules of Zanthoxylum bungeanum
Vol. 3, line 60 Lowest Grade

味辛，溫，有毒。主邪氣、咳逆，溫中，逐骨節皮膚死肌，寒濕痹痛，下氣。久服之，頭不白、輕身、增年。生川谷。

Flavor: Acrid
Nature: Warm
Toxicity: Toxic
Alt. names: n/a

Actions and Indications:
Indicated for evil *qì*, cough with counterflow, warming the center, expelling dead flesh from the bones, joints, and skin, [treating] cold-damp impediment pain, and precipitating *qì*.

Additional Information:
Taken for a long time, it prevents whitening of the head, lightens the body, and increases the years.
Grows in valleys with streams.

Translator's note:
Common Name: Sì-Chuān zanthoxylum.
Family: Rue (Rutaceae).

Native to Sì-Chuān. Although the *Zhōng Yào Dà Cí Diǎn* lists it together with 秦椒 *qín jiāo* (Shǎn-Xī zanthoxylum) as synonyms for 花椒 *huā jiāo* and identifies all of these as Zanthoxylum bungeanum, Sūn Sī-Miǎo distinguishes between the two. Since Z. bungeanum is native to western China, 蜀椒 *shǔ jiāo* seems to refer to another variety, maybe Z. schinifolium, a variety common in the low mountains of China, Southern Japan, and Korea, which is usually called 青椒 *qīng jiāo* and has similar medicinal uses to 花椒 *huā jiāo*. It also needs to be distinguished from 食茱萸 *shí zhū yú* (ailanthes zanthoxylum, which is sometimes called 辣椒 *là jiāo*), the fruit of the species Zanthoxylum ailanthoides.
《中藥大辭典》#2084.

黍米 *shǔ mǐ*
Seed of the non-glutinous variety of Panicum miliaceum
Vol. 2, line 109 Middle Grade

In the *Shén Nóng Běn Cǎo Jīng*, under the entry for 黍米.

味甘，溫，無毒。主益氣補中，多熱、令人煩。

Flavor: Sweet
Nature: Warm
Toxicity: Non-toxic
Alt. names: n/a

Actions and Indications:
Indicated for boosting *qì* and supplementing the center, and for profuse heat causing vexation in the person.

Translator's note:
Also known as broomcorn, which however refers strictly speaking to 高粱 *gāo liáng*, Sorghum vulgare of the True Grass family (Poaceae). Distinguish from the glutinous variety, which is called 秫米 *shú mǐ* (see entry above).
《中藥大辭典》#4152.

黍粘根 *shǔ nián gēn*
Root of Arctium lappa

Translator's note:
Common Name: Burdock root.
Family: Aster.
Usually called 牛蒡 *niú bàng*, *shǔ nián*, written either as 鼠黏 or as 黍黏, is a common synonym for this plant. While the *Zhōng Yào Dà Cí Diǎn* does not list the written form 黍粘 *shǔ nián*, the characters 黏 and

粘 are homophones and used interchangeably. For more information, see the entry on 牛蒡 niú bàng above.
《中藥大辭典》#0928.

蜀漆 shǔ qī
Foliage of Dichroa febrifuga

Translator's note:
Common Name: Dichroa leaf.
Family: Hydrangea (Hydrangeaceae).
For a description of the plant and root, and the translation of the relevant passage from the *Shén Nóng Běn Cǎo Jīng*, see the entry, a common synonym, on *cháng shān* above, which refers to the root of the same plant, and 《中藥大辭典》#3282.
《中藥大辭典》#4344.

黍穰 shǔ ráng
Stalk of Panicum miliaceum

Translator's note:
Common Name: Broomcorn millet stalk.
Family: True Grass (Poaceae).
For the plant description and a translation of the relevant passage from the *Shén Nóng Běn Cǎo Jīng*, see the entry on 黍米 shǔ mǐ above and 《中藥大辭典》#4152. For the stalk, see 《中藥大辭典》#4154, where it is listed under its more common name, 黍莖 shǔ jīng.

鼠壤 shǔ rǎng
Rat detritus
Vol. 2, line 88 Middle Grade

In the *Shén Nóng Běn Cǎo Jīng*, under the entry for 天鼠屎.

味辛，寒，無毒。主面癰腫，皮膚洒洒時痛，腸中血氣，破寒熱積聚，除惊悸。生山谷。

Flavor: Acrid
Nature: Cold
Toxicity: Non-toxic
Alt. names: 鼠法, 石肝

Actions and Indications:
Indicated for welling-abscess swelling in the face, shivering and periodic pain in the skin, and blood and

qì in the intestines.
Breaks up cold and heat accumulations and gatherings, and eliminates fright palpitations.

Additional Information:
Lives in mountain valleys.

Translator's note:
Sifted soil from a rat burrow. The *Běn Cǎo Gāng Mù* states that it must be soft and without lumps (《本草綱目》7:78). Also see Harper, *Early Chinese Medical Literature*, p. 294, MS1.E 23 and note 8. For a description of the animal, see 《中藥大辭典》#4415.
《中藥大辭典》#1737.

鼠頭 shǔ tóu
Head of Rattus norvegicus
(Norway, barn, sewer, or wharf rat)

Translator's note:
Common Name: Rat head.
Family: Murid (Muridae).
Other species used: Rattus rattus (black, roof, or gray rat), or R. flavipectus.
Also used medicinally in the *Qiān Jīn Fāng* 千金方 are the cranium (鼠頭骨 shǔ tóu gǔ), which is not listed in either the *Zhōng Yào Dà Cí Diǎn* or the *Běn Cǎo Gāng Mù*, and the entire body of a dead rat (死鼠 sǐ shǔ, see entry below).
《中藥大辭典》#4415, which also contains the general description of the animal.

薯蕷 shǔ yù
Root of Dioscorea opposita
Vol. 1, line 36 Highest Grade

味甘，溫，無毒。主傷中，補虛羸，除寒熱邪氣，補中，益氣力，長肌肉。長肌肉。久服，耳目聰明，輕身、不飢、延年。生山谷。

Flavor: Sweet
Nature: Warm
Toxicity: Non-toxic
Alt. names: 山芋; In *Qín* 秦 and *Chǔ* 楚, called 玉延; In *Zhèng* 鄭 and *Yuè* 越, called 土諸; In *Qí* 齊 and *Zhào* 趙, called 山羊.

Actions and Indications:
Indicated for damage to the center.
Supplements vacuity emaciation and eliminates the evil *qì* of cold and heat.
Supplements the center, boosts *qì* and strength, and grows flesh.

Additional Information:
Taken over a long time, it sharpens the ears and eyes, lightens the body, prevents hunger, and extends the years.
Grows in mountain valleys.

Translator's note:
Common Name: Potato yam.
Family: Yam (Dioscoreaceae).
Other species used: Dioscorea batatas.
More commonly known as 山藥 shān yào.
《中藥大辭典》#0426.

水銀 shuǐ yín
Mercury
Vol. 2, line 4 Middle Grade

味辛，寒，有毒。主疥瘻痂瘍、白禿，殺皮膚中蟲，墮胎，除熱，殺金、銀、銅、錫毒。熔化還復為丹。久服，神仙、不死。生平土，出于丹砂。

Flavor: Acrid
Nature: Cold
Toxicity: Toxic
Alt. names: n/a

Actions and Indications:
Indicated for crusts, fistulas, scabs, and itch, and for whitening and balding [of the head].
Kills worms within the skin, [treats] miscarriage, eliminates heat, and kills gold, silver, bronze, and tin toxin.

Additional Information:
Melt and then return it to its original state to make pills.
Taken for a long time, it turns the person into a spirit immortal and prevents death.
Grows in flat ground and comes out of 丹砂 dān shā.

Translator's note:
Liquid metal extracted from cinnabar (辰砂 chén shā) through roasting and condensation.
《中藥大辭典》#0770.

水蛭 shuǐ zhì
Dried body of Whitmania pigra
Vol. 3, line 86 Lowest Grade

味咸，平，有毒。主逐惡血、瘀血、月閉，破血瘕積聚，無子，利水道。生池澤。

Flavor: Salty

Nature: Neutral
Toxicity: Toxic
Alt. names: 至掌

Actions and Indications:
Indicated for expelling malign blood, static blood, menstrual block, breaking up blood conglomerations, accumulations, and gatherings, for [treating] infertility, and for disinhibiting the water ways.

Additional Information:
Lives in ponds and marshes.

Translator's note:
Common Name: Leech.
Family: Hirudinidae.
Other species used: Whitmania agranulata or Hirudo nipponia.
《中藥大辭典》#0767.

死鼠 sǐ shǔ
Entire body of Rattus norvegicus
(Norway, barn, sewer, or wharf rat)

Translator's note:
Common Name: Dead rat.
Family: Murid (Muridae).
Other species used: Rattus rattus (black, roof, or gray rat), or R. flavipectus.
《中藥大辭典》#4415.

松脂 sōng zhī
Rosin of Pinus massoniana
Vol. 1, line 94 Highest Grade

味苦，溫，無毒。主疽，惡創，頭瘍，白禿，疥瘙風氣。安五臟，除熱。久服，輕身、不老、延年。生山谷。

Flavor: Bitter
Nature: Warm
Toxicity: Non-toxic
Alt. names: 松膏, 松肪

Actions and Indications:
Indicated for flat-abscesses, malign wounds, head sores, whitening and balding, and scabs and itching with wind qì.
Quiets the five viscera and eliminates heat.

Additional Information:
Taken for a long time, it lightens the body, prevents aging, and extends the years.
Grows in mountain valleys.

Translator's note:
Common Name: Rosin.
Family: Pine (Pinaceae).
《中藥大辭典》#1943, where it is listed as 松香 *sōng xiāng*.

溲疏 *sōu shū*
Fruit of Deutzia scabra
Vol. 3, line 71   Lowest Grade

味辛，寒，無毒。主身皮膚中熱，除邪氣，止遺溺。可作浴湯。生山谷及田野、故邱虛地。

Flavor: Acrid
Nature: Cold
Toxicity: Non-toxic
Alt. names: n/a

Actions and Indications:
Indicated for heat stroke all over the skin.
Eliminates evil *qì* and stops enuresis.

Additional Information:
Can be made into a bath infusion.
Grows in mountain valleys and open fields, old hills and vacant land.

Translator's note:
Common Name: Scabrous deutzia fruit.
Family: Hydrangea (Hydrangeacea).
《中藥大辭典》#4243.

酥 *sū*
Butter

Translator's note:
The explanation in the *Zhōng Yào Dà Cí Diǎn* states that 酥 *sū* is the fat won by shaking fresh milk in a bag until the fat and milk separate, similar to modern butter. The *Běn Cǎo Gāng Mù*, however, describes a different product, won by scalding milk repeatedly, cooling it, taking the skin that floats on the top, boiling this again until the fat comes out, and finally separating it into solids and pure oil. This constitutes the end product, called 酥油 *sū yóu*. The *Běn Cǎo Gāng Mù* further stresses that the highest grade is made from cow's milk and is a cooling medicinal, while sheep and water buffalo milk are of inferior quality and have a heating nature. 酥油 *Sū yóu* is further refined into 醍醐 *tí hú*, which I translate as "ghee," the pure liquid extracted from 酥 *sū* by heating. See 《本草綱目》50:1785-6. 酥 *sū* is also called 酥膏 *sū gāo*, in reference to its paste-like texture.

《中藥大辭典》#4004.

酥膏 *sū gāo*
Butter

Translator's note:
See explanation in the entry above on 酥 *sū*, to which it is identical.

蘇葉 *sū yè*
Foliage of Perilla frutescens var. crispa

Translator's note:
Common Name: Perilla leaf.
Family: Mint (Lamiaceae).
Other species used: Perilla frutescens var. acuta (often called shiso by its Japanese name).
《中藥大辭典》#3436, where it is listed as 紫蘇葉 *zǐ sū yè*.

酸棗 *suān zǎo*
Seed of Ziziphus spinosa
Vol. 1, line 100   Highest Grade

味酸，平，無毒。主心腹寒熱，邪結氣聚，四肢酸疼，濕痺。久服，安五臟，輕身、延年。生川澤。

Flavor: Sour
Nature: Neutral
Toxicity: Non-toxic
Alt. names: n/a

Actions and Indications:
Indicated for cold and heat in the heart and abdomen, evil bindings and gatherings of *qì*, soreness and pain in the four limbs, and damp impediment.

Additional Information:
Taken for a long time, it quiets the five viscera, lightens the body, and extends the years.
Grows in streams and marshes.

Translator's note:
Common Name: Spiny jujube.
Family: Buckthorn (Rhamnaceae).
According to the *Zhōng Yào Dà Cí Diǎn*, 酸棗 *suān zǎo* is also used as a synonym for 五眼果樹皮 *wǔ yǎn guǒ shù pí* (the tree bark of Choreospondias axillaries,

《中藥大辭典》#0583), for 山楂 *shān zhā* (the seed of Crataegus pinnatifida or Chinese hawthorne, and several related species of the Rose family, Rosaceae, 《中藥大辭典》#0421), for 枳椇子 *zhǐ jǔ zǐ* (the seed or fruit of Hovenia dulcis or Japanese raisin tree of the Buckthorn family, Rhamnaceae, 《中藥大辭典》#2363), and for 緬棗 *miǎn zǎo* (the tree bark of Ziziphus mauritiana, Indian or cottony jujube, of the Buckthorn family, Rhamnaceae, 《中藥大辭典》#4745).

《中藥大辭典》 #4637, where it is listed as 酸棗仁 *suān zǎo rén*.

蒜 *suàn*
Stalk of Allium sativum

Translator's note:
Common Name: Garlic stalk.
Family: Lily (Liliaceae).
Alternatively, it might sometimes refer to the stalk of Allium scorodoprasum ("sandleek"), which is usually called 小蒜 *xiǎo suàn* and is listed as such in 《中藥大辭典》#0198.
《中藥大辭典》#0329, where it is listed as 大蒜 *dà suàn*.

太一餘糧 *tài yī yú liáng*
Limonite
Vol. 1, line 13 Highest Grade

味甘，平，無毒。主咳逆上氣，症瘕、血閉、漏下，除邪氣。久服，耐寒暑、不飢，輕身、飛行千里、神仙。生山谷。

Flavor: Sweet
Nature: Neutral
Toxicity: Non-toxic
Alt. names: 石腦

Actions and Indications:
Indicated for cough with counterflow and ascent of *qì*, concretions and conglomerations, blood blockage, and [vaginal] spotting.
Eliminates evil *qì*.

Additional Information:
Taken over a long time, it allows the person to endure cold and summerheat, prevents hunger, lightens the body, and lets the person fly a thousand miles and [become like] a spirit immortal.
Grows in mountain valleys.

Translator's note:
In modern times, this name is used interchangeably with 禹餘糧 *yǔ yú liáng*, (see entry on that substance below). Nevertheless, in early and medieval times, these two substances were treated differently, as evidenced by the fact that they have separate entries in the *Shén Nóng Běn Cǎo Jīng*. According to Lǐ Shí-Zhēn, 禹餘糧 *yǔ yú liáng* comes from ponds and marshes, while 太一餘糧 *tài yī yú liáng* comes from mountain valleys.
《中藥大辭典》#2472.

桃花 *táo huā*
Flower of Prunus persica

Translator's note:
Common Name: Peach flower.
Family: Rose (Rosaceae).
Other species used: Prunus davidiana.
For information on the medicinal properties of peach and peach fuzz, and a translation of the relevant passage from the *Shén Nóng Běn Cǎo Jīng*, see the entry below on 桃仁 *táo rén*.
《中藥大辭典》#2840.

桃膠 *táo jiāo*
Sap emerging from the bark of the trunk of Prunus persica

Translator's note:
Common Name: Peach resin.
Family: Rose (Rosaceae).
Other species used: Prunus davidiana.
《中藥大辭典》#2843.

桃仁 *táo rén*
Seed of Prunus persica
Vol. 3, line 98 Lowest Grade

味苦，平，無毒。主瘀血、血閉瘕，邪氣，殺小蟲。桃花，殺疰惡鬼，令人好顏色。桃梟，微溫。主殺百鬼精物。桃毛，主下血瘕寒熱，積寒，無子。桃蠹，殺鬼邪惡不祥。生川谷。

Flavor: Bitter
Nature: Neutral
Toxicity: Non-toxic
Alt. names: n/a

Actions and Indications:
Indicated for static blood, blood blockage and conglomerations, evil *qì*, and for killing small worms.

Additional Information:
Peach blossom: Kills infixation by malign ghosts and gives the person a good facial complexion.
Peach: Slightly warm and indicated for killing the hundred ghosts and spectral things.
Peach fuzz: Indicated for precipitating blood and [treating] concretions with [aversion to] cold and heat [effusion], accumulations of cold, and infertility.
Peach grubs: Kills ghosts, and evil, malign, and inauspicious things.
Grows in valleys with streams.

Translator's note:
Common Name: Peach kernel.
Family: Rose (Rosaceae).
Other species used: Prunus davidiana.
《中藥大辭典》#2838.

醍醐 *tí hú*
Ghee

Translator's note:
The pure liquid extracted from 酥 *sū* (butter, see entry above) by heating (《本草綱目》50:1786).
《中藥大辭典》#5000, where it is simply explained as "fat produced from cows milk."

天麻 *tiān má*
Rhizome of Gastrodia elata

Translator's note:
Common Name: Gastrodia rhizome.
Family: Orchid (Orchidaceae).
《中藥大辭典》#0622.

天門冬 *tiān mén dōng*
Tuber of Asparagus cochinchinensis
Vol. 1, line 22　Highest Grade

味苦，平，無毒。主諸暴風濕偏痹。強骨髓，殺
三蟲，去伏尸。久服，輕身、益氣、延年。生山
谷。

Flavor: Bitter
Nature: Neutral
Toxicity: Non-toxic
Alt. names: 顛勒

Actions and Indications:
Indicated for all sudden wind-damp deviation and impediment.
Strengthens the bones and marrow, kills the three types of worms, and removes hidden corpse [syndrome].

Additional Information:
Taken over a long time, it lightens the body, boosts *qi*, and extends the years.
Grows in mountain valleys.

Translator's note:
Common Name: Asparagus.
Family: Lily (Liliaceae).
《中藥大辭典》#0633.

天雄 *tiān xióng*
Mature root of Aconitum carmichaeli
Vol. 3, line 12　Lowest Grade

味辛，溫，有大毒。主大風，寒濕痹，歷節痛，
拘攣，緩急，破積聚，邪氣，金創，強筋骨，輕
身健行。生山谷。

Flavor: Acrid
Nature: Warm
Toxicity: Greatly toxic
Alt. names: 白幕

Actions and Indications:
Indicated for severe wind, wind-cold impediment, joint-running pain, and hypertonicity.
Relaxes tension, breaks accumulations and gatherings, [treats] evil *qi* and incised wounds, strengthens the sinews and bones, lightens the body, and fortifies the gait.

Additional Information:
Grows in mountain valleys.

Translator's note:
Common Name: Tiānxióng aconite root.
Family: Buttercup (Ranunculaceae).
Mature root of Aconitum carmichaeli, 川烏 *chuān wū* (the species from which 附子 *fù zǐ* is made; see entry above) or of Aconitum kusnezoffii (草烏 *cǎo wū*, wild aconite). See 《中藥大辭典》#3098 for information on the plant.
《中藥大辭典》#0623.

铁精 *tiě jīng*
Blast furnace ash
Vol. 2, line 11 Middle Grade

味辛，平，無毒。主明目，化銅。鐵落:味辛，平，無毒。主風熱，惡創，瘍疽創痂，疥氣在皮膚中。鐵:主堅肌，耐痛。生平澤。

Flavor: Acrid
Nature: Neutral
Toxicity: Non-toxic
Alt. names: n/a

Actions and Indications:
Indicated for brightening the eyes and transforming bronze.

Additional Information:
Iron flakes: Acrid flavor, neutral nature, non-toxic. Indicated for wind heat, malign wounds, open sores, flat-abscesses, wounds with scabs, and scabies qì inside the skin.
Iron ore: Indicated for hardening muscle and allowing the person to endure pain.
Grows in flatlands and marshes.

Translator's note:
Ashes created as a byproduct when smelting iron.
《中藥大辭典》#5503.

亭長 *tíng cháng*
Dried body of Epicauta Gorhami

Translator's note:
Common Name: Epicauta.
Family: Blister Beetle (Meloidae).
The medicinally active ingredient is cantharidin, a skin irritant also found in the related species Mylabris and Lytta viesicatoria (commonly called Spanish fly). The substance was a common ingredient in European aphrodisiacs and is also used for wart treatments. In 《中藥大辭典》 #4328 and in this index above, it is listed as 葛上亭長 *gé shàng tíng cháng*. See that entry for more information.

葶藶 *tíng lì*
Seed of Lepidium apetalum
Vol. 3, line 17 Lowest Grade

味辛，寒，無毒。主症瘕、積聚、結氣，飲食寒熱，破堅，逐邪，通利水道。生平澤及田野。

Flavor: Acrid

Nature: Cold
Toxicity: Non-toxic
Alt. names: 大室, 大適

Actions and Indications:
Indicated for concretions and conglomerations, accumulations and gatherings, bound *qì*, and [aversion to] cold and heat [effusion] when eating and drinking. Breaks up hardenings, expels evil, and frees and disinhibits the water ways.

Additional Information:
Grows in flat marshes and open fields.

Translator's note:
Common Name: Pepperwort or descurainia (Tansy mustard) seed.
Family: Mustard (Brassicaceae).
《中藥大辭典》#4342.

通草 *tōng cǎo*
Pith in the stalk of
Tetrapanax papyriferus
Vol. 2, line 22 Middle Grade

味辛，平，無毒。主去惡蟲，除脾胃寒熱，通利九竅、血脈、關節，令人不忘。生山谷及山陽。

Flavor: Acrid
Nature: Neutral
Toxicity: Non-toxic
Alt. names: 附支

Actions and Indications:
Indicated for removing malign worms.
Eliminates cold and heat in the spleen and stomach, frees and disinhibits the nine orifices, blood vessels, and joints, and causes people not to forget.

Additional Information:
Grows in mountain valleys and on the sunny side of mountains.

Translator's note:
Common Name: Rice-paper plant pith.
Family: Ivy (Araliaceae).
Most commonly used for making rice paper.
《中藥大辭典》#3528.

銅鏡鼻 *tóng jìng bí*
Bronze mirror knob
Vol. 3, line 4 Lowest Grade

In the *Shén Nóng Běn Cǎo Jīng*, under the entry for 粉

錫 (powdered tin, the closest entry to this).

味辛，寒，無毒。主伏尸毒螫，殺三蟲。錫鏡鼻，主女子血閉，症瘕腹腸，絕孕。生山谷。

Flavor: Acrid
Nature: Cold
Toxicity: Non-toxic
Alt. names: 解錫

Actions and Indications:
Indicated for latent corpse toxin stings, and killing the three types of worms.

Additional Information:
Tin mirror knob is indicated for women's blood blockage, concretions and conglomerations in the abdomen and intestines, and interruption of childbearing. Grows in mountain valleys.

Translator's note:
The *Běn Cǎo Gāng Mù* contains a full entry on "ancient mirrors" (古鏡 *gǔ jìng*) and explains there that in ancient times, bronze was never pure but always mixed with tin (《本草綱目》8:131). The medicinal use of bronze (red, white, or green) is fairly widespread. For a description of the medicinal properties of bronze, see 《中藥大辭典》#1804 (entry on 赤銅屑 *chì tóng xiè*, "red bronze filings).

筒桂 *tǒng guì*
Bark of Cinnamomum cassia

Translator's note:
Common Name: Tube cinnamon.
Family: Laurel (Lauraceae).
Cinnamon bark that has been rolled into tubes.
《中藥大辭典》#1579 is the entry on 肉桂 *ròu guì*.
See also the entries on 桂心 *guì xīn* and 桂枝 *guì zhī* above, the latter of which contains a translation of the relevant passage from the *Shén Nóng Běn Cǎo Jīng*.

土瓜 *tǔ guā*
Fruit of Trichosanthes cucumerina
Vol. 2, line 48　Lowest Grade

In the *Shén Nóng Běn Cǎo Jīng*, under the entry for 王瓜.

味苦，寒，無毒。主消渴，內痹，瘀血，月閉，寒熱，酸疼，益氣，愈聾。生平澤田野及人家坦牆間。

Flavor: Bitter
Nature: Cold
Toxicity: Non-toxic
Alt. names: 土瓜

Actions and Indications:
Indicated for dispersion thirst, internal impediment, static blood, menstrual block, [aversion to] cold and heat [effusion], and soreness and pain.
Boosts *qì* and heals deafness.

Additional Information:
Grows in flatlandss, marshes, open fields, and between walls and level places in people's houses.

Translator's note:
Common Name: Cucumber gourd.
Family: Gourd (Cucurbitaceae).
More commonly known as 王瓜 *wáng guā*, it needs to be distinguished from 栝樓 *guā lóu* (Trichosanthes kirilowii, Trichosanthes).
《中藥大辭典》#0946.

土瓜根 *tǔ guā gēn*
Root of Trichosanthes cucumerina

Translator's note:
Common Name: Cucumber gourd root.
Family: Gourd (Cucurbitaceae).
For the plant and a translation of the relevant passage from the *Shén Nóng Běn Cǎo Jīng*, see the preceding entry on 土瓜 *tǔ guā*.
《中藥大辭典》#0949, where it is listed as 王瓜根 *wáng guā gēn*.

兔骨 *tù gǔ*
Bones of Oryctolagus domesticus

Translator's note:
Common Name: Hare's or rabbit's bone.
Family: Rabbit and Hare (Leporidae).
Other species used: Lepus tolai and related members.
For a description of the animal, see 《中藥大辭典》#1838, which is the entry on 兔肉 *tù ròu*.
《中藥大辭典》#1841.

兔屎 *tù shǐ*
Feces of Oryctolagus domesticus

Translator's note:
Common Name: Hare's or rabbit's droppings.
Family: Rabbit and Hare (Leporidae).
Other species used: Lepus tolai and related members.
See 《中藥大辭典》 #1838 on 兔肉 *tù ròu* for a description of the animal, but the feces are not included as a medicinal ingredient in this reference. For the medicinal use of the feces, see the entry on hare, subsection "droppings," in 《本草綱目》 51:1834.

菟絲子 *tù sī zǐ*
Seed of Cuscuta chinensis
Vol. 1, line 26 Highest Grade

味辛，平，無毒。主續絕傷，補不足，益氣力，
肥健。汁去面䵟。久服，明目、輕身、延年。生
川澤田野，蔓延草木之上。

Flavor: Acrid
Nature: Neutral
Toxicity: Non-toxic
Alt. names: 菟蘆

Actions and Indications:
Indicated for joining damage from severance, supplementing insufficiencies, boosting *qì* and strength, and fattening and fortifying.

Additional Information:
The juice removes black spots from the face.
Taken over a long time, it brightens the eyes, lightens the body, and extends the years.
Grows in streams and marshes, and open fields, on top of sprawling plants.

Translator's note:
Common Name: Chinese or Japanese dodder seed.
Family: Morning Glory (Convolvulaceae).
Other species used: Cuscuta japonica.
《中藥大辭典》 #3939.

萎蕤 *wěi ruí*
Rhizome of Polygonatum odoratum

Translator's note:
Common Name: Solomon's seal.
Family: Lily (Liliaceae).
Other species used: Polygonatum macropodium,
P. involucratum, or P. inflatum, or for P. sibiricum, P. cyrtonema, P. kingianum and similar varieties (《中藥大辭典》 #4037, where it is listed as a synonym for 黄

精 *huáng jīng*).
《中藥大辭典》 #1033, where it is listed as a synonym for 玉竹 *yù zhú*.

蝟皮 *wèi pí*
Skin of Erinaceus europaeus
Vol. 2, line 89 Middle Grade

味苦，平，無毒。主五痔，陰蝕，下血，赤白，
五色血汁不止，陰腫、痛引腰背。酒煮殺之。生
川谷、田野。

Flavor: Bitter
Nature: Neutral
Toxicity: Non-toxic
Alt. names: n/a

Actions and Indications:
Indicated for the five types of hemorrhoids, genital erosion, precipitation of blood, red and white vaginal discharge, incessant five-colored bloody fluid, and genital swelling with pain stretching to the lumbus and back.

Additional Information:
Boil it in liquor to kill it.
Lives in valleys with streams and open fields.

Translator's note:
Common Name: Skin of the common or long-eared hedgehog.
Family: Hedgehog and Gymnure (Erinaceidae).
Other species used: Hemiechinus dahuricus.
《中藥大辭典》 #1877, where it is listed as 刺蝟皮 *cì wèi pí*.

烏豆 *wū dòu*
Black seed of Glycine max

Translator's note:
Common Name: Black soybean.
Family: Pea (Fabaceae).
《中藥大辭典》 #4156, where it is listed as 黑大豆 *hēi dà dòu*.

烏喙 wū huì
Main tuber of
Aconitum carmichaeli

Translator's note:
Common Name: Aconite main tuber.
Family: Buttercup (Ranunculaceae).
Other species used: Aconite kusneoffii (草烏頭 cǎo wū tóu) or (北烏頭 běi wū tóu, wild monkshood).
烏喙 wū huì refers specifically to the main tuber of 川烏頭 chuān wū tóu, Sì-Chuǎn monkshood. See the entry below on 烏頭 wū tóu for information on that medicinal and a translation of the relevant passage from the Shén Nóng Běn Cǎo Jīng.
《中藥大辭典》#3098.

烏梅 wū méi
Unripe fruit of Prunus mume

Translator's note:
Common Name: Mume.
Family: Rose (Rosaceae).
《中藥大辭典》#2929.

烏牛尿 wū niú niào
Urine of a black cow

Translator's note:
Not listed in the Zhōng Yào Dà Cí Diǎn or Běn Cǎo Gāng Mù. Perhaps the closest equivalent discussed in the Běn Cǎo Gāng Mù, the dirt on which a dog has urinated (犬尿泥 quǎn niào ní), is indicated for cold damage diseases in pregnancy and prevention of miscarriage by rubbing it on the abdomen and letting it dry. See 《本草綱目》 7:87.

屋上散草 wū shàng sǎn cǎo
Rooftop grass

Translator's note:
Literally, "grasses scattered on the rooftop." Not listed in the Zhōng Yào Dà Cí Diǎn or Běn Cǎo Gāng Mù. Nevertheless, the Zhōng Yào Dà Cí Diǎn lists 屋上無根草 wū shàng wú gēn cǎo (lit. "root-less grass on the rooftop") as a synonym for 瓦松 wǎ sōng. This refers to several varieties of stonecrop, esp. Orostachys (Sedum) fimbriatus and O. erudescens of the Orpine family (Crassulaceae), of which the whole

plant is used medicinally. See 《中藥大辭典》#1052. In the Běn Cǎo Gāng Mù, 瓦松 wǎ sōng is described as growing on roof tiles and is used medicinally to "increase the flow in women's channels" and to "free the menses and breaks blood." These functions are certainly related to the function of inducing the descent of blocked up breast milk, the context in which this medicinal is used in the Qiān Jīn Fāng.

烏頭 wū tóu
Main tuber of Aconitum carmichaeli
Vol. 3, line 11 Lowest Grade

味辛，溫，有大毒。主中風惡風，洒洒出汗，除寒濕痹，咳逆上氣，破積聚、寒熱。其汁，煎之，名射罔，殺禽獸。生山谷。

Flavor: Acrid
Nature: Warm
Toxicity: Greatly toxic
Alt. names: 奚毒，即子，烏喙

Actions and Indications:
Indicated for wind strike and malign wind with shivering and sweating.
Eliminates cold-damp impediment and cough with counterflow and ascent of qì, and breaks accumulations and gatherings with [aversion to] cold and heat [effusion].

Additional Information:
The simmered juice is called shè wǎng ("shooting deception") and kills wild birds and beasts.
Grows in mountain valleys.

Translator's note:
Common Name: Aconite main tuber.
Family: Buttercup (Ranunculaceae).
Other species used: Aconitum kusneoffii (草烏頭 cǎo wū tóu or 北烏頭 běi wū tóu, wild monkshood, 《中藥大辭典》#3098). See also the entries on 烏喙 wū huì (a synonym) and on 附子 fù zǐ (aconite) above.
《中藥大辭典》 #0454.

烏賊[魚]骨 wū zéi [yú] gǔ
Calcified shell of Sepiella maindroni
Vol. 2, line 95 Middle Grade

味咸，微溫，無毒。主女子漏下赤白，經汁血閉，陰蝕腫痛，寒熱症瘕，無子。生東海池澤。

Flavor: Salty
Nature: Slightly warm
Toxicity: Non-toxic

Alt. names: n/a

Actions and Indications:
Indicated for women's and girls' vaginal spotting of red or white fluid, blockage of menstrual fluid and blood, genital erosion with swelling and pain, [aversion to] cold and heat [effusion], concretions and conglomerations, and infertility.

Additional Information:
Lives in ponds and marshes in Dōng-Hǎi.

Translator's note:
Common Name: Cuttlefish bone.
Family: Cuttlefish (Sepiidae).
Other species used: Sepia esculenta (Golden cuttlefish).
The medicinal product is also called 海螵蛸 hǎi piāo xiāo.
《中藥大辭典》#2920.

蕪菁根 wú jīng gēn
Root of Brassica rapa

Translator's note:
Common Name: Turnip root.
Family: Mustard (Brassicaceae).
《中藥大辭典》#4933 is a description of the plant and the medicinal use of the root and leaves.

蕪菁子 wú jīng zǐ
Seed of Brassica rapa

Translator's note:
Common Name: Turnip seed.
Family: Mustard (Brassicaceae).
This drug is also called 蔓菁子 màn jīng zǐ, which needs to be distinguished from a drug with the identical pronunciation, 蔓荊子 màn jīng zǐ, the fruit of Vitex rotundifolia or V. trifolia of the Verbena family (Verbenaceae), which is also called 蔓青子 màn qīng zǐ (《中藥大辭典》#4768).
《中藥大辭典》#4935.

梧桐子 wú tóng zǐ
Seeds of Firmiana simplex

Translator's note:
Common Name: Firmiana seed (parasol, Chinese scholar, or varnish tree).
Family: Cacao (Sterculiaceae).
While also used as a medicinal ingredient, 梧桐子 wú tóng zǐ occurs in the Qiān Jīn Fāng primarily as a standard measurement for sizing pills.
《中藥大辭典》#3340.

蕪荑 wú yí
Processed fruit of Ulmus macrocarpa
Vol. 2, line 67 Middle Grade

味辛，平，無毒。主五內邪氣，散皮膚骨節中淫淫溫行毒，去三蟲，化食，逐寸白，散腹中溫溫喘息。生川谷。

Flavor: Acrid
Nature: Neutral
Toxicity: Non-toxic
Alt. names: 無姑, 蔽瑭

Actions and Indications:
Indicated for the five types of internal evil qi. Dissipates warm moving toxin spreading in the skin, bones, and joints, removes the three types of worms, transforms food, expels inch whiteworm, and dissipates warmth in the center of the abdomen with panting.

Additional Information:
Grows in valleys with streams.

Translator's note:
Common Name: Elm cake.
Family: Elm (Ulmaceae).
《中藥大辭典》#4932.

吳茱萸 wú zhū yú
Unripe fruit of Evodia rutaecarpa
Vol. 2, line 65 Middle Grade

味辛，溫，有小毒。主溫中，下氣，止痛，咳逆，寒熱，除濕、血痺，逐風邪，開腠理。根殺三蟲。生山谷。

Flavor: Acrid
Nature: Warm
Toxicity: Slightly toxic
Alt. names: 藙

Actions and Indications:
Indicated for warming the center, precipitating qi, relieving pain, and for [treating] cough with counterflow and [aversion to] cold and heat [effusion].

Eliminates damp and blood impediment, expels wind evil, and opens the interstices.

Additional Information:
The root kills the three types of worms.
Grows in mountain valleys.

Translator's note:
Common Name: Evodia.
Family: Rue (Rutaceae).
《中藥大辭典》#1642.

五加皮 *wǔ jiā pí*
Root bark of
Acanthopanax gracilistylus
Vol. 1, line 103 Highest Grade

味辛，溫，無毒。主心腹疝氣，腹痛，益氣，療躄，小儿不能行，疽創陰蝕。

Flavor: Acrid
Nature: Warm
Toxicity: Non-toxic
Alt. names: 豺漆

Actions and Indications:
Indicated for mounting *qì* in the heart and abdomen and abdominal pain.
Boosts *qì*, and cures sprains, small children's inability to walk, jaundice wounds, and genital erosion.

Translator's note:
Common Name: Acanthopanax root bark.
Family: Ivy (Araliaceae).
Other species used: Acanthopanax sessiliflorus, A. senticosus (Siberian ginseng), A. henryi, or A. verticillatus.
Regionally, this name is used as a synonym for other medicinals, such as 走遊草 *zǒu yóu cǎo* (the whole plant or root of Tetrastigma obtectum, 《中藥大辭典》#1813), 刺三甲 *cì sān jiǎ* (the root or root bark of Acanthopanax trifoliatus, 《中藥大辭典》#1863), or 楓荷梨 *fēng hé lí* (the root and rhizome of Dendropanax chevalieri, 《中藥大辭典》#4215), but it seems highly unlikely that Sūn Sī-Miǎo would have referred to any other plant besides Acanthopanax.

五味子 *wǔ wèi zǐ*
Fruit of Schisandra chinensis
Vol. 1, line 71 Highest Grade

味酸，溫，無毒。主益氣，咳逆上氣，勞傷羸瘦。補不足，強陰，益男子精。生山谷。

Flavor: Sour
Nature: Warm
Toxicity: Non-toxic
Alt. names: n/a

Actions and Indications:
Indicated for boosting *qì*, for cough with counterflow and ascent of *qì*, and for taxation damage and marked emaciation.
Supplements insufficiencies, strengthens *yīn*, and boosts male essence.

Additional Information:
Grows in mountain valleys.

Translator's note:
Common Name: Schisandra fruit.
Family: Magnolia (Magnoliaceae).
《中藥大辭典》#0558.

菥蓂子 *xī míng zǐ*
Seed of Thlaspi arvense
Vol. 1, line 48 Highest Grade

味辛，微溫，無毒。主明目，目痛，淚出，除痹，補五臟，益精光。久服，輕身，不老。生川澤及道旁。

Flavor: Acrid
Nature: Slightly warm
Toxicity: Non-toxic
Alt. names: 蔑析，大蕺，馬辛

Actions and Indications:
Indicated for brightening the eyes, for eye pain, and tearing.
Eliminates impediment, supplements the five viscera, and boosts essence and light.

Additional Information:
Taken over a long time, it lightens the body and prevents aging.
Grows in streams and marshes and along road sides.

Translator's note:
Common Name: Pennycress seed.
Family: Mustard (Brassicaceae).
《中藥大辭典》#3944.

細辛 *xì xīn*
Complete plant including root of Asarum heteropoides
Vol. 1, line 41 Highest Grade

味辛，溫，無毒。主咳逆，頭痛，腦動，百節拘
攣，風濕痺痛、死肌。久服，明目、利九竅，輕
身、長年。生山谷。

Flavor: Acrid
Nature: Warm
Toxicity: Non-toxic
Alt. names: 小辛

Actions and Indications:
Indicated for cough with counterflow, headache, stirring in the brain, hypertonicity in the hundred joints,
wind-damp impediment pain, and dead flesh.

Additional Information:
Taken over a long time, it brightens the eyes, disinhibits the nine orifices, lightens the body, and lengthens
the years.
Grows in mountain valleys.

Translator's note:
Common Name: Asarum, wild ginger.
Family: Birthwort (Aristolochiaceae).
Other species used: Asarum heteropoides Fr. Schm.
var. mandshuricum or A. sieboldii, but many other species can be substituted.
《中藥大辭典》#3454.

香豉 *xiāng chǐ*
Preparation of Glycine max

Translator's note:
Common Name: Fermented soybean.
Family: Pea (Fabaceae).
Also called 豆豉 *dòu chǐ*. For more information, see
the entry on 豆豉 *dòu chǐ* above and 《中藥大辭
典》#3361, where it is listed as 淡豆豉 *dàn dòu chǐ*.

消石 *xiāo shí*
Niter
Vol. 1, line 6 Highest Grade

味苦，寒，無毒。主五臟積熱，胃脹閉，滌去蓄
結飲食，推陳致新，除邪氣。煉之如膏，久服輕
身。生山谷。

Flavor: Bitter
Nature: Cold
Toxicity: Non-toxic
Alt. names: 芒硝

Actions and Indications:
Indicated for accumulated heat in the five viscera, and
distention and blockage in the stomach.
Flushes out amassed and bound food and drink,
pushes out the old and institutes the new, and eliminates evil *qì*.

Additional Information:
Refine it into a paste-like substance.
Taken over a long time, it lightens the body.
Grows in mountain valleys.

Translator's note:
The high-grade processed form of a naturally occuring sulfate mineral. It needs to be distinguished
from a lower-grade product called 朴硝 *pò xiāo*
low-grade sodium sulfate or impure mirabilite, 《中藥
大辭典》#1440), as well as the natural unprocessed
product, called 寒水石 *hán shuǐ shí* (glauberite). See
the entry above on 朴硝 *pò xiāo* for information on that
substance as well as for a translation of the relevant
entry in the *Shén Nóng Běn Cǎo Jīng*. 消石 *xiāo shí* is
also called 礵硝 *máng xiāo* (see entry above).
《中藥大辭典》#2927.

小草 *xiǎo cǎo*
Stalk and foliage of Polygala tenuifolia

Translator's note:
Common Name: Polygala herb (Snakeroot).
Family: Milkwort (Polygalaceae).
The common name of the plant is 遠志 *yuǎn zhì*, which
is used in medical literature to refer to the root. See
entry below on 遠志 *yuǎn zhì*, which also includes
a translation of the relevant passage from the *Shén
Nóng Běn Cǎo Jīng*. For a description of the plant
and root, see《中藥大辭典》#4629. The *Zhōng Yào
Dà Cí Diǎn* also records *xiǎo cǎo* as a synonym for 百
蕊草 *bǎi ruǐ cǎo*, the entire plant of Thesium chinense
of the Sandalwood family (Santalaceae,《中藥大辭
典》#1463).
《中藥大辭典》#0327

小薊根 *xiǎo jì gēn*
Root of Cephalanopsis segetum

Translator's note:
Common Name: Field thistle root.
Family: Aster (Asteraceae).
Other species used: Cephalanoplos, Cirsium segetum.

《中藥大辭典》 #0331, which is the entry on 小薊 *xiǎo jì* and describes the medicinal use of the root and entire plant.

小麥 *xiǎo mài*
Seed or flour of Triticum aestivum

Translator's note:
Common Name: Wheat.
Family: True Grass (Poaceae).
《中藥大辭典》 #0328.

薤白 *xiè bái*
Stalk of Allium macrostemon
Vol. 2, line 112 Middle Grade

味辛，溫，無毒。主金創，創敗，輕身、不飢、耐老。生平澤。

Flavor: Acrid
Nature: Warm
Toxicity: Non-toxic
Alt. names: n/a

Actions and Indications:
Indicated for incised wounds and wound vanquishing.
Lightens the body, prevents hunger, and allows the person to endure aging.

Additional Information:
Grows in flatlandss and marshes.

Translator's note:
Common Name: Chinese chive.
Family: Lily (Liliaceae).
Other species used: Allium chinense (most commonly known by its Japanese name, rakkyō).
Also called 小根蒜 *xiǎo gēn suàn* "small-bulbed garlic."
《中藥大辭典》 #5144.

蟹爪 *xiè zhǎo*
Claw of Eriocheir sinensis
Vol. 2, line 92 Middle Grade

In the *Shén Nóng Běn Cǎo Jīng*, under the entry for 蟹.

味咸，寒，有毒。主胸中邪氣、熱結痛，喎僻面

腫。敗漆。燒之，致鼠。生池澤。

Flavor: Salty
Nature: Cold
Toxicity: Toxic
Alt. names: n/a

Actions and Indications:
Indicated for evil *qì* in the chest, heat bind and pain, and deviation and swelling in the face.
Vanquishes lacquer.

Additional Information:
Burning it makes mice come out.
Lives in ponds and marshes.

Translator's note:
Common Name: Chinese mitten crab.
Family: Shore Crab (Grapsidae).
For a description of the animal, see 《中藥大辭典》 #5360.
《中藥大辭典》 #5361.

辛夷 *xīn yí*
Flower of Magnolia liliflora
Vol. 1, line 105 Highest Grade

味辛，溫，無毒。主五臟身体寒，風頭，腦痛，面皯。久服，下氣、輕身、明目、增年、耐老。生川谷。

Flavor: Acrid
Nature: Warm
Toxicity: Non-toxic
Alt. names: 辛矧, 侯桃, 房木

Actions and Indications:
Indicated for cold in the five viscera and the body, wind in the head, pain in the brain, and black spots in the face.

Additional Information:
Taken for a long time, it precipitates *qì*, lightens the body, brightens the eyes, increases the years, and allows the person to endure aging.
Grows in valleys with streams.

Translator's note:
Common Name: Lily magnolia flower.
Family: Magnolia (Magnoliaceae).
Other species used: Magnolia denudata (玉蘭 *yù lán*, yùlán magnolia).
Note that a different species (Magnolia officinalis) is used for the medicinal 厚朴 *hòu pò* (official magnolia bark).
《中藥大辭典》 #1822.

杏仁 *xìng rén*
Dried seed of Prunus armeniaca
Vol. 3, line 99 Lowest Grade

味甘，溫，有毒。主咳逆上氣，腸中雷鳴，喉痹，下氣，產乳，金創、寒心、賁豚。生川谷。

Flavor: Sweet
Nature: Warm
Toxicity: Toxic
Alt. names: n/a

Actions and Indications:
Indicated for cough with counterflow and ascent of *qì*, thunderous rumbling in the intestines, throat impediment, precipitating *qì*, for childbearing, for incised wounds, cold in the heart, and for running piglet.

Additional Information:
Grows in valleys with streams.

Translator's note:
Common Name: Apricot kernel.
Family: Rose (Rosaceae).
《中藥大辭典》#1688.

芎藭 *xiōng qióng*
Root of Ligusticum wallichii
Vol. 1, line 53 Highest Grade

味辛，溫，無毒。主中風入腦，頭痛，寒痹，筋攣，緩急，金創，婦人血閉無子。生川谷。

Flavor: Acrid
Nature: Warm
Toxicity: Non-toxic
Alt. names: n/a

Actions and Indications:
Indicated for wind strike entering the brain, headache, cold impediment, hypertonicity of the sinews, for relaxing tension, for incised wounds, and for women's blockage of blood and infertility.
Additional Information:
Grows in valleys with streams.

Translator's note:
Common Name: Chuānxiōng (lovage).
Family: Carrot (Apiaceae).
Commonly known as 川芎 *chuān xiōng*. In English TCM literature, it is often translated as "ligusticum," but it needs to be distinguished from other Ligusticum species used in Chinese medicine, such as 槁本 *gǎo běn* (Ligusticum sinense/jeholense, Chinese lovage), and 蛇床子 *shé chuáng zǐ* (Ligusticum monnieri, cnidium). For the leaves and sprouts of 芎藭 *xiōng qióng*, see entry above on 蘼蕪 *mí wú*.

《中藥大辭典》#0540.

雄黃 *xióng huáng*
Realgar
Vol. 2, line 1 Middle Grade

味苦，平、寒，有毒。主寒熱，鼠瘻，惡創，疽痔，死肌，殺精物、惡鬼、邪氣、百蟲毒腫，胜五兵。煉食之，輕身、神仙。生山谷，山之陽。

Flavor: Bitter
Nature: Neutral, cold
Toxicity: Toxic
Alt. names: 黃食石

Actions and Indications:
Indicated for cold and heat, mouse fistulas, malign wounds, flat-abscesses, hemorrhoids, and dead flesh. Kills spectral things, malign ghosts, and evil *qì*, [treats] swelling from the toxin of the hundred worms, prevails over the five types of weaponry.

Additional Information:
Eaten as an alchemical preparation, it lightens the body and transforms the person into a spirit immortal. Grows in mountain valleys, on the sunny side of the mountain.

Translator's note:
《中藥大辭典》#4016.

雄雞 *xióng jī*
Complete body of male Gallus gallus domesticus
Vol. 1, line 119 Highest Grade

In the *Shén Nóng Běn Cǎo Jīng*, under the entry for 丹雄雞.

味甘，微溫，無毒。主女人崩中漏下赤白沃，補虛溫中，止血，通神，殺毒，辟不祥。頭:主殺鬼，東門上者尤良。肪:主耳聾。腸:主遺溺。膍胵裹黃皮:主泄利。尿白:主消渴，傷寒寒熱。黑雌雞:主風寒濕痹，五緩六急，安胎。翮羽:主下血閉。雞子:主除熱，火瘡癇痓，可作虎魄神物。雞白蠹:肥脂。生平澤。

Flavor: Sweet
Nature: Slightly warm
Toxicity: Non-toxic
Alt. names: n/a

Actions and Indications:

Indicated for women's center flooding and vaginal spotting of red and white moisture.
Supplements vacuity and warms the center, stanches bleeding, frees the spirit, kills toxin, and repels inauspicious things.

Additional Information:
Head: Indicated for killing ghosts. The head of a rooster from the eastern gate is especially good.
Fat: Indicated for deafness.
Intestines: Indicated for enuresis.
Yellow skin from inside the gizzard: Indicated for diarrhea.
White in the excrement: Indicated for dispersion thirst and cold damage with [aversion to] cold and heat [effusion].
Black hen: Indicated for wind-cold-damp impediment, for the five types of retardation and six types of hypertonicity, and for quieting the fetus.
Feathers: Iindicated for precipitating blood blockage.
Eggs: Indicated for eliminating heat, fire sores, epilepsy and tetany, and can be turned into the wondrous substance amber.
White open-ended sack of the chicken: Fat.
Lives in flatlands and marshes.

續斷 *xù duàn*
Root of Dipsacus asper
Vol. 1, line 63 Highest Grade

味苦，微溫，無毒。主傷寒，補不足，金創，癰傷，折跌，續筋骨，婦人乳難、崩中、漏血。久服，益氣力。生山谷。

Flavor: Bitter
Nature: Slightly warm
Toxicity: Non-toxic
Alt. names: 龍豆, 屬折

Actions and Indications:
Indicated for cold damage, supplementing insufficiencies, treating incised wounds, welling-abscess damage, and fractures and falls, and for joining sinews and bones.
[Treats] women's breastfeeding difficulties, center flooding, and vaginal spotting of blood.

Additional Information:
Taken over a long time, it boosts *qì* and strength.
Grows in mountain valleys.

Translator's note:
Common Name: Dipsacus root.
Family: Teasel (Dipsacaceae).
Other species used: Dipsacus japonicus
《中藥大辭典》#5480.

續骨木 *xù gǔ mù*
Stems of Sambucus williamsii

Translator's note:
Common Name: Elder wood (Elderberry).
Family: Moschatel (Adoxaceae).
《中藥大辭典》#3295, where it is listed under the synonym 接骨木 *jiē gǔ mù*.

旋覆花 *xuán fù huā*
Flowerhead of Inula britannica
Vol. 3, line 21 Lowest Grade

味咸，溫，有小毒。主結氣、脅下滿、惊悸，除水，去五臟間寒熱，補中，下氣。生平澤、川谷。

Flavor: Salty
Nature: Warm
Toxicity: Slightly toxic
Alt. names: 金沸草, 盛椹

Actions and Indications:
Indicated for bound *qì*, fullness below the rib-sides, and fright palpitations.
Eliminates water, removes cold and heat in the five viscera, supplements the center, and precipitates *qì*.

Additional Information:
Grows in flat marshes and valleys with streams.

Translator's note:
Common Name: Inula flower.
Family: Aster (Asteraceae).
Other species used: Inula linariaefolia.
A close relative is elecampane (Inula helenium), the root of which is used for similar medicinal purposes in Western herbal medicine (D. J. Mabberley, *The Plantbook*, p. 362, and M. Grieve, *A Modern Herbal*, vol. 1, pp. 278-281). In addition, *xuán fù huā* is sometimes used to refer to 水朝陽 *shuǐ zhāo yáng*, the flower of Inula helianthus-aquatilis (《中藥大辭典》#0822).
《中藥大辭典》#3312.

玄參 *xuán shēn*
Root of Scrophularia ningpoensis
Vol. 2, line 26 Middle Grade

In the *Shén Nóng Běn Cǎo Jīng*, under the entry for 元參.

味苦，微寒，無毒。主腹中寒熱積聚，女子產乳餘疾，補腎氣，令人目明。生川谷。

Flavor: Bitter
Nature: Slightly cold
Toxicity: Non-toxic
Alt. names: 重台

Actions and Indications:
Indicated for accumulations and gatherings of cold and heat in the abdomen and for women's diseases left over from bearing and rearing children. Supplements kidney *qì* and brightens the person's eyes.

Additional Information:
Grows in valleys with streams.

Translator's note:
Common Name: Scrophularia root.
Family: Figwort (Scrophulariaceae).
Other species used: Scrophularia buergeriana in northeastern China.
《中藥大辭典》 #1030.

楊柳 *yáng liǔ*
Twigs of Salix babylonica

Translator's note:
Common Name: Weeping willow twigs.
Family: Willow (Salicaceae).
《中藥大辭典》 #2414, where it is listed as 柳枝 *liǔ zhī*.

陽起石 *yáng qǐ shí*
Actinolite
Vol. 2, line 8 Middle Grade

味咸，微溫，無毒。主崩中漏下，破子藏中血，症瘕結氣，寒熱，腹痛，無子，陰痿不起，補不足。生山谷。

Flavor: Salty
Nature: Slightly warm
Toxicity: Non-toxic
Alt. names: 白石

Actions and Indications:
Indicated for center flooding and vaginal spotting. Breaks up blood inside the uterus and concretions, conglomerations, and bound *qì*, with [aversion to] cold and heat [effusion] and abdominal pain.
[Treats] infertility and *yīn* wilt with inability to raise [the penis], and supplements insufficiencies.

Additional Information:

Grows in mountain valleys.

Translator's note:
Compounded actinolite or actinolite asbestos (amphibole asbestos).
《中藥大辭典》 #4007.

羊肉 *yáng ròu*
Meat of Capra hircus (common goat) or Ovis aries (domestic sheep)

Translator's note:
Common Name: Sheep or goat's meat.
Family: Bovine (Bovidae).
Often, Sūn Sī-Miǎo specifies to use fat sheep or goat meat (肥羊肉 *féi yáng ròu*).
《中藥大辭典》 #1514.

羊胰 *yáng yí*
Pancreas of
Capra hircus (common goat)
or Ovis aries (domestic sheep)

Translator's note:
Common Name: Sheep or goat's pancreas.
Family: Bovine (Bovidae).
For a description of the animal, see 《中藥大辭典》 #1514.
《中藥大辭典》 #1521.

羊脂 *yáng zhī*
Unrendered fat of
Capra hircus (common goat)
or Ovis aries (domestic sheep)

Translator's note:
Common Name: Common goat or sheep fat.
Family: Bovine (Bovidae).
For a description of the animal, see 《中藥大辭典》 #1514. For a discussion of the different types of animal fat used by Sūn Sī-Miǎo, see entry on 脂 *zhī* below.

飴 *yí*
Malt syrup

Translator's note:
Thick gelatinous syrup made from sprouted wheat or other grains. Listed in the *Zhōng Yào Dà Cí Diǎn* (and occasionally in Sūn Sī-Miǎo's prescriptions) as 飴糖 *yí táng* (malt sugar). The *Běn Cǎo Gāng Mù* describes it as a moist sugar of a consistency like thick honey or soft candy (《本草綱目》25:950). In a harder consistency, it is called 膠飴 *jiāo yí* (malt candy). 《中藥大辭典》#4663.

宜男草花 *yí nán cǎo huā*
Flower of Hemerocallis fulva

Translator's note:
Common Name: Day lily flower.
Family: Lily (Liliaceae).
Other species used: Hemerocallis flava, H. minor.
For a description of the original plant, see 《中藥大辭典》#4290 on 萱草根 *yí cǎo gēn*. The flower is more commonly called 金針菜 *jīn zhēn cài* and is listed as such in 《中藥大辭典》#2158.

蟻垤土 *yǐ dié tǔ*
Ant hill dirt

Translator's note:
Not listed in the *Zhōng Yào Dà Cí Diǎn*, but in *Běn Cǎo Gāng Mù* 7:81.

薏苡仁 *yì yǐ rén*
Seed kernel of Coix lachryma-jobi
Vol. 1, line 37 Highest Grade

味甘，微寒，無毒。主筋急拘攣，不可屈神，風濕痹，下氣。久服，輕身、益氣。其根，下三蟲。生平澤及田野。

Flavor: Sweet
Nature: Slightly cold
Toxicity: Non-toxic
Alt. names: 解蠡

Actions and Indications:
Indicated for hypertonicity of the sinews and inability to bend or stretch, and wind-damp impediment.

Precipitates *qì*.
Additional Information:
Taken over a long time, it lightens the body and boosts *qì*.
Its root precipitates the three [types of] worms.
Grows in flatlands and marshes and open fields.

Translator's note:
Common Name: Job's tears.
Family: True Grass (Poaceae).
The root and leaves are also used medicinally, but *yì yǐ* alone is used to refer to the seed.
《中藥大辭典》#5127, where it is listed as 薏苡仁 *yì yǐ rén*.

茵芋 *yīn yù*
Foliage and stalk of Skimmia reevesiana
Vol. 3, line 35 Lowest Grade

味苦，溫，有毒。主五臟邪氣，心腹寒熱，羸瘦，如瘧狀，發作有時，諸關節風濕痹痛。生川谷。

Flavor: Bitter
Nature: Warm
Toxicity: Toxic
Alt. names: n/a

Actions and Indications:
Indicated for evil *qì* in the five viscera, cold and heat in the heart and abdomen, marked emaciation, an appearance like malaria with regularly occurring episodes, and wind-damp impediment pain in all joints.

Additional Information:
Grows in valleys with streams.

Translator's note:
Common Name: Chinese skimmia leaf.
Family: Rue (Rutaceae).
《中藥大辭典》#3074.

榆白皮 *yú bái pí*
The fibrous inner bark of the root or trunk of Ulmus pumila
Vol. 1, line 99 Highest Grade

In the *Shén Nóng Běn Cǎo Jīng*, under the entry for 榆皮.

味甘，平，無毒。主大小便不通，利水道，除邪氣。久服，輕身、不飢。其實尤良。生山谷。

Flavor: Sweet
Nature: Neutral
Toxicity: Non-toxic
Alt. names: 零榆

Actions and Indications:
Indicated for stopped defecation and urination.
Disinhibits the water ways and eliminates evil *qì*.

Additional Information:
Taken for a long time, it lightens the body and prevents hunger.
Its fruit is particularly good.
Grows in mountain valleys.

Translator's note:
Common Name: Dwarf elm bark, Siberian elm, Bast.
Family: Elm (Ulmaceae).
《中藥大辭典》#4228.

禹餘糧 *yǔ yú liáng*
Limonite
Vol. 1, line 12 Highest Grade

味甘，寒，無毒。主咳逆，寒熱，煩滿，下利赤
白，血閉，症瘕，大熱。煉餌服 之，不飢、輕
身、延年。生東海、池澤及山島中。

Flavor: Sweet
Nature: Cold
Toxicity: Non-toxic
Alt. names: 白餘糧

Actions and Indications:
Indicated for cough with counterflow, [aversion to]
cold and heat [effusion], vexation and fullness, red
and white diarrhea, blood blockage, concretions and
conglomerations, and great heat.

Additional Information:
Taken as an alchemical preparation, it prevents hunger, lightens the body, and extends the years.
Grows in Dōng Hǎi in ponds and marshes, and on
mountainous islands.

Translator's note:
In modern times, this is equated with 太一餘糧 *tài
yī yú liáng* (see entry on that substance above).
Nevertheless, in early and medieval times, these two
substances were treated differently, as evidenced by
the fact that they have separate entries in the *Shén
Nóng Běn Cǎo Jīng*. According to Lǐ Shí-Zhēn, 禹餘糧
yǔ yú liáng comes from ponds and marshes, while 太
一餘糧 *tài yī yú liáng* comes from mountain valleys.
《中藥大辭典》#2472.

原蠶矢 *yuán cán shǐ*
Excrement of Bombyx mori

Translator's note:
Common Name: Silkworm droppings.
Family: Silkworm (Bombycidae).
《中藥大辭典》#2777, where it is listed as 原蠶沙
yuán cán shā.

遠志 *yuǎn zhì*
Root of Polygala tenuifolia
Vol. 1, line 39 Highest Grade

味苦，溫，無毒。主咳逆，傷中，補不足，除邪
氣，利九竅，益智慧，耳目聰明，不忘，強志倍
力。久服，輕身、不老。生川谷。

Flavor: Bitter
Nature: Warm
Toxicity: Non-toxic
Alt. names: 棘菀，葽繞，細草. Leaves are called 小草.

Actions and Indications:
Indicated for cough with counterflow, and damage to
the center.
Supplements insufficiencies, eliminates evil *qì*, disinhibits the nine orifices, boosts wisdom, sharpens the
ears and eyes, prevents forgetfulness, strengthens
the will, and doubles strength.

Additional Information:
Taken over a long time, it lightens the body and
prevents aging.
Grows in valleys with streams.

Translator's note:
Common Name: Polygala (Snakeroot).
Family: Milkwort (Polygalaceae).
The stalk and foliage are also used medicinally under
the name of 小草 *xiǎo cǎo* (see entry above).
《中藥大辭典》#4629.

月經衣 *yuè jīng yī*
Menstrual cloth

Translator's note:
Not listed in the *Zhōng Yào Dà Cí Diǎn* or *Běn Cǎo
Gāng Mù*. The *Běn Cǎo Gāng Mù* contains an entry
on "women's menstrual blood," in which Lǐ Shí-Zhēn
himself points out: "The gentleman stays far away
when women enter the month because the malign
fluid is rotten and polluted and because of its unclean
nature is able to harm *yáng* and cause illness." There-

fore, he states that it should be avoided by anybody who is compounding medicines. On the other hand, it is used in his times by evil persons for the purposes of black magic, in which case it is referred to as 紅鉛 *hóng qiān* (lit. "red lead" or "minium"). Nevertheless, only "fools place their faith in it" (愚人信之 *yú rén xìn zhī*). He does, however, quote seven old and five new prescriptions in his section on "appended prescriptions."

雲母 *yún mǔ*
Muscovite
Vol. 1, line 2 Highest Grade

味甘，平，無毒。主身皮死肌，中風寒熱，如在車船上，除邪氣，安五臟，益子精，明目，久服輕身、延年。生山谷山石間。

Flavor: Sweet
Nature: Neutral
Toxicity: Non-toxic
Alt. names: 云珠，云華，云英，云液，云沙，磷石

Actions and Indications:
Indicated for dead flesh in the body's skin, wind stroke with [aversion to] cold and heat [effusion], and [a feeling] as if on a cart or boat.
Eliminates evil *qì*, quiets the five viscera, boosts child essence [i.e. sperm], and brightens the eyes.
Taken for a long time, it lightens the body and extends the years.

Additional Information:
Grows in mountain valleys between mountains and rocks.

Translator's note:
《中藥大辭典》#4019.

蕓苔 *yún tái*
Foliage and stalk of Brassica campestris var. oleifera

Translator's note:
Common Name: Oil rape.
Family: Mustard (Brassicaceae).
Other species used: Brassica rapa, the variety of mustard from which rapeseed oil is produced, also called sarson.
《中藥大辭典》#4937.

皂莢 *zào jiá*
Fruit of Gleditsia sinensis
Vol. 3, line 61 Lowest Grade

味辛、鹹，溫，有小毒。主風痹、死肌、邪氣，風頭、淚出，利九竅，殺精物。生川谷。

Flavor: Acrid, salty
Nature: Warm
Toxicity: Slightly toxic
Alt. names: n/a

Actions and Indications:
Indicated for wind impediment, dead flesh, evil *qì*, wind in the head, and tearing.
Disinhibits the nine orifices and kills spectral things.

Additional Information:
Grows in valleys with streams.

Translator's note:
Common Name: Honey locust fruit.
Family: Pea (Fabaceae).
《中藥大辭典》#1743.

灶突墨 *zào tú mò*
Stove-pipe soot

Translator's note:
Soot that adheres to the stove-pipe after roasting herbs.
《中藥大辭典》#1461, where it is listed as 百草霜 *bǎi cǎo shuāng*.

灶屋上墨 *zào wū shàng mò*
Stove top soot

Translator's note:
Not listed in the *Zhōng Yào Dà Cí Diǎn* or Běn Cǎo Gāng Mù. See the following entry for similar substances related to stove ashes.

灶屋炱煤 *zào wū tái méi*
Kitchen soot

Translator's note:
Not listed in the *Zhōng Yào Dà Cí Diǎn*. Presumably it refers to the soot from all over the kitchen, as op-

posed to 灶突墨 *zào tú mò*, the soot adhering to the stove-pipe (see the entry above). The *Běn Cǎo Gāng Mù* has separate entries for 百草霜 *bǎi cǎo shuāng* (stove-pipe soot), 釜底墨 *fǔ dǐ mò* (pot soot), 伏龍肝 *fú lóng gān* (oven earth), and 梁上塵 *liáng shàng chén* (wall dust), but does not describe kitchen soot in general (《本草綱目》7:107, 106, 97, and 108, respectively).

澤蘭 *zé lán*
Foliage and stalk of Lycopus lucidus
Vol. 2, line 51 Middle Grade

味苦，微溫，無毒。主乳婦內衄，中風餘疾，大腹水腫，身面四肢浮腫，骨節中水，金創、癰腫、創膿。生大澤傍。

Flavor: Bitter
Nature: Slightly warm
Toxicity: Non-toxic
Alt. names: 虎蘭, 龍棗

Actions and Indications:
Indicated for nosebleed in childbearing women, residual diseases from wind strike, severe abdominal water swelling, puffy swelling in the body, face, and four limbs, water in the bones and joints, incised wounds, welling-abscess swelling, and wounds with pus.

Additional Information:
Grows alongside large marshes.

Translator's note:
Common Name: Lycopus or bugleweed leaf.
Family: Mint (Lamiaceae).
Other species used: Related species of lycopus. Occasionally, Sūn Sī-Miǎo uses the seed, in which case he specifies it as 澤蘭子 *zé lán zǐ*. 澤蘭 *zé lán* can also occasionally refer to Gynura segatum (usually called 三七草 *sān qī cǎo*, 《中藥大辭典》 #0098) or Eupatorium heterophyllum and related species (usually called 紅升麻 *hóng shēng má*, 《中藥大辭典》 #2499). In both cases it is the foliage and stalk, not the seeds, that are used medicinally.
《中醫大辭典》 #4883, which does not mention the medicinal use of the seed.

澤漆 *zé qī*
Entire plant of Euphorbia helioscopia
Vol. 3, line 34 Lowest Grade

味苦，微寒，無毒。主皮膚熱，大腹水氣，四肢面目浮腫，丈夫陰氣不足。生川澤。

Flavor: Bitter
Nature: Slightly cold
Toxicity: Non-toxic
Alt. names: n/a

Actions and Indications:
Indicated for heat in the skin, water *qì* in the greater abdomen, puffy swelling in the four limbs, face, and eyes, and for men's insufficiency of *yīn qì*.

Additional Information:
Grows in streams and marshes.

Translator's note:
Common Name: Sun spurge.
Family: Spurge (Euphorbiaceae).
《中藥大辭典》 #4881.

澤瀉 *zé xiè*
Rhizome of Alisma plantago-aquatica
Vol. 1, line 38 Highest Grade

味甘，寒，無毒。主風寒濕痹，乳難。消水，養五臟，益氣力，肥健。久服，耳目聰明，不飢、延年、輕身，面生光，能行水上。生池澤。

Flavor: Sweet
Nature: Cold
Toxicity: Non-toxic
Alt. names: 水瀉，芒芋，鵠瀉

Actions and Indications:
Indicated for wind-cold-damp impediment and breast-feeding difficulties.
Disperses water, nourishes the five viscera, boosts *qì* and strength, and fattens and fortifies.

Additional Information:
Taken over a long time, it sharpens the ears and eyes, prevents hunger, extends the years, lightens the body, engenders luster on the face, and makes the person able to walk on water.
Grows in ponds and marshes.

Translator's note:
Common Name: Alisma rhizome.
Family: Water Plantain (Alismataceae).
《中藥大辭典》 #4882.

甑帶 *zèng dài*
Steamer lining

Translator's note:
The material that is used to line the top of a cooking

pot used for steaming (《中華醫學大辭典》 p. 1568).
Not listed in the *Zhōng Yào Dà Cí Diǎn*. The *Běn Cǎo
Gāng Mù*, however, contains a detailed discussion
in a subsection to the entry on 甑 *zèng* ("steamers").
There we find the following quotation from *Mǎ Zhì* 馬
志, a medical official from around 975 CE: "In Jiāng-
Nán [i.e., the area south of the Yangzi River], steamer
linings are made from cattail. If you can get ones that
have been used for a long time and are rotten and broken, use those. They are able to dissipate *qì* because
they have been steamed by *qì* for a long time" (《本草
綱目》 38:1435).

獐骨 *zhāng gǔ*
Bones of Hydropotes inermis

Translator's note:
Common Name: Water deer's bone.
Family: Deer (Cervidae).
《中藥大辭典》 #4514.

爪甲 *zhǎo jiǎ*
Finger nails

Translator's note:
According to the *Zhōng Yào Dà Cí Diǎn*, they are
prepared either by washing and drying them, or by
roasting them with talcum powder until yellow.
《中藥大辭典》 #0065 lists this substance as 人指甲
rén zhǐ jiǎ.

蟅蟲 *zhè chóng*
Entire dried body of the female of
Eupolyphaga sinensis
Vol. 2, line 104 Middle Grade

味咸，寒，有毒。主心腹寒熱洒洒，血積症瘕，
破堅，下血閉，生子大良。生川澤及沙中、人家
牆壁下、土中濕處。

Flavor: Salty
Nature: Cold
Toxicity: Toxic
Alt. names: 土鱉

Actions and Indications:
Indicated for cold and heat in the heart and abdomen
with shivering, and for blood accumulations, concretions, and conglomerations.

Breaks hardenings, precipitates blocked blood, and is
excellent for engendering children.

Additional Information:
Lives in streams and marshes and in the sand, under
walls in people's houses, and in the ground in moist
places.

Translator's note:
Common Name: Wingless cockroach.
Other species used: Opisthoplatia orientalis or (regionally also Polyphaga plancyi).
Often translated in English TCM literature as ground
beetle.
《中藥大辭典》 #5152.

真珠 *zhēn zhū*
Pearl

Translator's note:
Other species used: Pteria margaritifera, P. marten-
sii, Hyriopsis cumingii, Cristaria plicata, or Anodonta
woodiana.
Calcium carbonate concretion formed by several species of salt-water or fresh-water mollusks. According
to Lǐ Shí-Zhēn, pearls need to be soaked in human
breast milk for three days and then cooked before
they can be used as a medicinal ingredient (《本草綱
目》 46:1674).
《中藥大辭典》 #2450, where it is listed as 珍珠 *zhēn
zhū*.

脂 *zhī*
Fat from horned animals

Translator's note:
Hard unrendered fat from horned animals of the
bovine family (Bovidae), particularly beef or mutton.
For more information on the difference between 脂
zhī and 膏 *gāo* (lard), see the entry on *gāo* above. In
general usage, 脂 *zhī* is commonly translated as "fat."
For beef fat, see 《中藥大辭典》 #0888; for sheep or
goat's fat, see 《中藥大辭典》 #1522 and the entry on
羊脂 *yáng zhī* above.

知母 *zhī mǔ*
Root of Anemarrhena asphodeloides
Vol. 2, line 29 Middle Grade

味苦，寒，無毒。主消渴熱中，除邪氣，肢体浮腫。下水，補不足，益氣。生川谷。

Flavor: Bitter
Nature: Cold
Toxicity: Non-toxic
Alt. names: 蚳母，連母，野蓼，地參，水參，水浚，貨母，蝭母

Actions and Indications:
Indicated for dispersion thirst with heat in the center, eliminating evil *qì*, and puffy swelling in the extremities and trunk.
Precipitates water, supplements insufficiencies, and boosts *qì*.

Additional Information:
Grows in valleys with streams.

Translator's note:
Common Name: Anemarrhena root.
Family: Lily (Liliaceae).
《中藥大辭典》 #2052.

栀子仁 *zhī zǐ rén*
Fruit of Gardenia jasminoides
Vol. 2, line 66 Middle Grade

In the *Shén Nóng Běn Cǎo Jīng*, under the entry for 卮子.

味苦，寒，無毒。主五內邪氣，胃中熱氣，面赤，酒皰皶鼻，白癩、赤癩，創瘍。生川谷。

Flavor: Bitter
Nature: Cold
Toxicity: Non-toxic
Alt. names: 木丹

Actions and Indications:
Indicated for the five types of internal evil *qì*, heat *qì* in the side stomach, redness of the face, drunkard's nose, and wounds and sores from white *lài* and red *lài*.

Additional Information:
Grows in valleys with streams.

Translator's note:
Common Name: Cape jasmine.
Family: Madder (Rubiaceae).
《中藥大辭典》 #3335, where it is listed as 栀子 *zhī zǐ*.

蜘蛛 *zhī zhū*
Entire body of Aranea ventricosa

Translator's note:
Common Name: Orb-weaver.
Family: Orb-Weaver (Araneidae).
Other species used: Similar spiders.
《中藥大辭典》 #4600.

枳實 *zhǐ shí*
Unripe fruit of Poncirus trifoliata
Vol. 2, line 68 Middle Grade

味苦，寒，無毒。主大風在皮膚中，如麻豆苦痒。除寒熱結，止利，長肌肉，利五臟，益氣、輕身。生川澤。

Flavor: Bitter
Nature: Cold
Toxicity: Non-toxic
Alt. names: n/a

Actions and Indications:
Indicated for severe wind in the skin and bitter itching as if in measles.
Eliminates cold and heat binds, checks diarrhea, makes the flesh grow, benefits the five viscera, boosts *qì*, and lightens the body.

Additional Information:
Grows in streams and marshes.

Translator's note:
Common Name: Chinese hardy orange.
Family: Rue (Rutaceae).
Other species used: Citrus aurantium (bitter orange) or C. wilsonii.
《中藥大辭典》 #2361.

豬膏 *zhū gāo*
Lard of Sus scrofa domestica

Translator's note:
Common Name: Pork lard.
Family: Pig (Suidae).
《中藥大辭典》 #4969.

豬腎 zhū shèn
Kidneys of Sus scrofa domestica

Translator's note:
Common Name: Pig kidney.
Family: Pig (Suidae).
《中藥大辭典》#4956.

豬蹄 zhū tí
Hooves of Sus scrofa domestica
Vol. 3, line 76 Lowest Grade

In the *Shén Nóng Běn Cǎo Jīng*, under the entry for 豬
卵 [piglet testicles].

味苦，溫，無毒。主驚癇、癲疾，鬼注、蠱毒，
除寒熱、賁豚、五癃、邪氣、攣縮。懸蹄，主五
痔、伏熱在腸、腸癰、內蝕。

Flavor: Bitter
Nature: Warm
Toxicity: Non-toxic
Alt. names: 豬顛

Actions and Indications:
Indicated for fright epilepsy, withdrawal disease, ghost
infixation, and *gǔ* toxin.
Eliminates cold and heat, running piglet, the five types
of dribbling urinary disease, evil *qì*, and contracture.

Additional Information:
The dewclaws are indicated for the five types of
hemorrhoids, latent heat in the intestines, intestinal
welling-abscesses, and internal erosion.

Translator's note:
Common Name: Pig Hooves
Family: Pig (Suidae).
In one instance, Sūn Sī-Miǎo specifies "pig's hind
hooves" (豬後懸蹄 *zhū hòu xuán tí*), probably for
reasons of sympathetic magic (a set of practices and
beliefs based on the premise that like produces like)
since the prescription is used for a treatment of hemorrhoids.
《中藥大辭典》#4960.

竹 zhú
Phyllostachys
Vol. 2, line 64 Middle Grade

In the *Shén Nóng Běn Cǎo Jīng*, under the entry for
竹葉.

味苦，平，無毒。主咳逆上氣，溢筋急惡瘍，殺
小蟲。根，作湯，益氣，止渴，補虛，下氣。
汁，主風痙。實，通神明，輕身、益氣。

Flavor: Bitter
Nature: Neutral
Toxicity: Non-toxic
Alt. names:

Actions and Indications:
Indicated for cough with counterflow and ascent of *qì*
and for spilling sinews and malign sores.
Kills small worms.

Additional Information:
The root, prepared as a decoction, boosts *qì*, relieves
thirst, supplements vacuity, and precipitates *qì*.
The juice is indicated for wind tetany.
The fruit frees the spirit light, lightens the body, and
boosts *qì*.

Translator's note:
Common Name: Bamboo leaf.
Family: True Grass (Poaceae).
Sūn Sī-Miǎo distinguishes between 淡竹 *dàn zhú*
(bland bamboo), 甘竹 *gān zhú* (sweet bamboo), 苦
竹 *kǔ zhú* (bitter bamboo), and 青竹 *qīng zhú* (green
bamboo). The leaves (葉 *yè*), root (根 *gēn*), sap (瀝
lì, i.e., the fluid that is excreted when bamboo stalks
are heated), and shavings (茹 *rú*, also called 皮 *pí*,
i.e., shavings of the stripped core of stalks) are used
medicinally. While the *Zhōng Yào Dà Cí Diǎn* gives 淡
竹 *dàn zhú*, 甘竹 *gān zhú*, and 青竹 *qīng zhú* as synonyms for bamboo and identifies them with Phyllostachys nigra (black bamboo), Sūn clearly distinguishes
between these varieties and uses them in different
prescriptions for different purposes, such as in volume
3, section 2 on "vacuity vexation," where a prescription
calling for 淡竹茹 *dàn zhú rú* (bland bamboo shavings) follows one calling for 甘竹茹 *gān zhú rú* (sweet
bamboo shavings). According to quotations in the *Běn
Cǎo Gāng Mù*, Táo Hóng-Jīng equates 甘竹 *gān zhú*
with 苦竹 *kǔ zhú* and distinguishes these from 甘竹
gān zhú (《本草綱目》37:1343). To reflect the specificity of the original prescriptions, I translate the terms
literally. The *Zhōng Yào Dà Cí Diǎn* states that when a
prescription simply calls for bamboo, this refers to 淡
竹 *dàn zhú*.
《中藥大辭典》#1471.

紫石英 zǐ shí yīng
Fluorite
Vol. 1, line 15 Highest Grade

味甘，溫，無毒。主心腹咳逆，邪氣，補不足，
女子風寒在子宮，絕孕十年無子。久服，溫中、
輕身、延年。生山谷。

Flavor: Sweet
Nature: Warm
Toxicity: Non-toxic
Alt. names: n/a

Actions and Indications:
Indicated for cough with counterflow in the heart and abdomen, and evil *qì*.
Supplements insufficiency and [treats] women's wind-cold in the uterus, interrupted pregnancies, and childlessness for ten years.

Additional Information:
Taken for a long time, it warms the center, lightens the body, and extends the years.
Grows in mountain valleys.

Translator's note:
《中藥大辭典》#3402.

紫菀 *zǐ wǎn*
Root and rhizome of Aster tataricus
Vol. 2, line 37 Middle Grade

味苦，溫，無毒。主咳逆上氣，胸中寒熱結氣，
去蠱毒，痿蹶，安五臟。生山谷。

Flavor: Bitter
Nature: Warm
Toxicity: Non-toxic
Alt. names: 青菀

Actions and Indications:
Indicated for cough with counterflow and ascent of *qì*, for cold and heat and bound *qì* in the chest, for removing *gǔ* poison, and for wilting reversal.
Quiets the five viscera.

Additional Information:
Grows in mountain valleys.

Translator's note:
Common Name: Aster root.
Family: Aster (Asteraceae).
《中藥大辭典》#3396.

紫葳 *zǐ wēi*
Flower of Campsis grandiflora
Vol. 2, line 73 Middle Grade

味酸，微寒，無毒。主婦人產乳餘疾，崩中，症
瘕血閉，寒熱，羸瘦，養胎。生西海川谷及山
陽。

Flavor: Sour
Nature: Slightly cold
Toxicity: Non-toxic
Alt. names:

Actions and Indications:
Indicated for women's residual diseases from child-bearing, flooding of the center, concretions, conglomerations, and blood blockage, [aversion to] cold and heat [effusion], and marked emaciation.
Nourishes the fetus.

Additional Information:
Grows in Xī-Hǎi in valleys with streams and on the sunny side of mountains.

Translator's note:
Common Name: Chinese trumpet flower.
Family: Trumpet Creeper (Bignoniaceae).
In a medical context, this substance is usually referred to as 凌霄花 *líng xiāo huā*.
《中藥大辭典》#2773.

酢梅 *zuò méi*
Fruit of Rhus sinensis

Translator's note:
Common Name: Sumac fruit.
Family: Rue (Rutaceae).
While this term is not recorded elsewhere, I interpret *zuò* as referring to 酢桶 *zuò tǒng*, which is a synonym for 鹽膚木 *yán fū mù*. Its fruit, which is used medicinally, is listed in the *Zhōng Yào Dà Cí Diǎn* as 鹽麩子 *yán fū zǐ*, but is also called 鹽梅子 *yán méi zǐ* (salty plum).
《中藥大辭典》#5722.

Appendix C: Formulary

艾葉湯 *ài yè tāng*
Mugwort Decoction

艾葉	ài yè	6g
丹參	dān shēn	6g
當歸	dāng guī	6g
麻黃	má huáng	6g
人參	rén shēn	9g
阿膠	ē jiāo	9g
甘草	gān cǎo	3g
生薑	shēng jiāng	18g
大棗	dà zǎo	12 pcs

Indications:
Decaying [fetus] and failure to complete [the pregnancy] due to increased cold, withered [fetus] due to heat, [fetal] stirring and agitation due to being struck by wind or cold, fullness in the heart, suspension and tension below the navel, rigidity and pain in the lumbus and back, suddenly appearing vaginal discharge, and abruptly alternating [aversion to] cold and heat [effusion].
Page: 105

安心湯 *ān xīn tāng*
Heart-Quieting Decoction

遠志	yuǎn zhì	6g
甘草	gān cǎo	6g
人參	rén shēn	9g
茯神	fú shén	9g
當歸	dāng guī	9g
芍藥	sháo yào	9g
麥門冬	mài mén dōng	24g
大棗	dà zǎo	30 pcs

Indications:
Postpartum surges, palpitations, and instability in the heart, severe abstraction, lack of self-awareness, deranged and false speech, vacuity vexation and shortness of breath, and instability of the will, all of which are caused by heart vacuity.
Page: 290

安中湯 *ān zhōng tāng*
Center-Quieting Decoction

黃芩	huáng qín	3g
當歸	dāng guī	6g
川芎	chuān xiōng	6g
人參	rén shēn	6g
乾地黃	gān dì huáng	6g
甘草	gān cǎo	9g
芍藥	sháo yào	9g
生薑	shēng jiāng	18g
麥門冬	mài mén dōng	24g
五味子	wǔ wèi zǐ	35ml
大棗	dà zǎo	35 pcs
大麻仁	dà má rén	35ml

Indications:
Damage to the fetus during the fifth month.
Page: 114

白堊丸 *bái è wán*
Chalk Pills

白堊	bái è	2.25g
龍骨	lóng gǔ	2.25g
芍藥	sháo yào	2.25g
黃連	huáng lián	1.5g
當歸	dāng guī	1.5g
茯苓	fú líng	1.5g
黃芩	huáng qín	1.5g
瞿麥	qú mài	1.5g
白蘞	bái liǎn	1.5g
石韋	shí wéi	1.5g
甘草	gān cǎo	1.5g
牡蠣	mǔ lì	1.5g
細辛	xì xīn	1.5g
附子	fù zǐ	1.5g
禹餘糧	yǔ yú liáng	1.5g
白石脂	bái shí zhī	1.5g
人參	rén shēn	1.5g
烏賊骨	wū zéi gǔ	1.5g

藁本	gǎo běn	1.5g
甘皮	gān pí	1.5g
大黃	dà huáng	1.5g

Indications:
Women's thirty-six diseases.
Page: 468

白堊丸 bái è wán
Chalk Pills

邯鄲白堊	hán dān bái è	1.5g
禹餘糧	yǔ yú liáng	1.5g
白芷	bái zhǐ	1.5g
白石脂	bái shí zhī	1.5g
乾薑	gān jiāng	1.5g
龍骨	lóng gǔ	1.5g
桂心	guì xīn	1.5g
瞿麥	qú mài	1.5g
大黃	dà huáng	1.5g
石韋	shí wéi	1.5g
白蘞	bái liǎn	1.5g
細辛	xì xīn	1.5g
芍藥	sháo yào	1.5g
甘草	gān cǎo	1.5g
黃連	huáng lián	1.5g
附子	fù zǐ	1.5g
當歸	dāng guī	1.5g
茯苓	fú líng	1.5g
鐘乳	zhōng rǔ	1.5g
蜀椒	shǔ jiāo	1.5g
黃芩	huáng qín	1.5g
牡蠣	mǔ lì	2.25g
烏賊骨	wū zéi gǔ	2.25g

Indications:
Women's thirty-six diseases [of vaginal discharge],
diseases in the uterus, and incessant vaginal spotting.
Page: 509

白堊丸 bái è wán
Chalk Pills

白堊	bái è	4.5g
白石脂	bái shí zhī	4.5g
牡蠣	mǔ lì	4.5g
禹餘糧	yǔ yú liáng	4.5g
龍骨	lóng gǔ	4.5g

細辛	xì xīn	4.5g
烏賊骨	wū zéi gǔ	4.5g
當歸	dāng guī	3g
芍藥	sháo yào	3g
黃連	huáng lián	3g
茯苓	fú líng	3g
乾薑	gān jiāng	3g
桂心	guì xīn	3g
人參	rén shēn	3g
瞿麥	qú mài	3g
石韋	shí wéi	3g
白芷	bái zhǐ	3g
白蘞	bái liǎn	3g
附子	fù zǐ	3g
甘草	gān cǎo	3g
蜀椒	shǔ jiāo	1.5g

Indications:
Women's menstrual period arriving twice in one
month, or failing to arrive every other month, or of an
excessive or scanty amount, or as incessant dribbling,
possibly with lumbar and abdominal pain at the onset
of menstruation; huffing and gasping, inability to eat,
heart and abdominal pain, possibly [vaginal discharge
of] blue-green, yellow, or black color, or like water, and
heaviness when lifting the limbs.
Page: 524

白馬蹄丸 bái mǎ tí wán
White Horse's Hoof Pills

白馬蹄	bái mǎ tí	3g
鱉甲	biē jiǎ	3g
鯉魚甲	lǐ yú jiǎ	3g
龜甲	guī jiǎ	3g
蜀椒	shǔ jiāo	3g
磁石	cí shí	6g
甘草	gān cǎo	6g
杜仲	dù zhòng	6g
萆薢	bì xiè	6g
當歸	dāng guī	6g
續斷	xù duàn	6g
川芎	chuān xiōng	6g
禹餘糧	yǔ yú liáng	6g
桑耳	sāng ěr	6g
附子	fù zǐ	6g

Indications:
Women's coldness in the lower burner, causing the formation of vaginal discharge like a red or white flood.
Page: 480

白馬毛散 *bái mǎ tuō sǎn*
White Horse's Mane Powder

白馬駐	bái mǎ tuō	6g
龜甲	guī jiǎ	12g
鱉甲	biē jiǎ	2.25g
牡蠣	mǔ lì	5.25g

Indications:
Vaginal discharge.
Page: 481

白石脂丸 *bái shí zhī wán*
Kaolin Pills

白石脂	bái shí zhī	2.25g
烏賊骨	wū zéi gǔ	2.25g
禹餘糧	yǔ yú liáng	2.25g
牡蠣	mǔ lì	2.25g
赤石脂	chì shí zhī	1.5g
乾地黃	gān dì huáng	1.5g
乾薑	gān jiāng	1.5g
龍骨	lóng gǔ	1.5g
桂心	guì xīn	1.5g
石韋	shí wéi	1.5g
白薟	bái liǎn	1.5g
細辛	xì xīn	1.5g
芍藥	sháo yào	1.5g
黃連	huáng lián	1.5g
附子	fù zǐ	1.5g
當歸	dāng guī	1.5g
黃芩	huáng qín	1.5g
蜀椒	shǔ jiāo	1.5g
鐘乳	zhōng rǔ	1.5g
白芷	bái zhǐ	1.5g
川芎	chuān xiōng	1.5g
甘草	gān cǎo	1.5g

Indications:
Women's thirty-six diseases with pain in the uterus and spotting of red or white vaginal discharge.
Page: 472

白頭翁湯 *bái tóu wēng tāng*
Pulsatilla Decoction

白頭翁	bái tóu wēng	6g
阿膠	ē jiāo	6g
秦皮	qín pí	6g
黃連	huáng lián	6g
甘草	gān cǎo	6g
黃檗	huáng bò	9g

Indications:
Postpartum diarrhea concurrent with vacuity extreme.
Page: 343

白薇丸 *bái wéi wán*
Black Swallowwort Pills

白薇	bái wéi	3g
細辛	xì xīn	3g
防風	fáng fēng	3g
人參	rén shēn	3g
秦椒	qín jiāo	3g
白薟	bái liǎn	3g
桂心	guì xīn	3g
牛膝	niú xī	3g
秦艽	qín jiāo	3g
蕪荑	wú yí	3g
沙參	shā shēn	3g
芍藥	sháo yào	3g
五味子	wǔ wèi zǐ	3g
白殭蠶	bái jiāng cán	3g
牡丹	mǔ dān	3g
蠐螬	qí cáo	3g
乾漆	gān qī	2.5g
柏子仁	bǎi zǐ rén	2.5g
乾薑	gān jiāng	2.5g
卷柏	juǎn bǎi	2.5g
附子	fù zǐ	2.5g
川芎	chuān xiōng	2.5g
紫石英	zǐ shí yīng	4.5g
桃仁	táo rén	4.5g
鍾乳	zhōng rǔ	6g
乾地黃	gān dì huáng	6g
白石英	bái shí yīng	6g
鼠婦	shǔ fù	1.5g
水蛭	shuǐ zhì	1.875g

虻蟲	méng chóng	1.875g
吳茱萸	wú zhū yú	2.25g
燒麻布叩	shāo má bù kòu	30cm
複頭	fù tóu	

Indications:
Causes a woman to bear children.
Page: 68

白薇丸 *bái wéi wán*
Black Swallowwort Pills

白薇	bái wéi	2.25g
紫石英	zǐ shí yīng	3.75g
澤蘭	zé lán	6g
太一餘糧	tài yī yú liáng	6g
當歸	dāng guī	3g
赤石脂	chì shí zhī	3g
白芷	bái zhǐ	4.5g
川芎	chuān xiōng	3g
藁本	gǎo běn	2.5g
石膏	shí gāo	2.5g
菴䕡子	ān lǘ zǐ	2.5g
卷柏	juǎn bǎi	2.5g
蛇床子	shé chuáng zǐ	3g
桂心	guì xīn	7.5g
細辛	xì xīn	9g
覆盆子	fù pén zǐ	7.5g
桃仁	táo rén	7.5g
乾地黃	gān dì huáng	2.25g
乾薑	gān jiāng	2.25g
蜀椒	shǔ jiāo	2.25g
車前子	chē qián zǐ	2.25g
蒲黃	pú huáng	7.5g
人參	rén shēn	4.5g
白龍骨	bái lóng gǔ	6g
遠志	yuǎn zhì	6g
麥門冬	mài mén dōng	6g
茯苓	fú líng	6g
橘皮	jú pí	1.5g

Indications:
Chronic infertility or interruption of the line of descent, heat above and cold below, and all the myriad diseases.
Page: 77

白玉湯 *bái yù tāng*
White Jade Decoction

白玉	bái yù	4.5g
白朮	bái zhú	15g
澤瀉	zé xiè	6g
蓯蓉	cōng róng	6g
當歸	dāng guī	15g

Indications:
Women's [conditions resulting from] excessive sexual activity, pain in the jade gate, and blocked urination.
Page: 394

白芷丸 *bái zhǐ wán*
Dahurian Angelica Pills

白芷	bái zhǐ	15g
乾地黃	gān dì huáng	12g
續斷	xù duàn	9g
乾薑	gān jiāng	9g
當歸	dāng guī	9g
阿膠	ē jiāo	9g
附子	fù zǐ	3g

Indications:
Postpartum [conditions of] excessive vaginal discharge and center flooding [from] injuries, exhaustion and shortage of *qì*, loss of color in the face and eyes, and pain in the center of the abdomen.
Page: 412

柏子仁丸 *bǎi zǐ rén wán*
Arborvitae Seed Pills

柏子仁	bǎi zǐ rén	6g
黃芪	huáng qí	6g
乾薑	gān jiāng	6g
紫石英	zǐ shí yīng	6g
蜀椒	shǔ jiāo	4.5g
杜仲	dù zhòng	5.25g
當歸	dāng guī	5.25g
甘草	gān cǎo	5.25g
川芎	chuān xiōng	5.25g
厚朴	hòu pò	3g
桂心	guì xīn	3g
桔梗	jié gěng	3g
赤石脂	chì shí zhī	3g
蓯蓉	cōng róng	3g

五味子	wǔ wèi zǐ	3g
白朮	bái zhú	3g
細辛	xì xīn	3g
獨活	dú huó	3g
人參	rén shēn	3g
石斛	shí hú	3g
白芷	bái zhǐ	3g
芍藥	sháo yào	3g
澤蘭	zé lán	6.75g
藁本	gǎo běn	2.25g
蕪荑	wú yí	2.25g
乾地黃	gān dì huáng	3.75g
烏頭	wū tóu	3.75g
防風	fáng fēng	3.75g
鐘乳	zhōng rǔ	6g
白石英	bái shí yīng	6g

Indications:
Women's five taxations and seven damages, thinness, coldness, marked emaciation, and whittling, lack of color in the face, deficient [intake of] food and drink, a lusterless appearance, as well as postpartum lack of descendants and infertility.
Page: 405

敗醬湯 *bài jiàng tāng*
Patrinia Decoction

敗醬	bài jiàng	9g
桂心	guì xīn	4.5g
川芎	chuān xiōng	4.5g
當歸	dāng guī	3g

Indications:
Chronic postpartum pain stretching to the lumbus and center of the abdomen, as if being stabbed with an awl or knife.
Page: 312

半夏茯苓湯 *bàn xià fú líng tāng*
Pinellia and Poria Decoction

半夏	bàn xià	3.75g
茯苓	fú líng	2.25g
乾地黃	gān dì huáng	2.25g
橘皮	jú pí	1.5g
細辛	xì xīn	1.5g
人參	rén shēn	1.5g
芍藥	sháo yào	1.5g
旋復花	xuán fù huā	1.5g

川芎	chuān xiōng	1.5g
桔梗	jié gěng	1.5g
甘草	gān cǎo	1.5g
生薑	shēng jiāng	3.75g

Indications:
Obstruction disease in pregnancy with confusion and oppression in the heart, empty vexation and counter-flow vomiting, aversion to the smell of food, dizziness and heaviness of the head, pain, vexation, and heaviness in the four limbs and hundred joints, lying down more and being up less, aversion to cold with sweating, and extreme tiredness and yellow emaciation.
Page: 92

半夏厚朴湯 *bàn xià hòu pò tāng*
Pinellia and Officinal Magnolia Bark Decoction

半夏	bàn xià	24g
厚朴	hòu pò	9g
茯苓	fú líng	12g
生薑	shēng jiāng	15g
蘇葉	sū yè	6g

Indications:
Women's fullness in the chest and hardness below the heart, and stickiness in the throat as if there were pieces of roasted meat [lodged there] that she can neither vomit up nor swallow down.
Page: 371

半夏湯 *bàn xià tāng*
Pinellia Decoction

半夏	bàn xià	15g
麥門冬	mài mén dōng	15g
吳茱萸	wú zhū yú	9g
當歸	dāng guī	9g
阿膠	ē jiāo	9g
乾薑	gān jiāng	3g
大棗	dà zǎo	12 pcs

Indications:
In the ninth month of pregnancy, for suddenly contracted diarrhea, abdominal fullness with a sensation of suspension and fullness, fetus surging up against the heart, lumbar and back pain with inability to turn or bend, and shortness of breath.
Page: 124

鱉甲湯 biē jiǎ tāng
Turtle Shell Decoction

鱉甲	biē jiǎ	an amount the size of a hand
當歸	dāng guī	6g
黃連	huáng lián	6g
乾薑	gān jiāng	6g
黃檗	huáng bò	30cm long, 3 cm wide

Indications:
Wind and cold strike caused by rising too early after childbirth, with diarrhea and vaginal discharge.
Page: 343

鱉甲丸 biē jiǎ wán
Turtle Shell Pills

鱉甲	biē jiǎ	4.5g
桂心	guì xīn	4.5g
防風	fáng fēng	1.5g
玄參	xuán shēn	2.25g
蜀椒	shǔ jiāo	2.25g
細辛	xì xīn	2.25g
人參	rén shēn	2.25g
苦參	kǔ shēn	2.25g
丹參	dān shēn	2.25g
沙參	shā shēn	2.25g
吳茱萸	wú zhū yú	2.25g
蟅蟲	zhè chóng	3g
水蛭	shuǐ zhì	3g
乾薑	gān jiāng	3g
牡丹	mǔ dān	3g
附子	fù zǐ	3g
皂荚	zào jiá	3g
當歸	dāng guī	3g
芍藥	sháo yào	3g
甘草	gān cǎo	3g
防葵	fáng kuí	3g
蠐螬	qí cáo	20 pcs
虻蟲	méng chóng	3.75g
大黃	dà huáng	3.75g

Indications:
Accumulations and gatherings in the center of the lower abdomen that are as big as the surface of a seven or eight cùn bowl and move up and down and around, unbearable pain, bitter coldness in the hands and feet, coughing and belching with fishy-smelling breath, heat in both rib-sides as if from a blazing fire,

coldness in the jade gate as if the wind was blowing in, and menstrual stoppage or early or late menstruation. After taking these [pills] for thirty days, she will recover and be pregnant.
Page: 443

補胎湯 bǔ tāi tāng
Fetus-Supplementing Decoction

細辛	xì xīn	3g
乾地黃	gān dì huáng	9g
白朮	bái zhú	9g
生薑	shēng jiāng	12g
大麥	dà mài	35ml
吳茱萸	wú zhū yú	35ml
烏梅	wū méi	24g
防風	fáng fēng	6g

Indications:
Damage to the fetus during the first month.
Page: 103

柴胡湯 chái hú tāng
Bupleurum Decoction

柴胡	chái hú	12g
白朮	bái zhú	6g
芍藥	sháo yào	6g
甘草	gān cǎo	6g
蓯蓉	cōng róng	3g
川芎	chuān xiōng	6g
麥門冬	mài mén dōng	6g
乾地黃	gān dì huáng	15g
大棗	dà zǎo	13 pcs
生薑	shēng jiāng	18g

Indications:
Damage to the fetus in the sixth month.
Page: 117

柴胡湯 chái hú tāng
Bupleurum Decoction

柴胡	chái hú	24g
桃仁	táo rén	50 pcs
當歸	dāng guī	9g
黃芪	huáng qí	9g
芍藥	sháo yào	9g
生薑	shēng jiāng	24g
吳茱萸	wú zhū yú	48g

Indications:
Alternating [aversion to] cold and heat [effusion] and incomplete elimination of malign dew after childbirth.
Page: 322

承澤丸 *chéng zé wán*
Luster-Granting Pills

梅核仁	méi hé rén	24g
辛夷	xīn yí	24g
葛上亭長	gé shàng tíng cháng	.875g
澤蘭子	zé lán zǐ	35ml
溲疏	sōu shū	6g
藁本	gāo běn	3g

Indications:
Women's thirty-six diseases of the lower burner, [resulting in] failure to become pregnant and interruption of childbearing.
Page: 71

赤散 *chì sǎn*
Red Powder

赤石脂	chì shí zhī	9g
桂心	guì xīn	3g
代赭	dài zhě	9g

Indications:
Postpartum diarrhea.
Page: 350

赤石脂丸 *chì shí zhī wán*
Halloysite Pills

赤石脂	chì shí zhī	9g
當歸	dāng guī	6g
白朮	bái zhú	6g
黃連	huáng lián	6g
乾薑	gān jiāng	6g
秦皮	qín pí	6g
甘草	gān cǎo	6g
蜀椒	shǔ jiāo	3g
附子	fù zǐ	3g

Indications:
Diarrhea from postpartum vacuity cold.
Page: 350

赤小豆散 *chì xiǎo dòu sǎn*
Azuki Bean Powder

| 赤小豆 | chì xiǎo dòu | 21pcs |

Indications:
Postpartum vexation and oppression with inability to eat and vacuity fullness.
Page: 264

蔥白湯 *cōng bái tāng*
Scallion White Decoction

蔥白	cōng bái	14 stalks
半夏	bàn xià	24g
生薑	shēng jiāng	24g
甘草	gān cǎo	9g
當歸	dāng guī	9g
黃芪	huáng qí	9g
麥門冬	mài mén dōng	24g
阿膠	ē jiāo	12g
人參	rén shēn	4.5g
黃芩	huáng qín	3g
旋復花	xuán fù huā	7ml

Indications:
In the seventh month of pregnancy, for sudden fright and fear [causing the fetus to] shake and stir, abdominal pain, sudden presence of vaginal discharge, reversal cold in the hands and feet, a pulse as if she was suffering from cold damage, vexing heat, abdominal fullness, shortness of breath, and constant complaints of rigidity in the nape and neck as well as lumbus and back.
Page: 118

蔥白湯 *cōng bái tāng*
Scallion White Decoction

蔥白	cōng bái	24g
阿膠	ē jiāo	6g
當歸	dāng guī	9g
續斷	xù duàn	9g
川芎	chuān xiōng	9g

Indications:
Stirring fetus with abdominal pain during pregnancy.
Page: 133

大補益當歸丸 *dà bǔ yì dāng guī wán*
Major Supplementing and Boosting Chinese Angelica Pills

當歸	dāng guī	12g
川芎	chuān xiōng	12g
續斷	xù duàn	12g
乾薑	gān jiāng	12g
阿膠	ē jiāo	12g
甘草	gān cǎo	12g
白朮	bái zhú	9g
吳茱萸	wú zhū yú	9g
附子	fù zǐ	9g
白芷	bái zhǐ	9g
桂心	guì xīn	6g
芍藥	sháo yào	6g
乾地黃	gān dì huáng	30g

Indications:
Postpartum vacuity emaciation and insufficiency, shortage of *qi* in the chest, hypertonicity and pain in the abdomen, possibly with pain stretching to the lumbus and back, or with excessive vaginal discharge, incessant bleeding, vacuity drain of *qi*, inability to sleep by day or night, as well as center flooding, loss of color in the face and eyes, and dry lips and mouth. It also treats men's injury[-related] expiry, whether due to a fall from a high place, the presence of internal injury, vacuity of the viscera and blood ejection, or a flesh injury from an incised wound.
Page: 411

大補中當歸湯 *dà bǔ zhōng dāng guī tāng*
Major Center-Supplementing Chinese Angelica Decoction

當歸	dāng guī	9g
續斷	xù duàn	9g
桂心	guì xīn	9g
川芎	chuān xiōng	9g
乾薑	gān jiāng	9g
麥門冬	mài mén dōng	9g
芍藥	sháo yào	12g
吳茱萸	wú zhū yú	24g
乾地黃	gān dì huáng	18g
甘草	gān cǎo	6g
白芷	bái zhǐ	6g
大棗	dà zǎo	40 pcs

Indications:
Postpartum vacuity detriment and insufficiency, tension in the center of the abdomen, possibly with bloody urine, bitter pain in the lower abdomen, internal assault [due to] falling from a high place, as well as excessive bleeding and internal damage from incised wounds. It is also suitable for men to take.
Page: 307

大豆湯 *dà dòu tāng*
Soybean Decoction

大豆	dà dòu	120g
葛根	gé gēn	24g
獨活	dú huó	24g
防己	fáng jǐ	18g

Indications:
Postpartum sudden wind strike with falling, oppression, and inability to recognize people when the condition erupts. Wind complications during pregnancy, and also various sicknesses when in childbed.
Page: 277

大豆紫湯 *dà dòu zǐ tāng*
Soybean Purple Decoction

大豆	dà dòu	120g
清酒	qīng jiǔ	700ml

Actions:
Eliminates vacuity wind [-related] cold, dampness and taxation damage.

Indications:
Wind strike with disablement and tetany, possibly with a rigid back and clenched mouth, or merely vexing heat or thirst, or heaviness of both head and body, or itching of the body, or in severe cases, retching counterflow and forward-staring eyes.
Page: 269

大黃干漆湯 *dà huáng gān qī tāng*
Rhubarb and Lacquer Decoction

大黃	dà huáng	6g
乾漆	gān qī	6g
乾地黃	gān dì huáng	6g
桂心	guì xīn	6g
乾薑	gān jiāng	6g

Indications:
[Continuing] presence of blood [in the uterus] right after childbirth with cutting pain in the center of the abdomen.
Page: 327

大黃朴硝湯 *dà huáng pò xiāo tāng*
Rhubarb and Impure Mirabilite Decoction

大黃	dà huáng	15g
牛膝	niú xī	15g
朴消	pò xiāo	9g
牡丹	mǔ dān	9g
甘草	gān cǎo	9g
紫菀	zǐ wǎn	9g
代赭	dài zhě	3g
桃仁	táo rén	6g
虻蟲	méng chóng	6g
水蛭	shuǐ zhì	6g
乾薑	gān jiāng	6g
細辛	xì xīn	6g
硭硝	máng xiāo	6g
麻仁	má rén	35ml

Indications:
Inhibited menstrual flow for several consecutive years, caused by the presence of wind-cold in the uterus.
Page: 527

大黃湯 *dà huáng tāng*
Rhubarb Decoction

大黃	dà huáng	9g
當歸	dāng guī	9g
甘草	gān cǎo	9g
生薑	shēng jiāng	9g
牡丹	mǔ dān	9g
芍藥	sháo yào	9g
吳茱萸	wú zhū yú	24g

Indications:
Incomplete elimination of malign dew after childbirth.
Page: 322

大黃丸 *dà huáng wán*
Rhubarb Pills

大黃	dà huáng	24g
柴胡	chái hú	24g
朴消	pò xiāo	24g
川芎	chuān xiōng	15g
乾薑	gān jiāng	24g
蜀椒	shǔ jiāo	6g
茯苓	fú líng	1 egg sized pc

Indications:
The hundred diseases below the girdle and infertility.
Page: 72

大虻蟲丸 *dà méng chóng wán*
Major Tabanus Pills

虻蟲	méng chóng	400 pcs
蠐螬	qí cáo	24g
乾地黃	gān dì huáng	12g
牡丹	mǔ dān	12g
乾漆	gān qī	12g
芍藥	sháo yào	12g
土瓜根	tǔ guā gēn	12g
桂心	guì xīn	12g
吳茱萸	wú zhū yú	9g
桃仁	táo rén	9g
黃芩	huáng qín	9g
牡蒙	mǔ méng	9g
茯苓	fú líng	15g
海藻	hǎi zǎo	15g
水蛭	shuǐ zhì	300 pcs
硭硝	máng xiāo	3g
人參	rén shēn	4.5g
葶藶	tíng lì	35ml

Indications:
Menstrual stoppage [that has lasted] for six or seven years, possibly with swelling, fullness, and *qi* counterflow, abdominal distention, conglomerations, and pain.
Page: 451

大牛角中仁散 *dà niú jiǎo zhōng rén sǎn*
Major Ox Horn Marrow Powder

牛角仁	niú jiǎo rén	1 pc
續斷	xù duàn	9g
乾地黃	gān dì huáng	9g
桑耳	sāng ěr	9g
白朮	bái zhú	9g
赤石脂	chì shí zhī	9g
礬石	fán shí	9g
乾薑	gān jiāng	9g
附子	fù zǐ	9g
龍骨	lóng gǔ	9g
當歸	dāng guī	9g
人參	rén shēn	3g

蒲黃	pú huáng	6g
防風	fáng fēng	6g
禹餘糧	yǔ yú liáng	6g

Indications:
Accumulated cold, center flooding, incessant hemorrhaging, lumbar and back pain, heaviness of the four limbs, and extreme vacuity.
Page: 497

大平胃澤蘭丸 *dà píng wèi zé lán wán*
Major Stomach-Calming Lycopus Pills

澤蘭	zé lán	9g
細辛	xì xīn	9g
黃芪	huáng qí	9g
鐘乳	zhōng rǔ	9g
柏子仁	bǎi zǐ rén	7.5g
乾地黃	gān dì huáng	7.5g
大黃	dà huáng	6g
前胡	qián hú	6g
遠志	yuǎn zhì	6g
紫石英	zǐ shí yīng	6g
川芎	chuān xiōng	4.5g
白朮	bái zhú	4.5g
蜀椒	shǔ jiāo	4.5g
白芷	bái zhǐ	3g
丹參	dān shēn	3g
栀子	zhī zǐ	3g
芍藥	sháo yào	3g
桔梗	jié gěng	3g
秦艽	qín jiāo	3g
沙參	shā shēn	3g
桂心	guì xīn	3g
厚朴	hòu pò	3g
石斛	shí hú	3g
苦參	kǔ shēn	3g
人參	rén shēn	3g
麥門冬	mài mén dōng	3g
乾薑	gān jiāng	3g
附子	fù zǐ	18g
吳茱萸	wú zhū yú	35ml
麥蘗	mài niè	35ml
陳麴	chén qū	24g
[大]棗	[dà] zǎo	50 pcs

Indications:
The five taxations and seven damages and the various insufficiencies in men and women, by stabilizing the will and eliminating vexing fullness [and by treating] vacuity cold in the hands and feet with marked emaciation, irregular onset and ending of the menses, and inability to move the body.
Page: 423

大五石澤蘭丸 *dà wǔ shí zé lán wán*
Major Five Stones and Lycopus Pills

鐘乳	zhōng rǔ	7.5g
禹餘糧	yǔ yú liáng	7.5g
紫石英	zǐ shí yīng	7.5g
甘草	gān cǎo	7.5g
黃芪	huáng qí	7.5g
石膏	shí gāo	6g
白石英	bái shí yīng	6g
蜀椒	shǔ jiāo	6g
乾薑	gān jiāng	6g
澤蘭	zé lán	6.75g
當歸	dāng guī	4.5g
桂心	guì xīn	4.5g
川芎	chuān xiōng	4.5g
厚朴	hòu pò	4.5g
柏子仁	bǎi zǐ rén	4.5g
乾地黃	gān dì huáng	4.5g
細辛	xì xīn	4.5g
茯苓	fú líng	4.5g
五味子	wǔ wèi zǐ	4.5g
龍骨	lóng gǔ	4.5g
石斛	shí hú	3.75g
遠志	yuǎn zhì	3.75g
人參	rén shēn	3.75g
續斷	xù duàn	3.75g
白朮	bái zhú	3.75g
防風	fáng fēng	3.75g
烏頭	wū tóu	3.75g
山茱萸	shān zhū yú	3g
紫菀	zǐ wǎn	3g
白芷	bái zhǐ	2.25g
藁本	gǎo běn	2.25g
蕪荑	wú yí	3.75g

Indications:
women's wind vacuity and cold strike, thunderous rumbling in the abdomen, [alternating] slackening and

tensing, wind headache, [aversion to] cold and heat [effusion], irregular menstruation, anguishing pain around the navel, possibly with glomus and hardness in the heart or abdomen, counterflow harming the ability to eat and drink, constant cold in the hands and feet, profuse confused dreams, impediment pain in the whole body, imbalance between defense and construction, vacuity and weakness [to the point of] being unable to move and stir, as well as postpartum vacuity detriment.
Page: 407

大下氣方 *dà xià qì fāng*
Major Qì-Precipitating Formula

烏頭	wū tóu	1.5g
黃芩	huáng qín	1.5g
巴豆	bā dòu	1.5g
半夏	bàn xià	9g
大黃	dà huáng	24g
戎鹽	róng yán	4.5g
䗪蟲	zhè chóng	2.25g
桂心	guì xīn	2.25g
苦參	kǔ shēn	2.25g
人參	rén shēn	3g
消石	xiāo shí	3g

Indications:
Women's taxation *qì* and food *qì*, fullness in the stomach and counterflow vomiting, and the [related] symptoms of heaviness and binding pain in the head and reddish or yellow urine.
Page: 364

大巖蜜湯 *dà yán mì tāng*
Major Rock Honey Decoction

乾地黃	gān dì huáng	6g
當歸	dāng guī	6g
獨活	dú huó	6g
甘草	gān cǎo	6g
芍藥	sháo yào	6g
桂心	guì xīn	6g
細辛	xì xīn	6g
小草	xiǎo cǎo	6g
吳茱萸	wú zhū yú	24g
乾薑	gān jiāng	9g

Indications:
Postpartum heart pain.
Page: 297

大遠志丸 *dà yuǎn zhì wán*
Major Polygala Pills

遠志	yuǎn zhì	9g
甘草	gān cǎo	9g
茯苓	fú líng	9g
麥門冬	mài mén dōng	9g
人參	rén shēn	9g
當歸	dāng guī	9g
白朮	bái zhú	9g
澤瀉	zé xiè	9g
獨活	dú huó	9g
菖蒲	chāng pú	9g
薯蕷	shǔ yù	6g
阿膠	ē jiāo	6g
乾薑	gān jiāng	12g
乾地黃	gān dì huáng	15g
桂心	guì xīn	9g

Actions:
Internally supplements injuries, boosts *qì*, and settles the heart spirit.

Indications:
Postpartum vacuity and insufficiency in the heart, vacuity palpitations below the heart, disquietude of the mind, severe abstraction, hypertonicity and pain in the center of the abdomen, disquieted sleep at night, and shortage of *qì* in the center of the chest in spite of heavy inhalations. This prescription It also treats vacuity detriment.
Page: 293

大澤蘭丸 *dà zé lán wán*
Major Lycopus Pills

澤蘭	zé lán	6.75g
藁本	gǎo běn	5.25g
當歸	dāng guī	5.25g
甘草	gān cǎo	5.25g
紫石英	zǐ shí yīng	9g
川芎	chuān xiōng	4.5g
乾地黃	gān dì huáng	4.5g
柏子仁	bǎi zǐ rén	4.5g
五味子	wǔ wèi zǐ	4.5g
桂心	guì xīn	3.75g
石斛	shí hú	3.75g
白朮	bái zhú	3.75g
白芷	bái zhǐ	3g

蓯蓉	cōng róng	3g
厚朴	hòu pò	3g
防風	fáng fēng	3g
薯蕷	shǔ yù	3g
茯苓	fú líng	3g
乾薑	gān jiāng	3g
禹餘糧	yǔ yú liáng	3g
細辛	xì xīn	3g
卷柏	juǎn bǎi	3g
蜀椒	shǔ jiāo	2.25g
人參	rén shēn	2.25g
杜仲	dù zhòng	2.25g
牛膝	niú xī	2.25g
蛇床子	shé chuáng zǐ	2.25g
續斷	xù duàn	2.25g
艾葉	ài yè	2.25g
蕪荑	wú yí	2.25g
楮實子	chǔ shí zǐ	6g
石膏	shí gāo	6g

Indications:
Vacuity detriment as well as residual wind strike diseases, mounting-conglomerations, and coldness and pain in the vagina; or wind in the head entering the brain, cold impediment, slackening and tensing of the sinews, blood blockage and infertility, intermittent roaming wind on the face, tearing of the eyes, increased sniveling and salivating, and confusion as if she was intoxicated; or coldness in the stomach counterflowing into the chest, incessant retching, diarrhea, and dribbling urination; or an imbalance of hot and cold in the five viscera and six bowels, glomus and tension below the heart, and evil *qì* cough counterflow; or white and red vaginal spotting, swelling and pain in the vagina, and propping fullness in the chest and rib-sides; or roughness of the skin all over the body resembling measles, uncomfortable itching, phlegm aggregations, and *qì* bind; or hypertonicity in the four limbs, wind circulating in the body, pain in the bones and joints, and blinding dizziness in the eyes; or *qì* ascent and aversion to cold, and shivering from cold as if in malaria; or throat impediment, nose congestion, and wind convulsions and topsy-turviness; or menstrual stoppage, instability of the *hún* and *pò* souls, and lack of appetite for food or drink; as well as treating postpartum internal spontaneous bleeding. Taking these [pills] will allow the patient to be with child.
Page: 416

丹參膏 *dān shēn gāo*
Salvia Paste

丹參	dān shēn	24g
川芎	chuān xiōng	9g
當歸	dāng guī	9g
蜀椒	shǔ jiāo	35ml

Indications:
Nourishes the fetus, lubricates the fetus and eases childbirth.
Page: 127

丹參酒 *dān shēn jiǔ*
Salvia Liquor

丹參	dān shēn	240g
艾葉	ài yè	240g
地黃	dì huáng	240g
忍冬	rěn dōng	240g
地榆	dì yú	240g

Indications:
Center flooding and bleeding, as well as residual diseases from childbirth.
Page: 504

丹參丸 *dān shēn wán*
Sage Pills

丹參	dān shēn	6g
續斷	xù duàn	6g
芍藥	sháo yào	6g
白膠	bái jiāo	6g
白朮	bái zhú	6g
柏子仁	bǎi zǐ rén	6g
人參	rén shēn	3.75g
川芎	chuān xiōng	3.75g
乾薑	gān jiāng	3.75g
當歸	dāng guī	5.25g
橘皮	jú pí	5.25g
吳茱萸	wú zhū yú	5.25g
白芷	bái zhǐ	3g
冠纓	guān yīng	3g
蕪荑	wú yí	2.25g
乾地黃	gān dì huáng	4.5g
甘草	gān cǎo	6g
乾犬卵	gān quǎn luǎn	1 set

| 東門上雄 | dōng mén shàng | 1 pc |
| 雞頭 | xióng jī tóu | |

Actions:
Nourishes the fetus and converts a female fetus into a male.

Indications:
For the beginning of pregnancy.
Page: 84

單行鬼箭湯 dān xíng guǐ jiàn tāng
Single Agent Winged Spindle Tree Decoction

| 鬼箭 | guǐ jiàn | 15g |

Indications:
Absence of breast milk.
Page: 228

單行石膏湯 dān xíng shí gāo tāng
Single Agent Gypsum Decoction

| 石膏 | shí gāo | 12g |

Indications:
Absence of breast milk.
Page: 220

單行竹瀝汁 dān xíng zhú lì zhī
Single Agent Bamboo Sap Juice

| 竹瀝 | zhú lì | |

Indications:
Patient's on the verge of death from being stirred by their husband during pregnancy.
Page: 396

淡竹茹湯 dān zhú rú tāng
Bamboo Shavings Decoction

生淡竹茹	shēng dàn zhú rú	24g
麥門冬	mài mén dōng	35ml
甘草	gān cǎo	3g
小麥	xiǎo mài	35ml
生薑	shēng jiāng	9g
大棗	dà zǎo	14 pcs

Indications:
Postpartum vacuity vexation with headache, shortness of breath verging on qì expiry, and oppression and turmoil in the center of the heart that fails to be resolved.
Page: 263

當歸散 dāng guī sǎn
Chinese Angelica Powder

當歸	dāng guī	6g
黃芩	huáng qín	6g
芍藥	sháo yào	3.75g
蝟皮	wèi pí	1.5g
牡蠣	mǔ lì	7.5g

Indications:
Vaginal prolapse.
Page: 380

當歸芍藥湯 dāng guī sháo yào tāng
Chinese Angelica and Peony Decoction

當歸	dāng guī	4.5g
芍藥	sháo yào	3g
人參	rén shēn	3g
桂心	guì xīn	3g
生薑	shēng jiāng	3g
甘草	gān cǎo	3g
大棗	dà zǎo	20 pcs
乾地黃	gān dì huáng	3g

Indications:
Postpartum vacuity detriment with counterflow, which is harming the [digestion of] food and drink.
Page: 248

當歸湯 dāng guī tāng
Chinese Angelica Decoction

當歸	dāng guī	6g
生薑	shēng jiāng	15g
芍藥	sháo yào	6g
羊肉	yáng ròu	48g

Indications:
Women's cold mounting, vacuity taxation and insufficiency, and gripping pain in the center of the abdomen after childbirth.
Page: 299

當歸湯 dāng guī tāng
Chinese Angelica Decoction

當歸	dāng guī	9g
乾薑	gān jiāng	6g
白尤	bái zhú	6g
川芎	chuān xiōng	7.5g

甘草	gān cǎo	3g
白艾	bái ài	3g
附子	fù zǐ	3g
龍骨	lóng gǔ	9g

Indications:
Red and white diarrhea after childbirth with abdominal pain.
Page: 342

當歸湯 *dāng guī tāng*
Chinese Angelica Decoction

當歸	dāng guī	6g
川芎	chuān xiōng	6g
黃芩	huáng qín	6g
芍藥	sháo yào	6g
甘草	gān cǎo	6g
生竹茹	shēng zhú rú	48g

Indications:
Center flooding with hemorrhaging and vacuity emaciation.
Page: 493

當歸丸 *dāng guī wán*
Chinese Angelica Pills

當歸	dāng guī	6g
葶藶	tíng lì	6g
附子	fù zǐ	6g
吳茱萸	wú zhū yú	6g
大黃	dà huáng	6g
黃芩	huáng qín	4.5g
桂心	guì xīn	4.5g
乾薑	gān jiāng	4.5g
牡丹	mǔ dān	4.5g
川芎	chuān xiōng	4.5g
細辛	xì xīn	3.75g
秦椒	qín jiāo	3.75g
柴胡	chái hú	3.75g
厚朴	hòu pò	3.75g
牡蒙	mǔ méng	3g
甘草	gān cǎo	3g
虻蟲	méng chóng	50 pcs
水蛭	shuǐ zhì	50 pcs

Indications:
Aggregations and binds below the navel, stabbing pain as if from biting insects or as if being stabbed with an awl or knife, possibly with red and white vaginal discharge, the twelve [concretion] diseases, pain in the lumbus and back, and early or delayed menstruation.
Page: 442

當歸丸 *dāng guī wán*
Chinese Angelica Pills

當歸	dāng guī	12g
川芎	chuān xiōng	12g
虻蟲	méng chóng	3g
烏頭	wū tóu	3g
丹參	dān shēn	3g
乾漆	gān qī	3g
人參	rén shēn	6g
牡蠣	mǔ lì	6g
土瓜根	tǔ guā gēn	6g
水蛭	shuǐ zhì	6g
桃仁	táo rén	50 pcs

Indications:
Lumbar and abdominal pain and menstrual stoppage or inhibition.
Page: 463

當歸洗湯 *dāng guī xǐ tāng*
Chinese Angelica Wash Decoction

當歸	dāng guī	9g
獨活	dú huó	9g
白芷	bái zhǐ	9g
地榆	dì yú	9g
敗醬	bài jiàng	6g
礬石	fán shí	6g

Indications:
Postpartum wind strike in the viscera and vaginal swelling and pain.
Page: 385

抵党湯 *dǐ dǎng tāng*
Tangut-Resisting Decoction

虎掌	hǔ zhàng	6g
大黃	dà huáng	6g
桃仁	táo rén	30 pcs
水蛭	shuǐ zhì	20 pcs

Indications:
Inhibited menstruation and fullness in the center of the abdomen that sometimes recedes spontaneously, as well as men's fullness and tension in the urinary bladder.
Page: 530

地黃酒 *dì huáng jiǔ*
Rehmannia Wine

地黃汁	dì huáng zhī	70ml
好麴	hǎo qū	700ml
好米	hǎo mǐ	48g

Indications:
The hundred postpartum diseases.
Page: 242

地黃羊脂煎 *dì huáng yáng zhī jiān*
Rehmannia and Sheep or Goat Fat Brew

生地黃汁	shēng dì huáng zhī	700ml
生薑汁	shēng jiāng zhī	350ml
羊脂	yáng zhī	96g
白蜜	bái mì	350ml

Actions:
Regulates [digestion of] food and drink.

Indications:
Childbirth.
Page: 241

獨活酒 *dú huó jiǔ*
Pubescent Angelica Wine

獨活	dú huó	48g
桂心	guì xīn	9g
秦芄	qín jiāo	15g

Indications:
Postpartum wind strike.
Page: 277

獨活湯 *dú huó tāng*
Pubescent Angelica Decoction

獨活	dú huó	15g
防風	fáng fēng	6g
秦椒	qín jiāo	6g
桂心	guì xīn	6g
白朮	bái zhú	6g
甘草	gān cǎo	6g
當歸	dāng guī	6g
附子	fù zǐ	6g
葛根	gé gēn	9g
生薑	shēng jiāng	15g
防己	fáng jǐ	3g

Indications:
Postpartum wind strike with clenched mouth and inability to speak.
Page: 272

獨活湯 *dú huó tāng*
Pubescent Angelica Decoction

獨活	dú huó	9g
當歸	dāng guī	9g
桂心	guì xīn	9g
芍藥	sháo yào	9g
生薑	shēng jiāng	9g
甘草	gān cǎo	6g
大棗	dà zǎo	20 pcs

Indications:
Postpartum abdominal pain with hypertonicity and pain stretching to the lumbus and back.
Page: 313

獨活紫湯 *dú huó zǐ tāng*
Pubescent Angelica Purple Decoction

獨活	dú huó	48g
大豆	dà dòu	15g
酒	jiǔ	940ml

Actions:
Supplements the kidneys.

Indications:
Wind strike tetany during the first hundred days postpartum with clenched mouth that cannot be opened, as well as for treating blood and *qì* pain and taxation damage.
Page: 270

阿膠湯 *ē jiāo tāng*
Ass Hide Glue Decoction

阿膠	ē jiāo	12g
旋復花	xuán fù huā	14ml
麥門冬	mài mén dōng	24g
人參	rén shēn	3g
吳茱萸	wú zhū yú	49ml
生薑	shēng jiāng	18g
當歸	dāng guī	6g
芍藥	sháo yào	6g
甘草	gān cǎo	6g
黃芩	huáng qín	6g

Indications:
In the fifth month of pregnancy, for dizziness in the head, a deranged heart, and retching and vomiting, which are related to the presence of heat; for abdominal fullness and pain, which are related to the presence of cold; and for frequent urination, sudden fear and panic, pain in the four limbs, [aversion to] cold and heat [effusion], stirring of the fetus in unusual places, abdominal pain, oppression that suddenly puts the patient on the verge of collapse, and sudden presence of vaginal discharge.
Page: 113

阿膠丸 *ē jiāo wán*
Ass Hide Glue Pills

阿膠	ē jiāo	12g
人參	rén shēn	6g
甘草	gān cǎo	6g
龍骨	lóng gǔ	6g
桂心	guì xīn	6g
乾地黃	gān dì huáng	6g
白朮	bái zhú	6g
黃連	huáng lián	6g
當歸	dāng guī	6g
附子	fù zǐ	6g

Indications:
Postpartum throughflux diarrhea from vacuity cold, with gripping pain in the heart and abdomen and concurrent incessant diarrhea.
Page: 345

防風酒 *fáng fēng jiǔ*
Saposhnikovia Wine

防風	fáng fēng	24g
獨活	dú huó	24g
女萎	nǚ wěi	6g
桂心	guì xīn	6g
茵芋	yīn yù	3g
石斛	shí hú	15g

Indications:
Postpartum wind strike.
Page: 284

防風湯 *fáng fēng tāng*
Saposhnikovia Decoction

防風	fáng fēng	15g
當歸	dāng guī	6g
芍藥	sháo yào	6g
人參	rén shēn	6g
甘草	gān cǎo	6g
乾薑	gān jiāng	6g
獨活	dú huó	15g
葛根	gé gēn	15g

Indications:
Postpartum wind strike with tension in the back and shortness of breath.
Page: 275

茯苓湯 *fú líng tāng*
Poria Decoction

茯苓	fú líng	15g
甘草	gān cǎo	6g
芍藥	sháo yào	6g
桂心	guì xīn	6g
生薑	shēng jiāng	18g
當歸	dāng guī	6g
麥門冬	mài mén dōng	24g
大棗	dà zǎo	30 pcs

Indications:
Fulminant discomfort from heart palpitations after childbirth with absurd and deranged speech, severe abstraction, and muddle-headedness in the center of the heart; all of which are caused by heart vacuity.
Page: 289

茯苓丸 *fú líng wán*
Poria Pills

茯苓	fú líng	3g
人參	rén shēn	3g
桂心	guì xīn	3g
乾薑	gān jiāng	3g
半夏	bàn xià	3g
橘皮	jú pí	3g
白朮	bái zhú	6g
葛根	gé gēn	6g
甘草	gān cǎo	6g
枳實	zhǐ shí	6g

Indications:
Obstruction disease in pregnancy with complaints of vexing oppression in the heart, dizziness and heaviness of the head, loathing of the smells of food and drink, subsequent retching, counterflow vomiting, oppression, and topsy-turviness, and drooping and weakness of the four limbs, [all of] which the patient cannot overcome by herself.
Page: 94

伏龍肝湯 *fú lóng gān tāng*
Stove Earth Decoction

伏龍肝	fú lóng gān	7 pcs
生地黃	shēng dì huáng	96g
生薑	shēng jiāng	15g
甘草	gān cǎo	6g
艾葉	ài yè	6g
楮實子	chǔ shí zǐ	6g
桂心	guì xīn	6g

Indications:
Center flooding with discharge of a red or white or bean juice-like fluid.
Page: 496

茯神湯 *fú shén tāng*
Root Poria Decoction

茯神	fú shén	3g
丹參	dān shēn	3g
龍骨	lóng gǔ	3g
阿膠	ē jiāo	6g
當歸	dāng guī	6g
甘草	gān cǎo	6g
人參	rén shēn	6g

赤小豆	chì xiǎo dòu	21 grains
大棗	dà zǎo	21 pcs

Indications:
Damage to the fetus during the third month.
Page: 109

茯神湯 *fú shén tāng*
Root Poria Decoction

茯神	fú shén	12g
人參	rén shēn	9g
茯苓	fú líng	9g
芍藥	sháo yào	3g
甘草	gān cǎo	3g
當歸	dāng guī	3g
桂心	guì xīn	3g
生薑	shēng jiāng	24g
大棗	dà zǎo	30 pcs

Indications:
Sudden discomfort from surging palpitations in the center of the heart after childbirth, possibly with instability of the will, severe abstraction, and deranged and absurd speech, all of which are caused by heart vacuity.
Page: 287

甘草散 *gān cǎo sǎn*
Licorice Powder

甘草	gān cǎo	6g
大豆黃卷	dà dòu huáng juǎn	9g
黃芩	huáng qín	9g
乾薑	gān jiāng	9g
桂心	guì xīn	9g
麻子仁	má zǐ rén	9g
大麥蘗	dà mài niè	9g
吳茱萸	wú zhū yú	9g

Indications:
Eases childbirth and prevents [postpartum] disease for the mother.
Page: 127

甘草散 *gān cǎo sǎn*
Licorice Powder

甘草	gān cǎo	3g
通草	tōng cǎo	3.75g
石鍾乳	shí zhōng rǔ	3.75g
雲母	yún mǔ	7.5g
屋上散草	wū shàng sǎn cǎo	2 handfuls

Indications:
Absence of breast milk.
Page: 229

甘草湯 *gān cǎo tāng*
Licorice Decoction

甘草	gān cǎo	6g
乾地黃	gān dì huáng	6g
麥門冬	mài mén dōng	6g
麻黃	má huáng	6g
川芎	chuān xiōng	9g
黃芩	huáng qín	9g
栝蔞根	guā lóu gēn	9g
杏仁	xìng rén	50 pcs
葛根	gé gēn	24g

Indications:
Wind strike in childbed with rigidity of the back and inability to turn or move, called wind tetany.
Page: 271

甘草湯 *gān cǎo tāng*
Licorice Decoction

甘草	gān cǎo	15g
芍藥	sháo yào	15g
通草	tōng cǎo	9g
羊肉	yáng ròu	144g

Indications:
Postpartum abdominal damage and expiry with [aversion to] cold and heat [effusion], abstraction, and manic speech and visions of ghosts. This condition is caused by wind strike [leading to] internal expiry and by a vacuity of visceral *qì*.
Page: 282

甘草湯 *gān cǎo tāng*
Licorice Decoction

甘草	gān cǎo	9g
芍藥	sháo yào	9g
桂心	guì xīn	9g
阿膠	ē jiāo	9g
大黃	dà huáng	12g

Indications:
Incomplete elimination of the residual blood after childbirth and nursing, [to the point where it] counterflows and prods the heart and chest, with counterflow cold in hands and feet, dried lips, abdominal distention, and shortness of breath.
Page: 321

甘草丸 *gān cǎo wán*
Licorice Pills

甘草	gān cǎo	9g
人參	rén shēn	6g
遠志	yuǎn zhì	9g
麥門冬	mài mén dōng	6g
菖蒲	chāng pú	9g
澤瀉	zé xiè	3g
桂心	guì xīn	3g
乾薑	gān jiāng	6g
茯苓	fú líng	6g
大棗	dà zǎo	50 pcs

Indications:
Postpartum vacuity and insufficiency in the heart, vacuity palpitations, disquieted heart spirit, lack of *qì* in spite of heavy inhalations, and possibly severe abstraction and lack of self-awareness.
Page: 291

干地黃當歸丸 *gān dì huáng dāng guī wán*
Dried Rehmannia and Chinese Angelica Pills

乾地黃	gān dì huáng	9g
當歸	dāng guī	4.5g
甘草	gān cǎo	4.5g
牛膝	niú xī	3.75g
芍藥	sháo yào	3.75g
乾薑	gān jiāng	3.75g
澤蘭	zé lán	3.75g
人參	rén shēn	3.75g
牡丹	mǔ dān	3.75g

丹參	dān shēn	3g
蜀椒	shǔ jiāo	3g
白芷	bái zhǐ	3g
黃芩	huáng qín	3g
桑耳	sāng ěr	3g
桂心	guì xīn	3g
䗪蟲	zhè chóng	40 pcs
川芎	chuān xiōng	5.25g
桃仁	táo rén	6g
水蛭	shuǐ zhì	70 pcs
虻蟲	méng chóng	70 pcs
蒲黃	pú huáng	14ml

Indications:
Menstrual stoppage or [menstruation] occurring twice in one month or failing to arrive in alternate months, an excessive or scanty menstrual flow, incessant dribbling, or its onset accompanied by unbearable stabbing pain in the lumbus and abdomen, [as well as] in the four limbs, huffing and gasping and failure to eat and drink, hardness and pain in the heart and abdomen, [vaginal] discharge of green, yellow, or black-colored fluid, or discharge like clear water, lack of interest in movement and activity, heaviness when lifting the limbs, only thinking of sleep and rest, desire to eat sour foods, and vacuity, jaundice, and emaciation.
Page: 435

干地黃湯 *gān dì huáng tāng*
Dried Rehmannia Decoction

乾地黃	gān dì huáng	9g
芍藥	sháo yào	9g
當歸	dāng guī	6g
蒲黃	pú huáng	6g
生薑	shēng jiāng	15g
桂心	guì xīn	18g
甘草	gān cǎo	3g
大棗	dà zǎo	20 pcs

Indications:
Postpartum fullness and pain in both ribsides, while simultaneously eliminating the myriad diseases.
Page: 298

干地黃湯 *gān dì huáng tāng*
Dried Rehmannia Decoction

乾地黃	gān dì huáng	9g
川芎	chuān xiōng	6g
桂心	guì xīn	6g

黃芪	huáng qí	6g
當歸	dāng guī	6g
人參	rén shēn	3g
防風	fáng fēng	3g
茯苓	fú líng	3g
細辛	xì xīn	3g
芍藥	sháo yào	3g
甘草	gān cǎo	3g

Actions:
Supplements insufficiencies, eliminates the various sicknesses, and myriad diseases.

Indications:
Incomplete elimination of malign dew after childbirth.
Page: 318

干地黃湯 *gān dì huáng tāng*
Dried Rehmannia Decoction

乾地黃	gān dì huáng	9g
白頭翁	bái tóu wēng	3g
黃連	huáng lián	3g
蜜蠟	mì là	7.5g
阿膠	ē jiāo	1 hand sized pc

Indications:
Postpartum diarrhea.
Page: 347

干薑丸 *gān jiāng wán*
Dried Ginger Pills

乾薑	gān jiāng	3g
川芎	chuān xiōng	3g
茯苓	fú líng	3g
消石	xiāo shí	3g
杏仁	xìng rén	3g
水蛭	shuǐ zhì	3g
虻蟲	méng chóng	3g
桃仁	táo rén	3g
蠐螬	qí cáo	3g
䗪蟲	zhè chóng	3g
柴胡	chái hú	6g
芍藥	sháo yào	6g
人參	rén shēn	6g
大黃	dà huáng	6g
蜀椒	shǔ jiāo	6g
當歸	dāng guī	6g

Indications:
[Aversion to] cold and heat [effusion], marked emaciation, soreness, whittling, and fatigue, propping fullness in the center of the chest, heaviness and pain in the shoulders, back, and spine, hardness, fullness, and accumulations in the abdomen possibly with unbearable pain, pain stretching to the lumbus and the lower abdomen, vexation and aching in the four limbs, reverse flow in the hands and feet, coldness up to the elbows and knees possibly with vexing fullness and vacuity heat in the hands and feet, causing her to want to toss herself into water, extreme pain in the hundred joints, constant discomfort and suspension pain below the heart, alternating [aversion to] cold and heat [effusion], nausea, tendency to drool and salivate, frequent love of salty, sour, sweet, or bitter substances, possibly an [appearance of] the body like chicken skin, menstrual stoppage, discomfort and difficulty during urination and defecation, and eating without engendering flesh.
Page: 429

干漆湯 *gān qī tāng*
Lacquer Decoction

乾漆	gān qī	3g
萎蕤	wěi ruí	3g
芍藥	sháo yào	3g
細辛	xì xīn	3g
甘草	gān cǎo	3g
附子	fù zǐ	3g
當歸	dāng guī	6g
桂心	guì xīn	6g
硭硝	máng xiāo	6g
黃芩	huáng qín	6g
大黃	dà huáng	9g
吳茱萸	wú zhū yú	24g

Indications:
Menstrual stoppage and lower abdominal hardness and pain so severe that she will not let anyone near her.
Page: 430

干漆丸 *gān qī wán*
Lacquer Pills

乾漆	gān qī	4.5g
土瓜根	tǔ guā gēn	4.5g
射干	shè gān	4.5g
芍藥	sháo yào	4.5g
牡丹	mǔ dān	3.75g
牛膝	niú xī	3.75g
黃芩	huáng qín	3.75g
桂心	guì xīn	3.75g
吳茱萸	wú zhū yú	3.75g
大黃	dà huáng	3.75g
柴胡	chái hú	3.75g
桃仁	táo rén	6g
鱉甲	biē jiǎ	6g
蟅蟲	zhè chóng	40 pcs
蠐螬	qí cáo	40 pcs
水蛭	shuǐ zhì	70 pcs
虻蟲	méng chóng	70 pcs
大麻仁	dà má rén	28ml
亂髮	luàn fà	2 egg sized pcs
菴蕳子	ān lǘ zǐ	14ml

Indications:
Menstrual stoppage and a hundred ailments that fail to improve.
Page: 439

甘竹茹湯 *gān zhú rú tāng*
Sweet Bamboo Shavings Decoction

甘竹茹	gān zhú rú	24g
人參	rén shēn	3g
茯苓	fú líng	3g
甘草	gān cǎo	3g
黃芩	huáng qín	9g

Indications:
Postpartum internal vacuity with vexation heat and shortness of breath.
Page: 260

葛根湯 *gé gēn tāng*
Pueraria Decoction

葛根	gé gēn	18g
生薑	shēng jiāng	18g
獨活	dú huó	12g
當歸	dāng guī	9g
甘草	gān cǎo	6g
桂心	guì xīn	6g
茯苓	fú líng	6g
石膏	shí gāo	6g
人參	rén shēn	6g
白朮	bái zhú	6g
川芎	chuān xiōng	6g

| 防風 | fáng fēng | 6g |

Indications:
Postpartum wind strike, clenched mouth, tetany, and impediment, distressed and rapid breathing, veiling dizziness and drowsiness, as well as the various [other] postpartum diseases.
Page: 283

栝樓湯 guā lóu tāng
Trichosanthes Decoction

栝蔞根	guā lóu gēn	6g
黃連	huáng lián	6g
人參	rén shēn	9g
大棗	dà zǎo	15 pcs
甘草	gān cǎo	6g
麥門冬	mài mén dōng	6g
桑螵蛸	sāng piāo xiāo	20 pcs
生薑	shēng jiāng	9g

Indications:
Postpartum urinary frequency concurrent with thirst.
Page: 354

栝樓湯 guā lóu tāng
Trichosanthes Decoction

栝蔞根	guā lóu gēn	12g
人參	rén shēn	9g
甘草	gān cǎo	6g
麥門冬	mài mén dōng	9g
大棗	dà zǎo	20 pcs
土瓜根	tǔ guā gēn	15g
乾地黃	gān dì huáng	6g

Indications:
Incessant strangury after childbirth.
Page: 361

桂蜜湯 guì mì tāng
Cinnamon and Honey Decoction

桂心	guì xīn	6g
米	mǐ	24g
附子	fù zǐ	3g
乾薑	gān jiāng	6g
甘草	gān cǎo	6g
當歸	dāng guī	6g
赤石脂	chì shí zhī	30g

Indications:
Postpartum residual cold and red or white diarrhea with pus and blood in the stool, dozens of bowel movements a day, abdominal pain, and recurring descent of blood.
Page: 339

桂心酒 guì xīn jiǔ
Cinnamon Bark Wine

| 桂心 | guì xīn | 9g |

Indications:
Postpartum chronic ailments and pain, as well as sudden heart and abdominal pain.
Page: 308

桂心酒 guì xīn jiǔ
Cinnamon Bark Wine

桂心	guì xīn	12g
牡丹	mǔ dān	12g
芍藥	sháo yào	12g
牛膝	niú xī	12g
乾漆	gān qī	12g
土瓜根	tǔ guā gēn	12g
牡蒙	mǔ méng	12g
吳茱萸	wú zhū yú	24g
大黃	dà huáng	9g
黃芩	huáng qín	6g
乾薑	gān jiāng	6g
蝱蟲	méng chóng	200 pcs
䗪蟲	zhè chóng	70 pcs
蠐螬	qí cáo	70 pcs
水蛭	shuǐ zhì	70 pcs
亂髮灰	luàn fà huī	3g
細辛	xì xīn	3g
殭蠶	jiāng cán	50 pcs
大麻仁	dà má rén	72g
灶突墨	zào tú mò	72g
乾地黃	gān dì huáng	18g
虎杖根	hǔ zhàng gēn	15g
鱉甲	biē jiǎ	15g
菴䕡子	ān lǘ zǐ	48g

Indications:
Menstrual stoppage and [blood] binding and forming concretions and conglomerations.
Page: 452

桂枝加附子湯 *guì zhī jiā fù zǐ tāng*
Cinnamon Twig Decoction Plus Aconite

桂枝	guì zhī	9g
芍藥	sháo yào	9g
甘草	gān cǎo	4.5g
附子	fù zǐ	2 pcs
生薑	shēng jiāng	9g
大棗	dà zǎo	12 pcs

Indications:
Postpartum wind vacuity with incessant sweating, difficult urination, and slight tension and difficulty to bend and stretch the four limbs.
Page: 256

黑散 *hēi sǎn*
Black Powder

麻黃	má huáng	3g
貫眾	guàn zhòng	3g
桂心	guì xīn	3g
甘草	gān cǎo	9g
乾漆	gān qī	9g
細辛	xì xīn	6g

Indications:
Postpartum diarrhea.
Page: 351

厚朴湯 *hòu pò tāng*
Official Magnolia Bark Decoction

厚朴	hòu pò	1 pc
桂	guì	30cm

Indications:
Women's taxation cold in the lower burner, detriment and weakness of bladder and kidney *qì*, and discharge of a white liquid with urination.
Page: 370

虎杖煎 *hǔ zhàng jiān*
Bushy Knotweed Brew

虎杖根	hǔ zhàng gēn	1 pc

Indications:
Accumulations and gatherings in the abdomen, vacuity distention and thunderous rumbling, heaviness of the four limbs, and menstrual stoppage. It also treats men's diseases.
Page: 454

滑石散 *huá shí sǎn*
Talcum Powder

滑石	huá shí	15g
通草	tōng cǎo	12g
車前子	chē qián zǐ	12g
葵子	kuí zǐ	12g

Indications:
Postpartum strangury.
Page: 360

黃連湯 *huáng lián tāng*
Coptis Decoction

黃連	huáng lián	3g
人參	rén shēn	3g
吳茱萸	wú zhū yú	35ml
生薑	shēng jiāng	9g
生地黃	shēng dì huáng	15g

Indications:
Damage to the fetus during the second month.
Page: 106

黃芩牡丹湯 *huáng qín mǔ dān tāng*
Scutellaria and Moutan Decoction

黃芩	huáng qín	6g
牡丹	mǔ dān	6g
桃仁	táo rén	6g
瞿麥	qú mài	6g
川芎	chuān xiōng	6g
芍藥	sháo yào	9g
枳實	zhǐ shí	9g
射干	shè gān	9g
海藻	hǎi zǎo	9g
大黃	dà huáng	9g
虻蟲	méng chóng	70 pcs
水蛭	shuǐ zhì	50 pcs
蠐螬	qí cáo	10 pcs

Indications:
Complete absence of menstruation from childhood to adulthood, a withered and yellow complexion, weakened *qì* and strength, and inability to taste food and drink.
Page: 438

黃芩散 *huáng qín sǎn*
Scutellaria Powder

黃芩	huáng qín	1.5g
蝟皮	wèi pí	1.5g
當歸	dāng guī	1.5g
芍藥	sháo yào	3g
牡蠣	mǔ lì	7.5g
竹皮	zhú pí	7.5g
狐莖	hú jīng	1 set

Indications:
Women's vaginal prolapse.
Page: 379

黃散 *huáng sǎn*
Yellow Powder

黃連	huáng lián	6g
黃芩	huáng qín	3g
蟅蟲	zhè chóng	3g
乾地黃	gān dì huáng	3g

Indications:
Postpartum diarrhea.
Page: 352

雞糞酒 *jī fèn jiǔ*
Chicken's Droppings Wine

雞糞	jī fèn	24g
烏豆	wū dòu	24g

Indications:
Postpartum wind strike and the [other] myriad [postpartum] diseases, as well as for every type of wind strike in men.
Page: 273

雞鳴紫丸 *jī míng zǐ wán*
Cockcrow Purple Pills

皂莢	zào jiá	.75g
藜蘆	lí lú	1.5g
甘草	gān cǎo	1.5g
礬石	fán shí	1.5g
烏喙	wū huì	1.5g
杏仁	xìng rén	1.5g
乾薑	gān jiāng	1.5g
桂心	guì xīn	1.5g
巴豆	bā dòu	1.5g

前胡	qián hú	3g
人參	rén shēn	3g
代赭	dài zhě	3.75g
阿膠	ē jiāo	4.5g
大黃	dà huáng	6g

Indications:
Women's concretions, conglomerations, accumulations, and gatherings.
Page: 459

雞脆胵湯 *jī pí zhì tāng*
Chicken Gizzard Lining Decoction

雞脆胵	jī pí zhì	2 or 3 sets
雞腸, 洗	jī cháng, xǐ	3 sets
乾地黃	gān dì huáng	6g
當歸	dāng guī	6g
甘草	gān cǎo	6g
麻黃	má huáng	12g
厚朴	hòu pò	9g
人參	rén shēn	9g
生薑	shēng jiāng	15g
大棗	dà zǎo	20 pcs

Indications:
Postpartum urinary frequency.
Page: 355

吉祥丸 *jí xiáng wán*
Auspicious Fortune Pills

天麻	tiān má	3g
五味子	wǔ wèi zǐ	6g
覆盆子	fù pén zǐ	24g
桃花	táo huā	6g
柳絮	liǔ xù	3g
白朮	bái zhú	6g
川芎	chuān xiōng	6g
牡丹	mǔ dān	3g
桃仁	tao rén	100 pcs
菟絲子	tù sī zǐ	24g
茯苓	fú líng	3g
楮實子	chǔ shí zǐ	24g
乾地黃	gān dì huáng	3g
桂心	guì xīn	3g

Indications:
Chronic lack of pregnancy.
Page: 73

鯽魚湯 jì yú tāng
Golden Carp Decoction

鯽魚	jì yú	21 cm
豬肪	zhū fǎng	24g
漏蘆	lòu lú	24g
石鍾乳	shí zhōng rǔ	24g

Indications:
Precipitates breast milk.
Page: 227

膠艾湯 jiāo ài tāng
Ass Hide Glue and Mugwort Decoction

阿膠	ē jiāo	6g
艾葉	ài yè	9g
川芎	chuān xiōng	6g
芍藥	sháo yào	6g
甘草	gān cǎo	6g
當歸	dāng guī	6g
乾地黃	gān dì huáng	12g

Indications:
For women from the second and third months of pregnancy up to the seventh and eighth months who have stumbled and fallen or lost [their balance] when kneeling, resulting in stirring fetus, injury, lumbar and abdominal pain so intense that [the patient] wants to die, if she shows visible symptoms, to the point of the fetus racing upwards and prodding the heart, and shortness of breath.
Page: 158

膠蠟湯 jiāo là tāng
Ass Hide Glue and Bee's Wax Decoction

阿膠	ē jiāo	3g
蠟	là	an amount the size of three chess pieces
當歸	dāng guī	4.5g
黃連	huáng lián	6g
黃檗	huáng bò	3g
陳廩米	chén lǐn mǐ	24g

Indications:
Five-color diarrhea in the first three days postpartum, with the discharge of various [substances] all mixed together.
Page: 338

金城太守白薇丸 jīn chéng tài shǒu bái wēi wán
Governor of Jīn-Chéng's Black Swallowwort Pills

白薇	bái wēi	3.75g
人參	rén shēn	2.25g
杜蘅	dù héng	2.25g
牡蒙	mǔ měng	2.25g
牛膝	niú xī	1.5g
細辛	xì xīn	3.75g
厚朴	hòu pò	2.25g
半夏	bàn xià	2.25g
沙參	shā shēn	1.5g
乾薑	gān jiāng	1.5g
白殭蠶	bái jiāng cán	2.25g
秦艽	qín jiāo	1.5g
蜀椒	shǔ jiāo	4.5g
當歸	dāng guī	2.25g
附子	fù zǐ	4.5g
防風	fáng fēng	4.5g
紫菀	zǐ wǎn	2.25g

Indications:
Inhibited and blocked menstrual flow and interruption of childbearing for eighteen years. Taking this medicine for twenty-eight days will [cause the patient] to be with child.
Page: 75

菊花湯 jú huā tāng
Chrysanthemum Decoction

菊花	jú huā	1 egg sized pc
麥門冬	mài mén dōng	24g
麻黃	má huáng	9g
阿膠	ē jiāo	9g
人參	rén shēn	4.5g
甘草	gān cǎo	6g
當歸	dāng guī	6g
生薑	shēng jiāng	15g
半夏	bàn xià	12g
大棗	dà zǎo	12 pcs

Indications:
In the fourth month of pregnancy, for seething below the heart and desire to retch, fullness in the chest and diaphragm, and lack of appetite, all of which are related to the presence of cold; for urinary difficulties, urinating very frequently like a dribble, and bitter tension below the navel, which are related to the presence of heat; and for sudden wind-cold, rigidity and

pain in the nape and neck, and [aversion to] cold and heat [effusion], [fetal] stirring, perhaps from fright, with intermittent and occasional pain in the lumbus, back, and abdomen, for the fetus ascending and distressing the chest, for heart vexation and inability to get rest, and for the sudden presence of vaginal discharge.
Page: 110

橘皮湯 *jú pí tāng*
Tangerine Peel Decoction

橘皮	jú pí	2.25g
竹茹	zhú rú	2.25g
人參	rén shēn	2.25g
白朮	bái zhú	2.25g
生薑	shēng jiāng	3g
厚朴	hòu pò	1.5g

Indications:
Retching and vomiting in pregnancy with failure to get food down.
Page: 96

葵根湯 *kuí gēn tāng*
Mallow Root Decoction

葵根	kuí gēn	6g
車前子	chē qián zǐ	24g
亂髮	luàn fà	3g
大黃	dà huáng	3g
冬瓜練	dōng guā liàn	49ml
通草	tōng cǎo	9g
桂心	guì xīn	3g
滑石	huá shí	3g
生薑	shēng jiāng	18g

Indications:
Postpartum strangury and rough urination.
Page: 358

葵子湯 *kuí zí tāng*
Mallow Seed Decoction

葵子	kuí zǐ	48g
生薑	shēng jiāng	18g
甘草	gān cǎo	6g
芍藥	sháo yào	12g
白朮	bái zhú	9g
柴胡	chái hú	9g
大棗	dà zǎo	20 pcs
厚朴	hòu pò	6g

Indications:
Damage to the fetus in the eighth month.
Page: 122

昆布丸 *kūn bù wán*
Kelp Pills

昆布	kūn bù	7.5g
海藻	hǎi zǎo	7.5g
芍藥	sháo yào	7.5g
桂心	guì xīn	7.5g
人參	rén shēn	7.5g
白石英	bái shí yīng	7.5g
款冬花	kuǎn dōng huā	7.5g
桑白皮	sāng bái pí	7.5g
茯苓	fú líng	7.5g
鐘乳	zhōng rǔ	7.5g
柏子仁	bǎi zǐ rén	7.5g
紫菀	zǐ wǎn	3g
甘草	gān cǎo	3g
乾薑	gān jiāng	3.75g
吳茱萸	wú zhū yú	4.5g
烏頭	wū tóu	4.5g
五味子	wǔ wèi zǐ	4.5g
細辛	xì xīn	4.5g
杏仁	xìng rén	100 pcs
橘皮	jú pí	35ml
蘇子	sū zǐ	35ml

Indications:
Women's latent *qì* in the center of the chest.
Page: 372

藍青丸 *lán qīng wán*
Indigo Residue Pills

藍青	lán qīng	4.5g
附子	fù zǐ	4.5g
鬼臼	guǐ jiù	4.5g
蜀椒	shǔ jiāo	4.5g
厚朴	hòu pò	6g
阿膠	ē jiāo	6g
甘草	gān cǎo	6g
艾葉	ài yè	9g
龍骨	lóng gǔ	9g
黃連	huáng lián	9g
當歸	dāng guī	9g
黃檗	huáng bò	3g

| 茯苓 | fú líng | 3g |
| 人參 | rén shēn | 3g |

Indications:
Postpartum diarrhea.
Page: 349

鯉魚湯 lǐ yú tāng
Carp Decoction

鯉魚	lǐ yú	96g
白朮	bái zhú	15g
生薑	shēng jiāng	9g
芍藥	sháo yào	9g
當歸	dāng guī	9g
茯苓	fú líng	12g

Indications:
Enlarged abdomen and water qì in the space for the fetus, during pregnancy.
Page: 176

鯉魚湯 lǐ yú tāng
Carp Decoction

鯉魚	lǐ yú	48g
蔥白	cōng bái	24g
[豆]豉	[dòu] chǐ	24g
乾薑	gān jiāng	6g
桂枝	guì zhī	6g

Indications:
Generalized vacuity with incessant flowing of sweat and occasional nightsweats.
Page: 255

遼東都尉所上丸 liáo dōng dū wèi suǒ shàng wán
Pills Presented by the Commander-in-Chief of Liáo-Dōng

恒山	héng shān	.75g
大黃	dà huáng	.75g
巴豆	bā dòu	.75g
天雄	tiān xióng	2 pcs
苦參	kǔ shēn	2.25g
白薇	bái wēi	2.25g
乾薑	gān jiāng	2.25g
人參	rén shēn	2.25g
細辛	xì xīn	2.25g
狼牙	láng yá	2.25g

龍膽	lóng dǎn	2.25g
沙參	shā shēn	2.25g
玄參	xuán shēn	2.25g
丹參	dān shēn	2.25g
芍藥	sháo yào	3.75g
附子	fù zǐ	3.75g
牛膝	niú xī	3.75g
茯苓	fú líng	3.75g
牡蒙	mǔ méng	3g
蓷蘆	guàn lú	4.5g

Indications:
Hard aggregations below the navel.
Page: 460

羚羊角散 líng yáng jiǎo sǎn
Antelope Horn Powder

| 羚羊角 | líng yáng jiǎo | 1 pc |

Indications:
Postpartum heart oppression.
Page: 189

硫磺散 liú huáng sǎn
Sulphur Pills

硫磺	liú huáng	1.5g
烏賊骨	wū zéi gǔ	1.5g
五味子	wǔ wèi zǐ	0.375g

Indications:
Women's vaginal prolapse.
Page: 367

龍骨散 lóng gǔ sǎn
Dragon Bone Powder

五色龍骨	wǔ sè lóng gǔ	4.5g
黃檗根皮	huáng bò gēn pí	4.5g
代赭	dài zhě	4.5g
赤石脂	chì shí zhī	4.5g
艾[葉]	ài [yè]	4.5g
黃連	huáng lián	6g

Indications:
Postpartum diarrhea.
Page: 352

龍骨散 *lóng gǔ sǎn*
Dragon Bone Powder

龍骨	lóng gǔ	9g
黃檗	huáng bò	6g
半夏	bàn xià	6g
竈中黃土	zào zhōng huáng tǔ	6g
桂心	guì xīn	6g
乾薑	gān jiāng	6g
石韋	shí wéi	3g
槐實	huái shí	3g
烏賊骨	wū zéi gǔ	12g
代赭	dài zhě	12g
白僵蠶	bái jiāng cán	5 pcs

Indications:
The twelve diseases of vaginal downpouring, which interrupt the ability to bear children.
Page: 474

龍骨丸 *lóng gǔ wán*
Dragon Bone Pills

龍骨	lóng gǔ	12g
乾薑	gān jiāng	6g
甘草	gān cǎo	6g
桂心	guì xīn	6g

Indications:
Postpartum vacuity cold with bloody and grain diarrhea that occurs innumerable times during the day and at night, as well as incessant [flow of] malign dew after childbirth.
Page: 344

漏蘆散 *lòu lú sǎn*
Rhaponticum Powder

漏蘆	lòu lú	1.5g
石鍾乳	shí zhōng rǔ	3g
栝樓根	guā lóu gēn	3g
蠐螬	qí cáo	21ml

Indications:
Absence of breast milk.
Page: 222

漏蘆湯 *lòu lú tāng*
Rhaponticum Decoction

漏蘆	lòu lú	6g
通草	tōng cǎo	6g
石鍾乳	shí zhōng rǔ	3g
黍米	shǔ mǐ	24g

Indications:
Absence of breast milk.
Page: 220

鹿肉湯 *lù ròu tāng*
Venison Decoction

鹿肉	lù ròu	192g
乾地黃	gān dì huáng	9g
甘草	gān cǎo	9g
川芎	chuān xiōng	9g
人參	rén shēn	6g
當歸	dāng guī	6g
黃芪	huáng qí	6g
芍藥	sháo yào	6g
麥門冬	mài mén dōng	6g
茯苓	fú líng	6g
半夏	bàn xià	24g
大棗	dà zǎo	20 pcs
生薑	shēng jiāng	6g

Indications:
Postpartum vacuity emaciation and taxation detriment.
Page: 246

鹿肉湯 *lù ròu tāng*
Venison Decoction

鹿肉	lù ròu	144g
芍藥	sháo yào	9g
半夏	bàn xià	24g
乾地黃	gān dì huáng	6g
獨活	dú huó	9g
生薑	shēng jiāng	18g
桂心	guì xīn	3g
川芎	chuān xiōng	3g
甘草	gān cǎo	3g
阿膠	ē jiāo	3g
人參	rén shēn	12g
茯苓	fú líng	12g

秦艽	qín jiāo	9g
黃芩	huáng qín	9g
黃芪	huáng qí	9g

Indications:
Postpartum wind vacuity with headache, vigorous heat [effusion], and evil and mean speech.
Page: 276

麻子酒 *má zǐ jiǔ*
Cannabis Fruit Wine

麻子	má zǐ	120g

Indications:
Failure to eliminate blood after childbirth.
Page: 328

馬蹄丸 *mǎ tí wán*
Horse's Hoof Pills

白馬蹄	bái mǎ tí	12g
禹餘糧	yǔ yú liáng	12g
龍骨	lóng gǔ	9g
烏賊骨	wū zéi gǔ	6g
白僵蠶	bái jiāng cán	6g
赤石脂	chì shí zhī	6g

Indications:
Continuous white spotting.
Page: 519

馬蹄屑湯 *mǎ tí xiè tāng*
Horse's Hoof Flakes Decoction

白馬蹄	bái mǎ tí	15g
赤石脂	chì shí zhī	15g
禹餘糧	yǔ yú liáng	12g
烏賊骨	wū zéi gǔ	12g
龍骨	lóng gǔ	12g
牡蠣	mǔ lì	12g
附子	fù zǐ	9g
乾地黃	gān dì huáng	9g
當歸	dāng guī	9g
甘草	gān cǎo	6g
白僵蠶	bái jiāng cán	3g

Indications:
Continuous white spotting.
Page: 518

馬通湯 *mǎ tǒng tāng*
Horse Dung Decoction

馬通汁	mǎ tōng zhī	70ml
乾地黃	gān dì huáng	12g
當歸	dāng guī	9g
阿膠	ē jiāo	12g
艾葉	ài yè	9g

Indications:
Fulminant bleeding of several *shēng* during pregnancy, after fleeing and running from a sudden scare or falling down from a high place.
Page: 158

馬通湯 *mǎ tǒng tāng*
Horse Dung Decoction

赤馬通汁	chì mǎ tōng zhī	24g
生艾葉	shēng ài yè	9g
阿膠	ē jiāo	9g
當歸	dāng guī	6g
乾薑	gān jiāng	6g
好墨	hǎo mò	half a ball

Indications:
Vaginal spotting of blood that has persisted incessantly for several months.
Page: 518

麥門冬散 *mài mén dōng sǎn*
Ophiopogon Powder

麥門冬	mài mén dōng	Equal amounts
石鍾乳	shí zhōng rǔ	
通草	tōng cǎo	
理石	lǐ shí	

Indications:
Absence of breast milk.
Page: 221

麥門冬湯 *mài mén dōng tāng*
Ophiopogon Decoction

麥門冬	mài mén dōng	24g
人參	rén shēn	6g
甘草	gān cǎo	6g
黃芩	huáng qín	6g
乾地黃	gān dì huáng	9g
阿膠	ē jiāo	12g
生薑	shēng jiāng	18g
大棗	dà zǎo	15 pcs

Indications:
In the sixth month of pregnancy, for sudden stirring [of the fetus], alternating [aversion to] cold and heat [effusion], intestinal fullness in the abdomen, swelling of the body, fright and fear, sudden presence of vaginal discharge, abdominal pain as if she was going into labor; and vexation and pain in the extremities.
Page: 116

硭硝湯 *máng xiāo tāng*
Mirabilite Decoction

硭硝	máng xiāo	6g
丹砂	dān shā	6g
當歸	dāng guī	6g
芍藥	sháo yào	6g
土瓜根	tǔ guā gēn	6g
水蛭	shuǐ zhì	6g
大黃	dà huáng	9g
桃仁	táo rén	24g

Indications:
Menstrual stoppage.
Page: 431

茅根湯 *máo gén tāng*
Imperata Decoction

白茅根	bái máo gēn	48g
瞿麥	qú mài	12g
地麥	dì mài	6g
桃膠	táo jiāo	3g
甘草	gān cǎo	3g
鯉魚齒	lǐ yú chǐ	100 pcs
人參	rén shēn	6g
茯苓	fú líng	12g
生薑	shēng jiāng	9g

Indications:
Postpartum strangury.
Page: 359

牡丹皮湯 *mǔ dān pí tāng*
Moutan Decoction

牡丹皮	mǔ dān pí	9g
乾地黃	gān dì huáng	9g
斛脈	hú mài	9g
柏葉	bǎi yè	6g
厚朴	hòu pò	6g
白芷	bái zhǐ	6g
伏龍肝	fú lóng gān	6g
青竹茹	qīng zhú rú	6g
川芎	chuān xiōng	6g
地榆	dì yú	6g
阿膠	ē jiāo	3g
芍藥	sháo yào	12g

Indications:
center flooding and blood exuberance.
Page: 505

牡丹丸 *mǔ dān wán*
Moutan Pills

牡丹	mǔ dān	9g
芍藥	sháo yào	6g
玄參	xuán shēn	6g
桃仁	táo rén	6g
當歸	dāng guī	6g
桂心	guì xīn	6g
虻蟲	méng chóng	50 pcs
水蛭	shuǐ zhì	50 pcs
蠐螬	qí cáo	20 pcs
瞿麥	qú mài	3g
川芎	chuān xiōng	3g
海藻	hǎi zǎo	3g

Indications:
Menstrual block, interruption, or stoppage in married women and virgins after the various diseases, as well as menstrual stoppage since childhood, and blood stagnation and non-dispersion right after childbirth.
Page: 437

牡蠣丸 *mǔ lì wán*
Oyster Shell Pills

牡蠣	mǔ lì	12g
大黃	dà huáng	48g
柴胡	chái hú	15g
乾薑	gān jiāng	9g
川芎	chuān xiōng	7.5g
茯苓	fú líng	7.5g
蜀椒	shǔ jiāo	30g
葶藶子	tíng lì zǐ	35ml
硭硝	máng xiāo	35ml
杏仁	xìng rén	35ml
水蛭	shuǐ zhì	1.5g
虻蟲	méng chóng	1.5g
桃仁	táo rén	70 pcs

Indications:
Menstrual block and stoppage with no desire for food and drink.
Page: 462

牡蒙丸 *mǔ méng wán*
Four-Leaved Paris Root Pills

牡蒙	mǔ méng	2.25g
厚朴	hòu pò	2.25g
消石	xiāo shí	2.25g
前胡	qián hú	2.25g
乾薑	gān jiāng	2.25g
蟅蟲	zhè chóng	2.25g
牡丹	mǔ dān	2.25g
蜀椒	shǔ jiāo	2.25g
黃芩	huáng qín	2.25g
桔梗	jié gěng	2.25g
茯苓	fú líng	2.25g
細辛	xì xīn	2.25g
葶藶	tíng lì	2.25g
人參	rén shēn	2.25g
川芎	chuān xiōng	2.25g
吳茱萸	wú zhū yú	2.25g
桂心	guì xīn	2.25g
大黃	dà huáng	7.5g
附子	fù zǐ	3.75g
當歸	dāng guī	1.5g

Indications:
Women's twelve postpartum concretion diseases, vaginal discharge, and infertility, all of which are [related to] the cold *qi* of cool wind. Perhaps the woman, prior to the conclusion of the hundred days postpartum and the complete elimination of malign blood from the uterine network vessels, squatted carelessly over the privy for a long time. [This allowed] dampness and cold to enter inside, to bind in the lower abdomen, to cause firmness and pain, and to form accumulations and gatherings, the smaller ones the size of a chicken egg, the larger ones the size of a fist, slippery and ungraspable when pressed down. [This condition can be accompanied by pain] as if gnawed by worms or stabbed by needles, *qi* intermittently prodding the heart, propping fullness in both rib-sides, inability to eat, failure to disperse and transform food and drink, causing it to flow up and down or to get stuck in the stomach duct, pain all the way from the jade gate to the back and arms, retching counterflow and shortness of breath, sweating, bitter coldness in the lower abdomen, wounds in the uterus, coughing with pain stretching to the genitals, spontaneous urination, a crooked vagina causing infertility, pain in the lumbus and hip, heaviness and random flailing of the four limbs, abruptly occuring extreme swelling all over the entire body, constipation, dribbling urination, a menstrual period that is either stopped or resembles rotten flesh, a blue-green, yellow, red, white, black, or other-colored [substance], or bean juice, and inauspicious dreams and thoughts.
Page: 448

木防己膏 *mù fáng jǐ gāo*
Woody Fangji Paste

木防己	mù fáng jǐ	12g
茵芋	yīn yù	15g

Indications:
Postpartum wind strike.
Page: 285

內補當歸建中湯 *nèi bǔ dāng guī jiàn zhōng tāng*
Internally Supplementing Chinese Angelica Center-Fortifying Decoction

當歸	dāng guī	12g
芍藥	sháo yào	18g
甘草	gān cǎo	6g
生薑	shēng jiāng	18g
桂心	guì xīn	9g
大棗	dà zǎo	10 pcs

Indications:
Postpartum vacuity emaciation and insufficiency with incessant gripping pain in the center of the abdomen,

shortage of *qì* in spite of heavy inhalations, possibly with hypertonicity and pain in the lower abdomen that stretches to the lumbus and back, and inability to eat or drink.
Page: 305

內補黃芪湯 *nèi bǔ huáng qí tāng*
Internally Supplementing Astragalus Decoction

黃芪	huáng qí	9g
當歸	dāng guī	9g
芍藥	sháo yào	9g
乾地黃	gān dì huáng	9g
半夏	bàn xià	9g
茯苓	fú líng	6g
人參	rén shēn	6g
桂心	guì xīn	6g
遠志	yuǎn zhì	6g
麥門冬	mài mén dōng	6g
甘草	gān cǎo	6g
五味子	wǔ wèi zǐ	6g
白朮	bái zhú	6g
澤瀉	zé xiè	6g
乾薑	gān jiāng	12g
大棗	dà zǎo	30 pcs

Indications:
The seven damages, pain in the body, tension and fullness in the lower abdomen, yellow or black face and eyes, inability to eat or drink, as well as the various [conditions of] vacuity, insufficiency, and shortage of *qì* with heart palpitations and disquietude.
Page: 253

內補芎藭湯 *nèi bǔ xiōng qióng tāng*
Internally Supplementing Chuānxiōng Decoction

川芎	chuān xiōng	12g
乾地黃	gān dì huáng	12g
芍藥	sháo yào	15g
桂心	guì xīn	6g
甘草	gān cǎo	9g
乾薑	gān jiāng	9g
大棗	dà zǎo	40 pcs

Indications:
Postpartum vacuity emaciation as well as excessive flooding damage, with vacuity exhaustion and gripping pain in the center of the abdomen.
Page: 306

牛膝湯 *niú xī tāng*
Achyranthes Decoction

牛膝	niú xī	3g
瞿麥	qú mài	3g
滑石	huá shí	6g
當歸	dāng guī	4.5g
通草	tōng cǎo	4.5g
葵子	kuí zǐ	12g

Indications:
Retained placenta in childbirth, which is causing the uterus to rot.
Page: 209

牛膝丸 *niú xī wán*
Achyranthes Pills

牛膝	niú xī	9g
芍藥	sháo yào	9g
人參	rén shēn	9g
大黃	dà huáng	9g
牡丹皮	mǔ dān pí	6g
甘草	gān cǎo	6g
當歸	dāng guī	6g
川芎	chuān xiōng	6g
桂心	guì xīn	3g
䗪蟲	zhè chóng	40 pcs
蠐螬	qí cáo	40 pcs
蜚蠊	fěi lián	40 pcs
虻蟲	méng chóng	70 pcs
水蛭	shuǐ zhì	70 pcs

Indications:
Intermittent menstruation after chidlbirth, abruptly fluctuating in the amount, then failing to flow when returning, constant pain, tension in the lower abdomen, downward pulling in the lumbus, and heaviness of the body.
Page: 536

朴消盪胞湯 *pò xiāo dàng bāo tāng*
Impure Mirabilite Uterus-Rinsing Decoction

朴消	pò xiāo	.375g
牡丹	mǔ dān	.375g
當歸	dāng guī	.375g
大黃	dà huáng	.375g
生桃仁	shēng tao rén	.375g
細辛	xì xīn	.125g

厚朴	hòu pò	.125g
桔梗	jié gěng	.125g
赤芍藥	chì sháo yao	.125g
人參	rén shēn	.125g
茯苓	fú líng	.125g
桂心	guì xīn	.125g
甘草	gān cǎo	.125g
牛膝	niú xī	.125g
橘皮	jú pí	.125g
虻蟲	méng chóng	1.25g
水蛭	shuǐ zhì	1.25g
附子	fù zǐ	.75g

Indications:
Infertility in women who have never given birth throughout their entire adult life or who have interrupted the thread [of descendants] and have not given birth for as long as thirty years.
Page: 63

蒲黃散 *pú huáng sǎn*
Typha Pollen Powder

蒲黃	pú huáng	7.5g

Indications:
Postpartum vexation and oppression.
Page: 264

蒲黃散 *pú huáng sǎn*
Typha Pollen Powder

蒲黃	pú huáng	12g
鹿茸	lù róng	6g
當歸	dāng guī	6g

Indications:
Incessant vaginal spotting.
Page: 521

蒲黃湯 *pú huáng tāng*
Typha Pollen Decoction

蒲黃	pú huáng	15g
桂心	guì xīn	3g
川芎	chuān xiōng	3g
桃仁	táo rén	20 pcs
硭硝	máng xiāo	3g
生薑	shēng jiāng	15g
生地黃	shēng dì huáng	15g
大棗	dà zǎo	15 pcs

Indications:
Residual disease after childbirth [such as] shortage of qì in the center of the chest, abdominal pain, headaches, and incomplete elimination of residual blood, by eliminating life-threatening distention and fullness in the center of the abdomen.
Page: 311

蒲黃湯 *pú huáng tāng*
Typha Pollen Decoction

蒲黃	pú huáng	1.5g
大黃	dà huáng	3g
硭硝	máng xiāo	3g
甘草	gān cǎo	3g
黃芩	huáng qín	3g
大棗	dà zǎo	30 pcs

Indications:
Residual sickness after childbirth, [such as] the presence of accumulated blood that fails to be removed, enlarged abdomen and shortness of breath, inability to eat and drink, upward surges [of qì] into the chest and ribsides; recurrent vexation, muddleheadedness, and counterflow fullness, soreness in the hands and feet, and heat bind in the center of the stomach.
Page: 323

七熬丸 *qī āo wán*
Seven Roasted [Ingredients] Pills

大黃	dà huáng	4.5g
前胡	qián hú	0.75g
硭硝	máng xiāo	0.75g
葶藶	tíng lì	0.75g
蜀椒	shǔ jiāo	0.75g
生薑	shēng jiāng	2.25g
川芎	chuān xiōng	2.25g
茯苓	fú líng	1.88g
杏仁	xìng rén	1.13g
桃仁	táo rén	20 pcs
虻蟲	méng chóng	3.5ml
水蛭	shuǐ zhì	3.5ml

Indications:
Inhibited menstruation, vexation and heat in the hands and feet, abdominal fullness, deep silence and unwillingness to wake up, and heart vexation.
Page: 530

七子散 *qī zǐ sǎn*
Seven Seeds Powder

五味子	wǔ wèi zǐ	1g
牡荆子	mǔ jīng zǐ	1g
菟絲子	tù sī zǐ	1g
車前子	chē qián zǐ	1g
菥蓂子	xī míng zǐ	1g
石斛	shí hú	1g
薯蕷	shǔ yù	1g
乾地黃	gān dì huáng	1g
杜仲	dù zhòng	1g
鹿茸	lù róng	1g
遠志	yuǎn zhì	1g
附子	fù zǐ	.75g
蛇床子	shé chuáng zǐ	.75g
川芎	chuān xiōng	.75g
山茱萸	shān zhū yú	.375g
烏頭	wū tóu	.375g
人參	rén shēn	.375g
茯苓	fú líng	.375g
黃芪	huáng qí	.375g
牛膝	niú xī	.375g
桂心	guì xīn	1.25g
巴戟天	bā jǐ tiān	1.5g
蓯蓉	cōng róng	1.25g
鍾乳粉	zhōng rǔ fěn	1g

Actions:
Supplements insufficiency.

Indications:
Husband's wind vacuity, with clouded vision, debilitation and scantness of essence and *qi*, and infertility.
Page: 60

千金丸 *qiān jīn wán*
Thousand Gold Pills

甘草	gān cǎo	.75g
貝母	bèi mǔ	.75g
秦椒	qín jiāo	.75g
乾薑	gān jiāng	.75g
桂心	guì xīn	.75g
黃芩	huáng qín	.75g
石斛	shí hú	.75g
石膏	shí gāo	.75g
粳米	jīng mǐ	.75g

大豆黃卷	dà dòu huáng juǎn	.75g
當歸	dāng guī	1.625g
麻子	fù zǐ	21ml

Indications:
Nourishes the fetus, treats birthing difficulties, upside down [presentation], and retained placenta. Also for a damaged or destroyed fetus that will not descend, and for such residual conditions as inability to sweat, incessant vexing fullness, and *qi* counterflow and fullness.
Page: 128

前胡牡丹湯 *qián hú mǔ dān tāng*
Peucedanum and Moutan Decoction

前胡	qián hú	6g
牡丹	mǔ dān	6g
玄參	xuán shēn	6g
桃仁	táo rén	6g
黃芩	huáng qín	6g
射干	shè gān	6g
旋覆花	xuán fù huā	6g
栝蔞根	guā lóu gēn	6g
甘草	gān cǎo	6g
芍藥	sháo yào	9g
茯苓	fú líng	9g
大黃	dà huáng	9g
枳實	zhǐ shí	9g

Indications:
Women's exuberant repletion, presence of heat in the abdomen, static, blocked, or stopped menstrual flow; as well as menstrual stoppage from taxation heat, after heat diseases, or due to contracting heat at the onset of menstruation.
Page: 434

秦椒丸 *qín jiāo wán*
Shǎn-Xī Zanthoxylum Pills

秦椒	qín jiāo	2.25g
烏頭	wū tóu	2.25g
玄參	xuán shēn	3g
人參	rén shēn	3g
白蘞	bái liǎn	3g
鼠婦	shǔ fù	3g
白芷	bái zhǐ	3g
黃芪	huáng qí	3g
桔梗	jié gěng	3g
露蜂房	lù fēng fáng	3g

白殭蠶	bái jiāng cán	3g
桃仁	táo rén	3g
蠐螬	qí cáo	3g
白薇	bái wēi	3g
細辛	xì xīn	3g
蕪荑	wú yí	3g
牡蒙	mǔ méng	2.5g
沙參	shā shēn	2.5g
防風	fáng fēng	2.5g
甘草	gān cǎo	2.5g
牡丹皮	mǔ dān	2.5g
牛膝	niú xī	2.5g
卷柏	juǎn bǎi	2.5g
五味子	wǔ wèi zǐ	2.5g
芍藥	sháo yào	2.5g
桂心	guì xīn	2.5g
大黃	dà huáng	2.5g
石斛	shí hú	2.5g
白朮	bái zhú	2.5g
柏子仁	bǎi zǐ rén	4.5g
茯苓	fú líng	4.5g
當歸	dāng guī	4.5g
乾薑	gān jiāng	4.5g
澤蘭	zé lán	5.25g
乾地黃	gān dì huáng	5.25g
川芎	chuān xiōng	5.25g
乾漆	gān qī	6g
白石英	bái shí yīng	6g
紫石英	zǐ shí yīng	6g
附子	fù zǐ	6g
鍾乳	zhōng rǔ	7.5g
水蛭	shuǐ zhì	70 pcs
虻蟲	méng chóng	100 pcs
燒麻布叩複頭	shāo má bù kòu fù tóu	21cm

Actions:
Scoures and flushes the viscera and bowels, causes the jade gate to receive the essence of the fetus.

Indications:
For women whose childbearing has been interrupted or who have never given birth at all.
Page: 79

慶雲散 *qìng yún sǎn*
Blessing Clouds Powder

覆盆子	fù pén zǐ	24g
五味子	wǔ wèi zǐ	24g
烏頭	wū tóu	3g
石斛	shí hú	6g
白朮	bái zhú	9g
桑寄生	sāng jì shēng	12g
天門冬	tiān mén dōng	15g
菟絲子	tù sī zǐ	24g
紫石英	zǐ shí yīng	6g

Actions:
Strengthens *yáng qì*.

Indications:
Male infertility.
Page: 69

人參當歸湯 *rén shēn dāng guī tāng*
Ginseng and Chinese Angelica Decoction

人參	rén shēn	3g
當歸	dāng guī	3g
麥門冬	mài mén dōng	3g
桂心	guì xīn	3g
乾地黃	gān dì huáng	3g
大棗	dà zǎo	20 pcs
粳米	jīng mǐ	24g
淡竹葉	dàn zhú yè	72g
芍藥	sháo yào	12g

Indications:
Postpartum vexation, oppression, and disquietude.
Page: 259

人參丸 *rén shēn wán*
Ginseng Pills

人參	rén shēn	9g
甘草	gān cǎo	9g
茯苓	fú líng	9g
麥門冬	mài mén dōng	6g
菖蒲	chāng pú	6g
澤瀉	zé xiè	6g
薯蕷	shǔ yù	6g
乾薑	gān jiāng	6g
桂心	guì xīn	3g
大棗	dà zǎo	50 pcs

Indications:
Serious postpartum vacuity heart palpitations, disquietude of the mind, lack of self-awareness, abstraction and panic, inability to sleep at night, and vacuity vexation and shortage of *qì*.
Page: 292

乳蜜湯 *rǔ mì tāng*
Milk and Honey Decoction

牛乳	niú rǔ	490ml
白蜜	bái mì	4.5g
當歸	dāng guī	9g
人參	rén shēn	9g
獨活	dú huó	9g
大棗	dà zǎo	20 pcs
甘草	gān cǎo	6g
桂心	guì xīn	6g

Actions:
Supplements and boosts the *qì*.

Indications:
The seven damages, vacuity detriment, shortage and insufficiency of *qì*, and kidney taxation and coldness in postpartum.
Page: 250

三石湯 *sān shí tāng*
Three Stones Decoction

紫石英	zǐ shí yīng	6g
白石英	bái shí yīng	7.5g
鐘乳	zhōng rǔ	7.5g
生薑	shēng jiāng	6g
當歸	dāng guī	6g
人參	rén shēn	6g
甘草	gān cǎo	6g
茯苓	fú líng	9g
乾地黃	gān dì huáng	9g
桂心	guì xīn	9g
半夏	bàn xià	15g
大棗	dà zǎo	15 pcs

Actions:
Supplements the kidneys and treats the myriad diseases.

Indications:
Postpartum vacuity cold, the seven damages, with periodic [aversion to] cold and heat [effusion], generalized pain, and lack of strength.
Page: 251

三石澤蘭丸 *sān shí zé lán wán*
Three Stones and Lycopus Pills

鐘乳	zhōng rǔ	12g
白石英	bái shí yīng	12g
紫石英	zǐ shí yīng	3.75g
防風	fáng fēng	3.75g
藁本	gǎo běn	3.75g
茯神	fú shén	3.75g
澤蘭	zé lán	6.75g
黃芪	huáng qí	6g
石斛	shí hú	6g
石膏	shí gāo	6g
甘草	gān cǎo	5.25g
當歸	dāng guī	5.25g
川芎	chuān xiōng	5.25g
白朮	bái zhú	4.5g
桂心	guì xīn	4.5g
人參	rén shēn	4.5g
乾薑	gān jiāng	4.5g
獨活	dú huó	4.5g
乾地黃	gān dì huáng	4.5g
白芷	bái zhǐ	3g
桔梗	jié gěng	3g
細辛	xì xīn	3g
柏子仁	bǎi zǐ rén	3g
五味子	wǔ wèi zǐ	3g
蜀椒	shǔ jiāo	3g
黃芩	huáng qín	3g
蓯蓉	cōng róng	3g
芍藥	sháo yào	3g
秦艽	qín jiāo	3g
防葵	fáng kuí	3g
厚朴	hòu pò	2.25g
蕪荑	wú yí	2.25g

Indications:
Wind vacuity and insufficiency by freeing the flow of blood in the channels and by supplementing [in] cold [conditions].
Page: 421

三物黃芩湯 *sān wù huáng qín tāng*
Three Agents Scutellaria Decoction

黃芩	huáng qín	6g
苦參	kǔ shēn	6g
乾地黃	gān dì huáng	12g

Indications:
Contracted wind while in childbed, possibly with discomfort, vexation, heat in the four limbs, and vexing heat.
Page: 281

桑根白皮湯 *sāng gēn bái pí tāng*
Mulberry Bark Decoction

桑根白皮	sāng gēn bái pí	1.5g
乾薑	gān jiāng	6g
桂心	guì xīn	3g
大棗	dà zǎo	20 pcs

Indications:
Damage by the husband, headache, tendency to retch, and heart oppression.
Page: 397

芍藥黃芪湯 *sháo yào huáng qí tāng*
Peony and Astragalus Decoction

芍藥	sháo yào	12g
黃芪	huáng qí	6g
白芷	bái zhǐ	6g
桂心	guì xīn	6g
生薑	shēng jiāng	6g
人參	rén shēn	6g
川芎	chuān xiōng	6g
當歸	dāng guī	6g
乾地黃	gān dì huáng	6g
甘草	gān cǎo	6g
茯苓	fú líng	9g
大棗	dà zǎo	10 pcs

Indications:
Postpartum heart and abdominal pain.
Page: 314

芍藥湯 *sháo yào tāng*
Peony Decoction

| 芍藥 | sháo yào | 12g |
| 生薑 | shēng jiāng | 12g |

厚朴	hòu pò	6g
甘草	gān cǎo	9g
當歸	dāng guī	9g
白朮	bái zhú	9g
人參	rén shēn	9g
薤白	xiè bái	24g

Indications:
In the eighth month of pregnancy, for wind or cold strike, offenses against prohibitions, pain all over the body, abruptly alternating [aversion to] cold and heat [effusion], stirring fetus, constant problems with dizziness and headaches, coldness below and around the navel, frequent urination of a white substance like rice juice or a green or yellow substance, or accompanied by cold shivering, bitter cold and pain in the lumbus and back, or blurred vision.
Page: 121

芍藥湯 *sháo yào tāng*
Peony Decoction

白芍藥	bái sháo yào	15g
乾地黃	gān dì huáng	15g
牡蠣	mǔ lì	15g
桂心	guì xīn	9g

Indications:
Postpartum vacuity heat with headache.
Page: 265

芍藥湯 *sháo yào tāng*
Peony Decoction

芍藥	sháo yào	18g
桂心	guì xīn	9g
甘草	gān cǎo	6g
膠飴	jiāo yí	24g
生薑	shēng jiāng	9g
大棗	dà zǎo	12 pcs

Indications:
Postpartum discomfort from pain in the lesser abdomen.
Page: 299

慎火草散 *shèn huǒ cǎo sǎn*
Stonecrop Powder

慎火草	shèn huǒ cǎo	6g
白石脂	bái shí zhī	6g
禹餘糧	yǔ yú liáng	6g
鱉甲	biē jiǎ	6g
乾薑	gān jiāng	6g
細辛	xì xīn	6g
當歸	dāng guī	6g
川芎	chuān xiōng	6g
石斛	shí hú	6g
芍藥	sháo yào	6g
牡蠣	mǔ lì	6g
黃連	huáng lián	12g
薔薇根皮	qiáng wēi gēn pí	12g
乾地黃	gān dì huáng	12g
熟艾	shú ài	3g
桂心	guì xīn	3g

Indications:
Center flooding and spotting of red, white, blue-green, and black discharge that is so foul-smelling that no one can get near her, [disease that is] causing the patient's face to be black and without color, and her skin to stick to the bones, an excessive menstrual period that comes and goes without constancy, bow-string tension in the lower abdomen, possibly with discomfort from gripping pain ascending all the way to the heart, swelling and distention in both rib-sides, eating without engendering flesh, causing her to [suffer from] hemilateral withering, lack of *qì* and breath, lumbar and back pain connecting to the rib-sides, inability to stand for a long period of time, and pervasive somnolence, encumbrance, and laziness.
Page: 485

慎火草散 *shèn huǒ cǎo sǎn*
Stonecrop Powder

慎火草	shèn huǒ cǎo	300g
當歸	dāng guī	12g
鹿茸	lù róng	12g
阿膠	ē jiāo	12g
龍骨	lóng gǔ	1.5g

Indications:
Vaginal spotting.
Page: 520

生地黃湯 *shēng dì huáng tāng*
Fresh Rehmannia Decoction

生地黃	shēng dì huáng	15g
生薑	shēng jiāng	6g
大黃	dà huáng	4.5g
芍藥	sháo yào	4.5g
茯苓	fú líng	4.5g
細辛	xì xīn	4.5g
桂心	guì xīn	4.5g
當歸	dāng guī	4.5g
甘草	gān cǎo	4.5g
黃芩	huáng qín	4.5g
大棗	dà zǎo	20 pcs

Indications:
Incomplete elimination of the residual blood in the abdomen with gripping pain, rigidity and fullness, and stopped breathing, during the third to seventh days postpartum.
Page: 327

生地黃湯 *shēng dì huáng tāng*
Fresh Rehmannia Decoction

生地黃	shēng dì huáng	15g
甘草	gān cǎo	3g
黃連	huáng lián	3g
桂心	guì xīn	3g
大棗	dà zǎo	20 pcs
淡竹葉	dàn zhú yè	48g
赤石脂	chì shí zhī	6g

Indications:
Suddenly occurring [aversion to] cold and heat [effusion] with diarrhea after childbirth.
Page: 348

生地黃湯 *shēng dì huáng tāng*
Fresh Rehmannia Decoction

生地黃	shēng dì huáng	48g
細辛	xì xīn	9g

Indications:
Center flooding and spotting, losing several *shēng* of blood per day.
Page: 499

升麻湯 *shēng má tāng*
Cimicifuga Decoction

升麻	shēng má	6g

Indications:
Incomplete elimination of malign substances after childbirth, whether a month, half a year, or one year have passed.
Page: 329

生牛膝酒 *shēng niú xī jiǔ*
Fresh Achyranthes Wine

生牛膝	shēng niú xī	9g

Indications:
Bitter postpartum pain in the center of the abdomen.
Page: 309

石斛地黃煎 *shí hú dì huáng jiān*
Dendrobium and Rehmannia Brew

石斛	shí hú	12g
生地黃汁	shēng dì huáng zhī	560ml
桃仁	táo rén	12g
桂心	guì xīn	6g
甘草	gān cǎo	12g
大黃	dà huáng	24g
紫菀	zǐ wǎn	12g
麥門冬	mài mén dōng	48g
茯苓	fú líng	48g
淳酒	chún jiǔ	560ml

Indications:
Vacuity emaciation, with shortness of breath, counterflow, fullness, and oppression in the chest, and wind *qì*.
Page: 240

石韋湯 *shí wéi tāng*
Pyrrosia Decoction

石韋	shí wéi	6g
榆[白]皮	yú [bái] pí	15g
黃芩	huáng qín	6g
大棗	dà zǎo	30 pcs
通草	tōng cǎo	6g
甘草	gān cǎo	6g
葵子	kuí zǐ	48g
白朮	bái zhú	9g

生薑	shēng jiāng	9g

Indications:
Sudden strangury after childbirth, *qì* strangury, blood strangury, and stone strangury.
Page: 357

拭湯 *shì tāng*
Wiping Decoction

麻黃	má huáng	24g
竹葉	zhú yè	24g
石膏	shí gāo	72g

Indications:
Cold damage in pregnancy, with headaches and high unremitting fever.
Page: 149

蜀椒湯 *shǔ jiāo tāng*
Sì-Chuān Zanthoxylum Decoction

蜀椒	shǔ jiāo	14ml
芍藥	sháo yào	3g
當歸	dāng guī	6g
半夏	bàn xià	6g
甘草	gān cǎo	6g
桂心	guì xīn	6g
人參	rén shēn	6g
茯苓	fú líng	6g
米	mǐ	24g
生薑汁	shēng jiāng zhī	35ml

Indications:
Postpartum heart pain, due to severe cold.
Page: 296

蜀漆湯 *shǔ qī tāng*
Dichroa Leaf Decoction

蜀漆葉	shǔ qī yè	3g
黃芪	huáng qí	15g
桂心	guì xīn	3g
甘草	gān cǎo	3g
黃芩	huáng qín	3g
知母	zhī mǔ	6g
芍藥	sháo yào	6g
生地黃	shēng dì huáng	48g

Indications:
Postpartum cases of intermittent vacuity heat, vexing fullness in the heart and chest, pain in the bones and

joints, as well as headache and vigorous heat that are always worst in the afternoon, and furthermore conditions that resemble mild malaria.
Page: 245

四石湯 *sì shí tāng*
Four Stones Decoction

紫石英	zǐ shí yīng	9g
白石英	bái shí yīng	9g
石膏	shí gāo	9g
赤石脂	chì shí zhī	9g
獨活	dú huó	18g
生薑	shēng jiāng	18g
葛根	gé gēn	12g
桂心	guì xīn	6g
川芎	chuān xiōng	6g
甘草	gān cǎo	6g
芍藥	sháo yào	6g
黃芩	huáng qín	6g

Indications:
Sudden postpartum wind strike with clenched mouth, tugging and slackening [of the channels], oppression and fullness, and inability to recognize people, when the disease erupts; as well as slackening and tensing in the various wind poison impediments, generalized tetany and rigidity, and lastly wind strike during pregnancy and the myriad diseases of women.
Page: 280

四順理中丸 *sì shùn lǐ zhōng wán*
Four [Ingredients] Center-Normalizing and -Rectifying Pills

甘草	gān cǎo	6g
人參	rén shēn	3g
白朮	bái zhú	3g
乾薑	gān jiāng	3g

Indications:
After delivery.
Page: 238

桃仁煎 *táo rén jiān*
Peach Kernel Brew

桃仁	táo rén	24g
虻蟲	méng chóng	24g
朴消	pò xiāo	15g
大黃	dà huáng	18g

Indications:
Vaginal discharge and menstrual block or stoppage.
Page: 455

桃仁煎 *táo rén jiān*
Peach Pit Brew

桃仁	táo rén	1,200 pcs

Actions:
Supplements and boosts the *qì*.

Indications:
The myriad diseases of women after childbirth.
Page: 239

桃仁散 *táo rén sǎn*
Peach Kernel Powder

桃仁	táo rén	50 pcs
蟅蟲	zhè chóng	20 pcs
桂心	guì xīn	5 cm
茯苓	fú líng	3g
薏苡仁	yì yǐ rén	6g
牛膝	niú xī	6g
代赭	dài zhě	6g
大黃	dà huáng	24g

Indications:
Arrival of the menses with pain around the navel, upsurging to the heart and chest, and alternating [aversion to] cold and heat [effusion] as in malaria or infixation.
Page: 532

桃仁芍藥湯 *táo rén sháo yào tāng*
Peach Kernel and Peony Decoction

桃仁	táo rén	12g
芍藥	sháo yào	6g
川芎	chuān xiōng	6g
當歸	dāng guī	6g
乾漆	gān qī	6g
桂心	guì xīn	6g
甘草	gān cǎo	6g

Indications:
Postpartum pain in the center of the abdomen.
Page: 300

桃仁湯 *táo rén tāng*
Peach Kernel Decoction

桃仁	táo rén	15g
吳茱萸	wú zhū yú	48g
黃芪	huáng qí	9g
當歸	dāng guī	9g
芍藥	sháo yào	9g
生薑	shēng jiāng	24g
醍醐	tí hú	24g
柴胡	chái hú	24g

Indications:
Alternating [aversion to] cold and heat [effusion] and incomplete elimination of malign dew after childbirth.
Page: 319

桃仁湯 *táo rén tāng*
Peach Kernel Decoction

桃仁	táo rén	9g
朴消	pò xiāo	9g
牡丹皮	mǔ dān pí	9g
射干	shè gān	9g
土瓜根	tǔ guā gēn	9g
黃芩	huáng qín	9g
芍藥	sháo yào	12g
大黃	dà huáng	12g
柴胡	chái hú	12g
牛膝	niú xī	6g
桂心	guì xīn	6g
水蛭	shuǐ zhì	70 pcs
虻蟲	méng chóng	70 pcs

Indications:
Menstrual stoppage.
Page: 428

桃仁湯 *táo rén tāng*
Peach Kernel Decoction

桃仁	táo rén	24g
當歸	dāng guī	6g
土瓜根	tǔ guā gēn	6g
大黃	dà huáng	6g
水蛭	shuǐ zhì	6g
虻蟲	méng chóng	6g
硭硝	máng xiāo	6g

牛膝	niú xī	9g
麻子仁	má zǐ rén	9g
桂心	guì xīn	9g

Indications:
Menstrual stoppage.
Page: 433

桃仁湯 *táo rén tāng*
Peach Kernel Decoction

桃仁	táo rén	50 pcs
澤蘭	zé lán	6g
甘草	gān cǎo	6g
川芎	chuān xiōng	6g
人參	rén shēn	6g
牛膝	niú xī	9g
桂心	guì xīn	9g
牡丹皮	mǔ dān pí	9g
當歸	dāng guī	9g
芍藥	sháo yào	12g
生薑	shēng jiāng	12g
半夏	bàn xià	12g
地黃	dì huáng	24g
蒲黃	pú huáng	49ml

Indications:
Menstrual irregularities after childbirth or miscarriage, possibly dribbling incessantly or recurring after it has stopped or like watery diarrhea, with huffing and gasping [that strains] the entire body, inability to eat, hardness and pain in the abdomen, inability to actively move around, a menstrual flow that is sometimes early and sometimes late or fails to arrive at all, heaviness when lifting the limbs, only wanting to rest and sleep, and excessive thought of sour foods.
Page: 525

調中湯 *tiáo zhōng tāng*
Center-Regulating Decoction

白芍藥	bái sháo yào	12g
續斷	xù duàn	3g
川芎	chuān xiōng	3g
甘草	gān cǎo	3g
白朮	bái zhú	9g
柴胡	chái hú	9g
當歸	dāng guī	4.5g
烏梅	wū méi	24g
生薑	shēng jiāng	12g

厚朴	hòu pò	9g
枳實	zhǐ shí	9g
生李根白皮	shēng lǐ gēn bái pí	9g

Indications:
Damage to the fetus during the fourth month.
Page: 111

銅鏡鼻湯 tóng jìng bí tāng
Bronze Mirror Knob Decoction

銅鏡鼻	tóng jìng bí	2.25g
大黃	dà huáng	7.5g
乾地黃	gān dì huáng	6g
芍藥	sháo yào	6g
川芎	chuān xiōng	6g
乾漆	gān qī	6g
硭硝	máng xiāo	6g
亂髮	luàn fà	a chicken egg sized amount
大棗	dà zǎo	30 pcs

Indications:
Residual sickness after childbirth, failure to eliminate malign dew, accumulations and gatherings that are causing disease, blood and qì binding and contending with each other, and pain in the heart and abdomen.
Page: 324

溫經湯 wēn jīng tāng
Menses-Warming Decoction

茯苓	fú líng	18g
芍藥	sháo yào	9g
薏苡仁	yì yǐ rén	12g
土瓜根	tǔ guā gēn	9g

Indications:
Women's pain in the lower abdomen.
Page: 370

烏雌雞湯 wū cí jī tāng
Black Hen Decoction

烏雌雞	wū cí jī	one bird
茯苓	fú líng	6g
吳茱萸	wú zhū yú	24g
芍藥	sháo yào	9g
白朮	bái zhú	9g
麥門冬	tiān mén dōng	35ml
人參	rén shēn	9g

阿膠	ē jiāo	6g
甘草	gān cǎo	3g
生薑	shēng jiāng	3g

Indications:
[During the first month of pregnancy,] for cases of pain due to increased cold; sudden panic due to increased heat; lumbar pain, abdominal fullness, and tightness in the uterus from heavy lifting; and the sudden appearance of vaginal discharge.
Page: 102

吳茱萸湯 wú zhū yú tāng
Evodia Decoction

吳茱萸	wú zhū yú	15g

Indications:
Postpartum vacuity emaciation with nightsweats and huddled aversion to cold.
Page: 254

吳茱萸湯 wú zhū yú tāng
Evodia Decoction

吳茱萸	wú zhū yú	6g
防風	fáng fēng	1.5g
桔梗	jié gěng	1.5g
乾薑	gān jiāng	1.5g
甘草	gān cǎo	1.5g
細辛	xì xīn	1.5g
當歸	dāng guī	1.5g
乾地黃	gān dì huáng	2.25g

Indications:
Women who prior [to childbirth suffered from] presence of cold, fullness and pain in the chest, possibly stabbing pain in the heart and abdomen, or retching and vomiting and reduced eating, swelling, coldness, or diarrhea, and faint and labored breathing verging on expiry, and whose symptoms have increased dramatically after childbirth.
Page: 310

五加酒 wǔ jiā jiǔ
Acanthopanax Liquor

五加皮	wǔ jiā pí	48g
枸杞子	gǒu qǐ zǐ	48g
乾地黃	gān dì huáng	6g
丹參	dān shēn	6g
杜仲	dù zhòng	48g
乾薑	gān jiāng	9g

天門冬	tiān mén dōng	12g
蛇床子	shé chuáng zǐ	24g
乳床	rǔ chuáng	24g

Indications:
Postpartum aggregations, emaciation, and cold in the jade gate.
Page: 376

五京丸 *wǔ jīng wán*
Five Jīng Pills

乾薑	gān jiāng	9g
蜀椒	shǔ jiāo	9g
附子	fù zǐ	3g
吳茱萸	wú zhū yú	24g
當歸	dāng guī	6g
狼毒	láng dú	6g
黃芩	huáng qín	6g
牡蠣	mǔ lì	6g

Indications:
Accumulations and gatherings in the center of the abdomen, nine pains and seven damages, as well as coldness in the center of the lumbus stretching to the lower abdomen, food damage, and vaginal discharge after contracting cold.
Page: 458

五石湯 *wǔ shí tāng*
Five Stones Decoction

紫石英	zǐ shí yīng	6g
鐘乳	zhōng rǔ	6g
白石英	bái shí yīng	6g
楮實子	chǔ shí zǐ	6g
石膏	shí gāo	6g
茯苓	fú líng	6g
白朮	bái zhú	6g
桂心	guì xīn	6g
川芎	chuān xiōng	6g
甘草	gān cǎo	6g
薤白	xiè bái	18g
人參	rén shēn	9g
當歸	dāng guī	9g
生薑	shēng jiāng	24g
大棗	dà zǎo	20 pcs

Actions:
Supplements the kidneys and treats the myriad diseases.

Indications:
Postpartum vacuity cold, the seven damages, with periodic [aversion to] cold and heat [effusion], generalized pain, and lack of strength.
Page: 251

五石湯 *wǔ shí tāng*
Five Stones Decoction

白石英	bái shí yīng	6g
鐘乳	zhōng rǔ	6g
赤石脂	chì shí zhī	6g
石膏	shí gāo	6g
紫石英	zǐ shí yīng	9g
牡蠣	mǔ lì	6g
人參	rén shēn	6g
黃芩	huáng qín	6g
白朮	bái zhú	6g
甘草	gān cǎo	6g
栝蔞根	guā lóu gēn	6g
川芎	chuān xiōng	6g
桂心	guì xīn	6g
防己	fáng jǐ	6g
當歸	dāng guī	6g
乾薑	gān jiāng	6g
獨活	dú huó	9g
葛根	gé gēn	12g

Indications:
Postpartum sudden wind strike with clenched mouth, falling, oppression, and foaming at the mouth, tugging and slackening [of the channels], veiling dizziness, and inability to recognize people, when the disease erupts; as well as for damp impediment with flaccidity, generalized tetany, and the myriad diseases of pregnancy.
Page: 278

硝石湯 *xiāo shí tāng*
Niter Decoction

消石	xiāo shí	9g
附子	fù zǐ	9g
虻蟲	méng chóng	9g
大黃	dà huáng	3g
細辛	xì xīn	3g
乾薑	gān jiāng	3g
黃芩	huáng qín	3g
芍藥	sháo yào	6g
土瓜根	tǔ guā gēn	6g

丹參	dān shēn	6g
代赭	dài zhě	6g
蠐螬	qí cáo	6g
大棗	dà zǎo	10 pcs
桃仁	táo rén	48g
牛膝	niú xī	48g
朴消	pò xiāo	12g

Indications:
Blood conglomerations, retained menses, and static blood [causing] enlargement and stoppage, by precipitating the disease and dissipating the hardened blood.
Page: 464

小柴胡湯 *xiǎo chái hú tāng*
Minor Bupleurum Decoction

柴胡	chái hú	24g
黃芩	huáng qín	9g
人參	rén shēn	9g
甘草	gān cǎo	9g
生薑	shēng jiāng	6g
大棗	dà zǎo	12 pcs
半夏	bàn xià	12g

Indications:
Contraction of wind while in childbed, possibly with discomfort, vexation, and heat in the four limbs and headache. This is always caused by the occurrence of [malign] dew.
Page: 281

小獨活湯 *xiǎo dú huó tāng*
Minor Pubescent Angelica Decoction

獨活	dú huó	24g
葛根	gé gēn	18g
甘草	gān cǎo	6g
生薑	shēng jiāng	18g

Actions:
Supplements the kidneys.

Indications:
Wind strike tetany during the first hundred days postpartum with clenched mouth that cannot be opened, as well as for treating blood and *qì* pain and taxation damage.
Page: 271

小牛角腮散 *xiǎo niú jiǎo sāi sǎn*
Minor Ox Horn Marrow Powder

牛角腮, 燒令赤	niú jiǎo sāi, shāo lìng chì	1 pc
鹿茸	lù róng	6g
禹餘糧	yǔ yú liáng	6g
當歸	dāng guī	6g
乾薑	gān jiāng	6g
續斷	xù duàn	6g
阿膠	ē jiāo	9g
烏賊骨	wū zéi gǔ	3g
龍骨	lóng gǔ	3g
赤小豆	chì xiǎo dòu	48g

Indications:
The five [types of] vaginal gushing.
Page: 473

小銅鏡鼻湯 *xiǎo tóng jìng bí tāng*
Minor Bronze Mirror Knob Decoction

銅鏡鼻, 燒末	tóng jìng bí, shāo mò	1.25g
大黃	dà huáng	6g
甘草	gān cǎo	6g
黃芩	huáng qín	6g
硭硝	máng xiāo	6g
乾地黃	gān dì huáng	6g
桃仁	táo rén	50 pcs

Indications:
Residual sickness after childbirth, failure to eliminate malign dew, accumulations and gatherings that are causing disease, blood and *qì* binding and contending with each other, and pain in the heart and abdomen.
Page: 325

小五石澤蘭丸 *xiǎo wǔ shí zé lán wán*
Minor Five Stones and Lycopus Pills

鐘乳	zhōng rǔ	4.5g
紫石英	zǐ shí yīng	4.5g
礬石	fán shí	4.5g
白石英	bái shí yīng	5.25g
赤石脂	chì shí zhī	5.25g
當歸	dāng guī	5.25g
甘草	gān cǎo	5.25g
石膏	shí gāo	6g

陽起石	yáng qǐ shí	6g
乾薑	gān jiāng	6g
澤蘭	zé lán	6.75g
蓯蓉	cōng róng	7.5g
龍骨	lóng gǔ	7.5g
桂心	guì xīn	7.5g
白朮	bái zhú	3.75g
芍藥	sháo yào	3.75g
厚朴	hòu pò	3.75g
人參	rén shēn	3.75g
蜀椒	shǔ jiāo	3.75g
山茱萸	shān zhū yú	3.75g
柏子仁	bǎi zǐ rén	3g
藁本	gǎo běn	3g
蕪荑	wú yí	2.25g

Indications:
Taxation cold and vacuity detriment, reduced [intake of] food and drink, lack of luster and color in the face, coldness and pain in the center of the abdomen, menstrual irregularities, and shortage of *qì* and lack of strength in spite of frequent inhalations, by supplementing and boosting and warming the center.
Page: 408

小澤蘭丸 *xiǎo zé lán wán*
Minor Lycopus Pills

澤蘭	zé lán	6.75g
當歸	dāng guī	5.25g
甘草	gān cǎo	5.25g
川芎	chuān xiōng	3g
柏子仁	bǎi zǐ rén	3g
防風	fáng fēng	3g
茯苓	fú líng	3g
白芷	bái zhǐ	2.25g
蜀椒	shǔ jiāo	2.25g
藁本	gǎo běn	2.25g
細辛	xì xīn	2.25g
白朮	bái zhú	2.25g
桂心	guì xīn	2.25g
蕪荑	wú yí	2.25g
人參	rén shēn	2.25g
食茱萸	shí zhū yú	2.25g
厚朴	hòu pò	2.25g
石膏	shí gāo	6g

Indications:
Postpartum vacuity emaciation, taxation cold, and a weak and emaciated body.
Page: 418

薤白湯 *xiè bái tāng*
Chinese Chive Decoction

薤白	xiè bái	6g
半夏	bàn xià	6g
甘草	gān cǎo	6g
人參	rén shēn	6g
知母	zhī mǔ	6g
石膏	shí gāo	12g
栝蔞根	guā lóu gēn	9g
麥門冬	mài mén dōng	24g

Indications:
Postpartum vexing heat in the chest and counterflow *qì*.
Page: 258

蟹爪湯 *xiè zhǎo tāng*
Crab's Claw Decoction

蟹爪	xiè zhǎo	24g
甘草	gān cǎo	60cm
桂心	guì xīn	60cm
阿膠	ē jiāo	6g

Indications:
Pregnant women who have fallen over or lost [their balance] when kneeling, [resulting in] the fetus stirring, turning and prodding the heart, in serious cases with bleeding from the mouth, counterflow and inability to breathe, and perhaps downpouring bleeding of [as much as] one *dǒu* and five *shēng*, failure of the fetus to emerge, [aversion to] cold if the fetus has died, [heat] as if another person were applying a heat compress in the center of her abdomen, tension as if in labor, vacuity and lack of *qì*, exhaustion and fatigue to the point of near-death, and alternating vexation and oppression.
Page: 160

杏仁湯 *xìng rén tāng*
Apricot Kernel Decoction

杏仁	xìng rén	6g
甘草	gān cǎo	6g
麥門冬	mài mén dōng	24g
吳茱萸	wú zhū yú	24g

鍾乳	zhōng rǔ	6g
乾薑	gān jiāng	6g
五味子	wǔ wèi zǐ	35ml
紫菀	zǐ wǎn	3g
粳米	jīng mǐ	35ml

Indications:
Damage to the fetus in the seventh month.
Page: 119

杏仁湯 xìng rén tāng
Apricot Kernel Decoction

杏仁	xìng rén	9g
橘皮	jú pí	9g
白前	bái qián	9g
人參	rén shēn	9g
桂心	guì xīn	12g
蘇葉	sū yè	24g
半夏	bàn xià	24g
生薑	shēng jiāng	30g
麥門冬	mài mén dōng	3g

Indications:
Postpartum vacuity of qì.
Page: 248

杏仁湯 xìng rén tāng
Apricot Kernel Decoction

杏仁	xìng rén	6g
桃仁	táo rén	3g
大黃	dà huáng	9g
水蛭	shuǐ zhì	30 pcs
虻蟲	méng chóng	30 pcs

Indications:
Menstrual irregularities, possibly arriving twice in one month, or once in two or three months, or prematurely or delayed, or menstrual stoppage.
Page: 527

芎藭湯 xiōng qióng tāng
Chuānxiōng Decoction

川芎	chuān xiōng	6g
甘草	gān cǎo	6g
蒲黃	pú huáng	4.5g
女萎	nǔ wěi	4.5g
芍藥	sháo yào	3.75g

大黃	dà huáng	3.75g
當歸	dāng guī	2.25g
桂心	guì xīn	3g
桃仁	táo rén	3g
黃芪	huáng qí	3g
前胡	qián hú	3g
生地黃	shēng dì huáng	24g

Indications:
Postpartum abdominal pain.
Page: 312

芎藭湯 xiōng qióng tāng
Chuānxiōng Decoction

川芎	chuān xiōng	6g
乾地黃	gān dì huáng	6g
黃芪	huáng qí	6g
芍藥	sháo yào	6g
吳茱萸	wú zhū yú	6g
甘草	gān cǎo	6g
當歸	dāng guī	9g
乾薑	gān jiāng	9g

Indications:
Incessant vaginal discharge and spotting of blood.
Page: 513

雄雞湯 xióng jī tāng
Rooster Decoction

雄雞	xióng jī	One Bird
甘草	gān cǎo	6g
人參	rén shēn	6g
茯苓	fú líng	6g
阿膠	ē jiāo	6g
黃芩	huáng qín	3g
白朮	bái zhú	3g
麥門冬	mài mén dōng	35ml
芍藥	sháo yào	12g
大棗	dà zǎo	12 pcs
生薑	shēng jiāng	3g

Indications:
Cold conditions with blue-green feces, heat conditions with difficult urination of red or yellow urine, sudden fright and fear, anxiety and worrying, flights of temper and rage, a tendency to stumble and fall, stirring in the vessels, abdominal fullness, bitter pain around the

navel or in the lumbus and back, and sudden presence of vaginal discharge.
Page: 107

旋覆花湯 *xuán fù huā tāng*
Inula Decoction

旋復花	xuán fù huā	3g
厚朴	hòu pò	9g
白朮	bái zhú	9g
黃芩	huáng qín	9g
茯苓	fú líng	9g
枳實	zhǐ shí	9g
半夏	bàn xià	6g
芍藥	sháo yào	6g
生薑	shēng jiāng	6g

Indications:
disquieted fetus in the sixth and seventh month of pregnancy.
Page: 135

陽起石湯 *yáng qǐ shí tāng*
Actinolite Decoction

陽起石	yáng qǐ shí	6g
甘草	gān cǎo	6g
續斷	xù duàn	6g
乾薑	gān jiāng	6g
人參	rén shēn	6g
桂心	guì xīn	6g
附子	fù zǐ	3g
赤石脂	chì shí zhī	9g
伏龍肝	fú lóng gān	15g
生地黃	shēng dì huáng	24g

Indications:
Menstrual irregularities, early or late, profuse or scanty, or now red now white.
Page: 534

羊肉當歸湯 *yáng ròu dāng guī tāng*
Sheep or Goat's Meat and Chinese Angelica Decoction

羊肉	yáng ròu	144g
當歸	dāng guī	6g
黃芩	huáng qín	6g
川芎	chuān xiōng	6g
甘草	gān cǎo	6g

防風	fáng fēng	6g
芍藥	sháo yào	9g
生薑	shēng jiāng	12g

Indications:
Postpartum cutting pain in the center of the abdomen and below the heart with inability to eat, alternating [aversion to] cold and heat [effusion], and lack of *qì* and strength as in wind strike.
Page: 302

羊肉杜仲湯 *yáng ròu dù zhòng tāng*
Sheep or Goat's Meat and Eucommia Decoction

羊肉	yáng ròu	192g
杜仲	dù zhòng	9g
紫菀	zǐ wǎn	9g
五味子	wǔ wèi zǐ	6g
細辛	xì xīn	6g
款冬花	kuǎn dōng huā	6g
人參	rén shēn	6g
厚朴	hòu pò	6g
川芎	chuān xiōng	6g
附子	fù zǐ	6g
萆薢	bì xiè	6g
甘草	gān cǎo	6g
黃芪	huáng qí	6g
當歸	dāng guī	9g
桂心	guì xīn	9g
白朮	bái zhú	9g
生薑	shēng jiāng	24g
大棗	dà zǎo	30 pcs

Indications:
Postpartum lumbar pain and cough.
Page: 303

羊肉黃芪湯 *yáng ròu huáng qí tāng*
Sheep or Goat's Meat and Astragalus Decoction

羊肉	yáng ròu	144g
黃芪	huáng qí	9g
大棗	dà zǎo	30 pcs
茯苓	fú líng	3g
甘草	gān cǎo	3g
當歸	dāng guī	3g
桂心	guì xīn	3g
芍藥	sháo yào	3g
麥門冬	mài mén dōng	3g

乾地黃   gān dì huáng   3g

Indications:
Postpartum vacuity.
Page: 245

羊肉生地黃湯 *yáng ròu shēng dì huáng tāng*
Sheep or Goat's Meat and Fresh Rehmannia
Decoction

羊肉	yáng ròu	144g
生地黃	shēng dì huáng	6g
桂心	guì xīn	6g
當歸	dāng guī	6g
甘草	gān cǎo	6g
川芎	chuān xiōng	6g
人參	rén shēn	6g
芍藥	sháo yào	9g

Actions:
Supplements the center, boosts the viscera, strengthens the *qì*, and disperses the blood.

Indications:
Postpartum abdominal pain [that lasts] for three days.
Page: 304

羊肉湯 *yáng ròu tāng*
Sheep or Goat's Meat Decoction

肥羊肉	féi yáng ròu	144g
當歸	dāng guī	3g
桂心	guì xīn	6g
芍藥	sháo yào	12g
甘草	gān cǎo	6g
生薑	shēng jiāng	12g
川芎	chuān xiōng	9g
乾地黃	gān dì huáng	15g

Indications:
Postpartum vacuity emaciation, with panting and lack of breath, perspiration of white sweat, and gripping pain in the center of the abdomen.
Page: 243

羊肉湯 *yáng ròu tāng*
Sheep or Goat's Meat Decoction

羊肉	yáng ròu	96g
大蒜	dà suàn	72g
香豉	xiāng chǐ	72g

Indications:
Postpartum wind strike with chronic infertility and failure to bear children, inhibited menstruation, and abruptly alternating red and white [vaginal discharge], as well as vacuity taxation and exuberant cold in men.
Page: 283

羊肉湯 *yáng ròu tāng*
Sheep or Goat's Meat Decoction

肥羊肉	féi yáng ròu	96g
茯苓	fú líng	9g
黃芪	huáng qí	9g
乾薑	gān jiāng	9g
甘草	gān cǎo	6g
獨活	dú huó	6g
桂心	guì xīn	6g
人參	rén shēn	6g
麥門冬	mài mén dōng	49ml
生地黃	shēng dì huáng	15g
大棗	dà zǎo	12 pcs

Indications:
Great vacuity, *qì* ascent, abdominal pain, and simultaneous slight wind that occur after child birth or as a result of physical damage.
Page: 301

禹餘糧丸 *yǔ yú liáng wán*
Limonite Pills

禹餘糧	yǔ yú liáng	7.5g
烏賊骨	wū zéi gǔ	7.5g
吳茱萸	wú zhū yú	7.5g
桂心	guì xīn	7.5g
蜀椒	shǔ jiāo	7.5g
當歸	dāng guī	3.75g
白朮	bái zhú	3.75g
細辛	xì xīn	3.75g
乾地黃	gān dì huáng	3.75g
人參	rén shēn	3.75g
芍藥	sháo yào	3.75g
川芎	chuān xiōng	3.75g
前胡	qián hú	3.75g
乾薑	gān jiāng	9g
礬石	fán shí	0.75g
白薇	bái wēi	2.25g
紫菀	zǐ wǎn	2.25g

黃芩	huáng qín	2.25g
䗪蟲	zhè chóng	3g

Indications:
Postpartum accumulation of cold, hardness, and aggregations.
Page: 446

禹餘糧丸 *yǔ yú liáng wán*
Limonite Pills

禹餘糧	yǔ yú liáng	15g
白馬蹄	bái mǎ tí	30g
龍骨	lóng gǔ	9g
鹿茸	lù róng	6g
烏賊骨	wū zéi gǔ	3g

Indications:
Center flooding, incessant red and white [vaginal discharge], and critical encumbrance.
Page: 487

遠志湯 *yuǎn zhì tāng*
Polygala Decoction

遠志	yuǎn zhì	6g
人參	rén shēn	6g
甘草	gān cǎo	6g
當歸	dāng guī	6g
桂心	guì xīn	6g
麥門冬	mài mén dōng	6g
芍藥	sháo yào	3g
茯苓	fú líng	3g
生薑	shēng jiāng	18g
大棗	dà zǎo	20 pcs

Indications:
Sudden discomfort from surging palpitations and instability in the center of the heart, a disquieted will, deranged and false speech, severe confusion and muddleheadedness, and lack of awareness of one's own affects.
Page: 288

雲母芎藭散 *yún mǔ xiōng qióng sǎn*
Muscovite and Chuānxiōng Powder

雲母	yún mǔ	3g
川芎	chuān xiōng	3g
代赭	dài zhě	3g
東門邊木	dōng mén biān mù	3g
白僵蠶	bái jiāng cán	0.75g

烏賊骨	wū zéi gǔ	0.75g
白堊	bái è	0.75g
蝟皮	wèi pí	0.75g
鱉甲	biē jiǎ	2.25g
桂心	guì xīn	2.25g
伏龍肝	fú lóng gān	2.25g
生鯉魚頭	shēng lǐ yú tóu	2.25g

Indications:
The five floodings, generalized emaciation, counterflow cough, vexation fullness and shortage of *qi*, pain below the heart, formation of sores in the face, inability to bend and stretch in the lumbus and back, swelling in the vagina as if there were sores, itching in the [pubic] hair and occasional pain that penetrates to the uterus, inhibited urination with constant hypertonicity, dizziness in the head, tension and pain in the neck, heat in the hands and feet, *qi* counterflow surging and tension, heart vexation and inability to rest, tension and pain in the abdomen, inability to get down food, acid regurgitation with bitter belching, rumbling in the upper and lower intestines, vaginal spotting of red, white, blue-green, yellow, or black liquid, and severe body odor and stains on the clothing as if dirtied by glue.
Page: 484

澤蘭散 *zé lán sǎn*
Lycopus Powder

澤蘭	zé lán	6.75g
禹餘糧	yǔ yú liáng	7.5g
防風	fǎng fēng	7.5g
石膏	shí gāo	6g
白芷	bái zhǐ	6g
乾地黃	gān dì huáng	6g
赤石脂	chì shí zhī	6g
肉蓯蓉	ròu cōng róng	6g
鹿茸	lù róng	6g
川芎	chuān xiōng	6g
藁本	gǎo běn	3.75g
蜀椒	shǔ jiāo	3.75g
白朮	bái zhú	3.75g
柏子仁	bǎi zǐ rén	3.75g
桂心	guì xīn	5.25g
甘草	gān cǎo	5.25g
當歸	dāng guī	5.25g
乾薑	gān jiāng	5.25g
蕪荑	wú yí	3g
細辛	xì xīn	3g
厚朴	hòu pò	3g

人參	rén shēn	2.25g

Indications:
Postpartum wind vacuity.
Page: 425

澤蘭湯 zé lán tāng
Lycopus Decoction

澤蘭	zé lán	6g
當歸	dāng guī	6g
生地黃	shēng dì huáng	6g
甘草	gān cǎo	4.5g
生薑	shēng jiāng	9g
芍藥	sháo yào	3g
大棗	dà zǎo	10 pcs

Indications:
Incomplete elimination of malign dew after childbirth, with abdominal pain that cannot be relieved, tension and pain in the lower abdomen, pain stretching to the lumbus and back, and shortage of *qì* and strength.
Page: 320

澤蘭湯 zé lán tāng
Lycopus Decoction

澤蘭	zé lán	3g
石膏	shí gāo	3g
當歸	dāng guī	2.25g
遠志	yuǎn zhì	3.75g
甘草	gān cǎo	2.25g
厚朴	hòu pò	2.25g
藁本	gǎo běn	1.875g
川芎	chuān xiōng	1.875g
乾薑	gān jiāng	1.5g
人參	rén shēn	1.5g
桔梗	jié gěng	1.5g
乾地黃	gān dì huáng	1.5g
白朮	bái zhú	1.125g
蜀椒	shǔ jiāo	1.125g
白芷	bái zhǐ	1.125g
柏子仁	bǎi zǐ rén	1.125g
防風	fáng fēng	1.125g
山茱萸	shān zhū yú	1.125g
細辛	xì xīn	1.125g
桑白皮	sāng bái pí	12g
麻子仁	má zǐ rén	12g

Indications:
Residual sickness after childbirth with cold discharge that is icy and contains pus, abdominal urgency, fullness and pain in the chest and rib-sides, coughing and vomiting of blood, [aversion to] cold and heat [effusion], red and yellow urine, and inhibited defecation.
Page: 346

增損禹餘糧丸 zēng sǔn yǔ yú liáng wán
Modified Limonite Pills

禹餘糧	yǔ yú liáng	6g
龍骨	lóng gǔ	6g
人參	rén shēn	6g
桂心	guì xīn	6g
紫石英	zǐ shí yīng	6g
烏頭	wū tóu	6g
寄生	jì shēng	6g
杜仲	dù zhòng	6g
五味子	wǔ wèi zǐ	6g
遠志	yuǎn zhì	6g
澤瀉	zé xiè	9g
當歸	dāng guī	9g
石斛	shí hú	9g
蓯蓉	cōng róng	9g
乾薑	gān jiāng	9g
蜀椒	shǔ jiāo	3g
牡蠣	mǔ lì	3g
甘草	gān cǎo	3g

Indications:
Women's center flooding due to taxation detriment that resembles a menstrual period, coming and going profusely, impossible to stop, and continuing incessantly for several days, emptiness vacuity in the five viscera, and loss of color, yellow complexion, and emaciation.
Page: 487

增損澤蘭丸 zēng sǔn zé lán wán
Modified Lycopus Pills

澤蘭	zé lán	5.25g
甘草	gān cǎo	5.25g
當歸	dāng guī	5.25g
川芎	chuān xiōng	5.25g
附子	fù zǐ	3g
乾薑	gān jiāng	3g
白朮	bái zhú	3g
白芷	bái zhǐ	3g

桂心	guì xīn	3g
細辛	xì xīn	3g
防風	fáng fēng	3.75g
人參	rén shēn	3.75g
牛膝	niú xī	3.75g
柏子仁	bǎi zǐ rén	4.5g
乾地黄	gān dì huáng	4.5g
石斛	shí hú	4.5g
厚朴	hòu pò	1.5g
藁本	gǎo běn	1.5g
蕪荑	wú yí	1.5g
麥門冬	mài mén dōng	6g

Actions:
Regulates blood and *qì*, supplements vacuity taxation

Indications:
The myriad postpartum diseases.
Page: 410

獐骨湯 *zhāng gǔ tāng*
Water Deer's Bone Decoction

獐骨	zhāng gǔ	1 set
遠志	yuǎn zhì	9g
黄芪	huáng qí	9g
芍藥	sháo yào	9g
乾薑	gān jiāng	9g
防風	fáng fēng	9g
茯苓	fú líng	9g
厚朴	hòu pò	9g
當歸	dāng guī	6g
橘皮	jú pí	6g
甘草	gān cǎo	6g
獨活	dú huó	6g
川芎	chuān xiōng	6g
桂心	guì xīn	12g
生薑	shēng jiāng	12g

Indications:
Postpartum vacuity, the five taxations and seven damages, vacuity detriment and insuffiency, and failure to regulate cold and heat in the viscera and bowels.
Page: 247

真朱湯 *zhēn zhū tāng*
Pearl Decoction

| 真朱 | zhēn zhū | 3g |
| 榆白皮 | yú bái pí | 24g |

Indications:
Fetal death in the abdomen.
Page: 196

蒸大黄丸 *zhēng dà huáng wán*
Steamed Rhubarb Pills

大黄	dà huáng	3.75g
枳實	zhǐ shí	2.25g
川芎	chuān xiōng	2.25g
白朮	bái zhú	2.25g
杏仁	xìng rén	2.25g
芍藥	sháo yào	1.5g
乾薑	gān jiāng	1.5g
厚朴	hòu pò	1.5g
吳茱萸	wú zhū yú	3g

Indications:
Nourishes the fetus during pregnancy and eases childbirth.
Page: 129

知母湯 *zhī mǔ tāng*
Anemarrhena Decoction

知母	zhī mǔ	9g
芍藥	sháo yào	6g
黄芩	huáng qín	6g
桂心	guì xīn	3g
甘草	gān cǎo	3g

Indications:
Abruptly alternating [aversion to] cold and heat [effusion] postpartum with vigorous warmth throughout the whole body and vexation and oppression in the chest and heart.
Page: 261

梔子湯 *zhī zǐ tāng*
Gardenia Decoction

梔子	zhī zǐ	30 pcs
當歸	dāng guī	6g
芍藥	sháo yào	6g
米	mǐ	35ml
生薑	shēng jiāng	15g
羊脂	yáng zhī	3g

Indications:
Postpartum emptiness in the place where the fetus was engendered with inexhaustible bleeding and gripping pain in the lower abdomen.
Page: 326

鍾乳湯 *zhōng rǔ tāng*
Stalactite Decoction

石鍾乳	shí zhōng rǔ	.75g
白石脂	bái shí zhī	.75g
通草	tōng cǎo	1.5g
桔梗	jié gěng	1.5g
消石	xiāo shí	.75g

Indications:
Absence of breast milk.
Page: 219

鍾乳澤蘭丸 *zhōng rǔ zé lán wán*
Stalactite and Lycopus Pills

鐘乳	zhōng rǔ	9g
澤蘭	zé lán	9.75g
防風	fáng fēng	5.25g
人參	rén shēn	4.5g
柏子仁	bǎi zǐ rén	4.5g
麥門冬	mài mén dōng	4.5g
乾地黃	gān dì huáng	4.5g
石膏	shí gāo	4.5g
石斛	shí hú	4.5g
川芎	chuān xiōng	3.75g
甘草	gān cǎo	3.75g
白芷	bái zhǐ	3.75g
牛膝	niú xī	3.75g
山茱萸	shān zhū yú	3.75g
當歸	dāng guī	3.75g
藁本	gǎo běn	3.75g

細辛	xì xīn	3g
桂心	guì xīn	3g
蕪荑	wú yí	1.5g
艾葉	ài yè	2.25g

Indications:
Myriad diseases of chronic vacuity emaciation, vexation and pain in the four limbs and all over the body, binding cold below the navel, inability to eat, bruises and black spots in the face and eyes, and anxiety, rage, and unhappiness.
Page: 414

豬膏煎 *zhū gāo jiān*
Pork Lard Jam

豬膏	zhū gāo	24g
清酒	qīng jiǔ	35ml
生薑汁	shēng jiāng zhī	70ml
白蜜	bái mì	70ml

Indications:
Postpartum generalized vacuity with [aversion to] cold and heat [effusion] and spontaneous sweating.
Page: 255

豬腎湯 *zhū shèn tāng*
Pig's Kidney Decoction

豬腎	zhū shèn	1 set
白朮	bái zhú	12g
茯苓	fú líng	9g
桑寄生	sāng jì shēng	9g
乾薑	gān jiāng	9g
乾地黃	gān dì huáng	9g
川芎	chuān xiōng	9g
麥門冬	mài mén dōng	24g
附子	fù zǐ	1 pc from center
大豆	dà dòu	21ml

Indications:
Damage to the fetus in the ninth month.
Page: 124

豬腎湯 *zhū shèn tāng*
Pig's Kidney Decoction

豬腎	zhū shèn	1 set
香豉	xiāng chǐ	700ml
白粳米	bái jīng mǐ	700ml
蔥白	cōng bái	700ml

Indications:
Postpartum vacuity emaciation with panting, lack of breath, and abruptly alternating [aversion to] cold and heat [effusion]. This condition resembles malaria and is called "childbed taxation."
Page: 244

茱萸虻蟲湯 zhū yú méng chóng tāng
Evodia and Tabanus Decoction

吳茱萸	wú zhū yú	9g
虻蟲	méng chóng	3g
水蛭	shuǐ zhì	3g
蟅蟲	zhè chóng	3g
牡丹	mǔ dān	3g
生薑	shēng jiāng	48g
小麥	xiǎo mài	24g
半夏	bàn xià	24g
大棗	dà zǎo	20 pcs
桃仁	táo rén	50 pcs
人參	rén shēn	9g
牛膝	niú xī	9g
桂心	guì xīn	18g
甘草	gān cǎo	4.5g
芍藥	sháo yào	6g

Indications:
Chronic cold-related inhibited menstruation, whether profuse or scanty.
Page: 528

竹根湯 zhú gēn tāng
Bamboo Root Decoction

甘竹根	gān zhú gēn	1050ml
小麥	xiǎo mài	140ml
大棗	dà zǎo	20 pcs
甘草	gān cǎo	3g
麥門冬	mài mén dōng	24g

Indications:
Postpartum vacuity vexation and shortness of breath.
Page: 259

竹瀝湯 zhú lì tāng
Bamboo Sap Decoction

竹瀝	zhú lì	24g
防風	fáng fēng	9g
黃芩	huáng qín	9g
麥門冬	mài mén dōng	9g

茯苓	fú líng	12g

Indications:
Constant suffering from vexation and oppression during pregnancy. This is child vexation.
Page: 139

竹茹湯 zhú rú tāng
Bamboo Shavings Decoction

竹茹	zhú rú	48g
乾地黃	gān dì huáng	12g
人參	rén shēn	3g
芍藥	sháo yào	3g
桔梗	jié gěng	3g
川芎	chuān xiōng	3g
當歸	dāng guī	3g
甘草	gān cǎo	3g
桂心	guì xīn	3g

Indications:
Women's sweating of blood, vomiting blood, bloody urine, and descent of blood.
Page: 366

竹葉湯 zhú yè tāng
Bamboo Leaves Decoction

生淡竹葉	shēng dàn zhú yè	24g
麥門冬	mài mén dōng	24g
甘草	gān cǎo	6g
生薑	shēng jiāng	9g
茯苓	fú líng	9g
大棗	dà zǎo	14 pcs
小麥	xiǎo mài	35ml

Indications:
Postpartum vexation and oppression in the heart that fails to be resolved.
Page: 262

竹葉湯 zhú yè tāng
Bamboo Leaves Decoction

淡竹葉	dàn zhú yè	1 handful
葛根	gé gēn	9g
防風	fáng fēng	6g
桔梗	jié gěng	3g
甘草	gān cǎo	3g
人參	rén shēn	3g
大附子	dà fù zǐ	1 big pc

生薑	shēng jiāng	15g
大棗	dà zǎo	15 pcs
桂心	guì xīn	3g

Indications:
Postpartum wind strike with fever, full red facial complexion, panting, and headache.
Page: 274

竹葉湯 zhú yè tāng
Bamboo Leaves Decoction

竹葉	zhú yè	9g
甘草	gān cǎo	3g
茯苓	fú líng	3g
人參	rén shēn	3g
小麥	xiǎo mài	35ml
生薑	shēng jiāng	9g
大棗	dà zǎo	14 pcs
麥門冬	mài mén dōng	9g
半夏	bàn xià	15g

Indications:
Postpartum vacuity thirst with lack of *qì* and strength.
Page: 360

紫石門冬丸 zǐ shí mén dōng wán
Fluorite and Asparagus Pills

紫石英	zǐ shí yīng	9g
天門冬	tiān mén dōng	9g
當歸	dāng guī	6g
川芎	chuān xiōng	6g
紫葳	zǐ wēi	6g
卷柏	juǎn bǎi	6g
桂心	guì xīn	6g
烏頭	wū tóu	6g
乾地黃	gān dì huáng	6g
牡蒙	mǔ měng	6g
禹餘糧	yǔ yú liáng	6g
石斛	shí hú	6g
辛夷	xīn yí	6g
人參	rén shēn	1.5g
桑寄生	sāng jì shēng	1.5g
續斷	xù duàn	1.5g
細辛	xì xīn	1.5g
厚朴	hòu pò	1.5g
乾薑	gān jiāng	1.5g
食茱萸	shí zhū yú	1.5g

牡丹	mǔ dān	1.5g
牛膝	niú xī	1.5g
柏子仁	bǎi zǐ rén	3g
薯蕷	shǔ yù	4.5g
烏賊骨	wū zéi gǔ	4.5g
甘草	gān cǎo	4.5g

Indications:
Complete inability to give birth and interruption of the thread.
Page: 66

紫石英柏子仁丸 zǐ shí yīng bǎi zǐ rén wán
Fluorite and Arborvitae Seed Pills

紫石英	zǐ shí yīng	9g
柏子仁	bǎi zǐ rén	9g
烏頭	wū tóu	6g
桂心	guì xīn	6g
當歸	dāng guī	6g
山茱萸	shān zhū yú	6g
澤瀉	zé xiè	6g
川芎	chuān xiōng	6g
石斛	shí hú	6g
遠志	yuǎn zhì	6g
寄生	jì shēng	6g
蓯蓉	cōng róng	6g
乾薑	gān jiāng	6g
甘草	gān cǎo	6g
蜀椒	shǔ jiāo	3g
杜蘅	dù héng	3g
蕪荑	wú yí	3g
細辛	xì xīn	4.5g

Indications:
Heat disease in the spring and summer after being exposed to unseasonably warm wind in the winter, headache, heat toxin wind vacuity, heaviness in the hundred channels, red and white vaginal discharge, no thought of food or drink, dizziness in the head and heart palpitations, distress, anxiety, and abstraction, and inability to [go on with their] daily life.
Page: 413

紫石英天門冬丸 zǐ shí yīng tiān mén dōng wán
Fluorite and Asparagus Pills

紫石英	zǐ shí yīng	9g
天門冬	tiān mén dōng	9g
禹餘糧	yǔ yú liáng	9g

蕪荑	wú yí	6g
烏頭	wū tóu	6g
蓯蓉	cōng róng	6g
桂心	guì xīn	6g
甘草	gān cǎo	6g
五味子	wǔ wèi zǐ	6g
柏子仁	bǎi zǐ rén	6g
石斛	shí hú	6g
人參	rén shēn	6g
澤瀉	zé xiè	6g
遠志	yuǎn zhì	6g
杜仲	dù zhòng	6g
蜀椒	shǔ jiāo	3g
卷柏	juǎn bǎi	3g
寄生	jì shēng	3g
石楠	shí nán	3g
雲母	yún mǔ	3g
當歸	dāng guī	3g
烏賊骨	wū zéi gǔ	3g

Indications:
Wind-cold in the infant's palace [causing] habitual mis-carriage [in women who do] become pregnant, or for discomfort from heart pain in recently married women, which can subsequently turn into heart racing; or for a complete absence of menstruation from childhood on. Taking these [pills] will make her fat and plump and cause her to be with child.
Page: 420

坐導藥 *zuò dǎo yào*
suppository

皂莢	zào jiá	3g
山茱萸	shān zhū yú	3g
當歸	dāng guī	3g
細辛	xì xīn	6g
五味子	wǔ wèi zǐ	6g
乾薑	gān jiāng	6g
大黃	dà huáng	1.5g
礬石	fán shí	1.5g
戎鹽	róng yán	1.5g
蜀椒	shǔ jiāo	1.5g

Indictaions:
Complete inability to give birth and interruption of the thread [of descendants to continue the family line].
Page: 65

Bibliography

D.1. Primary Sources

Anon.《敦煌醫藥文獻輯校》. 編者：馬繼興、王淑民、陶廣正、樊正倫.
南京：江蘇古籍出版社，1998.

Anon.《敦煌中醫藥全書》. 主編：叢春雨. 北京：中醫古籍出版社，1994.

Anon.《黃帝內經》Ca. first century BCE. See the following editions:
—.《黃帝內經素文》. 編者：任應秋. 北京：人民衛生出版社，1986.
—.《黃帝內經素文譯釋》. 主編：孟景春、王新華. 上海：上海科學技術出版社，1997
.
—.《靈樞讀本》. 編者：李政育. 臺北：新文豐出版公司，1977.
巢元方 (fl. 605-616)《巢氏諸病源候論校注》. 主編：丁光迪. 北京：人民衛生出版
社，2000 (4th edition).

Anon.《難經》Ca. second century CE. Edition：Paul U. Unschuld, editor, translator and annotator. Berkeley：University of California Press, 1986.

Anon.《神農本草經輯注》西漢. 主編：馬繼興. 北京：人民衛生出版社，1995.

Anon.《胎產書》Terminus ante quem 168 BCE.《馬王堆漢墓帛書》，vol. 4., pp.
136 ff. 北京：文物出版社，1985.

陳延之《小品方》南北朝 (317-589 CE). 編者：祝新年. 上海：上海中醫學院出版
社，1993.

陳自明《婦人大全良方》1284. 主編：余瀛鰲. 北京：人民衛生出版社，1985.

李時珍《本草綱目》1596. 劉衡如、劉山永校注. 北京：華夏出版社, 1998

劉昉《幼幼新書》1150. 編者：馬繼興. 北京：人民衛生出版社，1987.

劉向《列女傳》西漢. 編者：黃清泉. 臺北：三民書局, 1996.

齊仲甫《女科百問》1220．《珍本醫書集成》, vol. 8：婦科類, pp. 1047-1093．上海：上海科學技術出版社，1985．

孫思邈《備急千金要方》Ca. 652 CE．See the following editions:
—．編者：張瑞賢，劉更生, et al.《千金方》Part I．北京：華夏出版社，1996．
—．李景榮等校釋《備急千金要方校釋》．北京：人民衛生出版社，1996．
—．主編：馬繼興《孫真人千金方》．北京：人民衛生出版社, 1995．

.孫思邈《千金翼方》Ca. 652 CE．編者：張瑞賢, 劉更生, et al.《千金方》Part II．北京：華夏出版社，1996．

丹波康賴《醫心方》984．高文鑄等校注研究．北京：華夏出版社，1996．

王懷隱《太平聖惠方》978-992．北京：人民衛生出版社，1958．

王燾《外台秘要》752．高文鑄校注．北京：華夏出版社，1993．

許慎 (died 146 CE)《說文解字》．主編：李恩江, 賈玉民．鄭州：中原農民出版社，2000.

咎殷 (fl. 897)《經效產寶》．《中國婦科名著集成》pp. 1-26．北京：華夏出版社，1997.

張機 (張仲景)《金匱要略》西漢．主編：李克光．上海：上海科學技術出版社，1991．

2.1　D.2. Secondary Sources

Ahern, Emily M. *"The Power and Pollution of Chinese Women." Women in Chinese Society.*
Margery Wolf and Roxane Witke, ed. Stanford, Ca: Stanford University Press, 1975. pp. 193- 214.
Andrews, Bridie. "*Tailoring Tradition: The Impact of Modern Medicine on Traditional Chinese
Medicine, 1887-1937.***"** *Notions Et Perceptions Du Changement En Chine.* Viviane Alleton
and Alexei Volkov, ed. College de France: Institut des Hautes Études Chinoises, 1994. pp.149-
166. Anon. 《漢語大辭典》 [*Great Dictionary of the Chinese Language*]. CD-Rom Version.
Hongkong: The Commercial Press, 1998.
—. 《紀念孫思邈逝世1300週年專輯》 [Special Issue in Commemoration of the 1300
Anniversary of Sūn Sī-Miǎo's Passing Away] 《中華醫史雜誌》 **13.1 (1983).**
—. 《中華本草》 [Chinese Materia Medica] 上海：上海科學技術出版公司, 1999.
—. 《中藥大辭典》 [Great Dictionary of Chinese Materia Medica]. 臺北：新文豐出版社, 1982.
Barlow, Tani E., and Angela Zito, editors. *Body, Subject, and Power in China.* Chicago: University
of Chicago Press, 1994.
Bensky, Dan, and Andrew Gamble, compilors and editors. *Chinese Herbal Medicine: Materia
Medica.* Revised Edition. Seattle: Eastland Press, 1993.
Berkowitz, Alan J. *Patterns of Disengagement. The Practice and Portrayal of Reclusion in Early
Medieval China.* Stanford, California: Stanford University Press, 2000.

"Spirit Possession Revisited: Beyond Instrumentality." *Annual Review of Anthropology 23* (1994): pp. 407-34.

Bordo, Susan. "Are Mothers Persons? Reproductive Rights and the Politics of Subject-ivity." *Unbearable Weight. Feminism, Western Culture and the Body*. Susan Bordo, ed. Berkeley: University of California Press, 1993. pp. 71-98.

Bray, Francesca. "A Deathly Disorder: Understanding Women's Health in Late Imperial China." *Knowledge and the Scholarly Medical Traditions*. Don Bates, ed. Cambridge: Cambridge University Press, 1995. pp. 235-250.

—. Technology and Gender. *Fabrics of Power in Late Imperial China*. Berkeley: University of California Press, 1997.

Buckley, Thomas and Alma Gottlieb, ed. *Blood Magic. The Anthropology of Menstruation*. Berkeley: University of California Press, 1988.

Cass, Victoria B. "Female Healers in the Ming and the Lodge of Ritual and Ceremony." *Journal of the American Oriental Society* 106.1 (1986): pp. 233-40.

Chang, Chia-feng. *Aspects of Smallpox and its Significance in Chinese History*. Unpublished doctoral dissertation: University of London School of Oriental and African Studies, 1996.

Chén Yǒng-Zhèng 陳永正. 《中國方術大辭典》 [Dictionary of Occult Arts in China]. 廣東: 中山大學出版社, 1991.

Chén Yuán-Péng 陳元朋. 《兩宋的尚醫士人與儒醫》 [Medical Scholars and Confucian Physicians in the Liǎng and Sòng Periods]. 臺北: 國立臺灣大學出版社, 1997.

Chu, Cordia. "Tso Yueh-Tzu (Sitting the Month) in Contemporary Taiwan." *Maternity and Reproductive Health in Asian Societies*. Pranee Liamputtong Rice and Lenore Manderson, ed. Amsterdam: Harwood Academic Publishers, 1996. pp. 191-204.

Cullen, Christopher. "Patients and Healers in Late Imperial China: Evidence from the Jinpingmei." *History of Science* 31 (1993): pp. 99-150.

Davis-Floyd, Robbie E. and Carolyn F. Sargent, ed. *Childbirth and Authoritative Knowledge. Crosscultural Perspectives*. Berkeley: University of California Press, 1997.

. "Autopsia, Historia and What Women Know: The Authority of Women in Hippocratic Gynaecology." *Knowledge and the Scholarly Medical Traditions*. Don Bates, ed. Cambridge: Cambridge University Press, 1995.

Delaney, Janice, et al. The Curse. *A Cultural History of Menstruation*. Urbana and Chicago: University of Illinois Press, 1988.

"Indian Influences on Early Chinese Ophthalmology: Glaucoma as a Case Study." *Bulletin of the School of Oriental and African Studies,* University of London 62, part 2 (1999): pp. 306-322.

—. "The Role of Foreign Medicine in Shaping Sui and Tang Gynecology." Unpublished paper, presented at the Annual Meeting of the Association of Asian Studies, March 4-7, 2004, in San Diego.

Despeux, Catherine. *Prescriptions D'Acuponcture Valant Mille Onces D'or: Traité D'Acuponcture De Sun Simiao Du VIIe Siécle*. Paris: Trédaniel, 1987.

— and Frédéric Obringer. *La Maladie Dans La Chine Médiévale*: La Toux. Paris: Editions l'Harmattan, 1997.

DeWoskin, Kenneth J. *Doctors, Diviners, and Magicians of Ancient China: Biographies of fangshi*. New York: Columbia University Press, 1983.

Duden, Barbara. *The Woman Beneath the Skin. A Doctor's Patients in 18th c. Germany*. Harvard: Harvard University Press, 1991.

Ebrey, Patricia Buckley. *The Inner Quarters. Marriage and the Lives of Chinese Women in the Sung Period*. Berkeley: University of California Press, 1993.

Elliott, Dyan. Fallen Bodies. *Pollution, Sexuality and Demonology in the Middle Ages*. Philadelphia: University of Pennsylvania Press, 1999.

Elpel, Thomas J. *Botany in a Day. Thomas J. Elpel's Field Guide to Plant Families*. Pony,

Montana: Hollowtop Outdoor Primitive School, 2000.

Engelhardt, Ute. "Die klassische Tradition der Qi-Übungen: Eine Darstellung anhand des Tang-zeitlichen Textes Fuqi Jingyi Lun von Sima Chengzhen." *Münchener Ostasiatische Studien, Band 44*. Wiesbaden: Franz Steiner Verlag, 1987.

—. "Dietetics in Tang China and the First Extant Works of Materia Medica." *Innovation in Chinese Medicine*. Elisabeth Hsu, ed. Cambridge: Cambridge University Press, 2001. pp. 173-91.

Farquhar, Judith. *Appetites: Food and Sex in Post-Socialist China*. Duke University Press, 2002.

—. Knowing Practice: the Clinical Encounter of Chinese Medicine. *Studies in the Ethnographic Imagination*. Boulder: Westview Press, 1994.

—. "Multiplicity, Point of View, and Responsibility in Traditional Chinese Healing." *Body, Subject, and Power in China*. Tani E. Barlow and Angela Zito, ed. Chicago: University of Chicago Press, 1994. pp. 78-99.

—. "Objects, Processes and Female Infertility in Chinese Medicine." *Medical Anthropology Quarterly* 5.4 (1991): pp. 370-99.

Faure, Bernard. The Red Thread. *Buddhist Approaches to Sexuality*. Princeton: Princeton University Press, 1998.

Foucault, Michel. *A History of Sexuality*. New York: Pantheon, 1978.

Furth, Charlotte. "Blood, Body, and Gender. Medical Images of the Female Condition in China, 1600-1850." *Chinese Science* (July, 1986): pp. 43-66.

—. "Concepts of Pregnancy, Childbirth, and Infancy in Ch'ing Dynasty China." *Jounal of Asian Studies* 46.1 (1987): pp. 7-35.

—. *A Flourishing Yin. Gender in China's Medical History, 960-1665*. Berkeley: University of California Press, 1999.

—. "From Birth to Birth: The Growing Body in Chinese Medicine." *Chinese Views of Childhood*. Anne Behnke Kinney, ed. Honolulu: University of Hawai'i Press, 1995. pp. 157-191.

—. "Rethinking Van Gulik: Sexuality and Reproduction in Traditional Chinese Medicine." *Engendering China*. C. Gilmartin et al., ed. Harvard: Harvard University Press, 1994. pp. 125-146.

Gān Zǔ-Wàng 干祖望. 《孫思邈評傳》 [A Critical Biography of Sūn Sī-Miǎo]. 江蘇: 南京大學出版社, 1995.

Ginsberg, Faye and Rapp Rayna. "The Politics of Reproduction." *Annual Revue of Anthropology* 20 (1991): pp. 311-343.

Grieve, M. *A Modern Herbal. The Medicinal, Culinary, Cosmetic and Economic Properties, Cultivation and Folk-lore of Herbs, Grasses, Fungi, Shrubs and Trees with All Their Modern Scientific Uses*. Republication of the 1931 edition by Harcourt, Brace & Company. New York: Dover Publications, 1971.

Guō Lì-Chéng 郭立誠. 《中國生育禮俗考》 [Investigation of Chinese Childbirth Rituals and Customs]. 臺北: 文史哲出版社, 1979.

Hā Xiào-Xián 哈孝賢. 《內經婦科輯文集義》 [Collection and Explanation of Gynecological Texts in the Nèijīng]. 北京: 中國醫藥科技出版社, 1996.

Hanson, Marta. "Robust Northerners and Delicate Southerners: The Nineteenth-Century Invention of a Southern Medical Tradition." *Positions* 6.3 (1998): pp. 515-50.

Harper, Donald. "The Conception of Illness in Early Chinese Medicine, As Documented in Newly Discovered 3rd and 2nd Century B.C. Manuscripts." *Sudhoffs Archiv* 74 (1990): pp. 210-35.

—. *Early Chinese Medical Literature. The Mawangdui Medical Manuscripts*. New York: Keagan Paul International, 1998.

Hay, John. "The Human Body As a Microcosmic Source of Macrocosmic Values in Calligraphy." *Theories of the Arts in China*. Susan Bush and Christian Murck, ed. Princeton, N.J.: Princeton University Press, 1983. pp. 74-102.

Hé Shí-Xī 何時希, 編者. 《珍本女科醫書輯佚八種》 [A Precious Compilation of Eight Lost

Medical Books on Female Diseases]. 上海：學林出版社, 1984.

Holmgren, Jennifer. "Widow Chastity in the Northern Dynasties: the Lie-Nu Biographies in the Weishu." *Papers on Far Eastern History* 23 (1981): pp. 165-86.

Holzman, Donald. "A Dialogue with the Ancients: Tao Qian's Interrogation of Confucius." Unpublished paper presented at the ACLS conference New Dimensions of Thought and Action in Early Medieval China. Bellingham, Washington: August 23-25, 1996.

Hou, Ching-lang. "The Chinese Belief in Baleful Stars." *Facets of Taoism. Essays in Chinese Religion.* Holmes Welch and Anna Seidel, ed. New Haven and London: Yale University Press, 1979. pp. 193-228.

Hsu, Elisabeth. "Change in Chinese Medicine: Bian and Hua, an Anthropologist's Approach." *Notions Et Perceptions Du Changement En Chine.* Viviane Alleton and Alexeï Volkov, ed. College de France: Institut des Hautes Études Chinoises, 1994. pp. 41-58.

—. "Pulse Diagnostics in the Western Han: how mai and qi determine bing." *Innovation in Chinese Medicine.* Elisabeth Hsu, ed. Cambridge: Cambridge University Press, 2001. pp. 51-91.

—. The Transmission of Chinese Medicine. *Cambridge Studies in Medical Anthropology* 7. Cambridge: Cambridge University Press, 1999.

Hucker, Charles O. A Dictionary of Official Titles in Imperial China. Taipei: SMC Publishing, 1995.

Jiāng Dá-Zhì 江達智. 《春秋戰國時代生育及婚喪禁忌之研究》 [Childbirth and Wedding Taboos in Early China]. Unpublished master's thesis: 國立成功大學, 1992.

Jiāng Huán 江萑 and Wèi Zhī-Xiù 魏之琇. 《名醫類案》 [Case Histories of Famous Physicians]. 北京: 中國中醫藥出版社, 1996.

Jordan, Brigitte. *Birth in Four Cultures. A Cross-Cultural Investigation of Childbirth in Yucatan, Holland, Sweden, and the United States.* Montréal - London: Eden Press, 1983.

Kalinowski, Marc. "La Divination Par Les Nombres Dans Les Manuscrits De Dunhuang." Nombres, Astres, Plantes Et Viscéres. *Sept Essais Sur L'Histoire Des Sciences Et Des Techniques En Asie Orientale.* Vol. 35. College de France. Institut des Hautes Etudes Chinoises, 1994.

—. 《馬王堆帛書『刑德』試探》 [Discussion of xíng dé in the Mǎwángduīsilk texts]. 《華學》 1 (1995): pp. 82-101.

Katz, Paul R. *Demon Hordes and Burning Boats. The Cult of Marshal Wen in Late Imperial Chekiang.* New York: State University of New York Press, 1995.

Kendall, Laurel. "Cold Wombs in Balmy Honolulu: Ethnogynecology Among Korean Immigrants." *Social Science and Medicine* 25.4 (1987): 367-376.

Kinney, Anne Behnke, *Representations of Childhood and Youth in Early China* (Stanford: Stanford University Press, 2004).

Kinoshita Harutsu 木下晴都. 《中國經絡學》 [Chinese Vessel Theory]. 臺北: 培琳出版社, 1998.

Ko, Dorothy. *Teachers of the Inner Chambers. Women and Culture in Seventeenth Century China.* Stanford, CA: Stanford University Press, 1994.

Kunitz, Stephen J. "Classifications in Medicine." *Grand Rounds. One Hundred Years of Internal Medicine.* Russell C. Maulitz and Diana E. Long, ed. Philadelphia: University of Pennsylvania Press, 1988. pp. 279-296.

Kuriyama, Shigehisa. "Interpreting the History of Bloodletting." *Journal of the History of Medicine and Allied Sciences* 50 (1995): pp. 11-46.

—. "The Imagination of Winds and the Development of the Chinese Conception of the Body." *Body, Subject, and Power in China.* Tani E. Barlow and Angela Zito, ed. Chicago: University of Chicago Press, 1994.

Laqueur, William. *Making Sex: Body and Gender From the Greeks to Freud.* Harvard: Harvard University Press, 1990.

Lee, Jender 李貞德 [Lǐ Zhēn-Dé]. "Childbirth in Early Imperial China." Nan Nü: Men, Women,

697

and Gender in Early and Imperial China. 7. 2 (2005), pp. 216-286.

—. "Gender and Medicine in Tang China." Paper presented at New Perspectives on the Tang: an International Conference, Princeton University, April 18-20, 2002.

—. "The Life of Women in the Six Dynasties." *Journal of Women and Gender Studies* 4 (1993): pp. 47-80.

—. *Women and Marriage in China During the Period of Disunion*. Unpublished doctoral dissertation: University of Washington, 1992.

—. 《漢唐之間的女性醫療照顧者》[Women Healers in Late Antiquity and Early Medieval China]. 《臺大歷史學報》23 (1999): pp. 123-156

—. 《漢唐之間求子醫方試探兼論婦疫濫觴與性別論述》[Reproductive Medicine in Late Antiquity and Early Medieval China: Gender Discourse and the Birth of Gynecology]. 《中央研究院歷史語言研究所集刊》68.2 (1997): pp. 283-367.

—. 《漢唐之間醫書中的生產之道》[Childbirth in Late Antiquity and Early Medieval China]. 《中央研究院歷史語言研究所集刊》67.3 (1996): pp. 533-654.

—. 《漢魏六朝的乳女》[Wetnurses in Late Antiquity and Early Medieval China]. 《中央研究院歷史語言研究所集刊》70. Part 2 (1999).

Lee, T'ao. "Ten Celebrated Physicians and Their Temple." *Chinese Medical Journal* 58 (1940): pp. 267-274.

Leung, Angela Kiche. "Autour De La Naissance: La Mere Et L'Enfant En Chine Aux XVIe Et XVII Siècles." *Cahiers Internationaux De Sociologie* 76 (1984): pp. 51-69.

Lǐ Jiàn-Mín 李建民. 《馬王堆漢幕帛書『禹藏埋胞圖』箋証》[Notes on the Placenta Burial Chart From Mǎ-Wáng-Duī]. 《中央研究院歷史語言研究所集刊》65.4 (1994): pp. 725-832.

—. 《明堂與陰陽-以五十二病方灸其泰陰泰陽為例》[Míngtáng and Yīnyáng: Examplified by the Wǔshíèrbìngfāng from Mǎ-Wáng-Duī]. 《中央研究院歷史語言研究所集刊》70.1 (1999): pp. 49-118.

—. 《養生，情色與房中術:中國早期房中數之探索》[Physical Cultivation, Sex, and the Arts of the Bedchamber]. 《北縣文化》38 (1993): pp. 18-23.

—. 《中國古代『禁方』考論》[The Transmission of Secret Techniques in Ancient China]. 《中央研究院歷史語言研究所集刊》68.1 (1997): pp. 117-66.

Lǐ Jīng-Wěi 李經緯, 主編. 《中醫大辭典》[Great Dictionary of Chinese Medicine], second edition. 北京: 人民衛生出版社, 2004.

—. 《孫思邈在發展藥學上的貢獻》[Sūn Sī-Miǎo's Contributions to the Development of Pharmacology]. 《中華醫史雜誌》13.1 (1983): pp. 20-25.

Liào Yù-Qún 廖育群. 《陳延之與『小品方』研究的新進展》[New Developments in the Study of Chén Yán-Zhī's Xiǎo Pǐn Fāng]. 《中華醫史雜誌》17.2 (1987): pp. 74-75.

Lin Fu-shih. Chinese Shamanism in the Chiang-Nan Area During the Six Dynasties Period (3rd-6th Century A.D.). Unpublished doctoral dissertation: Princeton University, 1994.

—. "Religious Taoism and Dreams: An Analysis of the Dream-Data Collected in the Yun-Chi Ch'i-Ch'ien." *Cahier D'Extréme-Asie* 8 (1995): pp. 95-112.

Lín Fù-Shì 林富士. 《中國六朝時期的巫覡與醫療》[Shamanism and Medicine in the Six Dynasties Period]. 《中央研究院歷史語言研究所集刊》70.1 (1999): pp. 1-47.

—. 《東漢晚期的疾疫與宗教》[Epidemics and Religion in Late Hàn China]. 《中央研究院歷史語言研究所集刊》66.3 (1995): pp. 695-745.

Lín Měi-Huì 林美慧. 《健康漂亮坐月子》[Sitting out the Month in Health and Beauty]. 臺北: 積木文化出版社, 2000.

Lloyd, Geoffrey, and Nathan Sivin. *The Way and the Word. Science and Medicine in Early China and Greece*. New Haven and London: Yale University Press, 2002.

Lomperis, Linda and Stanbury Sarah, editors. *Feminist Approaches to the Body in Medieval Literature*. Philadelphia: University of Pennsylvania Press, 1993.

Loewe, Michael, ed. Early Chinese Texts. A Biographical Guide. Berkeley: *The Society for the*

Study of Early China, 1993.

Luó Yuán-Kǎi 羅元愷, 編者.《中醫婦科學》[Gynecology in Chinese Medicine].《高等中醫研究參考叢書》vol. 3. 臺北: 知音出版社, 1997.

Maciocia, Giovanni. *Obstetrics and Gynecology in Chinese Medicine.* New York: Churchill Livingstone, 1998.

Mǎ Dà-Zhèng 馬大正.《中國婦產科發展史》[A History of the Development of Gynecology and Obstetrics in China]. 西安: 陝西科學教育出版社, 1991.

Mǎ Jì-Xìng 馬繼興, 編者.《馬王堆古醫書考釋》[Explanation of Ancient Medical Documents from Mǎ-Wáng-Duī]. 長沙: 湖南科學技術出版社, 1992.

—.《醫心方中的古醫學文獻初探》[Preliminary Investigation of the Ancient Medical Records in the Yī Xīn Fāng]《日本醫學雜誌》31.1 (1985): pp. 326-371.

Mabberley, D.J. *The Plant Book.* Cambridge, U.K.: Cambridge University Press, 2000.

Manderson, Lenore. "Roasting, Smoking and Dieting in Response to Birth: Malay Confinement in Cross-Cultural Perspective." *Social Science and Medicine* 153 (1981): pp. 509-520.

Martin, Emily. "Medical Metaphors of Women's Bodies, Menstruation and Menopause." *Writing on the Body. Female Embodiment and Feminist Theory.* Katie Conboy, Nadia Medina, and Sarah Stanbury, ed. New York: Columbia University Press, 1997. pp. 15-41.

—. *The Woman in the Body.* Beacon Press, 1992.

McGavin, C. George. *Essential Entomology. An Order-by-Order Introduction.* New York: Oxford University Press, 2001.

McMullen, David. *State and Scholars in T'ang China.* Cambridge: Cambridge University Press, 1988.

Mark S. Micale, Approaching Hysteria. *Disease and its Interpretations.* Princeton, NJ: Princeton University Press, 1995.

Mitchell, Craig, Féng Yè, and Nigel Wiseman. Shang Han Lun. *On Cold Damage. Translation and Commentaries.* Brookline, Massachusetts: Paradigm Publications, 1999.

Miyashita Sanrô 宮下三郎.《孫思邈在日本》[Sūn Sī-Miǎo in Japan].《中華醫史雜誌》13.1 (1983): pp. 56-60.

Morohashi Tetsuji 諸橋轍次, 主編.《大漢和辭典》[Great Chinese-Japanese Dictionary]. 臺北: 北一出版社, 1987.

Nichter, Mark, editor. *Anthropological Approaches to the Study of Ethnomedicine.* Amsterdam: Gordon and Breach Science Publishers, 1992.

—. "The Mission Within the Madness: Self-Initiated Medicalization As Expression of Agency." *Pragmantic Women and Body Politics.* Margaret Kaufert and Patricia A. Lock, ed. Cambridge: Cambridge University Press, 1998. pp. 327-353.

— and Nichter Mimi. "Hype and Weight." Medical Anthropology 13 (1991): pp. 249-284.

Niú Bīng-Zhān 牛兵占, 編者.《中國婦科名著集成》[Collection of Famous Works in Chinese Gynecology]. 北京: 華夏出版社, 1998.

Okanishi Tameto 岡西為人.《宋以前醫籍考》[The Study of Medical Books of the Sòng Dynasty and Earlier]. 北京: 人民衛生出版社, 1958.

Paschold, Chris E. Die Frau und ihr Körper im medizinischen und didaktischen Schrifttum des französischen Mittelalters. *Würzburger Medizinhistorische Forschungen* 47. Würzburg: Königshausen & Neumann, 1989.

Pillsbury, Barbara L. K. "'Doing the Month': Confinement and Convalescence of Chinese Women after Childbirth." *Social Science and Medicine* 12 (1978): pp. 11-22.

Preus, Anthony. "Galen's Criticism of Aristotle's Conception Theory." *Journal of the History of Biology* 10 (1977): pp. 78-84.

Ráo Zōng-Yí 饒宗頤.《雲夢秦簡日書研究》[Study of the Yún-Mèng Qín Bamboo slip Almanac]. 香港: 中文大學出版社, 1982.

Raphals, Lisa. *Sharing the Light. Representations of Women and Virtue in Early China.* Albany:

State University of New York, 1998.

Read, Bernard E. *Botanical, Chemical, and Pharmacological Reference List to Chinese Materia Medica.* Beijing: Peking Union Medical College, 1923.
—. *Chinese Materia Medica. Avian Drugs.* Beijing: Peking Natural History Bulletin, 1932.
—. *Chinese Medicinal Plants From the Pen Ts'Ao Kang Mu. Botanical, Chemical and Pharmacological Reference List.* Beijing: Peking Natural History Bulletin, 1936.
Rice, Pranee Liamputtong and Manderson Lenore, editors. *Maternity and Reproductive Health in Asian Societies.* Amsterdam: Harwood Academic Publishers, 1996.
Robertson, Elisabeth. "Medieval Medical Views of Women and Spirituality in the Ancrene Wisse and Julian of Norwich's Showings." *Feminist Approaches to the Body in Medieval Literature.* Linda Lomperis and Sarah Stanbury, ed. Philadelphia: University of Pennsylvania Press, 1993. pp. 142-167.
Scheid, Volker. *Chinese Medicine in Contemporary China. Plurality and Synthesis.* Durham & London: Duke University Press, 2002.
Scheper-Hughes, Nancy, and Margaret M. Lock. "The Mindful Body: a Prolegomenon to Future Work in Medical Anthropology." *Medical Anthropology Quarterly* 1.1 (1987): pp. 6-41.
Shail, Andrew and Gillian Howie, ed. *A Cultural History of Menstruation.* Palgrave MacMillan, 2005.
Shǎn xī wèi shēng zhì biān zuǎn wěi yuán huì bàn gōng shì 陝西衛生志編纂委員會辦公室.《藥王孫思邈》[The King of Medicine, Sūn Sī-Miǎo]. 西安: 陝西科學技術出版社, 1990.
Sich, Dorothea. "Traditional Concepts and Customs on Pregnancy, Birth and Post Partum Period in Rural Korea." *Social Science and Medicine* 15B (1981): pp. 65-69.
Simons, Ronald C., and Charles C. Hughes, ed. *The Culture-bound Syndromes: Folk Illnesses of Psychiatric and Anthropological Interest.* Dordrecht; Boston: Kluwer Academic Publishers, 1985.
Sivin, Nathan. *Chinese Alchemy: Preliminary Studies.* Cambridge: Harvard University Press, 1968.
—. *Medicine, Philosophy and Religion in Ancient China.* Brookfield, VT: Variorum, 1995.
—. "Text and Experience in Classical Chinese Medicine." *Knowledge and the Scholarly Medical Traditions.* Don Bates, ed. Cambridge: Cambridge University Press, 1995. pp. 177-184.
Sobo, Elisa J. ""Unclean Deeds": Menstrual Taboos and Binding 'Ties' in Rural Jamaica." *Anthropological Approaches to the Study of Ethnomedicine.* Mark Nichter, ed. Amsterdam: Gordon and Breach Science Publishers, 1992. pp. 101-126.
Sontag, Susan. *Illness as Metaphor.* New York: Vintage, 1979.
Stein, Stephan. Zwischen Heil und Heilung. *Zur frühen Tradition des Yangsheng in China.* Ülzen: Medizinisch Literarische Verlagsgesellschaft, 1999.
Strickman, Michel. *Chinese Magical Medicine.* Stanford: Stanford University Press, 2002.
Symonds, Patricia V. "Journey to the Land of Light: Birth among Hmong Women." *Maternity and Reproductive Health in Asian Societies.* Pranee Liamputtong Rice and Lenore Manderson, ed. Amsterdam: Harwood Academic Publishers, 1996. pp. 103 ff.
Tanba no Mototane 丹波元胤.《中國醫籍考》[Study of China's Medical Records]. 北京: 人民衛生出版社, 1983.
Táng Lì-Fāng 唐儷芳.《做月子對產婦的意義》[The Meaning of "Doing the Month" for Postpartum Women]. Unpublished Master's Thesis: Guofang Medical College 國防醫學院, 1994.
Táo Yù-Fēng 陶御風, 主編.《歷代筆記醫事別錄》[An Informal Record of Medical Matters From Historical Anecdotes]. 天津: 天津科學技術出版社, 1988.
Ukena, Peter. "Solutus cum Soluta: Alexander Seitz' Thesen über die Notwendigkeit des Geschlechtverkehrs zwischen Unverheirateten." *Fachprosa-Studien: Beiträge zur mittelalterlichen Wissenschafts- und Geistesgeschichte.* Gundolf Keil, ed. Berlin: Erich Schmidt Verlag, 1982. pp. 278-290.

Unschuld, Paul U. "Der Chinesische 'Arzneikönig' Sun Simiao: Geschichte - Legende - Ikonographie." *Monumenta Serica* 42: pp. 217-257.

—. "Approaches to Traditional Chinese Medical Literature." *Proceedings of an International Symposium on Translation Methodologies and Terminologies.* Dordrecht: Kluwer Academic Publishers, 1989.

—. *Huang Di Nei Jing Su Wen. Nature, Knowledge, Imagery in an Ancient Chinese Medical Text* (Berkeley, University of California Press, 2003).

—. *Medical Ethics in Imperial China.* Berkeley: University of California Press, 1979.

—. *Medicine in China. A History of Ideas.* Berkeley: University of California Press, 1985.

—. *Medicine in China. Historical Artifacts and Images.* Sabine Wilms, translator. New York: Prestel-Verlag, 2000.

Van de Valle, Etienne, and Elisha P. Renne. *Regulating Menstruation. Beliefs, Practices, Interpretations.* Chicago: University of Chicago Press, 2001.

Wáng Shào-Zéng 王紹增, 主編.《醫古文百篇釋譯》[Ancient medical writings, annotated and explained]. 哈尔滨: 黑龍江科學技術出版社, 1995.

Wèi Zǐ-Xiào 魏子孝, 主編.《中醫中藥史》[The History of Chinese Medicine and Pharmacology]. 臺北: 文津出版社, 1994.

Whittaker, Andrea. "White Blood and Falling Wombs: Ethnogynecology in Northeast Thailand." *Maternity and Reproductive Health in Asian Societies.* Pranee Liamputtong Rice and Lenore Manderson, ed. Amsterdam: Harwood Academic Publishers, 1996. pp. 207 ff.

Wilms, Sabine. *Childbirth Customs in Early China.* MA Thesis, University of Arizona, 1992.

—"Ten Times More Difficult to Treat: Female Bodies in Medical Texts from Early Imperial China." *Nan Nü: Men, Women, and Gender in Early and Imperial China.* 7. 2 (2005), pp. 182-215.

— "The Art and Science of Menstrual Balancing in Medieval China." Andrew Shail, ed. *A Cultural History of Menstruation.* Palgrave: 2005.

— "The Transmission of Medical Knowledge on 'Nurturing the Fetus' in Early China." *Asian Medicine: Tradition and Modernity* 2 (2005).

Wiseman, Nigel, and Féng Yè. *A Practical Dictionary of Chinese Medicine.* Brookline, MA: Paradigm Publications, 1998.

—. English-Chinese, Chinese English Dictionary of Chinese Medicine. 長沙: 湖南科學技術出版社, 1996.

Wu, Yi-li. "A Vessel of Blood, a Gate of Life: Metaphors of Uterine Function and the Construction of Female Illness in Ming-Qing Gynecology." Unpublished paper, presented at the Annual Meeting of the Association of Asian Studies, March 4-7, 2004, in San Diego.

—. "Ghost fetuses, false pregnancies, and the parameters of medical uncertainty in classical Chinese gynecology." *Nan Nü: Men, Women, and Gender in Early and Imperial China,* 4.2 (2002): pp. 170-206.

—. "The Bamboo Grove Monastery and Popular Gynecology in Qing China." Late Imperial China 21.1 (2000): pp. 41-76.

—. *Transmitted Secrets: The Doctors of the Lower Yangzi Region and Popular Gynecology in Late Imperial China.* Unpublished doctoral dissertation, Yale University, 1998.

Wú Zé-Yán 吳澤炎, 主編.《辭源》[Origin of Words]. 臺北: 臺灣商務印書館, 2001.

Xiè Guān 謝觀, 主編.《中華醫學大辭典》[Great Dictionary of Chinese Medicine]. 沈陽: 遼寧科學出版社, 1994.

Yáng Jí-Chéng 楊吉成, 編者.《中國飲食辭典》[Dictionary of Chinese Foods and Drinks]. 臺北: 長春樹書坊, 1989.

Yī Ruò-Lán 衣若蘭.《從三姑六婆看明代婦女與社會》[Women in Míng Society from the Perspective of sān gū liù pó]. Unpublished master's thesis: 國立師範大學, 1997.

Zhāng Dēng-Běn 張登本, 主編.《內經辭典》[Dictionary of the Nèi Jīng]. 北京: 人民衛生出版社, 1990.

Zhāng Lù 張璐. 《千金方衍義》 [Expanded Meaning of the Qiān Jīn Fāng]. 北京: 中國中醫藥出版社, 1995.

Zhāng Qí-Wén 張奇文, 主編. 《婦科雜病》 [Various Gynecological Diseases]. 北京: 人民衛生出版社, 1995.

—, 主編. 《胎產病証》 [Childbirth-Related Disease Patterns]. 北京: 人民衛生出版社, 1995.

—, 主編. 《月經病証》 [Menstruation-Related Disease Patterns]. 北京: 人民衛生出版社, 1995.

Zháng Zhì-Bīn 張志斌 《古代中國婦產科疾病史》 [History of Gynecological and Obstetrical Illnesses in Ancient China]. 北京: 中醫古籍出版社, 2000.

Zhōu Yī-Móu 周一謀. 《壽星孫思邈攝生精要》 [Essentials for Preserving Life by the Star of Longevity Sūn Sī-Miǎo]. 福州: 福建科學出版社, 1994.

Text Index

Pinyin Index

崩中極重者	bēng zhōng jí zhòng zhě	extremely critical cases of center flooding	506
鼻齆	bí wèng	a pathology of nose blockage	391
閉	bì	blockage	
痺	bì	impediment	
扁鵲	Biǎn Què		38, 190
病	bìng	disease (also: condition)	
不安	bù ān	disquietude	159
不定	bù dìng	unstable	
不利	bù lì	inhibition [of menstruation]	148, 428
不通	bù tōng	stopped	428
不足	bù zǔ	insufficiency	
蠶連	cán lián	paper used in silkworm production for collecting the eggs laid by the silkworm moths in order to raise further silkworms	374
蠶紙	cán zhǐ	silkworm paper	374
蠶子故紙	cán zǐ gù zhǐ		374
廁	cè	An outdoor structure, the use of which would make her susceptible to an invasion of wind from below.	237
側生	cè shēng	side-ways (i.e., face) presentation	183
產防運法	chǎn fáng yùn fǎ	method for preventing [the fetus'] turning during birth	190
產後百日	chǎn hòu bǎi rì	a hundred days post-partum	271, 306
產後乳結癰	chǎn hòu rǔ jié yōng	postpartum binding and abscesses in the breasts	
產後滿月	chǎn hòu mǎn yuè	fulfilling one month postpartum	285
產後乳結癰方論	chǎn hòu rǔ jié yōng fāng lùn	discussion and prescriptions for postpartum binding and abscesses in the breasts	218
產後乳無汁候	chǎn hòu rǔ wú zhī	postpartum absence of breast milk	32, 218
產後乳汁溢	chǎn hòu rǔ zhī yì	postpartum spillage of breast milk	32, 218
產後上氣	chǎn hòu shàng qì	postpartum qì ascent	235
產後心痛	chǎn hòu xīn tòng	postpartum heart pain	235
產後中風	chǎn hòu zhòng fēng	postpartum wind strike	236
產門	chǎn mén	"birth gate," that is, vagina	81
產難	chǎn nàn	birthing difficulties	184
產圖	chǎn tú	"birth charts:" This term originally included three different types of charts, for setting up the birth hut (outdoors) or screen (indoors), for the position of the woman during labor, and for the burial of the placenta.	181
巢元方	Cháo Yuán-Fāng		218, 339, 353
炒令微焦	chǎo lìng wēi jiāo	fried until lightly scorched	
陳麴	chén qū	aged leaven	
沉重	chén zhòng	heaviness	

疹	chèn	chronic ailment	309
疹痛	chèn tòng	chronic pain	
痴	chī	feeble-mindedness	
尺	chǐ	cubit position for taking the pulse	88
赤白痢	chì bái lì	red and white diarrhea	340
赤痢	chì lì	red diarrhea	170, 339
瘛瘲	chì zòng	tugging and slackening	279
衝	chòng	surging	
衝心	chòng xīn	surging upwards to the heart	
衝悸	chòng jì	surging palpitations	
喘	chuǎn	panting	
喘乏	chuǎn fá	panting and lack of breath	
瘡	chuāng	sore (n) (also: wound. Syn. 瘈 yí)	449
淳	chún	concentrated/pure	475
脣褰	chún qiān	sealed lips	134
脣塞	chún sài	sealed lips	134
疵	cī	blemish	
刺	cì	stabbing	18
刺痛	cì tòng	stabbing pain	
悴	cuì	haggard	
寸	cùn	inch position for taking the pulse, the position located closest to the elbow	88
寸白蟲	cùn bái chóng	Inch white-worm: one of the nine worm diseases. In modern TCM equated with tape worm infestation.	100
剉	cuò	broken up	
大便青	dà biàn qīng	blue-green feces that have not been transformed [i.e., eliminated] are associated with infant convulsions.	108
大如揲面	dà rǔ shé miàn	the size of a surface for counting yarrow stalks [in divination]	444
大升	dà shēng	Large shēng: the equivalent of three regular shēng.	172
怠	dài	fatigue	
怠惰	dài duò	fatigue	
帶下	dài xià	vaginal discharge (also in the literal sense of "below the girdle" and in the more general sense of "women's diseases")	37, 38, 41, 72, 73, 477
帶下三十六疾	dài xià sān shí liù jí	The thirty-six diseases of vaginal discharge	71
帶下五賁	dài xià wǔ bēn	five [types of] vaginal gushing	
淡	dàn	bland/thin	91
當溫臥	dāng wēn wò	[The medicine] should [be taken] heated and when lying down	108
刀圭	dāo guī	knife tip -- the equivalent of one tenth of a square-inch spoon.	203, 533
刀環	dāo huán	The ring at the end of the knife.	188
倒產	dǎo chǎn	breech presentation	
導藥	dǎo yào	abducting medicine, suppository	60

倒出	dào chū	This refers to the child being born in breech presentation with the head first.	100
盜汗	dào hàn	night sweats	
德	dé	1) Potency 2) Virtue, that is, proper behavior	59
等分	děng fēn	equal amounts	456
顛倒	diān dǎo	topsy-turviness (in one context also: upside down [presentation of the fetus], fainting)	94, 95
顛狂疾	diān kuáng jí	mania and withdrawal disease	94
動胎	dòng tāi	stirring fetus	396
洞	dòng	throughflux	
洞下	dòng xià	throughflux diarrhea	345
洞泄	dòng xiè	most severe diarrhea until [the contents of the stomach] are emptied out and nothing is left	345
豆汁	dòu zhī	bean juice: this could refer either to the liquid in which beans have been simmered, to soy milk, or to a fermented drink made from soy beans.	81
毒腫	dú zhǒng	toxic swelling (i.e., toxemia in pregnancy)	177
短氣	duán qì	shortness of breath	
斷產	duàn chǎn	interrupt childbirth: this means that it is intended to induce sterility for birth control, which in this case is permanent as the concluding sentence states.	374
頓服之	dùn fú zhī	quaff in a single dose	198
遁尸	dùn shī	vanishing corpse	326
惰	duò	laziness	
墮身	duò shēn	Litterally fall of the body	320, 526
墮胎	duò tāi	miscarriage (in modern usage, mostly "abortion").	55, 320, 526
惡	è	malign	468
惡露	è lù	malign dew (also called 惡血 malign blood)	35, 55, 162, 237, 281
惡露不盡	è lù bù jìn	incomplete elimination of malign dew	318
惡物	è wù	malign substance	237, 318
惡心	è xīn	nausea	143
惡血	è xuè	malign blood: blood that remains in a woman's body after childbirth	55, 237
惡阻	è zǔ	malign obstruction (i.e., morning sickness)	144
二十四節	èr shí sì jié	twenty-four nodes	56
發露	fā lù	This refers to "malign dew" (惡露 è lù) or lochia	281
乏	fá	lack	
乏氣	fá qì	lack of qi	
煩	fán	vexation	
反支月	fǎn zhī yuè	Determining the opposite branch month is based on a variety of calendrical and hemerological calculations that is explained in iatromantic literature.	180

方	fāng	formula, prescription: in this context, the term fāng clearly refers not only to the narrow meaning of medicinal formulas and acupuncture prescriptions, but to its broader meaning of the various types of technical advice, such as ritual instructions, astrological rules, alchemical secrets, and household recipes.	237
方寸匕	fāng cùn bǐ	square-inch spoon: defined by Sūn Sī-Miǎo in this way: "As for a full square-inch spoon, make a spoon of a perfect one-inch square, scatter and disperse [the powder on it] and measure it by the amount that doesn't fall down."	62
放溫	fàng wēn	This means to let it cool off a little. Alternatively, it could mean to "keep it warm."	103
痱	féi	disablement: name of a disorder characterized by flaccidity of the four limbs, inability to move, and slight turmoil in the spirit and will.	269
肥白	féi bái	fat and white: a sign of great health	73
分三服	fēn sān fú	divide into three doses	298
風	fēng	wind	236
風痱候	fēng féi hòu	symptoms of wind disablement	269
膚革	fū gé	the thick layer on the inside of the skin	120
服	fú	to take	462
伏	fú	latent	
伏氣	fú qì	latent qi: this term could refer to a condition caused by dampness and heat lying latent in the channels. It could also quite literally refer to "deep-lying [i.e., shallow] breathing."	373
咀咬	fǔ jǔ	to chew	64
腹	fù	abdomen	462
傅母之徒	fù mǔ zhī tú	elderly men and women charged with rearing and guiding the sons and daughters in elite households in ancient times.	57
婦人	fù rén	wives	408, 517
婦人方	fù rén fāng	prescriptions for women	4, 24, 517
婦人將產病	fù rén jiāng chǎn bìng	diseases [that arise] when delivery is pending	22, 208
婦人三十六病	fù rén sān shí liù bìng	women's thirty-six diseases	38, 55
腹中冷熱不調	fù zhōng lěng rè bù tiáo	imbalance of hot and cold in the abdomen	471
腹中急	fù zhōng jí	tension in the abomen	306
泔	gān	rice water	220
感	gǎn	contract	
感病	gǎn bìng	contract disease	
膏	gāo	Usually translated as "lard," that is, the soft fat from animals without horns, most often pigs	83, 104, 467
羹	gēng	fancy broth	101
功	gōng	work	57
蠱	gǔ	gǔ venom	145
穀道	gǔ dào	pathway of grains: this is a reference to the anus.	206
骨立	gǔ lì	a sign of extreme wasting and emaciation.	451

穀氣	gǔ qì	Grain qì: this is a reference to yáng qì, derived from the consumption of food.	262
骨蝕	gǔ shí	bone erosion	388
痼	gù	intractable disease	
故蠶子布	gù cán zǐ bù	old silkworm cloth	374
故舡上竹茹	gù chuán shàng zhú rú	More often called 敗船茹 bài chuán rú, these are shavings of entangled bamboo roots used to fix leaks in boats.	167
刮	guā	shaved	
關	guān	bar section of the pulse	88
關元	guān yuán	Pass Head (CV-4)	82, 250, 522
歸來	guī lái	ST-29	401
鬼氣	guǐ qì	ghost qì	369
害食	hài shí	food damage: damage to the body in general, but especially the spleen and stomach, caused by the improper intake or digestion of food.	459
害吐	hài tù	injury from vomiting, that is, tendency to vomit	468
寒熱	hán rè	[aversion to] cold and heat [effusion]	92
寒疝	hán shān	cold mounting	
寒下	hán xià	this refers to discharge caused by contracting cold after birth	347
漢	Hàn		15, 16, 19, 20, 28, 31, 56, 61, 64, 459, 543
豪毛	háo máo	filament hairs	123
橫生	héng shēng	transverse (i.e., cross) presentation	183
厚衣居堂	hòu yí jū táng	wear thick clothes and remain inside the house	113
惚	hū	confusion	
槲葉脈	hú yè mài	oak leaf veins	506
戶注	hù zhù	corpse influx	532
緩	huǎn	flaccidity	
緩弱	huǎn ruò	flaccidity and weakness	
黃痢	huáng lì	yellow diarrhea	339
恍	huǎng	disorientation (in Wiseman and Féng: abstraction)	
灰	huī	ash	
毀	huǐ	destroy	
恚	huì	rage	
火籠	huǒ lóng	a portable basket-shaped heater.	64
霍亂	huò luàn	sudden turmoil	
積	jī	accumulation	
積聚	jī jù	accumulations and gatherings	
箕舌	jī shé	the tongue of a winnowing basket	540
積血	jī xuè	blood accumulations	
疾	jí	racing (in other contexts: disease, sickness)	
疾脈	jí mài	racing pulse	

九竅	jiǔ qiào	nine orifices: this expression can be understood either as referring to the seven upper orifices of the ears, eyes, nostrils, and mouth, in conjunction with the lower orifices of the posterior and anterior yīn (urethra and anus) or only to the orifices in the head, that is, the ears, eyes, nostrils, mouth, tongue, and throat.	33, 121, 467
九痛七害	jiǔ tòng qī hài	nine pains and seven harms	459
酒浸一宿，熬	jiǔ jìn yī xiǔ, āo	soaked in liquor overnight and heated slowly	
疽	jū	flat abscess	
拘	jū	hypertonicity (also: gripping, in the sense of cramping)	
拘痛	jū tòng	hypertonicity and pain	
倦	juàn	fatigue	
絹裏	juàn lǐ	wrapped in silk	490
絕	jué	expire (also: interrupt, cut off)	
絕產	jué chǎn	interruption of childbearing, infertility	72, 335, 471
絕無子	jué wú zǐ	total infertility	471
厥	jué	reversal	
咳	ké	cough	
咳嗽	ké sòu	cough	
渴	kě	thirst	164
可治	kě zhì	treatable	457
客熱	kè rè	visiting heat. Kè "visiting" refers to the termporary or seasonal nature of a condition	93
口噤	kǒu jìn	clenched jaw	
枯	kū	desiccated	
苦	kǔ	discomfort (depending on context, also: bitter, suffering).	
駃藥	kuài yào	galloping medicines: this refers to harsh purgatives	235
狂	kuāng	mania	
憒	kuì	muddleheadedness	
憒悶	kuì mèn	muddleheadedness and oppression	
困	kùn	encumbered	
困頓	kùn dùn	encumbrance and fatigue	
藍黑色	lán hēi sè	of blue-black color	108
爛	làn	ulcerated	
勞	láo	taxation	
勞氣食氣	láo qì shí qì	qì conditions due to taxation and qì conditions due to food.	365
勞傷氣血	láo shāng qì xuè	taxation damage of qì and blood	234
羸	léi	marked emaciation	
羸瘦	léi shòu	marked emaciation	
冷痢	lěng lì	cold diarrhea	347
冷熱	lěng rè	Conditions characterized by either an aversion to cold and chills or by heat effusion and fever.	92
離經	lí jīng	the channels are being separated	111

裏急	lǐ jí	tension in the digestive organs	
李時珍	Lǐ Shí-Zhēn		196, 201
痢	lì	diarrhea	170
利	lì	uninhibited [bowel movements]	170
瀝	lì	dripping	
淋	lín	dribbling (also: strangury in the context of urinary problems)	164
淋瀝	lín lì	painful and inhibited urination	
淋渴	lín kě	strangury and thirst	
留	liú	retained	
留血	liú xuè	retained blood	
留熱	liú rè	retained heat	
流	liú	drifting (Litterally to flow, stream)	
流產	liú chǎn	miscarriage (abortion)	
流火	liú huǒ	drifting fire	286
流痧	liú shā	drifting sand syndrome	286
流形	liú xíng	flowing into form	101
流腫	liú zhǒng	drifting swelling	286
流疰	liú zhù	drifting infixation	
六極	liù jí	six extremes	121
聾	lóng	deafness	
龍門	lóng mén	"dragon gate," used to refer to the vagina of married women who have not yet given birth	81, 401
漏	lòu	spotting	37, 41, 54
漏胞	lòu bāo	uterine spotting	137
漏赤白	lòu chì bái	red and white spotting	
漏下	lòu xià	vaginal spotting	40
漏下黑血	lòu xià hēi xuè	vaginal leaking [spotting] of black [or red, or yellow etc.] blood	514
漏陰	lòu yīn	Leaky Yīn KI-6	522
瘺	lòu	fistula	
攣	luán	contractions	
亂	luàn	derangement (In a more general sense: disorder), turmoil	
滿	mǎn	fullness	
毛髮初生	máo fà chū shēng	the hair begins to grow	114
冒	mào	veiling	
悶	mèn	oppression	
米宿漬	mǐ sù zì	soak rice overnight	220
蜜炙令焦	mì zhì lìng jiāo	mixfried in honey until burnt	352
綿裡	mián lǐ	wrapped in thin silk cloth	244
面目脫色	miàn mù tuō sè	loss of color in the face and eyes	
末	mò	pulverized	
目瞑	mù míng	blurred vision	
難產	nán chǎn	difficult delivery	184

內象成子	nèi xiàng chéng zǐ	inner imaging to complete the child	83
逆	nì	counterflow	
逆產	nì chǎn	breech birth	183
溺血	niào xuè	bloody urine	
膿	nóng	pus	
齊		Northern Qí	10, 101
女人	nǚ rén	women	517
衄	nǜ	nosebleed	
瘧	nüè	malaria	150
嘔	ǒu	retching	
疲	pí	tired	
否澀	pǐ sè	blocked and inhibited	
癖	pì	aggregation	
迫	pò	distress (v)	
破如豆粒	pò rú dòu lì	broken into grain-sized pieces	
破如米豆	pò rú mǐ dòu	broken into pieces the size of grains or beans	
迫胸	pò xiōng	distress the chest	
臍下	qí xià	below the navel	477
氣海	qì hǎi	Sea of Qì CV-6	174
氣候	qì hòu	qì symptoms	365
氣極	qì jí	qì extreme, caused by vacuity detriment to the lung, causes extreme shortage of qì and breath, distention of the chest and ribs, inability to speak, and rage	121
氣絕	qì jué	qì expiry	190
氣厥	qì jué	qì reversal	
氣淋	qì lín	qì strangury	357
氣門	qì mén	Qì Gate, 3 cùn to either side of (CV-4)	82
氣脫	qì tuō	qì desertion	379
氣息迫急	qì xī pò jí	distressed and rapid breathing	
強	qiáng	rigid	
竅孔	qiào kǒng	referring generally to the body's nine orifices	467
切	qiē	chopped	
切痛	qiē tòng	cutting pain	
琴瑟	qín sè	Two kinds of fretted string instruments, the first with five or seven strings, the second with fifty or later twenty-five strings and movable bridges.	99
輕	qīng	lightly/carelessly	235
清黃汁	qīng huáng zhī	green-yellow liquid	73
青痢	qīng lì	green-blue diarrhea	339
窮端	qióng duān	coccyx	468
窮骨	qióng gǔ	sacrum	468
窮孔	qióng kǒng	extremity hole	468

疝	shān	mounting	
傷	shāng	damage	
傷丈夫	shāng zhàng fū	damaged by the husband	396
燒	shāo	charred	
燒作末	shāo zuò mò	charred and pulverized	
少氣	shǎo qì	shortage of qi	
深其居處	shēn qí jū chù	withdraw deep inside the house	113
生不乳	shēng bù rǔ	agalactia	471
盛	shèng	exuberant (in the sense of pathologically overabundant)	
濕	shī	dampness	
濕痹	shī bì	damp impediment	279
尸病	shī bìng	corpse disease	326
施化	shī huà	This is an abbreviation of the common phrase 陽施陰化 yáng bestows and yīn transforms	70
尸疾	shī jí	corpse disease	325
實	shí	repletion	
十二癥	shí èr zhēng	twelve concretions: a standard expression for the twelve varieties of women's vaginal discharge	75
石淋	shí lín	stone strangury	358
石門	shí mén	Stone Gate, CV-5	64
始胞	shǐ bāo	beginning fetus: the name suggests that the third month was an important turning point, when a woman's pregnancy and the presence of a fetus in her uterus was recognized medically	126
始脂	shǐ zhī	beginning hard fat	107
嗜	shì	predilection	
手太陽小腸經	shǒu tài yáng xiǎo cháng jīng	hand greater yáng small intestine channel	90
手太陰肺經	shǒu tài yīn fèi jīng	hand greater yīn lung channel	89
手足先出	shǒu zú xiān chū	birth with hands or feet first	183
瘦	shòu	emaciation	
受胎	shòu tāi	conception of the fetus	26, 78
受胎三月	shòu tāi sān yuè	The first three months of pregnancy	98
熟者	shú	cooked	
鼠辱	shǔ rǔ	wart	
數試有驗	shù shì yǒu yàn	It has achieved good results in numerous tests	497
水穀痢	shuǐ gǔ lì	water and grain diarrhea	339, 344
水穀之道	shuǐ gǔ zhī dào	pathways of water and grains	55
水氣	shuǐ qì	water qi: defined by Wiseman and Féng as "pathological excesses of water in the body and, specifically, water swelling provoked by it. The main cause is impairment of movement and transformation of water due to spleen-kidney yáng vacuity" (*Practical Dictionary*, p. 668).	164
水腫	shuǐ zhǒng	water swelling (i.e., edema)	
四德	sì dé	four womanly virtues	57

微下	wēi xià	This refers to a slight vaginal discharge, a common symptom of cold-related conditions.	307
萎	wěi	withered	
萎悴	wěi cuì	withered	
文王	Wén Wáng	King Wén, the father of the founder of the Zhōu dynasty	99
梧桐子	wú tóng zǐ	parasol tree seeds: A measurement that refers to an amount that equals two soybeans or four azuki beans.	67
無御丈夫	wú yù zhàng fū	Do not engage in sexual intercourse with the husband	101
無子	wú zǐ	infertility	471
五崩	wǔ bēng	five-colored flooding	41, 55, 485
五更	wǔ gēng	fifth watch: the time of the last nightwatch, i.e., right before dawn.	528
五勞七傷	wǔ láo qī shāng	five taxations and seven damages: A standard expression for debilitating conditions of vacuity taxation	60
五色痢	wǔ sè lì	five-colored diarrhea: this refers to a subcategory of lì that is a combination of the other types of diarrhea,	339
五邪	wǔ xié	five evils	459
五心	wǔ xīn	five hearts: a technical term referring to the soles of the feet, palms of the hands, and the center of the chest.	156
五嶽	wǔ yuè	five sacred peaks	235
勿使得汗	wù shǐ dé hàn	do not make her sweat	274
瘜肉	xí ròu	polyp	
洗	xǐ	washed	
喜吐	xǐ tù	tendency to vomit	468
細切	xì qiē	finely chopped	
下赤白	xià chì bái	red and white discharge: this refers to a discharge containing blood and pus.	340
下焦三十六疾	xià jiāo sān shí liù jí	thirty-six diseases of the lower burner, that is, the thirty-six diseases of vaginal discharge	71
下脫	xià tuō	downward prolapse (of the genitals or uterus)	379
下血及穀下	xià xuè jí gǔ xià	descent of blood as well as grain discharge	344
下重痢不止	xià/chóng lì bù zhǐ	repeated diarrhea that will not stop	
癇	xián	convulsions (in modern TCM, epilepsy)	
消	xiāo	wasting (Litterally to disperse)	
削	xiāo	whittling away	
挾	xié	complicated by	
挾風	xié fēng	complicated by wind	
邪思洩利	xié sī xiè lì	evil thought diarrha: refers to diarrhea induced by evil thoughts	468
瀉	xiè	drain: a technical term referring to a specific needling method which is described in the *Sù Wèn*	189
瀉泄	xiè	diarrhea (characters are used interchangeably or together)	
懈	xiè	fatigue	

陰陽不交	yīn yáng bù jiāo	lack of sex	369
蔭	yìn	shaded, sheltered, covered	475
蔭胎	yìn tāi	a medical term denoting a fetus that has stopped growing in the uterus, due to the mother's physical weakness, insufficiency of yīn blood, and subsequent inability to nurture the fetus sufficiently.	475
癰	yōng	abscess (specifically an ulcerating welling-abscess)	
憂	yōu	anxiety	
瘀	yū	stasis/static	428
瘀血	yū xuè	static blood	
余疾	yú jí	Residual conditions: I interpret this literally as referring to conditions that were caused by and are left over from the taxation and exhaustion of childbirth.	323
余血	yú xuè	residual blood, conditions caused by residual blood after childbirth	324
魚目	yú mù	fish eyes	254
與鬼交通	yǔ guǐ jiāo tōng	intercourse with ghosts: explained in terms very similar to wind evil, it is caused by vacuity in the internal organs, which has weakened the hold of the spirit, allowing ghosts to invade.	48, 369
御	yù	to drive a chariot, and its frequent use in sexual cultivation literature to refer to a man's action of mounting a woman in sexual intercourse	101
玉門	yù mén	"jade gate" or vagina of virgins	81, 377, 378
玉泉	yù quán	Jade Spring: not a standard acupuncture point name	401
月閉	yuè bì	menstrual blockage	428
月浣	yuè huàn	monthly rinse: a reference to menstruation that apparently emphasizes the physiological function of flushing the uterus of stale blood.	467
月經不利	yuè jīng bù lì	inhibited menstruation	
月經不調	yuè jīng bù tiáo	menstrual irregularities	37
月經不通	yuè jīng bù tóng	stopped menstrual flow	
月經來過期	yuè jīng lái guò qī	a menstrual period that arrives in excess of its time	495
暈	yūn	dizziness	190
暈厥	yūn jué	fainting expiry	
慍	yùn	seething	
躁	zào	agitation	
燥	zào	dry	
燥胎	zào tāi	dried-out fetus	
再作	zào zuò	make it again	198
賊風	zéi fēng	bandit wind	297
張仲景	Zhāng Zhòng-Jǐng		4, 13, 19, 20, 39, 41, 309, 468
脹	zhàng	distention	
疹	zhěn	papules	309
振	zhèn	quivering	
振寒	zhèn hán	quivering with cold	

蒸	zhēng	steamed	130, 476
癥	zhēng	concretion	75
癥瘕	zhēng jiǎ	concretions and aggregations	75
蒸三斗米下	zhēng sān dǒu mǐ xià	steamed under three dǒu of rice	476
支滿	zhī mǎn	propping fullness	418
炙	zhì	roasted	
痔	zhì	hemorrhoids	489
滯	zhì	stagnation	
治如食法	zhì rú shí fǎ	prepared as for cooking	102, 107
治篩下	zhì shāi xià	finely pestle and sift	62
中極	zhōng jí	Central Pole, CV-3	401
腫	zhǒng	swelling	
中	zhòng	strike	
中惡	zhòng è	malignity strike	144
中風	zhòng fēng	wind strike	
周	Zhōu		6, 7, 9, 99, 542, 545, 546
主	zhǔ	govern, in the pharmaceutical context also "indicated for" when referring to the actions of a medicinal or formula.	69
煮米飲服	zhǔ mǐ yǐn fú	cook rice and take [the medicine] ... in its liquid.	350
疰	zhù	infixation	532
疰蟲	zhù chóng	worm infixation	532
疰夏	zhù xià	summer infixation	532
注	zhù	downpour	532
注下	zhù xià	downpour diarrhea	
注陰	zhù yīn	flooding of the vagina	
住	zhù	to lodge, stay	532
轉筋	zhuǎn jīn	cramping	
壯熱	zhuàng rè	strong fever	261
淳	zhūn	to irrigate, pour water	475
子	zǐ	"sons", "seeds", child	60, 212
子宮	zǐ gōng	infant's palace	421
子門	zǐ mén	infant's gate	81
子門閉	zǐ mén bì	infant's gate blockage	376. 378
子女	zǐ nǚ	This expression is ambiguous and could be interpret either as "sons and daughters" or as "female offspring"	57
子懸	zǐ xuán	fetal suspension	
紫蓋丸	zǐ gài wán	Purple canopy pills. The purple canopy is one of the emperor's insignia and therefore denotes something of great value.	449
紫湯	zǐ tāng	purple decoction: due to its location within this prescription, this could mean to make the infusion by mixing the charred chicken feathers into a base of hēi dòu 黑豆 decoction rather than salt water.	286

瘲	zòng	slackening	
阻	zǔ	obstruction	
坐草	zuò cǎo	sitting on grass: a standard expression in early medical literature, connoting the time spent in active labor.	184
作膏	zuò gāo	processed into a paste	
坐藥	zuò yào	sitting medicine	60
坐月子	zuò yuè zǐ	sitting out the month	33, 236

Materia Medica Index English

黍粘根	Arctium lappa, Root	315, 597, 612
檳榔	Areca catechu, Fruit	70, 557
防己	Aristolochia fangchi, Root	174, 273, 278, 279, 568, 597
鼠婦	Armadillidium vulgare, Dried body	69, 79, 612
艾葉	Artemisia argyi, Dry-roasted foliage	105, 132, 134, 158, 172, 174, 340, 349, 353, 415, 417, 486, 489, 492, 497, 505, 518, 548
菴閭子	Artemisia keiskeana, Fruit	77, 440, 441, 453, 458, 548
杜衡	Asarum forbesii, Rhizome and root, or whole plant	76, 375, 414, 567
細辛	Asarum heteropoides, Complete plant including root	63, 65, 67, 68, 70, 76, 77, 79, 93, 103, 249, 297, 303, 310, 319, 327, 346, 351, 367, 373, 374, 383, 405, 407, 410, 414, 415, 417, 422, 423, 426, 431, 432, 442, 444, 446, 447, 449, 453, 461, 464, 469, 472, 477, 486, 499, 503, 510, 524, 528, 567, 624
天門冬	Asparagus cochinchinensis, Tuber	66, 67, 70, 102, 376, 420, 617
貫眾	Aspidium crassirhizoma, Rhizome	351, 367, 575
紫菀	Aster tataricus, Root and rhizome	76, 120, 240, 303, 372, 375, 408, 447, 528, 636
黃芪	Astragalus membranaceus, Root	61, 79, 118, 245 - 247, 253, 265, 276, 301 - 303, 308, 313, 314, 318, 319, 322, 390, 405, 407, 422, 423, 489, 492, 513, 581
白朮	Atractylodes macrocephala, Rhizome	70, 74, 80, 84, 94, 96, 102, 103, 108, 112, 117, 122, 125, 130, 135, 143, 175, 176, 182, 239, 251, 254, 273, 279, 284, 287, 292, 294, 303, 342, 345, 346, 350, 357, 395, 405, 408 - 411, 417, 419, 422, 424, 425, 446, 497, 515, 536, 553
槐耳	Auricularia auricula (sophora wood ear)	489, 580
大麥麴	Barley leaven	201, 562
射干	Belamcanda chinensis, Rhizome	428, 434, 438, 440, 441, 608
冬瓜汁	Benincasa hispida, Juice	359
冬瓜練	Benincasa hispida, Pulp	358, 565
瓜瓣	Benincasa hispida, Seed	212, 574
蜚蠊	Blatta orientalis, Whole body	537, 569
白龍骨	Bleached fossilized vertebra and bone of mammals	78, 511
白芨	Bletilla striata, Rhizome	384, 550
白僵蠶	Bombyx mori, Dried 4th or 5th stage larva of the moth	68, 76, 79, 475, 484, 519, 550
殭蠶	Bombyx mori, Dried 4th or 5th stage larva of the moth	446, 453, 583
牛乳	Bos taurus domesticus, Milk	250, 598
牛角䚡	Bos taurus domesticus, Ossified marrow in the center of the horn	473, 489, 491, 497, 506, 598
敗鼓皮	Bos taurus domesticus, Skin	554
牛屎	Bos taurus domesticus, Excrement	598
蕪菁子	Brassica rapa, Seeds	165, 622
蕪菁根	Brassica rapa, Root	176, 622
蔓菁根	Brassica rapa, Root	595
銅鏡鼻	Bronze mirror knob	324, 325, 618

大薊根	Cirsium japonicum, Root	413, 562
薊根	Cirsium japonicum, Root	507, 582
肉蓯蓉	Cistanche salsa, Fleshy stalk	425, 604
蓯蓉	Cistanche salsa, Stalk	61, 117, 335, 395, 405, 409, 414, 417, 420, 423, 488, 492, 561
橘皮	Citrus reticulata, Peel	96, 173, 247, 248, 373, 489, 584
清酒	Clear liquor	255, 269, 602
女萎	Clematis apiifolia, Stalk	284, 312, 599
蛇床子	Cnidium monnieri, Fruit	61, 77, 376, 378, 381, 383, 388, 390, 417, 607
木防己	Cocculus trilobus, Root	285, 568, 597
薏苡	Coix lachryma-jobi, Seed kernel	370, 532, 629
黃連	Coptis chinensis, Rhizome	78, 106, 171, 173, 174, 338, 342, 343, 345, 347 - 350, 352 - 354, 373, 390, 391, 393, 418, 468, 472, 480, 486, 510, 515, 525, 580
山茱萸	Cornus officinalis, Fruit	61, 65, 346, 367, 373, 408, 409, 413, 415, 503, 606
白艾	Crossostephium chinense, Foliage	342, 549
巴豆	Croton tiglium, Seed	335, 364, 450, 460, 461, 549
菟絲子	Cuscuta chinensis, Seed	61, 70, 74, 206, 378, 620
白薇	Cynanchum atratum, Root	68, 76, 77, 79, 167, 447, 461, 515, 516, 553
白前	Cynanchum stauntoni, Root and rhizome	248, 552
鯉魚	Cyprinus carpio, Meat or whole body	176, 256, 359, 480, 484, 589
石斛	Dendrobium nobile, Whole plant	61, 66, 70, 80, 129, 240, 284, 405, 407, 410, 413, 415, 417, 420, 422, 424, 486, 488, 609
溲疏	Deutzia scabra, Fruit	71, 615
瞿麥	Dianthus superbus, Entire plant, including flowers	184, 198, 209, 210, 359, 437, 438, 468, 509, 525, 603
蜀漆	Dichroa febrifuga, Foliage	265, 613
恒山	Dichroa febrifuga, Root	150, 155, 156, 461, 577
常山	Dichroa febrifuga, Root	558
萆薢	Dioscorea hypoglauca, Rhizome	303, 481, 556
薯蕷	Dioscorea opposita, Root	61, 67, 293, 294, 367, 417, 556, 613
續斷	Dipsacus asper, Root	67, 84, 111, 134, 308, 408, 411, 412, 417, 474, 480, 481, 489 - 492, 497, 535, 627
茯苓	Dried fungus of Poria cocos	61, 63, 73, 74, 78, 80, 93 - 95, 102, 108, 109, 125, 128, 135, 139, 163, 175, 176, 240, 245 - 247, 251, 253, 260, 262, 263, 276, 284, 288, 289, 292, 293, 296, 301, 314, 319, 327, 349, 359, 370 - 372, 406, 407, 417, 419, 429, 434, 449 - 451, 461, 462, 468, 476, 478, 489, 492, 510, 525, 531, 532, 534, 569
鬼臼	Dysosma versipellis, Root	349, 576
蛇蛻皮	Elaphe taeniurus, Sloughed snake skin	203, 204, 607
麻黃	Ephedra sinica, Stalk	105, 110, 119, 150, 272, 290, 351, 355, 514, 592
葛上亭長	Epicauta Gorhami, Dried body	71, 573
亭長	Epicauta Gorhami, Dried body	618

桑螵蟲矢	Mulberry worm excrement	162, 606
雲母	Muscovite	229, 421, 484, 631
消石	Niter	74, 219, 365, 429, 449, 450, 464, 624
麥門冬	Ophiopogon japonicus, Tuber	78, 108, 110, 113, 115 - 117, 119, 124, 125, 139, 222, 223, 240, 244 - 246, 249, 254, 258, 259, 262, 263, 272, 289 - 293, 301, 308, 354, 361, 368, 374, 410, 415, 418, 424, 494, 594
雌黃	Orpiment	86, 560
兔骨	Oryctolagus domesticus, Bones	495, 619
兔屎	Oryctolagus domesticus, Feces	388, 399, 620
糯米	Oryza glutinosa, Seed	129, 564, 599
米粉	Oryza sativa, Flour	386, 596
陳廩米	Oryza sativa, Seed	338, 558
米	Oryza sativa, Seed	296, 297, 326, 339, 596
粳米	Oryza sativa, Seed of the non-glutinous variety	120, 128, 129, 149, 156, 170, 244, 260, 262, 341, 564, 584
米飲	Oryza sativa, Water after cooking	73, 203, 350, 478, 514, 516, 596
龍骨	Os draconis	109, 165, 252, 342, 344, 345, 349, 352, 406, 407, 409, 418, 468, 472, 474, 479, 485, 487, 488, 498, 504, 509, 519, 520, 524, 590
牡蠣	Ostrea rivularis, Shell	168, 266, 278, 379, 381, 386, 414, 458, 462, 463, 469, 472, 480, 482, 486, 488, 495, 500, 503, 510, 511, 516, 519, 524, 597
芍藥	Paeonia albiflora, Root	68, 80, 84, 93, 102, 108, 111, 113, 114, 117, 121, 122, 130, 135, 143, 158, 167, 176, 243, 245 - 249, 253, 256, 260, 261, 265, 276, 280, 282, 289, 291, 296 - 300, 302, 304, 305, 307, 308, 312 - 314, 319 - 322, 324, 326, 327, 330, 333, 340, 358, 366, 370, 372, 373, 379, 381, 386, 388, 390, 394, 398, 406, 409, 412, 419, 423, 424, 428, 430 - 432, 434, 436 - 438, 440, 444, 447, 451, 453, 461, 464, 468, 472, 486, 493, 494, 506, 510, 513, 525, 526, 529, 535, 536, 559, 607
白芍藥	Paeonia lactiflora	111, 266, 596, 607
赤芍	Paeonia rubra, Root	63, 559
牡丹	Paeonia suffruticosa, Bark of the root	63, 67, 68, 74, 80, 322, 331, 428, 434, 436 - 438, 440, 442, 444, 449, 451, 452, 494, 505, 526, 528, 529, 531, 534, 536, 596, 607
人參	Panax ginseng, Root	61, 63, 67, 68, 76, 78, 79, 84, 93, 94, 96, 102, 104 - 106, 108, 109, 111, 113, 114, 116, 119, 122, 170, 182, 238, 241, 245, 246, 248, 250, 252, 253, 258 - 260, 262, 263, 274 - 276, 278, 281, 284, 288, 290 - 292, 294, 296, 301 - 304, 314, 318, 322, 341, 344 - 346, 349, 354, 355, 359 - 361, 365, 366, 372, 375, 405, 407, 409, 410, 4215, 417, 419, 420, 422, 426, 430, 436, 444, 447, 449, 452, 460, 461, 463, 469, 477, 488, 489, 492, 494, 498, 504, 513, 525, 526, 529, 534 - 536, 603
黍米	Panicum miliaceum, Seed of the non-glutinous variety	220, 611 - 613
桑螵蛸	Paratenodera sinensis, Cocoon-like egg capsules	354, 605
牡蒙	Paris quadrifolia, Root	66, 76, 80, 335, 442, 448, 451, 453, 461, 476, 597
敗醬	Patrinia villosa, Whole plant with root	312, 385, 554
真珠	Pearl	196, 213, 633

桃膠	Prunus persica, Sap emerging from the bark of the trunk	359, 616
桃仁	Prunus persica, Seed	63, 74, 77, 79, 239, 240, 300, 311, 313, 319, 322, 325, 329, 331, 385, 428, 430, 432 - 434, 436 - 438, 440, 441, 451, 455, 457, 458, 462 - 464, 501, 526 - 532, 534, 616
李根白皮	Prunus salicina, Shavings from the bark of the root	112, 588, 609
乾葛根	Pueraria lobata, Dried root	263, 485
葛根	Pueraria lobata, Root	94, 154, 252, 253, 271 - 275, 278 - 280, 283, 290, 573
白頭翁	Pulsatilla chinensis, Root	229, 343, 344, 347, 552
石榴皮	Punica granatum, Rind of the fruit	170 - 172, 174, 341, 610
醇酒	Pure grain spirit	240, 560
石韋	Pyrrosia lingua, Foliage	357, 367, 469, 472, 475, 480, 509, 525, 611
㺓牛屎	Qín buffalo dung	177, 602
蝦蟆	Rana limnocharis, Whole body	388, 577
鼠頭	Rattus norvegicus, Head	399, 613
雄黃	Realgar	369, 391, 626
乾地黃	Rehmannia glutinosa, Dried root	61, 66, 69, 74, 78, 80, 84, 93, 103, 114, 116, 117, 125, 138, 157 - 159, 243, 245, 246, 248, 250, 253, 260, 266, 272, 276, 281, 294, 297, 298, 306, 308, 310, 314, 318, 324, 325, 328, 340, 345 - 347, 352, 355, 361, 366, 376, 406, 407, 410, 412, 415, 416, 422, 424, 425, 432, 436, 445, 447, 451, 453, 472, 486, 489, 491, 492, 496, 497, 503, 505, 513, 515, 519, 571
生地黃	Rehmannia glutinosa, Fresh root	106, 137, 142, 159, 261, 265, 301, 304, 311, 313, 320, 327, 330, 348, 394, 479, 490, 497 - 499, 565
生地黃汁	Rehmannia glutinosa, Juice from the fresh root	138, 183, 186, 211, 240 - 242, 334, 377, 456, 537
地黃	Rehmannia glutinosa, Root	146, 161, 305, 505, 526, 565
漏蘆	Rhaponticum uniflorum, Root	220, 222, 223, 226, 227, 229, 591
大黃	Rheum palmatum, Root	63, 65, 72, 80, 93, 130, 240, 244, 250, 313, 321 - 325, 327 - 329, 331, 344, 358, 364, 368, 374, 383, 390, 398, 424, 428, 430 - 434, 439, 440, 442, 444, 449, 450, 453, 455, 460 - 462, 464, 469, 476, 478, 509, 515, 516, 527, 530 - 536, 561
乾漆	Rhus verniciflua, Dried sap	68, 80, 300, 324, 328, 351, 377, 399, 430, 440, 450, 451, 453, 456, 463, 514, 536, 572
薔薇根皮	Rosa multiflora, Bark of the root	486, 601
覆盆子	Rubus chingii, Fruit	62, 70, 74, 77, 570
乳床	rǔchuáng	376
甘皮	Saccharum sinensis, Bark	469, 572
羚羊角	Saiga tatarica, Horn of male	189, 333, 589
柳絮	Salix babylonica, Seed	74, 590
鹽	Salt (sodium chloride)	143, 200, 202, 206, 186, 315, 604
丹參	Salvia miltiorrhiza, Root	84, 105, 109, 127, 161, 375, 376, 390, 424, 436, 444, 445, 450, 461, 463, 454, 470, 491, 505, 563
續骨木	Sambucus williamsii, Stems	332, 627
地榆	Sanguisorba officinalis, Root	171, 341, 385, 388, 490, 491, 502, 505, 506, 565
海藻	Sargassum fusiforme, Whole plant	372, 438, 452, 577

小麥	Triticum aestivum, Seed	212, 259, 262, 263, 341, 361, 529, 625
款冬花	Tussilago farfara, Flower	303, 372, 586
蒲黃	Typha angustata, Pollen	78, 129, 186, 199, 213, 264, 298, 311, 312, 323, 341, 389, 395, 412, 413, 436, 489, 492, 498, 512, 521, 526, 600
蕪荑	Ulmus macrocarpa, Processed fruit	68, 79, 84, 391, 406, 408 - 410, 414, 415, 417, 419, 420, 423, 426, 503, 622
榆白皮	Ulmus pumila, fibrous inner bark of the root or trunk	146, 157, 163, 184, 196, 210, 357, 629
藜蘆	Veratrum nigrum, Root and rhizome	335, 459, 588
桑寄生	Viscum coloratum, Branches and foliage	67, 70, 109, 125, 414, 421, 488, 605
牡荊子	Vitex negundo L. var. cannabifolia, Fruit	60, 596
狐莖	Vulpes vulpes, Penis	379, 578
白玉	White jade, Fine slivers	394, 395, 553
白石英	White quartz	69, 80, 251, 252, 278, 280, 372, 406, 407, 409, 422, 552
水蛭	Whitmania pigra, Dried body	63, 69, 80, 331, 429 - 433, 436, 437, 439, 440, 442, 444, 450, 452, 453, 462, 463, 513, 527 - 531, 534, 536, 614
東門邊木	Wood from the side of the eastern gate	484, 566
食茱萸	Zanthoxylum ailanthoides, Fruit	67, 400, 419, 611
秦椒	Zanthoxylum bungeanum, Seed capsule	68, 79, 128, 129, 272, 442, 601, 602, 611, 612
蜀椒	Zanthoxylum bungeanum, Seed capsules	65, 72, 76, 78, 127, 296, 346, 349, 350, 383, 384, 405, 407, 409, 414, 417, 419, 420, 422, 424, 425, 430, 436, 444, 446, 447, 449, 450, 458, 462, 469, 470, 472, 477, 478, 480, 486, 488, 503, 510, 525, 531, 533, 535, 612
欅皮	Zelkova schneideriana, Bark	170, 585
乾薑	Zingiber officinale, Dried root	65 - 68, 72, 76, 78, 80, 84, 94, 95, 120, 124, 125, 128 - 130, 138, 174, 239, 247, 250, 254, 256, 275, 279, 292 - 294, 297, 301, 305, 307, 308, 310, 328, 335, 336, 339, 342 - 344, 346, 348, 350, 367, 372, 375, 376, 397, 405, 407, 409 - 412, 414, 417, 419, 422, 424, 426, 429, 432, 436, 442, 444, 445, 447, 449, 450, 453, 458, 460 - 462, 464, 470, 472, 474, 475, 477, 478, 486, 488, 498, 503, 509, 513, 518, 525, 528, 533, 535, 536, 571
生薑	Zingiber officinale, Fresh root	93, 96, 103, 105, 106, 108, 111 - 118, 121, 122, 135, 150, 157, 173, 176, 186, 243, 246 - 249, 252, 256, 262, 263, 271, 273, 274, 276, 280, 281, 283, 287 - 290, 296, 298, 299, 302, 303, 305, 311, 313, 314, 319, 320, 322, 326, 327, 354, 355, 357 - 359, 361, 371, 374, 394, 398, 494, 497, 526, 529, 531, 583
生薑汁	Zingiber officinale, Juice from the fresh root	186, 241, 255, 296
大棗	Ziziphus jujuba, Mature fruit	105, 108, 109, 111, 115 - 117, 122, 124, 142, 154, 223, 245, 246, 248, 251 - 254, 256, 259, 260, 262, 263, 274, 279, 281, 288 - 293, 298, 299, 301, 303 - 305, 307, 308, 311, 314, 320, 323, 325, 327, 348, 354, 355, 357, 358, 361, 397, 424, 464, 529, 562

Materia Medica Index Pinyin

覆盆子	fù pén zǐ	62, 70, 74, 77, 570
附子	fù zǐ	61, 63, 69, 80, 125, 129, 174, 256, 273, 287, 303, 307, 339, 342, 345, 349, 350, 386, 391, 410, 412, 413, 420, 431, 442, 444, 446, 449, 458, 461, 463, 464, 469, 472, 476, 481, 486, 498, 510, 512, 519, 525, 535, 570
甘草	gān cǎo	63, 67, 80, 84, 93, 94, 102, 105, 107, 109, 111, 113, 114, 116 - 119, 121, 122, 128, 132, 133, 155, 159, 160, 182, 195, 199, 223, 226, 229, 238, 240, 243, 245 - 249, 251, 252, 254, 256, 258 - 263, 265, 271 - 276, 279 - 283, 288, 289, 291 - 293, 296 - 305, 307, 308, 310, 312, 314, 319 - 323, 325, 327, 330, 331, 339 - 346, 348 - 351, 354, 355, 357, 359 - 361, 366, 372, 388, 390, 391, 393, 394, 398, 405, 407, 409 - 411, 414 - 416, 419, 420, 422, 425, 431, 432, 434, 436, 442, 444, 446, 460, 469, 473, 481, 491, 493, 494, 497, 503, 510, 513, 514, 519, 525, 526, 528, 529, 534 - 536, 571
乾地黃	gān dì huáng	61, 66, 69, 74, 78, 80, 84, 93, 103, 114, 116, 117, 125, 138, 157 - 159, 243, 245, 246, 248, 250, 253, 260, 266, 272, 276, 281, 294, 297, 298, 306, 308, 310, 314, 318, 324, 325, 328, 340, 345 - 347, 352, 355, 361, 366, 376, 406, 407, 410, 412, 415, 416, 422, 424, 425, 432, 436, 445, 447, 451, 453, 472, 486, 489, 491, 492, 496, 497, 503, 505, 513, 515, 519, 571
乾葛根	gān gé gēn	263, 485
乾薑	gān jiāng	65 - 68, 72, 76, 78, 80, 84, 94, 95, 120, 124, 125, 128 - 130, 138, 174, 239, 247, 250, 254, 256, 275, 279, 292 - 294, 297, 301, 305, 307, 308, 310, 328, 335, 336, 339, 342 - 344, 346, 348, 350, 367, 372, 375, 376, 397, 405, 407, 409 - 412, 414, 417, 419, 422, 424, 426, 429, 432, 436, 442, 444, 445, 447, 449, 450, 453, 458, 460 - 462, 464, 470, 472, 474, 475, 477, 478, 486, 488, 498, 503, 509, 513, 518, 525, 528, 533, 535, 536, 571
甘皮	gān pí	469, 572
乾漆	gān qī	68, 80, 300, 324, 328, 351, 377, 399, 430, 440, 450, 451, 453, 456, 463, 514, 536, 572
甘竹根	gān zhú gēn	259, 572
甘竹茹	gān zhú rú	260, 572
藁本	gǎo běn	71, 77, 346, 406, 408 - 410, 415, 416, 419, 422, 425, 469, 503, 572, 626
葛根	gé gēn	94, 154, 252, 253, 271 - 275, 278 - 280, 283, 290, 573
葛上亭長	gé shàng tíng cháng	71, 573
狗脊	gǒu jǐ	516, 573
枸杞	gǒu qǐ	376, 573
枸杞根	gǒu qǐ gēn	479, 574
羖羊角	gǔ yáng jiǎo	190, 557
瓜瓣	guā bàn	212, 574
栝蔞根	guā lóu gēn	104, 222, 223, 225, 226, 258, 272, 279, 331, 354, 361, 368, 434, 574
栝樓實	guā lóu shí	224, 575
栝樓子	guā lóu zǐ	225
冠纓	guān yīng	84, 575
萑蘆	guàn lú	461, 471, 575
貫眾	guàn zhòng	351, 367, 575
龜甲	guī jiǎ	480, 481, 485, 491, 500, 575
鬼箭	guǐ jiàn	228, 576
鬼臼	guǐ jiù	349, 576

桔梗	jié gěng	63, 76, 78, 79, 93, 219, 250, 274, 310, 346, 366, 375, 405, 422, 424, 449, 476, 569, 583
粳米	jīng mǐ	120, 128, 129, 149, 156, 170, 244, 260, 262, 341, 564, 584
酒	jiǔ	270
菊花	jú huā	110, 584
橘皮	jú pí	96, 173, 247, 248, 373, 489, 584
櫸皮	jǔ pí	170, 585
卷柏	juǎn bǎi	66, 68, 77, 80, 417, 421, 585
苦參	kǔ shēn	281, 365, 424, 444, 461, 585
款冬花	kuǎn dōng huā	303, 372, 586
葵根莖	kuí gēn jīng	160, 164, 358, 586
葵子	kuí zǐ	122, 157, 159, 163, 164, 198, 209, 210, 244, 356, 357, 586
昆布	kūn bù	372, 587
蠟	là	338, 587
藍青	lán qīng	349, 587
狼毒	láng dú	458, 569, 587
狼牙	láng yá	391, 461, 588
藜蘆	lí lú	335, 459, 588
李根白皮	lǐ gēn bái pí	112, 588, 609
理石	lǐ shí	222, 223, 589
鯉魚	lǐ yú	176, 256, 359, 480, 484, 589
羚羊角	líng yáng jiǎo	189, 333, 589
硫磺	liú huáng	367, 368, 378, 380, 389, 610
柳絮	liǔ xù	74, 590
龍膽	lóng dǎn	368, 461, 590
龍骨	lóng gǔ	109, 165, 252, 342, 344, 345, 349, 352, 406, 407, 409, 418, 468, 472, 474, 479, 485, 487, 488, 498, 504, 509, 519, 520, 524, 590
漏蘆	lòu lú	220, 222, 223, 226, 227, 229, 591
露蜂房	lù fēng fáng	79, 330, 591
蘆根	lú gēn	363, 575, 591
鹿角	lù jiǎo	162, 166, 333, 501, 537, 591
鹿角膠	lù jiǎo jiāo	240
鹿茸	lù róng	61, 425, 446, 473, 487, 491, 492, 500, 512, 516, 520, 521, 591
鹿肉	lù ròu	246, 276, 592
亂髮	luàn fà	166, 324, 358, 440, 453, 500, 592
麻黃	má huáng	105, 110, 119, 150, 272, 290, 351, 355, 514, 592
麻油	má yóu	211, 593
麻子仁	má zǐ rén	109, 128, 145, 328, 346, 433, 457, 458, 477, 528, 593
馬蹄	mǎ tí	593
馬通	mǎ tōng	490
馬通汁	mǎ tōng zhī	158, 488, 518, 594

Formula Index English - Pinyin

Formula Index Pinyin - English

大平胃澤蘭丸	dà píng wèi zé lán wán	Major Stomach-Calming Lycopus Pills	423, 647
大五石澤蘭丸	dà wǔ shí zé lán wán	Major Five Stones and Lycopus Pills	406, 407, 647
大下氣方	dà xià qì fāng	Major Qì-Precipitating Formula	364, 648
大嚴蜜湯	dà yán mì tāng	Major Rock Honey Decoction	297, 648
大遠志丸	dà yuǎn zhì wán	Major Polygala Pills	293, 648
大澤蘭丸	dà zé lán wán	Major Lycopus Pills	416, 648
丹參膏	dān shēn gāo	Salvia Paste	126, 127, 649
丹參酒	dān shēn jiǔ	Salvia Liquor	504, 649
丹參丸	dān shēn wán	Sage Pills	84, 649
單行鬼箭湯	dān xíng guǐ jiàn tāng	Single Agent Winged Spindle Tree Decoction	228, 650
單行石膏湯	dān xíng shí gāo tāng	Single Agent Gypsum Decoction	220, 650
單行竹瀝汁	dān xíng zhú lì zhī	Single Agent Bamboo Sap Juice	396, 650
淡竹茹湯	dān zhú rú tāng	Bamboo Shavings Decoction	260, 262, 263, 366, 650
當歸散	dāng guī sǎn	Chinese Angelica Powder	380, 650
當歸芍藥湯	dāng guī sháo yào tāng	Chinese Angelica and Peony Decoction	247, 248, 650
當歸湯	dāng guī tāng	Chinese Angelica Decoction	299, 342, 493, 650, 651
當歸丸	dāng guī wán	Chinese Angelica Pills	441, 442, 463, 651
當歸洗湯	dāng guī xǐ tāng	Chinese Angelica Wash Decoction	385, 651
抵党湯	dǐ dǎng tāng	Tangut-Resisting Decoction	530, 652
地黃酒	dì huáng jiǔ	Rehmannia Wine	242, 652
地黃羊脂煎	dì huáng yáng zhī jiān	Rehmannia and Sheep or Goat Fat Brew	241, 652
獨活酒	dú huó jiǔ	Pubescent Angelica Wine	277, 652
獨活湯	dú huó tāng	Pubescent Angelica Decoction	270, 272, 313, 652
獨活紫湯	dú huó zǐ tāng	Pubescent Angelica Purple Decoction	270, 652
阿膠湯	ē jiāo tāng	Ass Hide Glue Decoction	113, 653
阿膠丸	ē jiāo wán	Ass Hide Glue Pills	345, 653
防風酒	fáng fēng jiǔ	Saposhnikovia Wine	284, 653
防風湯	fáng fēng tāng	Saposhnikovia Decoction	275, 653
茯苓湯	fú líng tāng	Poria Decoction	289, 653
茯苓丸	fú líng wán	Poria Pills	92 - 94, 653, 654
伏龍肝湯	fú lóng gān tāng	Stove Earth Decoction	496, 654
茯神湯	fú shén tāng	Root Poria Decoction	108, 109, 287, 654
甘草散	gān cǎo sǎn	Licorice Powder	127, 229, 654, 655
甘草湯	gān cǎo tāng	Licorice Decoction	271, 282, 321, 655
甘草丸	gān cǎo wán	Licorice Pills	291, 655
干地黃當歸丸	gān dì huáng dāng guī wán	Dried Rehmannia and Chinese Angelica Pills	435, 655
干地黃湯	gān dì huáng tāng	Dried Rehmannia Decoction	298, 318, 347, 656
干薑丸	gān jiāng wán	Dried Ginger Pills	429, 656
干漆湯	gān qī tāng	Lacquer Decoction	430, 657
干漆丸	gān qī wán	Lacquer Pills	439, 657
甘竹茹湯	gān zhú rú tāng	Sweet Bamboo Shavings Decoction	260, 657
葛根湯	gé gēn tāng	Pueraria Decoction	283, 657

麥門冬散	mài mén dōng sǎn	Ophiopogon Powder	221, 665
麥門冬湯	mài mén dōng tāng	Ophiopogon Decoction	116, 666
硭硝湯	máng xiāo tāng	Mirabilite Decoction	66, 431, 666
茅根湯	máo gén tāng	Imperata Decoction	359, 666
牡丹皮湯	mǔ dān pí tāng	Moutan Decoction	505, 666
牡丹丸	mǔ dān wán	Moutan Pills	437, 508, 666
牡蠣丸	mǔ lì wán	Oyster Shell Pills	462, 667
牡蒙丸	mǔ méng wán	Four-Leaved Paris Root Pills	448, 667
木防己膏	mù fǎng jǐ gāo	Woody Fangji Paste	285, 667
內補大當歸丸	nèi bǔ dà dāng guī wán	Internally Supplementing Major Chinese Angelica Pills	412
內補當歸建中湯	nèi bǔ dāng guī jiàn zhōng tāng	Internally Supplementing Chinese Angelica Center-Fortifying Decoction	305, 667
內補黃芪湯	nèi bǔ huáng qí tāng	Internally Supplementing Astragalus Decoction	253, 668
內補芎藭湯	nèi bǔ xiōng qióng tāng	Internally Supplementing Chuānxiōng Decoction	306, 668
牛膝湯	niú xī tāng	Achyranthes Decoction	209, 668
牛膝丸	niú xī wán	Achyranthes Pills	536, 668
朴消盪胞湯	pò xiāo dàng bāo tāng	Impure Mirabilite Uterus-Rinsing Decoction	62, 63, 668
蒲黃散	pú huáng sǎn	Typha Pollen Powder	264, 521, 669
蒲黃湯	pú huáng tāng	Typha Pollen Decoction	311, 323, 669
七熬丸	qī āo wán	Seven Roasted [Ingredients] Pills	530, 669
七子散	qī zǐ sǎn	Seven Seeds Powder	60, 670
千金丸	qiān jīn wán	Thousand Gold Pills	128, 670
前胡牡丹湯	qián hú mǔ dān tāng	Peucedanum and Moutan Decoction	434, 670
秦椒丸	qín jiāo wán	Shǎn-Xī Zanthoxylum Pills	79, 670
慶雲散	qìng yún sǎn	Blessing Clouds Powder	69, 671
人參當歸湯	rén shēn dāng guī tāng	Ginseng and Chinese Angelica Decoction	259, 671
人參丸	rén shēn wán	Ginseng Pills	292, 671
乳蜜湯	rǔ mì tāng	Milk and Honey Decoction	250, 672
三石湯	sān shí tāng	Three Stones Decoction	251, 252, 672
三石澤蘭丸	sān shí zé lán wán	Three Stones and Lycopus Pills	421, 672
三物黃芩湯	sān wù huáng qín tāng	Three Agents Scutellaria Decoction	281, 673
桑根白皮湯	sāng gēn bái pí tāng	Mulberry Bark Decoction	397, 673
芍藥黃芪湯	sháo yào huáng qí tāng	Peony and Astragalus Decoction	314, 673
芍藥湯	sháo yào tāng	Peony Decoction	121, 265, 299, 673
慎火草散	shèn huǒ cǎo sǎn	Stonecrop Powder	485, 520, 674
生地黃湯	shēng dì huáng tāng	Fresh Rehmannia Decoction	327, 348, 499, 674
升麻湯	shēng má tāng	Cimicifuga Decoction	329, 675
生牛膝酒	shēng niú xī jiǔ	Fresh Achyranthes Wine	309, 675
石斛地黃煎	shí hú dì huáng jiān	Dendrobium and Rehmannia Brew	240, 675
石韋湯	shí wéi tāng	Pyrrosia Decoction	357, 675
拭湯	shì tāng	Wiping Decoction	149, 675
蜀椒湯	shǔ jiāo tāng	Si-Chuān Zanthoxylum Decoction	296, 675

澤蘭散	zé lán sǎn	Lycopus Powder	425, 685
澤蘭湯	zé lán tāng	Lycopus Decoction	320, 346, 686
增損禹餘糧丸	zēng sǔn yǔ yú liáng wán	Modified Limonite Pills	487, 686
增損澤蘭丸	zēng sǔn zé lán wán	Modified Lycopus Pills	410, 686
獐骨湯	zhāng gǔ tāng	Water Deer's Bone Decoction	247, 687
真朱湯	zhēn zhū tāng	Pearl Decoction	196, 687
蒸大黃丸	zhēng dà huáng wán	Steamed Rhubarb Pills	129, 687
知母湯	zhī mǔ tāng	Anemarrhena Decoction	261, 687
梔子湯	zhī zǐ tāng	Gardenia Decoction	326, 688
鍾乳湯	zhōng rǔ tāng	Stalactite Decoction	219, 688
鍾乳澤蘭丸	zhōng rǔ zé lán wán	Stalactite and Lycopus Pills	414, 688
豬膏煎	zhū gāo jiān	Pork Lard Jam	255, 688
豬腎湯	zhū shèn tāng	Pig's Kidney Decoction	124, 244, 688
茱萸虻蟲湯	zhū yú méng chóng tāng	Evodia and Tabanus Decoction	528, 689
竹根湯	zhú gēn tāng	Bamboo Root Decoction	259, 689
竹瀝湯	zhú lì tāng	Bamboo Sap Decoction	139, 689
竹茹湯	zhú rú tāng	Bamboo Shavings Decoction	366, 689
竹葉湯	zhú yè tāng	Bamboo Leaves Decoction	262, 274, 360, 689, 690
紫石門冬丸	zǐ shí mén dōng wán	Fluorite and Asparagus Pills	66, 690
紫石英柏子仁丸	zǐ shí yīng bǎi zǐ rén wán	Fluorite and Arborvitae Seed Pills	413, 690
紫石英天門冬丸	zǐ shí yīng tiān mén dōng wán	Fluorite and Asparagus Pills	420, 690
坐導藥	zuò dǎo yào	suppository	65, 691

Indications Index

The Chinese Medicine Database
www.cm-db.com

The Chinese Medicine Database is a clinical resource for Chinese medicine practitioners, students, and scholars. It is updated daily and provides it's users with information on:

587+ Single herbs
1329+ Formulas
The 361 regular points
15,000 Western Diagnoses with corresponding ICD-9 Codes
and translations of Classical texts such as:

The Bèi Jí Qiān Jīn Yào Fāng
The Nán Jīng
The Qí Jīng Bā Mài Kǎo
The Shāng Hán Lái Sū Jí
The Shāng Hán Míng Lǐ Lùn
The Shén Nóng Běn Cǎo Jīng
The Zàng Fǔ Biāo Běn Hán Rè Xū Shí Yòng Yào Shì
and 47 other texts that have yet to be translated

Subscribers to the Chinese Medicine Database can also:

Participate in our online forum
Keep notes on the database
Blog
Upload pictures
Find and make friends all over the world
Share and compare their notes with their friends' notes

Subscribers also receive store discounts on books and NCCAOM approved lectures at our online store: www.cm-dbcart.com

The CM-DB believes that access to the Classics is fundamental to our further understanding of Chinese medicine. We invest 50% of each online subscription into the translation of Classical texts. Our hope is that by making this service available online, it will allow the international community access to thousands of texts which would not have otherwise been translated into English. The CM-DB believes that together, we have the resources to afford this massive amount of translation, and we hope that you will join us in the pursuit of this knowledge.

,